Clinical Microbiology: A Practical Approach

Clinical Microbiology: A Practical Approach

Edited by Erika Tanner

AMERICAN
MEDICAL PUBLISHERS
www.americanmedicalpublishers.com

American Medical Publishers,
41 Flatbush Avenue,
1st Floor, New York,
NY 11217, USA

Visit us on the World Wide Web at:
www.americanmedicalpublishers.com

ISBN: 978-1-63927-259-4

Cataloging-in-Publication Data

Clinical microbiology : a practical approach / edited by Erika Tanner.
p. cm.
Includes bibliographical references and index.
ISBN 978-1-63927-259-4
1. Diagnostic microbiology. 2. Medical microbiology. 3. Communicable diseases.
4. Pathogenic microorganisms. I. Tanner, Erika.
QR67 .C55 2022
616.904 1--dc23

Table of Contents

Preface

Clinical microbiology is the discipline of medical science that focuses on the prevention, diagnosis and treatment of infectious diseases. Numerous clinical applications of microbes for better health are studied in this domain. Clinical microbiology is also characterized as one of the largest sub-fields of microbiology that is applied to medicine. This field commonly focuses on the treatment of infection caused by various bacteria, fungus, viruses and parasites. The treatment of diseases caused by these pathogens is advised after studying their characteristics such as mechanisms of infection, growth and modes of transmission. The most important part of clinical microbiology is epidemiology, which studies the patterns, causes and effects of health and disease in people. The clinical aspect of the field aims to focus on the presence and growth of microbial infections in individuals, their effects on the human body, and the methods of treating these infections. This book unravels the recent studies in the field of clinical microbiology. It traces the progress of this field and highlights some of its key concepts and applications. This book is a resource guide for experts as well as students.

This book is the end result of constructive efforts and intensive research done by experts in this field. The aim of this book is to enlighten the readers with recent information in this area of research. The information provided in this profound book would serve as a valuable reference to students and researchers in this field.

At the end, I would like to thank all the authors for devoting their precious time and providing their valuable contribution to this book. I would also like to express my gratitude to my fellow colleagues who encouraged me throughout the process.

Editor

1

Prevalence of class 1 and 2 integrons in multi-drug resistant *Escherichia coli* isolated from aquaculture water in Chaharmahal Va Bakhtiari province, Iran

Elahe Tajbakhsh[1*], Faham Khamesipour[2], Reza Ranjbar[3] and Ifeoma Chinyere Ugwu[4]

Abstract

Background: Integrons play important role in the spread and maintenance of antimicrobial resistance among strains of *Escherichia coli* (*E. coli*) and other species of *Enterobacteriaceae*. This study investigated the prevalence of class 1 and 2 integrons among *E. coli* strains isolated from aquaculture water of fish fields in Iran.

Methods: One hundred and fifty water samples from different geographical regions in Chaharmahal Va Bakhtiari province were examined over a 2 months period. Isolation was through culture and biochemical tests. Integrons were identified through polymerase chain reaction (PCR) using oligonucleotide primers specific for class 1 and 2 integrons. Antimicrobial susceptibility testing was carried out using disc diffusion methods.

Results: Eighteen percent of the water samples were positive for *E. coli*. All the strains were multi-drug resistant; 100% to ciprofloxacin, chloramphenicol, gentamycin, ampicillin and tetracycline and least resistant to imipenem (7.2%). Ten (50%) of the most resistant strains were positive for class 1 (40%) and class 2 (10%).

Conclusions: *Escherichia coli* in aquaculture in Iran carried integrons class 1 and 2 which could be of public health concern since they could play a role in the spread and maintenance of antimicrobial resistance among bacterial population in the region and should be constantly monitored.

Keywords: Antimicrobial resistance, Aquaculture, *E. coli*, Integrons, Iran

Background

Development of antimicrobial resistance in microorganisms has been attributed to indiscriminate use of antibiotics which poses serious public health concern worldwide [1]. Multi drug resistant strains of *Escherichia coli* (*E. coli*) can be found in both human and animal isolates worldwide [2] with multiple drug resistant non-pathogenic *E. coli* found in the intestine implicated as important reservoir of resistance genes [3]. Acquired multi-drug resistance to antimicrobial agents creates an extensive trouble in case of the management of intra and extra intestinal infections caused by *E. coli*, which are a major source of diseases, mortality and increased production costs [4]. Pathogenic *E. coli* strains could acquire resistance genes through horizontal gene transfer of mobile genetic elements like integrons which have been reported to house resistance genes. Mobile genetic elements like plasmids and transposons are known to carry integrons which can contain genes for sit-specific recombination and are capable of capturing and mobilizing gene cassettes [5, 6]. Integrons are categorized into types, the super-integrons and the antibiotic resistance integrons (ARIs) [7, 8]. Dissemination of antibiotic resistance genes among bacteria can occur by mobile genetic elements containing the ARIs (5, 7, 9). There are four classes of integrons namely classes 1, 2, 3 and 4 which are known to carry multi-drug resistance genes [7, 9, 10]. Class 1 integrons are the most

*Correspondence: ee_tajbakhsh@yahoo.com
[1] Department of Microbiology, Faculty of Basic Sciences, Shahrekord Branch, Islamic Azad University, Shahrekord, Iran
Full list of author information is available at the end of the article

widespread and have been frequently found in ESBL producing clinical isolates of *Enterobacteriaceae* [11, 12]. Class 2 integrons occur less frequently in ESBL producing *E. coli* and *Klebsiella pneumoniae* while class 3 integrons are rarely found [13]. Class 4 integrons have only been described in *Vibrio cholerae* strain [10]. The Prevalence of class 1 and 2 integrons in multi-drug resistant *E. coli* isolated from aquaculture water was investigated in this study.

Methods

Sample collection

A total of 150 water samples from different fish fields from different geographical regions in Chaharmahal Va Bakhtiari province, Iran were examined over a period of 2 months, from October 2013 to November 2013. Water from each fish field was collected in 1,000 mL glass bottles and was taken to the laboratory immediately for bacterial isolation. All samples were labeled to show serial number, place of water, type of water as well as time and date of collection.

Bacterial isolation and biochemical tests for the identification of *E. coli*

Examination of the water samples was completed within 24 h after collection using Standard Total Coliform Multiple-Tube (MPN) Fermentation Techniques. After determination of MPN the tubes showing growth were inoculated onto MacConkey agar and positive ones subcultured on Eosin-methylene blue (EMB) plates (Merck). After 24 h incubation at 35 ± 0.5°C for 24 ± 2 h g negative microorganisms were isolated from MacConkey and EMB agar and determined at the species level using cytochrome oxidase, triple sugar iron agar, urea and indole tests as putatively *E. coli.*

DNA extraction and polymerase chain reaction (PCR) conditions for detection of integrons

Purification of DNA directly from water samples filtered was achieved using a Genomic DNA purification kit (Fermentas, Germany) according to the manufacturer's instructions. Oligonucleotide primers specific for the *E. coli* are presented in Additional file 1: Table S1 [13, 14].

The PCR reactions were performed in a total volume of 25 μL, including 1.5 mM $MgCl_2$, 50 mM KCl, 10 mM Tris–HCl (pH 9.0), 0.1% Triton X-100, 200 μM dNTPs each (Fermentas), 50 pmoL of each of the *E. coli* specific primers, 1.5 U of Taq DNA polymerase (Fermentas), and 3 μL (40–260 ng/μL) of DNA.

Amplification reactions were carried out using a DNA thermo-cycler (Eppendorf Mastercycler 5330, Eppendorf-Nethel-Hinz GmbH, Hamburg, Germany) and are listed in Additional file 1: Table S1 [13, 14]. Amplified samples were analyzed by electrophoresis in a 1.5% agarose gel in 1× TBE buffer at 80 V for 30 min, stained with solution of Ethidium Bromide and examined under Ultra Violet illumination (Uvitec, UK). Twenty most resistant strains out of the 27 isolates were tested for presence of integrons in their genome using PCR technique described above. For each set of PCR reactions, was positive control for class 1 integrons.

PCR conditions for detection of resistance genes

The presence of genes associated with choramphenicol [*cml*A], gentamicin [*aac*(*3*)-IIa, tetracycline-[*tet*(A), ciprofloxacin, norfloxacin and nalidixic acid resistance-(*qnrA*), and sulphonamides (*Sul 1* and *Sul 2*) was determined by PCR using specific primers are presented in Additional file 2: Table S2 [15–18].

Antimicrobial Susceptibility Testing

Antimicrobial susceptibility tests were performed by the Kirby-Bauer disc diffusion method using Mueller–Hinton agar (HiMedia Laboratories, Mumbai, India, MV1084), according to the Clinical and Laboratory Standards Institute guidelines [19]. After incubating the inoculated plate aerobically at 37°C for 18–24 h in an aerobic atmosphere, the susceptibility of the *E. coli* isolates to 12 antimicrobial agents was determined, and the results were interpreted in accordance with interpretive criteria provided by CLSI [19]. *E. coli* ATCC 25922 was used as quality control organisms in antimicrobial susceptibility determination.

The following antibiotic disks (Padtan-Teb, Iran) were used: ceftazidime (CAZ) (30 μg), tetracycline (TE) (30 μg), chloramphenicol (C) (30 μg), imipenem (IMP) (10 μg), ciprofloxacin (CRO) (5 μg), norfloxacin (NOR) (10 μg), cefalotin (CF) (30 μg), nalidixic acid (NA) (30 μg), nitrofurantoin (FM) (300 μg), trimethoprim/sulfamethoxazole (SXT) (30 μg) and gentamicin (GM) (10 μg).

Results

Out of the 150 water samples, 27 harboured *E. coli* after culture and biochemical tests. Hence the prevalence of *E. coli* in aquaculture was 18%.

Antimicrobial resistance

All isolates exhibited multi-drug resistance phenotypically. They were most resistant to ciprofloxacin, chloramphenicol, gentamycin, ampicillin and tetracycline (100%) and were least resistant to imipenem (7.4%) Additional file 3: Table S3.

Detection of integrons

Out of these *E. coli* isolates, 10 (37%) carried integrons presumably in their plasmids. Eight isolates carried Class

1 integrons while 2 isolates carried class 2 integrons. Class 1 and 2 integrons were not found in any single isolate Additional file 4: Table S4. The results show in Fig. 1.

Detection of resistance genes and integrons

Of the 27 strains that were resistant to chloramphenicol and gentamicin, 23 (85.2%) contained the *cmlA and aac(3)IIa* genes respectively while 22 (81.5%) contained *tetA* gene. *qnrA* gene that is responsible for ciprofloxacin, norfloxacin and nalidixic acid resistance was detected in one (3.7%) of the strains tested. *Sul1*gene was found in 9 (33.3%) strains while *sul 2* gene was present in 7 (25.9%) of the strains (Additional file 5: Table S5, Additional file 6: Table S6).

Discussion

It was observed that aquaculture in Chaharmahal Va Bakhtiari province, Iran provided enabling environment for the growth and survival of microorganisms since 18% of aquaculture samples haboured *E. coli*. This could be as a result of direct contamination of the water by feacal content due to the abundance of *E. coli* in mammalian colon [20]. Fecal content could be from the intestine of the fish [21] or from manure feeding which have been reported to increase incidence of *E. coli* in aquaculture [22]. These organisms could be dangerous to the fish grown in such aquaculture thereby reducing the quantity and quality of the produce. Since *E. coli* causes disease for both fish and other mammals [23, 24], fish farmers and aquaculture attendants are at the danger of exposure to these organisms since working in aquaculture involves high degree physical contact with the water. This could lead to aquatic infections spreading to the community since *E. coli* in seafood have been implicated as a source of diarrheagenic infections [25]. To safeguard cross-infections in this instance, microbial water quality maintenance, post-harvest care, handling hygiene and adequate sanitation during processing must be adhered to strictly [25].

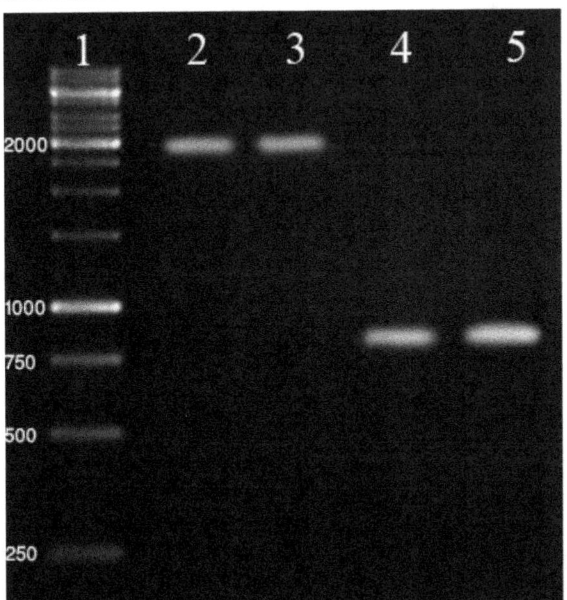

Fig. 1 Agarose gel electrophoresis of class 1 and 2 integrons in *E. coli* strains. *Lane 1* 1,000 bp DNA Ladder, *Lane 2* positive control, *Lane 3* class 1 integrons (1,900 bp), *Lane 4 and 5* class 2 integrons (789 bp).

The *E. coli* isolated were found to be multi-drug resistant, being resistant to more than five antimicrobials commonly used for feed additives and or therapeutics; suggesting a linkage between antibiotic usage and development of resistance [26, 27]. Although these isolates were not proven to be pathogenic, their antimicrobial resistance attributes also make them dangerous as potential source of resistance dissemination among bacterial population in the region. They could constitute environmental hazard since aquaculture water when discarded could become available to other animals and could contaminate sources of water for domestic, industrial and animal husbandry use. Since these resistance attributes have been reported elsewhere to be mediated by specific genes [28] which may be transferable horizontally [29], the possibility of resistance transfer to other *E. coli* species and other bacterial organisms in a multi culture environment is high. Molecular studies on the underlying resistance mechanisms in these multi-resistant *E. coli* revealed that resistance phenotypes were mediated by several different genes. This finding suggests that the presence of these multi-resistant *E. coli* in these aquaculture water were probably due to the acquisition of resistance genes by different isolates from different sources.

This antimicrobial resistance is encoded oftentimes by integrons that occur on plasmids or that are integrated into the bacterial chromosome. We found 50% of the most resistant isolates positive for integrons, class 1 (40%) and class 2 (10%) which was similar to the report of Goldstein et al. [10] that class 1 integrons were present in approximately 46% of the isolates from the family *Enterobacteriaceae*. In that report, class 2 integrases were present only among *E. coli* and *Salmonella* isolates. Kang et al. [30] also reported 44% integrons among *E. coli* isolates in Korea. Our result was however, lower than 76% occurrence of class 1 integrons reported by van Essen-Zandbergen et al. [31] among isolates of *E. coli* in Netherlands. Again, our finding goes contrary to the report of Bass et al. [32] which previously determined that multiple-drug resistance exhibited by avian *E. coli* isolates correlated with the incidence of class 1 integrons. The presence of integrons in these isolates may not have contributed to the multidrug resistance attributes of the isolates since the isolates without class 1 or 2 integrons exhibited nearly the same phenotypic resistance pattern with the isolates that carried class 1 or 2 integrons. However, most of the genes found in the isolates seem to be carried by class 1 integrons which is expected since class 1 type occurred more with isolates. Multi-drug resistance may also have been conferred by other genetic elements like plasmids, transposons or individual gene cassettes. Among those integron negative strains, with exception of one that was resistant to all the antimicrobials tested, all were resistant to the same class of antimicrobials and none was resistant to naldixic acid, sulfamethoxazole-trimethoprim, nitrofurantoin, imipenem and cephalotin. It seems class 2 integron do not carry the genetic basis for resistance to naldixic acid, sulfamethoxazole-trimethoprin, nitrofurantoin, and imipenem since the class 2 positive strains were susceptible to them.

Although integrons were detected in the strains of *E. coli*, their carriage did not seem to play a major role in the ability of the strains to become resistant. Similar finding was reported by Gallego and Towner [33] among clinical isolates of *Acinetobacter baumannii* in Northern Spain. However, the role of integrons in the spread and maintenance of resistance factors among the *E. coli* population and other species of the *Enterobaceriacae* cannot be overemphasized [6, 34].

Conclusion

In conclusion, the *E. coli* strains from aquaculture in Iran carried class 1 and 2 integrons which may be contributing to the resistance of these organisms to common antimicrobials. The potential for horizontal gene transfer among bacterial population is hereby highlighted. There is therefore need for adequate monitoring to forestall perpetuation of antimicrobial resistance in the region.

Additional files

Additional file 1: Table S1. Primers used for the PCR to detect integrons.

Additional file 2: Table S2. Primers used for the PCR to detect Resistance genes.

Additional file 3: Table S3. Antimicrobial resistance profile of *E. coli* strains from aquaculture.

Additional file 4: Table S4. Antimicrobial resistance pattern and integron carriage among *E. coli* strains from aquaculture water.

Additional file 5: Table S5. Antimicrobial resistance of *E. coli* strains from aquaculture by PCR and by antibiotic disks methods.

Additional file 6: Table 6. Multiple drug resistance (MDR), Antimicrobial resistance gene and integron carriage among *E. coli* strains from aquaculture water.

Abbreviations

E. coli: *Escherichia coli*; PCR: polymerase chain reaction; ARIs: antibiotic resistance integrons; MPN: Standard Total Coliform Multiple-Tube; EMB: Eosin-methylene blue; CLSI: Clinical and Laboratory Standards Institute; BP: base pair; CAZ: ceftazidime; TE: tetracycline; CP: chloramphenicol; IMP: imipenem; CF: ciprofloxacin; NOR: norfloxacin; C: cefalotin; NA: nalidixic acid; NF: nitrofurantoin; SXT: trimethoprim/sulfamethoxazole; GM: gentamicin.

Authors' contributions

All authors contributed equally to this work. All authors read and approved the final manuscript.

Author details

[1] Department of Microbiology, Faculty of Basic Sciences, Shahrekord Branch, Islamic Azad University, Shahrekord, Iran. [2] Young Researchers and Elite Club, Shahrekord Branch, Islamic Azad University, Shahrekord, Iran. [3] Molecular Biology Research Center, Baqiyatallah University of Medical Sciences, Tehran, Iran. [4] Department of Veterinary Pathology and Microbiology, University of Nigeria, Nsukka, Enugu State, Nigeria.

Acknowledgements

The authors would like to thanks Professor Ebrahim Rahimi and Dr. Chidozie Clifford for their support.

Competing interests

The authors declare that they have no competing interests.

References

1. World Health Organisation (2010) WHO global strategy for containment of antimicrobial resistance. WHO, Geneva, Switzerland, p 105
2. Amara A, Ziani Z, Bouzoubaa K (1995) Antibioresistance of *Escherichia coli* strains isolated in Morocco from chickens with colibacillosis. Vet Microbiol 43:325–330
3. Osterblad M, Hakanen A, Manninen R, Leistevuo T, Peltonen R, Meurman O et al (2000) A between-species comparison of antimicrobial resistance in enterobacteria in faecal flora. Antimicrob Agents Chemother 44:1479–1484
4. Gupta K, Hooton TM, Stamm WE (2001) Increasing antimicrobial resistance and the management of uncomplicated community-acquired urinary tract infections. Ann Int Med 135:41–50
5. Hall RM, Collis CM (1995) Mobile gene cassettes and integrons: capture and spread of genes by site-specific recombination. Mol Microbiol 15:593–600
6. Stokes HW, Hall RM (1989) A novel family of potentially mobile DNA elements encoding site-specific gene-integration functions: integrons. Mol Microbiol 3:1669–1683
7. Cambray G, Guerout AM, Mazel D (2010) Integrons. Annu Rev Genet 44:141–166
8. Fluit AC, Schmitz FJ (2004) Resistance integrons and super-integrons. Clin Microbiol Infect 10:272–288
9. Hall RM (1997) Mobile gene cassettes and integrons: moving antibiotic resistance genes in gram-negative bacteria. Ciba Found Symp 207:192–205
10. Goldstein C, Lee MD, Sanchez S, Hudson C, Phillips B, Register B et al (2001) Incidence of class 1 and 2 integrases in clinical and commensal bacteria from livestock, companion animals, and exotics. Antimicrob Agents Chemother 45:723–726
11. Jones LA, McIver CJ, Rawlinson WD, White PA (2003) Polymerase chain reaction screening for integrons can be used to complement resistance surveillance programs. Commun Dis Intel 27:103–110
12. Yao F, Quian Y, Chen S, Wang P, Huang Y (2007) Incidence of extended spectrum β-lactamases and characterization of integrons in extended spectrum β-lactamase producing *Klebsiella pneumoniae* isolated in Shantou, China. Acta Biochim Biophys Sin 39:527–532
13. Machado E, Cantón R, Baquero F, Galán JC, Rollán A, Peixe L et al (2005) Integron content of extended spectrum β-lactamase producing

Escherichia coli strains over 12 years in a single hospital in Madrid, Spain. Antimicrob Agents Chemother 49:1823–1829
14. Li D, Liu B, Chen M, Guo D, Guo X, Liu F et al (2010) A multiplex PCR method to detect 14 *Escherichia coli* serogroups associated with urinary tract infections. J Microbiol Methods 82(1):71–77
15. Maynard C, Bekal S, Sanschagrin F, Levesque RC, Brousseau R, Masson L et al (2004) Heterogeneity among virulence and antimicrobial resistance gene profiles of extraintestinal *Escherichia coli* isolates of animal and human origin. J Clin Microbiol 42(12):5444–5452
16. Ahmed MO, Clegg PD, Williams NJ, Baptiste KE, Bennett M (2010) Antimicrobial resistance in equine faecal *Escherichia coli* isolates from North West England. Ann Clin Microbiol Antimicrob 9:12
17. Soleimani-Asl Y, Zibaei M, Firoozeh F (2013) Detection of *qnrA* gene among quinolone-resistant *Escherichia coli* isolated from urinary tract infections in Khorram Abad during 2011-2012. Feyz 17(5):488–495
18. Kerrn MB, Klemmensen N, Frimodt-Møller N, Espersen F (2002) Susceptibility of Danish *Escherichia coli* strains isolated from urinary tract infections and bacteraemia, and distribution of *sul* genes conferring sulphonamide resistance. J Antimicrob Chemotherapy 50:513–516
19. Clinical and laboratory standards institute (CLSI) (ed) (2012) Performance standards for antimicrobial susceptibility testing: twenty-second informational supplement M100-S21. CLSI, Wayne
20. Kaper JB, Nataro JP, Mobley HLT (2004) Pathogenic *Escherichia coli*. Nat Rev 2:123–140
21. Carson CA, Shear BL, Ellersieck MR, Asfaw A (2001) Identification of fecal *Escherichia coli* from humans and animals by ribotyping. Appl Environ Microbiol 67(4):1503–1507
22. Dang ST, Dalsgaard A (2012) *E. coli* contamination of fish raised in integrated pig-fish aquaculture systems in Vietnam. J Food Prot 75(7):1317–1319
23. Nataro J, Pand Kaper JB (1998) Diarrheagenic *Escherichia coli*. Clin Microbiol Rev 11(1):142–201
24. Guerra B, Junker E, Schroeter A, Malorny B, Lehmann S, Helmuth R (2003) Phenotypic and genotypic characterization of antimicrobial resistance in German *Escherichia coli* isolates from cattle, swine and poultry. J Antimicrob Chemother 52:489–492
25. Renata AC (2013) Escherichia coli in seafood: a brief review. Adv Biosci Biotechnol 4:450–454
26. Carneiro DO, Figueiredo HCP, Pereira Júnior DJ, Leal AG, Logato PVR (2007) Perfil de susceptibilidade a antimicrobianos de bactérias isoladas em diferentes sistemas de cultivo de tilápia-do-Nilo (*Oreochromis niloticus*). Arq Bras Med Vet Zootec 59(4):869–876
27. Kemper N (2008) Veterinary antibiotics in the aquatic and terrestrial environment. Ecol Indic 8(1):1–13
28. Recchia GD, Hall RM (1995) Gene cassettes—a new class of mobile element. Microbiology 141:3015–3027
29. Leverstein-vanHall MA, Paauw A, Box ATA, Blok HEM, Verhoef J, Fluit AC (2002) Presence of integrons-associated with resistance in the community is widespread and contributes to multidrug resistance in the hospital. J Clin Microbiol 40:3038–3040
30. Kang HY, Jeong YS et al (2005) Characterization of antimicrobial resistance and class 1 integrons found in *Escherichia coli* isolates from humans and animals in Korea. J Antimicrob Chemother 55(5):639–644
31. van Essen-Zandbergen A, Smith H, Veldman K, Mevius D (2007) Occurrence and characteristics of class 1, 2 and 3 integrons in *Escherichia coli*, *Salmonella* and *Campylobacter* spp. in the Netherlands. J Antimicrob Chemother 59(4):746–750
32. Bass L, Liebert CA, Lee MD, Summers AO, White DG, Thayer SG, Maurer JJ (1999) Incidence and characterization of integrons, genetic elements mediating multiple-drug resistance, in avian *Escherichia coli*. Antimicrob Agents Chemother 43:2925–2929
33. Gallego L, Towner K (2001) Carriage of class 1 integrons and antibiotic resistance in clinical isolates of *Acinetobacter baumannii* from northern Spain. J Med Microbiol 50:71–77
34. Chah KF, Agbo IC, Eze DC, Somalo S, Estapa V, Torres C (2010) Antimicrobial resistance, integrons and plasmid replicon typing in multi-resistant clinical *E. coli* strains fron Enugu state, Nigeria. J Basic Microbiol 50:1–7

2

Antibiotic consumption in laboratory confirmed vs. non-confirmed bloodstream infections among very low birth weight neonates in Poland

A. Różańska[1*], J. Wójkowska-Mach[1], P. Adamski[2], M. Borszewska-Kornacka[3], E. Gulczyńska[4], M. Nowiczewski[4], E. Helwich[5], A. Kordek[6], D. Pawlik[7] and M. Bulanda[1]

Abstract

Background: Newborns are a population in which antibiotic consumption is extremely high. Targeted antibiotic therapy should help to reduce antibiotics consumption. The aim of this study was an assessment of antibiotic usage in bloodstream infections treatment in the Polish Neonatology Surveillance Network (PNSN) and determining the possibility of applying this kind of data in infection control, especially for the evaluation of standard methods of microbiological diagnostics.

Methods: Data were collected between 01.01.2009 and 31.12.2013 in five teaching NICUs from the PNSN. The duration of treatment in days (DOT) and the defined daily doses (DDD) were used for the assessment of antibiotics consumption.

Results: The median DOT for a single case of BSI amounted to 8.0 days; whereas the median consumption expressed in DDD was 0.130. In the case of laboratory confirmed BSI, median DOT was 8 days, and consumption—0.120 DDD. Median length of therapy was shorter for unconfirmed cases: 7 days, while the consumption of antibiotics was higher—0.140 DDD ($p < 0.0001$). High consumption of glycopeptides expressed in DOTs was observed in studied population, taking into account etiology of infection.

Conclusions: Even application of classical methods of microbiological diagnostics significantly reduces the consumption of antibiotics expressed by DDD. However, the high consumption of glycopeptides indicates the necessity of applying rapid diagnostic assays. Nevertheless, the assessment of antibiotic consumption in neonatal units represents a methodological challenge and requires the use of different measurement tools.

Keywords: Antimicrobial consumption, Infection surveillance, Bloodstream infections, Neonatal infections

Background

Infection control in neonatal intensive care units (NICUs) should have high priority, because its incidence is among the highest in different patient populations. Bloodstream infections (BSI) are the most common clinical form of infections in NICUs. The incidence of early-onset BSI (diagnosed <3 days after delivery) is 7% in Poland [1] and in Norway [2], 6% in the USA [3] and 2.4% in Israel [4].

In contrast, risk of late-onset BSI reaches 14.9/1000 patient days (pds) worldwide [5]; in the German NeoKISS: 8.3/1000 pds [6] and in Poland—6.7/1000 pds [7]. However, in the USA (for infants born at 28 weeks gestation or earlier)—36% [8], while in Israel, 39% [9].

Numerous studies show that newborns are a population in which antibiotic usage is extremely high [10, 11]. Those studies were performed mainly in West European

*Correspondence: rozanska@ifb.pl
[1] Chair of Microbiology, Jagiellonian University Medical College, 18 Czysta Street, 31-121 Krakow, Poland
Full list of author information is available at the end of the article

countries and in the United States, but there are no such reports from Poland or Central Europe.

Assessment of antibiotic usage in neonatal intensive care units encounters significant difficulties connected with the lack of standardized methods for this specific patient population. Defined daily dose (DDD), an international standard measure used for drug consumption assessment, is a technical unit of measurement which reflects the average maintenance dose per day for a drug used for its main indication in adults [12]. For this reason, this parameter has certain limitations for the analysis in the child population. However, defined daily dose was used in some studies, especially for comparative purposes in homogenous patient population [13]. Other parameters used for antibiotic usage assessment are as follows: LOT—the number of days during which at least one dose of any antibiotic was received, DOT—the aggregate sum of LOT or PDD—prescribed daily dose or proportion of patients with antibiotic treatment in a specific period [14–16].

Antibiotics consumption assessment can have numerous implications. In the area of infection control it can serve as a relatively simple indicator for assessing the effectiveness of methods of microbiological diagnostics. Microbiological diagnostics of blood stream infections in hospital practice still remains a challenge.

The aims of this study were:

- an assessment of antibiotic usage in bloodstream infection (BSI) treatment, taking into account etiology, in the Polish Neonatal Surveillance Network wards using two kinds of parameters, that is DDD and DOT,
- determining the possibility of applying this kind of data in infection control, especially for the evaluation of standard methods of microbiological diagnostics.

Methods

Data were collected prospectively between 01.01.2009 and 31.12.2013 in five teaching neonatal intensive care units (NICU) that took part in the Polish Neonatology Surveillance Network (PNSN). The PNSN is a prospective national surveillance system for the most relevant infections in the group of very low birth weight (birth weight <1500 g, VLBW) infants in Poland. The PNSN recorded severe infections, including BSI, observed during hospitalization: from admission to discharge, transfer or death. Participation in PNSN was voluntary and confidential for wards. Detailed description of data collection system, study wards, epidemiology of early- and late-onset BSI and its microbiology have been already published elsewhere [1, 7]. The study was approved by the Bioethics Committee of Jagiellonian University Medical College—no. KBET/221/B/2011. All data entered into the electronic database and analyzed retrospectively during the preparation of this article were previously de-identified. BSI (both: early- and late-onset) were defined according to Gastmeier et al. [17] with modifications. BSI was detected when at least two of the following signs were observed:

Temperature >38 or <36.5 °C or temperature instability, tachycardia or bradycardia, apnea, prolonged capillary refill, metabolic acidosis, hyperglycemia, the other sign of bloodstream infections, such as: lethargy; and one of the following criteria: C-reactive protein (CRP) >2.0 mg/dL, immature/total neutrophil ratio (I/T ratio) >0.2, leukocytes <5000/μL, platelets <10,000/μL.

Early-onset BSI was defined as septicemia diagnosed <3 days after delivery.

Laboratory confirmed BSI (LC-BSI) were those cases in which positive results of the microbiological testing were obtained, that means etiological factor was isolated. All blood specimens of at least 1 mL (taken prior to implementing antibiotic treatment) were injected into an aerobic blood culture bottle. Isolates were identified by the automated identification system (VITEK 2, bioMérieux, Poland). In the studied wards, molecular methods for identification of etiological factors were not used. BSI cases in which samples for microbiological testing were not collected or etiological factor was not isolated were classified as not confirmed ones.

Antibiotic usage for BSI treatment (until cure) was assessed for 767 cases. The analysis of antibiotic use included only the cases in which treatment was successful—13 records concerning infants who had died within 7 days of starting the therapy were excluded from the study (all of them were laboratory confirmed).

Two kinds of indicators were used for the description of antibiotic usage:

1. DOT, expressed in days—the aggregate (for every separate type of antibiotics) sum of number of days during which at least one dose of any antibiotic was received, and
2. DDD, expressed in grams—the defined daily dose, according to the ATC/DDD system of the World Health Organization (Anatomical Therapeutic Chemical, group "J01") [12].

Both measures were taken into account in reference to one case of infection. Data on the medicine type, dose, and the length of therapy were derived from individual records in the chart of each individual patient.

Antibiotic consumption were calculated for all antimicrobials used in therapy, and for the following classes: beta-lactams (ampicillin, cloxacillin, piperacillin, cefotaxime, ceftriaxone, ceftazidime, meropenem, imipenem), aminoglycosides (amikacin, netilmicin, gentamicin), glycopeptides (vancomycin), antimycotics (fluconazole, amphotericin B) and others (ciprofloxacin, clindamycin, erythromycin, clarithromycin, sulfamethoxazole with trimethoprim). Etiological factors were assigned to the following groups: Gram-negative (*Enterobacteriaceae* and other rods), Gram-positive (staphylococci, streptococci), candida. While conducting treatment with the application of drugs from several groups, used in parallel or consecutively, all of them were included into analysis. When, during treatment, positive microbiological cultures were obtained from different samples, or samples taken at different times (within 5 days), growth of microorganisms belonging to various groups (e.g. *Escherichia coli* and *Candida albicans*) was defined as cases of changing etiology (group "changing").

Due to DDD and DOT distribution significantly different from the normality, the statistical analysis based on the Kruskal–Wallis test. If the significance had been obtained, analysis was suplemented by the post hoc Steel–Dwass test, with critical value $p = 0.05$. All analysis were provided with SAS JMP package.

Results

In the study period, records of 2003 VLBW newborns and 780 BSI cases (regardless of the date of recognition of first BSI symptoms) were filled with all data.

Laboratory confirmed BSI (LC-BSI) constituted 84.9% (662) of all recognized cases of BSI.

In the analyzed population of VLBW neonates with BSI, in whom the etiological agent was isolated, combination therapy was used in 67% of cases, while in the group without microbiological confirmation, in 74% of cases.

The total duration of antibiotic therapy for 767 cases of BSI, which are incorporated into the present analysis, amounted to 14,056 DOTs or 381.6 DDDs. The median length of antibiotic therapy for a single case of BSI, regardless of microbiological confirmation or its lack, amounted to 8.0 days; whereas the median consumption expressed in DDD was 0.130. In the case of LC-BSI, median DOT was also 8.0 days, and consumption—0.120 DDD. Median length of therapy was shorter for unconfirmed cases: 7.0 days, while the consumption of antibiotics was higher—0.140 DDD ($p < 0.0001$) (Table 1).

Antibiotic consumption expressed by the DDD index was higher in the case of BSI caused by Gram-positive cocci than Gram-negative bacilli (0.140 vs. 0.136 DDD, Table 2), and the differences concerned 2× higher consumption of aminoglycosides (0.109 vs. 0.056 DDD, Table 2; $p = 0.0092$, Table 3).

Highest DOT values for beta-lactams concerned fungal infections and for the "changing" group, similarly to the consumption of antibiotics expressed by DDD.

Median length of therapy for BSI infections caused by Gram-positive cocci was longer than the ones caused by Gram-negative bacilli (9.0 vs. 7.5 DOT, Table 2), and the differences were mainly associated with the employment of glycopeptides (8.0 vs. 10.0 DOT, Table 2, $p = 0.0004$, Table 3).

Detailed data on antibiotic consumption expressed by DDD and DOT (values of medians per one infection case), taking into account groups of antibiotics, are presented in Table 2.

The results of statistical analysis regarding the consumption of the individual groups of antibiotics depending on the etiology of infection are shown in Table 3.

Depending on the applied indicator assessing the consumption of antibiotics in the treatment of BSI: DOT or DDD, the percentage share for individual groups of antibiotics varied.

Table 1 Values (median) of DOT and DDD in bloodstream infections treatment in microbiologically confirmed (LC) vs. unconfirmed cases (Not-LC)

Antimicrobial group	DOT (days)		p value	DDD		p value
	Microbiologically confirmed N = 649	Microbiologically unconfirmed N = 118		Microbiologically confirmed N = 649	Microbiologically unconfirmed N = 118	
	Median (IQR)	Median (IQR)		Median (IQR)	Median (IQR)	
Aminoglycosides	7.0 (5.0; 9.3)	7.0 (6.0;7.0)	0.5265	0.101 (0.050; 0.171)	0.095 (0.045; 0.179)	<0.0001
Antimycotic	12.5 (9.0;16.0)	10.0 (7.8;14.3)		0.210 (0.132; 0.040)	0.198 (0.073; 0.463)	
Beta-lactams	8.0 (5.0;11.0)	7.0 (6.8;8.8)		0.254 (0.136; 0.438)	0.300 (0.210; 0.420)	
Glycopeptides	10.0 (8.0;11.0)	9.0 (7.0;11.0)		0.120 (0.080; 0.168)	0.120 (0.083; 0.146)	
Other	9.0 (6.0;14.8)	8.0 (5.0;15.5)		0.210 (0.105; 0.530)	0.098 (0.060; 0.410)	
Total	8.0 (5.0; 16.0)	7.0 (5.0; 15.5)		0.120 (0.050; 0.530)	0.143 (0.045; 0.463)	

DOT days of therapy (per one infection case), *DDD* defined daily dose (per one infection case), *IQR* interquartile range, *N* number of BSI cases

Table 2 Values (median) of DOT and DDD in bloodstream infections treatment according to etiological factors

Etiology	DOT (days) Median (IQR)	DDD Median (IQR)
Gram+ N = 452		
Aminoglycosides	7.0 (5.0; 9.0)	0.109 (0.560; 0.180)
Antimycotics	12.0 (9.3; 16.0)	0.195 (0.131; 0.341)
Beta-lactams	7.0 (5.0; 10.0)	0.252 (0.180; 0.420)
Glycopeptides	10.0 (8.0; 11.0)	0.128 (0.088; 0.168)
Other	9.0 (5.0; 15.0)	0.211 (0.096; 0.452)
Total	9.0 (5.0; 15.0)	0.140 (0.056; 0.453)
Gram− N = 103		
Aminoglycosides	6.0 (4.3; 8.0)	0.056 (0.036; 0.137)
Antimycotics	12.0 (8.2; 17.0)	0.228 (0.131; 0.360)
Beta-lactams	8.0 (4.0; 11.0)	0.244 (0.096; 0.448)
Glycopeptides	8.0 (4.0; 9.0)	0.098 (0.039; 0.149)
Other	8.5 (5.3; 10.8)	0.229 (0.099; 0.608)
Total	7.5 (4.0; 17.0)	0.136 (0.036; 0.447)
Changing N = 76		
Aminoglycosides	7.0 (5.0; 10.0)	0.105 (0.061; 0.180)
Antimycotics	12.0 (10.0; 16.0)	0.250 (0.158; 0.735)
Beta-lactams	7.0 (6.5; 11.0)	0.281 (0.169; 0.495)
Glycopeptides	10.0 (7.0; 11.0)	0.085 (0.056; 0.167)
Other	9.0 (6.0; 14.5)	0.187 (0.120; 2.580)
Total	9.0 (5.0; 16.0)	0.149 (0.056; 2.580)
Candida N = 18		
Aminoglycosides	8.5 (4.8; 12.8)	0.140 (0.070; 0.210)
Antimycotics	10.5 (9.0; 15.8)	0.225 (0.092; 0.353)
Beta-lactams	12.0 (9.0; 19.5)	450 (192.9; 2175)
Glycopeptides	10.0 (7.3; 10.8)	0.087 (0.063; 0.161)
Other	13.5 (10.0; 17.0)	3.276 (0.153; 6.400)
Total	10.0 (4.8; 19.5)	0.164 (0.063; 6.400)

Changing—when, during treatment, positive microbiological cultures were obtained from different samples, or samples taken at different times (within 5 days), growth of microorganisms belonging to various groups (e.g. *Escherichia coli* and *Candida albicans*) was defined as cases of changing etiology (group "changing")

DOT days of therapy (per one case), *DDD* defined daily dose (per one case), *IQR* interquartile range, *N* number of cases

In treatment of BSI as a whole, according to the DOT index, glycopeptides were used the longest: 42.1%, and, after taking into account the etiology of infection, it was the predominant group also in infections caused by Gram-positive cocci: 51%, in the event of changes in the etiological agent: 40.6%. In treatment of microbiologically unconfirmed BSI, glycopeptides were used in 33.8% DOT (Fig. 1).

The largest share in total consumption of antibiotics in all analyzed cases of BSI expressed by DDD was represented by beta-lactams: 32.6%, especially with microbiologically unconfirmed BSI: 53.2% (Fig. 2).

In the event when antibiotic consumption was evaluated by DDD, antifungal medication constituted almost one-fourth of the applied drugs, and when the unit of measurement was DOT—13.3% (Figs. 1, 2).

Discussion

BSI represent a critical complication associated with hospitalization of very low birth weight (VLBW) infants, contributing to longer stay, and different long-term adverse outcomes. This phenomenon is well-understood and described [3, 7, 18–21], contrary to the subject under discussion, in which, unfortunately, data concerning antibiotic consumption are sparse and incomplete.

The proportion of microbiologically confirmed cases of BSI observed in the present study indicates similarity, but not identicalness, with other national programs. In the analysis of differences, attention should be paid to the applied definition of infections and different significance of microbiological findings for various types of surveillance. In American NHSN, in which to confirm LC-BSI, it was necessary to obtain at least 2 identical blood cultures, clinical sepsis was observed in 6.7–12.7% of infections [22], i.e. twice less frequently than in this study—significantly less restrictive in evaluating microbiological results. It unfortunately, indicates too rare application of the capabilities of contemporary microbiology in everyday clinical practice of the studied NICUs. This is confirmed by the results of a Cypriot study, in which LC-BSI constituted 96% of all BSIs [23]. Another matter is the debated problem of legitimacy of repeated blood drawing for cultures from VLBW newborns. Currently, it is more and more frequently assumed that, in this patient population, it is more justifiable to draw a single full-volume sample than to take two or more—even in the event of a result revealing typical skin contaminants, i.e. coagulase-negative staphylococci [24]. This is confirmed by the definitions adopted in the Netherlands [25], in NICHD Vermont Oxford Network [3] and the ones employed in the German national program called Neo-KISS [17].

The obtained data show that the use of diagnostics, even based on the standard, basic level, meaning culture, is a proceeding effectively affecting the consumption of antibiotics, and therefore, the costs of therapy, i.e. they reduce the consumption of antibiotics expressed by DDD.

The indicator most commonly used to assess the consumption of drugs, including antibiotics, is defined daily dose. This recognized international standard applicable in measuring the consumption of antibiotics is based on the average dose for the treatment of adults. For this reason, it is an indicator which, in relation to children, should be used with caution and one should take into account its limitations [26, 27].

Table 3 Statistical significance of antibiotic consumption expressed in DOT and DDD in bloodstream infections treatment according to etiological factor

	Candida	Gram–	Gram+	Changing
DOT aminoglycosides (H = 6.5939, df = 4; p = 0. 590)				
Not LC	0.7346	0.4524	0.9929	0.2733
Candida	na	0.6917	0.9235	0.9962
Gram–		na	0.4358	0.2780
Gram+			na	0.8323
Total DDD aminoglycosides (H = 31.7944, df = 4; p < 0.0137)				
Not LC	0.7980	0.3370	0.5284	0.9576
Candida	na	0.3438	0.9582	0.9757
Gram–		na	0.0092	0.3480
Gram+			na	1.0000
DOT antifungals (H = 2.5563, df = 4; p = 0.6346)				
Not LC	0.9978	0.9978	0.8403	0.7241
Candida	na	0.9995	0.9155	0.8539
Gram–		na	0.9885	0.8474
Gram+			na	0.9753
Total DDD antifungals (H = 16.5505, df = 4; p = 0.4042)				
Not LC	0.1485	0.7166	0.9926	0.7086
Candida	na	0.3429	0.4524	0.9454
Gram–		na	0.2909	0.9236
Gram+			na	0.1509
DOT beta-lactams (H = 15.0687, df = 4; p = 0.0046)				
Not LC	0.0286	0.8176	0.7340	0.0039
Candida	na	0.2451	0.1935	0.3721
Gram–		na	0.9978	0.2494
Gram+			na	0.1390
Total DDD beta-lactams (H = 11.2708, df = 4; p = 0.1930)				
Not LC	0.6238	0.3438	0.2861	0.3044
Candida	na	0.9999	0.9852	1.0000
Gram–		na	0.6380	1.0000
Gram+			na	0.7880
DOT glycopeptides (H = 19.0396, df = 4; p = 0.0008)				
Not LC	0.9986	0.0481	0.4925	0.9997
Candida	na	0.4196	0.9989	0.9992
Gram–		na	0.0004	0.1049
Gram+			na	0.6125
Total DDD glycopeptides (H = 0.4767, df = 4; p = 0.0010)				
Not LC	0.8227	0.5865	0.4612	0.5951
Candida	na	1.0000	0.4731	0.9998
Gram–		na	0.0498	0.9802
Gram+			na	0.0157
DOT other (H = 2.2959, df = 4; p = 0.6815)				
Not LC	0.6828	0.9978	0.9220	0.9922
Candida	na	0.7617	0.8871	0.9772
Gram–		na	0.9735	0.9984
Gram+			na	0.9999
Total DDD other (H = 3.8955, df = 4; p = 0.3787)				
Not LC	0.9707	0.9538	0.8169	0.9981
Candida	na	0.9986	0.4667	0.5815
Gram–		na	0.8990	0.9884
Gram+			na	0.9910

p values for each pair of etiological factor groups are given in the table cells

Changing—when, during treatment, positive microbiological cultures were obtained from different samples, or samples taken at different times (within 5 days), growth of microorganisms belonging to various groups (e.g. *Escherichia coli* and *Candida albicans*) was defined as cases of changing etiology (group "changing")

DOT days of therapy, *DDD* defined daily dose, *IQR* interquartile range, *na* not applicable, *Not LC* not laboratory confirmed

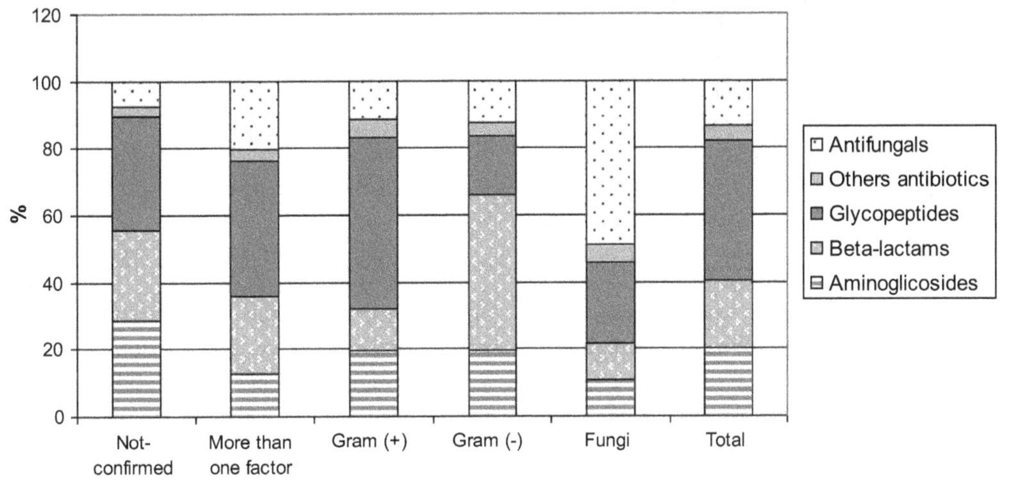

Fig. 1 Distribution of antibiotic groups used in the treatment of BSI according to etiology, expressed in DOT

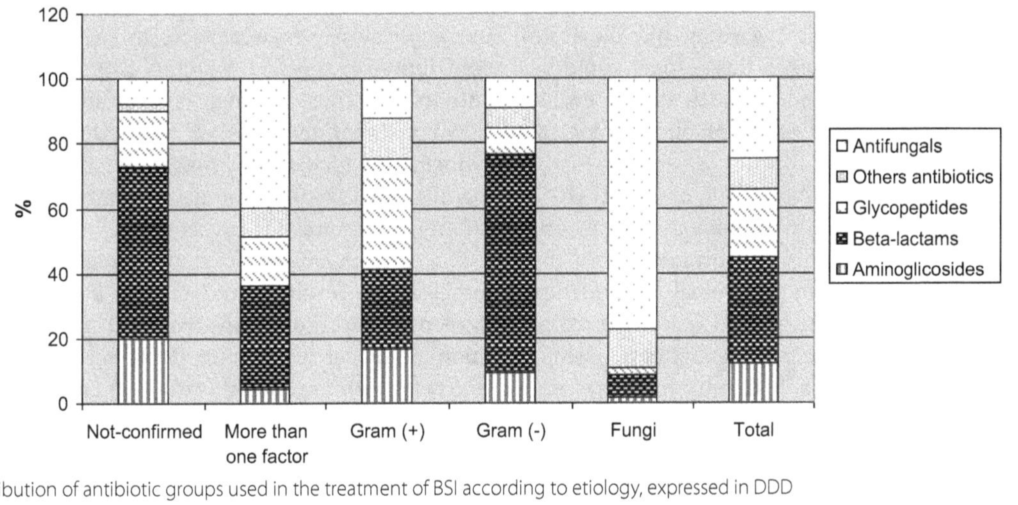

Fig. 2 Distribution of antibiotic groups used in the treatment of BSI according to etiology, expressed in DDD

Howether, both measures: DDD and the length of therapy were used by different authors with the application of various denominators—the number of admissions, number of person days or with respect to the treatment of a single patient [13, 15].

To evaluate the consumption of antibiotics in pediatric wards, particularly neonatal units, Gerber et al. employed DOT [15]. Depending on the type of neonatal unit, they found the length of treatment to be in the range from 5.7 in medical NICUs to 34.3 DOT in surgical NICUs. Median DOT in this study was about forty percent higher than in the medical NICUs in the study by Gerber; however, due to distinct populations and different degrees of detail, it is difficult to explicitly compare these values. Studies concerning antibiotic consumption in the neonatal population are not numerous, but what is more important: the published papers present a differentiated approach to the subject and are carried out with the use of diverse methodology and for various needs [5, 11, 13, 26, 28].

However, the main objective of this study was the analysis of the evaluation of antibiotic consumption in the treatment of one form of infection in a narrow and specific patient population, giving special consideration to the possibility of its use in the evaluation of the effectiveness and accuracy of microbiological diagnostics as an element of surveillance of infections in NICU.

And so, in NICUs covered by the study, significantly lower consumption of antibiotics expressed by DDD was observed in the case of LC-BSI treatment, compared to those in which the etiological agent was not isolated. On this basis, it can be concluded that the microbiological diagnosis of BSI in newborns treated in NICU was conducted properly and the results of microbiological tests were used in targeted therapy, what made it possible to obtain a reduction in the consumption of antimicrobial drugs and, consequently, the cost of treatment. In Polish NICUs, costs of medication account for nearly one-fifth of the total cost of treatment, the amount of which is inversely proportional to a child's birth weight and directly proportional to the length of hospitalization [20].

A different situation was observed in the population of the PNSN neonates, who developed necrotising enterocolitis, wherein the length of therapy and consumption rates were not affected by the isolation of the potential etiological agent [29]. But with NEC, difficulties present themselves as regards obtaining material for microbiological examination, which would enable the isolation of the etiological agent. The quoted results concerning antibiotic consumption in NEC cases and the ones demonstrated in the present study regarding BSI illustrate the possibilities of how analyses in this respect could be utilized in infection control and, in particular, in evaluation of adequacy and effectiveness of microbiological diagnostics.

On the other hand, no significant differences in DOT values in cases of LC-BSI and microbiologically unconfirmed BSI were observed. This is contradictory to the current approach to modern antimicrobial stewardship: in newborn population, with suspected BSI, it is recommended to terminate antibiotic treatment after 48 h since the identification of symptoms, if the infection was not confirmed microbiologically. Even traditional diagnostics based on the culture method ensures obtaining a positive result (information on microbial etiology of infection) within 48 h [30, 31].

For antimicrobial stewardship to efficiently and effectively influence the reduction of antibiotic consumption, but not to decrease patient safety, in neonatal units, a principle of daily detailed review of the situation of neonates treated with antibiotics should be introduced, so as to minimize the intake of antibiotics in children, whose blood cultures and other clinical specimens tested negative and symptoms of infection are no longer observed or infectious origin of the disease was excluded. The lack of significant differences in DOT values of laboratory confirmed vs. not-confirmed BSI cases would point to the fact that these recommendations are not applied in the PNSN wards.

It should also be noted that rapid diagnostic molecular methods (which enable rapid assessment of the need to implement or discontinue therapy with vancomycin) could be implemented to decrease glycopeptides consumption, because glycopeptides are not easy to use in neonates [32, 33]. For it has been observed that the use of glycopeptides in the case of BSI caused by *Enterobacteriaceae* was lower by only approx. 20% in comparison with BSI caused by Gram-positive cocci. Generally, in our study, in treatment of BSI as a whole glycopeptides were used the longest. Similar situation was reported in study of Sameer et al. [34].

As for aminoglycosides, only the use of the DDD indicator permitted the demonstration of their significantly increased consumption in BSI caused by Gram-positive cocci (109 DDD), in comparison with BSI that were caused by Gram-negative bacilli (56.1 DDD).

Also noteworthy is the fact that there is a large share of antifungal drugs in the treatment of the analyzed cases of BSI, 25% of the entire consumption expressed by DDD (13.3% DOT), with simultaneous, lower than anticipated, participation of yeast-like fungi isolated in microbiological testing [35, 36]. This coincides with the trends observed in other studies. According to Fridkin, the application of fluconazole in infection prophylaxis contributed to this fact, which is also confirmed by other authors [6]. Thus, the high level of antimycotic medication consumption in PNSN wards fulfilled the task of reducing the incidence of fungal infections.

Antibiotic consumption assessment using at least two different measures, as presented in our study, can be a useful tool in antibiotic stewardship [27]. In presenting case, the results of the analysis indicate the need of implementing more sensitive and faster methods of microbiological diagnostics (PCR and/or MALDI-TOF) as a first step of reducing antibiotics consumption due to faster identification of etiological factor of infection. PCR increases the sensitivity of diagnostics test and shortens the time of identification of microorganisms without culture. MALDI-TOF improves the specificity and shortens the time of identification after receiving microorganism grow in culture method [37, 38]. These diagnostics techniques are still very rarely used in Polish hospital. They are considered as expensive procedures by hospitals' management, because complex cost-effectiveness analysis in the field of infection control, taking into account at least the cost of prolonged hospital stay, are not performed. In the study patient population occurrence of BSI significantly increases length of stay in NICU, by approximately 20 days [21].

Conclusions

Analysis of antibiotic consumption is an essential component of infection control, especially for NICU patients—for effective planning and reliable evaluation of interrelationships between individual elements of control programs.

Application of classical methods of microbiological diagnostics based on blood cultures significantly reduces the consumption of antibiotics expressed by DDD.

High consumption of glycopeptides marked by DOT indicates the necessity of applying rapid diagnostic assays.

Nevertheless, the assessment of antibiotic consumption in neonatal units represents a methodological challenge and requires the use of different measurement tools.

Abbreviations
BSI: bloodstream infection; DOT: days of therapy; DDD: defined daily dose; LC-BSI: laboratory confirmed bloodstream infection; LOT: length of therapy; NICU: neonatal intensive care unit; PDD: prescribed daily dose; PNSN: Polish Neonatal Surveillance Network; VLBW: very low birth weight; PCR: polymerase chain reaction; MALDI-TOF: matrix assisted laser desorption ionisation, MALDI; time of flight, TOF.

Authors' contributions
AR designed the study and was a major contributor in writing the manuscript; JWM drafted the first version of this manuscript; PA performed statistical analysis; MBK, EG, MN, AK, DP collected the data on the wards; MB have given final approval of the version to be published. All authors read and approved the final manuscript.

Author details
[1] Chair of Microbiology, Jagiellonian University Medical College, 18 Czysta Street, 31-121 Krakow, Poland. [2] Institute of Nature Conservation Polish Academy of Sciences, Krakow, Poland. [3] Clinic of Neonatology and Intensive Neonatal Care, Warsaw Medical University, Warsaw, Poland. [4] Clinic of Neonatology, Polish Mother's Memorial Hospital-Research Institute, Lodz, Poland. [5] Clinic of Neonatology and Intensive Neonatal Care, Institute of Mother and Child, Warsaw, Poland. [6] Department of Neonatal Diseases, Pomeranian Medical University, Szczecin, Poland. [7] Clinic of Neonatology, Jagiellonian University Medical College, Krakow, Poland.

Acknowledgements
Not applicable.

Competing interests
The authors declare that they have no competing interests.

Funding
The project of the Polish Neonatology Surveillance Network was funded by the Polish Ministry of Science and Higher Education (Decision No. 669/E-215-BSWN-0180/2008). The funder had no impact on the design of the study and collection, analysis and interpretation of data and writing the manuscript.

References

1. Wójkowska-Mach J, Borszewska-Kornacka M, Domańska J, Gadzinowski J, Gulczyńska E, Helwich E, et al. Early-onset Infections of very-low-birth-weight infants in Polish neonatal intensive care units. Pediatr Infect Dis J. 2012;31(7):691–5.
2. Ronnestad A, Abrahamsen TG, Medbo S, Reigstad H, Lossius K, Kaaresen PI, et al. Septicemia in the first week of life in a Norwegian National Cohort of extremely premature infants. Pediatrics. 2005;115:e262–8. doi:10.1542/peds.2004-1834.
3. Stoll BJ, Hansen NI, Bell EF, Shankaran S, Laptook AR, Walsh MC, et al. The Eunice Kennedy Shriver National Institute of Child Health and Human Development Neonatal Research Network: neonatal outcomes of extremely preterm infants from the NICHD Neonatal Research Network. Pediatrics. 2010;123(3):443–56. doi:10.1542/peds.2009-2959.
4. Klinger G, Levy I, Sirota L, Boyko V, Lerner-Geva L, Reichman B. Outcome of early-onset sepsis in a national cohort of very low birth weight infants. Pediatrics. 2010;125(4):e736–40. doi:10.1542/peds.2009-2017.
5. Versporten A, Sharland M, Bielicki J, Drapier N, Vankerckoven V, Goossens H. The antibiotic resistance and prescribing in European children project. A neonatal and pediatric antimicrobial web-based point prevalence survey in 73 hospitals worldwide. Pediatr Infect Dis J. 2013;32(6):242–53.
6. Fridkin SK, Kaufman D, Edwards JR, Shetty S, Horan T. Changing incidence of Candida bloodstream infections among NICU patients in the United States: 199502994. Padiatrics. 2006;117(5):1680–7.
7. Wojkowska-Mach J, Borszewska-Kornacka M, Domanska J, Gadzinowski J, Gulczynska E, Nowiczewski M, et al. Late-onset bloodstream infections of very-low-birth-weight infant. Data from the Polish Neonatology Surveillance Network in 2009–2011. J BMC Infect Dis. 2014;14(1):339. doi:10.1186/1471-2334-14-339.
8. Schwab F, Geffers C, Barwolff S, Ruden H, Gastmeier P. Reducing neonatal nosocomial bloodstream infections through participation in a national surveillance system. J Hosp Infect. 2007;65:319–25.
9. Makhoul IR, Sujov P, Smolkin T, Lusky A, Reichman B. Pathogen-specific early mortality in very low birth weight infants with late-onset sepsis: a national survey. Clin Infect Dis. 2005;40:218–24.
10. Grohskopf LA, Huskins WC, Sinkowitz-Cochran RL, Levine GL, Goldmann DA, Jarvis WR. Use of antimicrobial agents in United States neonatal and pediatric intensive care patients. Pediatr Infect Dis J. 2005;24:766–73.
11. Liem Y, van den Hoogen A, Rademaker C, Egberts TC, Fleer F, Krediet TG. Antibiotic weight-watching: slimming down on antibiotic use in a NICU. Acta Peadiatr. 2010;99:1900–2.
12. WHO Collaborating Centre for Drug Statistics Methodology, Guidelines for ATC classification and DDD assignment 2010. Oslo, 2009. ISSN 1726-4898, ISBN 978-82-8082-369-4
13. Porta A, Hsia Y, Doerholt K, Menson E, Spyridis N, Bielicki J, et al. Comparing neonatal and paediatric antibiotic prescribing between hospitals: a new algorithm to help international benchmarking. J Antimicrob Chemother. 2012;67:1278–86.
14. Berrington A. Antimicrobial prescribing in hospitals: be careful what you measure. J Antimicrob Chemother. 2010;65:163–8.
15. Gerber JS, Kronman MP, Ross RK, Hersh AL, Newland JG, Metjian TA, et al. Identifying targets for antimicrobial stewardship in children's hospitals. Infect Control Hosp Epidemiol. 2013;34(12):1252–8.
16. Haug JB, Reikvam A. WHO defined daily doses versus hospital-adjusted defined daily doses: impact on results of antibiotic use surveillance. J Antimicrob Chemother. 2013;68:2940–7.
17. Gastmeier P, Geffers C, Schwab F, Fitzner J, Oblader M, Ruden H. Development of a surveillance system for nosocomial infections: the component for neonatal intensive care in Germany. J Hosp Infect. 2004;57:126–31.
18. Brodie SB, Sands KE, Gray JE, Parker RA, Goldmann DA, Davis RB, Richardson DK. Occurrence of nosocomial bloodstream infections in six neonatal intensive care units. Pediatr Infect Dis J. 2000;19:56–65.
19. Drews MB, Ludwig AC, Leititis JU, Daschner FD. Low birth weight and nosocomial infection of neonates in a neonatal intensive care unit. J Hosp Infect. 1995;30:65–72.
20. Krawczyk-Wyrwicka I, Piotrowski A, Rydlewska-Liszkowska I, Hanke W. Costs of intensive care of newborns born prematurely. Prz Epidemiol. 2006;60:155–62.
21. Różańska A, Wójkowska-Mach J, Adamski P, Borszewska-Kornacka M, Gulczyńska E, Nowiczewski M, et al. Infections and risk-adjusted length of stay and hospital mortality in Polish neonatology intensive care units. Int J Infect Dis. 2015;35:87–92.
22. Edwards JR, Peterson KD, Mu Y, Banwrjee S, Allen-Bridson K, Morrell G, et al. National healthcare safety network (nhsn) report: data summary for 2006 through 2008, issued december 2009. Am J Infect Control. 2009;37:783–805. doi:10.1016/j.ajic.2009.10.001.

23. Gikas A, Roumbelaki M, Bagatzouni-Pieridou D, Alexandrou M, Zinieri V, Dimitriadis I, et al. Device-associated infections in the intensive care units of Cyprus: results of the first national incidence study. Infection. 2010;38:165–71.
24. Huang YC, Wang YH, Chou YH, Lien RI. Significance of coagulase-negative staphylococci isolated from a single blood culture from neonates in intensive care. Ann Trop Paediatr. 2006;26(4):311–8.
25. Van der Zwet WC, Kaiser AM, van Elburg RM, Berkhof J, Fetter WP, Parlevliet GA, et al. Nosocomial infections in a Dutch neonatal intensive care unit: surveillance study with definitions for infection specifically adapted for neonates. J Hosp Infect. 2005;61:300–11.
26. Liem Y, Heerdink A, Egberts A, Rademaker CM. Quantifying antibiotic use in peadiatrics: a proposal for neonatal DDDs. Eur J Clin Microbiol Infect Dis. 2010;29:1301–3.
27. Barlam T, Cosgrove S, Abbo L, MacDougall C, Schuetz AN, Septimus EJ, et al. Implementing an antibiotic stewardship program: guidelines by the Infectious Diseases Society of America and the Society for Healthcare Epidemiology of America. Clin Infect Dis. 2016;62(10):e51–77.
28. Różańska A, Wójkowska-Mach J, Borszewska-Kornacka M, Ćmiel A, Gadzinowski J, Gulczyńska E, et al. Antibiotic consumption and its costs of purchase in Polish Neonatology Networks Units. Przegl Epidemiol. 2012;66:513–9.
29. Wójkowska-Mach J, Różańska A, Borszewska-Kornacka M, Domańska J, Gadzinowski J, Gulczyńska E, et al. Necrotizing enterocolitis in preterm infants: epidemiology and antibiotic consumption in the Polish Neonatology Network neonatal intensive care units in 2009. PLoS ONE. 2014;9(3):e92865. doi:10.1371/journal.pone.0092865.
30. Garcia-Prats JA, Cooper TR, Schneider VF, Stager CE, Hansen TN. Rapid detection of microorganisms in blood cultures of newborn infants utilizing an automated blood culture system. Pediatrics. 2000;105(3):523–7.
31. Kaiser JR, Cassat JE, Lewno MJ. Should antibiotics be discontinued at 48 hours for negative late-onset sepsis evaluations in the neonatal intensive care unit? J Perinatol. 2002;22(6):445–7.
32. Lim HS, Chong YP, Noh YH, Jung JA, Kim YS. Exploration of optimal dosing regimens of vancomycin in patients infected with methicillin-resistant *Staphylococcus aureus* by modeling and simulation. J Clin Pharm Ther. 2014;16.39(2):196–203.
33. Ampe E, Delaere B, Hecq JD, Tulkens PM, Glupczynski Y. Implementation of a protocol for administration of vancomycin by continuous infusion: pharmacokinetic, pharmacodynamic and toxicological aspects. Int J Antimicrob Agents. 2013;41(5):439–46.
34. Sameer J, Oshoudi A, Prasad P, Delamona P, Larson E, Zaoutis T, et al. Antibiotic use in neonatal intensive care units and adherence with Centers for Disease Control and Prevention 12 step campaign to prevent antimicrobial resistance. Pediatr Infect Dis J. 2009;28(12):1047–51.
35. Friedman S, Richardson SE, Jacobs SE, O'Brien K. Systemic Candida infection in extremely low birth weight infants: short term morbidity and long term neurodevelopmental outcome. Pediatr Infect Dis J. 2000;19:499–504.
36. Manzoni P, Stolfi I, Pugni L, Decembrio L, Magnani C, Vetrano G, et al. A multicenter, randomized trial of prophylactic fluconazole in preterm neonates. N Engl J Med. 2007;356:2483–95.
37. Nieman AE, Savelkoul PH, Beishuizen A, Henrich B, Lamik B, MacKenzie CR, et al. A prospective multicenter evaluation of direct molecular detection of blood stream infection from a clinical perspective. BMC Infect Dis. 2016;16:314. doi:10.1186/s12879-016-1646-4.
38. Chen Y, Porter V, Mubareka S, Kotowich L, Simor AE. Rapid identification of bacteria directly from positive blood cultures by use of a serum separator tube, smudge plate preparation, and matrix-assisted laser desorption ionization-time of flight mass spectrometry. J Clin Microbiol. 2015;53(10):3349–52. doi:10.1128/JCM.01493-15.

3

Outbreak of plasmid-mediated NDM-1-producing *Klebsiella pneumoniae* ST105 among neonatal patients in Yunnan, China

Rui Zheng[1,2,3†], Qian Zhang[4†], Yidan Guo[5], Yue Feng[1,2], Li Liu[1,2], Amei Zhang[1,2], Yue Zhao[1,2], Xiaoyu Yang[1,2] and Xueshan Xia[1,2*]

Abstract

Background: In the past decade, the carbapenemase-producing *Enterobacteriaceae* (CPE) have been reported worldwide. Emergence of carbapenemase-producing strains among *Enterobacteriaceae* has been a challenge for treatment of clinical infection. The present study was undertaken to investigate the characteristics of carbapenem-resistant *Klebsiella pneumoniae* recovered from an outbreak that affected 17 neonatal patients in neonatal intensive care unit (NICU) of Kunming City Maternal and Child health Hospital, which is located in the Kunming city in far southwest of China.

Methods: Minimum inhibitory concentrations (MICs) for antimicrobial agents were determined according to the guidelines of the Clinical and Laboratory Standards Institute (CLSI); Modified Hodge test and Carba-NP test were preformed to identified the phenotypes of carbapenemases producing; To determine whether carbapenem resistance was transferable, a conjugation experiment was carried out in mixed broth cultures; Resistant genes were detected by using PCR and sequencing; Plasmids were typed by PCR-based replicon typing method; Clone relationships were analyzed by using multilocus-sequence typing (MLST) and pulsed field gel electrophoresis (PFGE).

Results: Eighteen highly carbapenem-resistant *Klebsiella pneumoniae* were isolated from patients in NICU and one carbapenem-resistant *K. pneumoniae* isolate was detected in incubator water. All these isolates harbored bla_{NDM-1}. Moreover, other resistance genes, viz., bla_{IMP-4}, bla_{SHV-1}, bla_{TEM-1}, $bla_{CTX-M-15}$, *qnrS1*, *qnrB4*, and *aacA4* were detected. The bla_{NDM-1} gene was located on a ca. 50 kb IncFI type plasmid. PFGE analysis showed that NDM-1-producing *K. pneumoniae* were clonally related and MLST assigned them to sequence type 105.

Conclusions: NDM-1 producing strains present in the hospital environment pose a potential risk and the incubator water may act as a diffusion reservoir of NDM-1- producing bacteria. Nosocomial surveillance system should play a more important role in the infection control to limit the spread of these pathogens.

Keywords: CPE, NDM-1, ST105, China

Background

Gram-negative bacilli are the most important cause of healthcare associated infections [1]. Among these, *Enterobacteriaceae* continue to be an important cause of such infections [2], particularly the carbapenemase-producing *Enterobacteriaceae* (CPE) in developing countries, such as China [3]. In the past decade, the CPEs have been reported worldwide, including KPC-, GES-, VIM-, IMP-, GIM-, NDM- and OXA- types [4]. Among them, the NDM-type carbapenemase is a novel metalo-beta-lactamase that was identified for the first time in 2008 [5]. NDM-1 carbapenemase belongs to class B of Ambler β-lactamases, and efficiently hydrolyses a broad range of β-lactams, including penicillins, cephalosporins, and

*Correspondence: oliverxia2000@aliyun.com
†Rui Zheng and Qian Zhang contributed equally to this paper
[2] Faculty of Life Science and Technology, Kunming University of Science and Technology, No. 727 Jing Ming Road, Chenggong District, Kunming, Yunnan, China
Full list of author information is available at the end of the article

carbapenems, except for aztreonam. Up to this day, the emergence of carbapenemase-producing strains among *Enterobacteriaceae* has been a challenge for treatment of clinical infection [6].

Plasmid-mediated drug resistance is one of the most serious problems in the treatment of infectious diseases due to the horizontal transfer of plasmids account for the dissemination of resistance genes and the emergence of drug resistant strains [7, 8]. Carbapenemase-producing strains are most often associated with many non-β-lactam-resistance genes, because of their locations on plasmids [9], which made therapeutic options for infections were very limited.

Klebsiella pneumoniae was a leading cause of nosocomial infections and spread rapidly in health care settings due to efficiency of colonization and rapid development of resistance to a wide range of antimicrobials [10]. Recently, *K. pneumoniae* harboring $bla_{\text{NDM-1}}$ were emergencing in China, which should pay great attention [11, 12]. Therefore, investigation of the molecular characteristics of NDM-1-producing *K. pneumoniae* is critical. Here, we identified 19 *K. pneumoniae* harboring $bla_{\text{NDM-1}}$, the transmission of these NDM-1-producing *K. pneumoniae* among neonatal patients at Kunming City Maternal and Child health Hospital was delineated in this study.

Methods

Bacterial isolates

Kunming City Maternal and Child health Hospital was a 200-bed tertiary care community health facility in the provincial capital, Kunming City. Carbapenem-resistant *Enterobacteriaceae* (CRE) isolates were rare in this facility prior to this outbreak. On January 22, 2014, one *K. pneumoniae* strain (M1) was isolated from a sputum specimen, obtained from a neonatal patient in the neonatal intensive care unit (NICU), this strain was resistant to carbapenems including imipenem and meropenem. On January 23, 2014, another carbapenem-resistant *K. pneumoniae* strain (M2) was isolated from a stool sample obtained from another neonate in the same ward. We screened the rectal swab samples taken from patients in the NICU ward; simultaneously, environmental swabs of bed linen, stethoscopes, doorknobs, and water in the neonatal incubator, and the hand swabs obtained from doctors and nurses, were also collected. All swabs were inoculated on the Mueller–Hinton plates containing 2 μg/mL meropenem. The colonies that grew on the selection medium and clinical isolates with decreased susceptibility to carbapenems were picked and identified using a VITEK 2 Compact (bioMérieux, Marcy l'Etoile, France).

Detection of phenotypes

The production of carbapenemases was evaluated in all isolates using a Modified Hodge test [13] and Carba NP test [14], as previously described.

Antimicrobial susceptibility testing

MICs for antimicrobial agents were determined by using the microdilution susceptibility testing method, according to the guidelines of the CLSI [15]. The antibiotics tested included imipenem, meropenem, ceftazidime, aztreonam, piperacillin, piperacillin/tazobactam, tigecycline, levofloxacin, and amikacin. MIC results were interpreted as specified by CLSI [13], except for tigecycline, which was interpreted as defined by the US Food and Drug Administration (susceptible: MIC $\leq$ 2 mg/L; resistant: MIC $\geq$ 8 mg/L). *Escherichia coli* ATCC 25922 was used as quality control.

Detection of drug-resistant genes

Bacterial chromosomal DNA was obtained from clinical strains and transconjugants with a TIANamp Bacterial DNA Kit according to the manufacturer's instructions (TIANGEN BIOTECH, Beijing, China). PCR and DNA sequence analysis were performed to confirm the presence of drug-resistant genes. The primers used in this study were described previously [3, 16]. β-lactamase genes, including, Ambler class A ($bla_{\text{CTX-M}}$, bla_{TEM}, bla_{SHV}, bla_{KPC}, bla_{IMI} and bla_{GES}), class B (bla_{VIM}, bla_{IMP}, bla_{NDM}, and bla_{SPM}), class C (bla_{CMY}, $bla_{\text{ACT-1}}$, and $bla_{\text{DHA-1}}$), and class D ($bla_{\text{OXA-48}}$) were detected in all clinical isolates and their transconjugants. Moreover, genes related to quinolone activity including *qnrA*, *qnrB*, and *qnrS*, *integron* genes and the *aac* gene were also detected. Products were sequenced on an ABI PRISM 3730AXL sequencer analyzer and compared with the reported sequences from GenBank.

Molecular typing

NDM-1-producing strains were genotyped by using MLST and PFGE. Seven housekeeping genes (*gapA*, *infB*, *mdh*, *pgi*, *phoE*, *rpoB*, and *tonB*) were amplified according to the protocol described on the MLST website [17]. PFGE were performed according to the procedure described by Pulse Net from the website of the Centers for Disease Control and Prevention [18]. *Salmonella enterica* serotype H9812 was used as a marker. The XbaI restriction patterns were analyzed and interpreted according to the criteria of Tenover et al. [19].

Analysis of plasmid and conjugation experiment

In order to determine whether carbapenem resistance was transferable, a conjugation experiment was carried out in mixed broth cultures. *Escherchia coli* J53 (Az^R) was used as the recipient strain. Test strains and the recipient strain were grown separately overnight in Luria–Bertani broth at 35 °C with shaking. Cultures (2 ml) of test strains and recipient strains were mixed in a tube and incubated at 35 °C for 4 h with shaking. Then, 50 μL of the mixture was placed on Mueller–Hinton agar containing 2 μg/mL meropenem and 200 mg/L sodium azide and incubated at 35 °C for 20 h. The colonies that grew on this medium were regarded as the products of successful conjugation and were picked up and identified using a VITEK 2 Compact. Plasmid DNA from donors and transformants were extracted with a TIANprep Plasmid Maxi Plasmid Kit according to the manufacturer's instructions (TIANGEN BIOTECH, Beijing, China) and was electrophoresed on 0.8 % agarose gels at 100 V for 4 h. The plasmid replicons of the bla_{NDM-1}-encoding plasmids were typed by using the PCR-based replicon typing method described previously [20].

Results

Bacterial isolates

Eighteen carbapenem-resistant *K. pneumoniae* strains (M1–M18) were isolated from 17 patients in a variety specimens including sputum, stool, and blood; and one carbapenem-resistant *K. pneumoniae* (M19) was detected in incubator water. The CRE outbreak was declared on March 31, 2014. Resistace screening was performed for all patients in the NICU until no further transmission was detected. All the 17 patients had received meropenem treatment as initial monotherapy, one patient died on February 10, 2014, while all others were recovered.

Phenotypes and drug-resistant genes

All strains (M1–M19) harbored bla_{NDM-1}, a carbapenemase-encoding gene. M3, M5, M8, M9, M17, M18, and M19 co-harbor another carbapenemase gene bla_{IMP-4}. Thirteen of 19 isolates showed positive phenotypic screening results for the Modified Hodge test, the positivity rate was 72 %, while the positive rate for the Carba-NP test was 100 %. Other β-lactamase genes were identified in 19 strains, including those of the bla_{TEM}, bla_{CTX-M}, and bla_{SHV}. The *qnr* and *aac* genes were also detected; no AmpC-like enzymes and *integron* genes were found. The remaining resistance genes that were evaluated were not detected. Details on these findings are shown in Table 1.

Antimicrobial susceptibility testing

Drug-resistance profiles were consistent between the 18 NDM-1-producing *K. pneumoniae* clinical isolates (M1–M18) and the one NDM-1-producing *K. pneumoniae* strain obtained from incubator water (M19). All the 19 strains were highly resistant to the tested carbapenems, including meropenem and imipenem. The MIC values for meropenem were in the range of 32–128 μg/mL and those of imipenem ranged from 4 to >128 μg/mL. Nineteen strains exhibited discrepant-level resistance to aztreonam, six isolates were sensitive, seven isolates were intermediate, and the rest six were resistant. The MIC values for the other tested β-lactam antibiotics were high (>128 μg/mL) in all tested strains. Tigecycline exhibited potent activity against all tested strains, none tigecycline reisitant strain was detected. All the isolates remained susceptible to ciprofloxacin and amikacin. These results are summarized in Table 1.

PFGE and MLST typing

PFGE patterns of the XbaI DNA digests of 19 *K. pneumoniae* isolates were obtained. Gel images were input into BioNumerics and phylogenetic tree was built for cluster analysis (Fig. 1). PFGE revealed four cluster among 19 *K. pneumoniae*. One cluster of 16 closely related isolates was found that exhibited >90 % similarities. MLST analysis showed that all the 19 *K. pneumoniae* strains identified here were defined as a single sequence type (ST105) with the allelic profile 2-3-2-1-1-4-18.

Plasmid analysis and bacterial conjugation

Carbapenems resistance was successfully transferred from all *K. pneumoniae* isolates to *E. coli* J53 (Az^R) by conjugation. The MIC values of the 19 transconjugants were tested, and all *E. coli* transconjugants exhibited significantly reduced carbapenem susceptibility to the tested carbapenems, including imipenem and meropenem, as compared to *E. coli* J53 (Az^R). Meanwhile, the transconjugants were resistant to β-lactam antibiotics, although not to aztreonam, and were susceptible to quinolones and aminoglycosides (Table 2). Analysis of plasmids harbored by M1–M19 and transconjugants revealed the presence of two plasmids (ca. 50 and ca. 2.3 kb), while the transconjugants only acquired the ca. 50-kb plasmid. PCR analysis confirmed that the plasmid present in transconjugants harbored both bla_{NDM-1} and bla_{SHV-1}. PCR-based inc/rep typing method showed that FIA, FIB, FIC, and F replicons were positive in all bla_{NDM-1}- encoding plasmids, which belonged to IncFI incompatibility group.

Discussion

Emergence of NDM-1-producing *Enterobacteriaceae* have disseminated worldwide from the Indian subcontinent brought about problems regarding therapy and control. In China, plasmids encoding bla_{NDM-1} have been identified in *Enterobacteriaceae* isolates in several regions including Beijing, Shanghai, Hong Kong, and

Table 1 Drug resistance profiles and resistance mechanisms of NDM-1-producing *K. pneumoniae*

Strains	Organism	Source	*NDM*	*IMP*	*CTX*	*SHV*	*TEM*	*QnrB*	*qnrS*	*aac*	MICs, μg/mL									
											MEM	IPM	CAZ	FOX	AMK	TIG	PIP	PIP/TZB	ATM	LEV
M1	KPN	Sputum	*NDM-1*	–	*CTX-M-15*	*SHV-1*	*TEM-1*	–	–	–	128	32	>128	>128	1	0.25	>128	>128/4	>128	<0.06
M2	KPN	Stool	*NDM-1*	–	*CTX-M-15*	*SHV-1*	–	*qnrB4*	–	*aacA4*	64	32	>128	>128	2	0.25	>128	>128/4	4	0.25
M3	KPN	Stool	*NDM-1*	*IMP-4*	*CTX-M-15*	*SHV-1*	–	–	*qnrS1*	*aacA4*	64	16	>128	>128	1	0.25	>128	>128/4	8	<0.06
M4	KPN	Stool	*NDM-1*	–	*CTX-M-15*	*SHV-1*	–	*qnrB4*	*qnrS1*	*aacA4*	128	32	>128	>128	2	0.25	>128	>128/4	4	<0.06
M5	KPN	Stool	*NDM-1*	*IMP-4*	*CTX-M-15*	*SHV-1*	–	*qnrB4*	*qnrS1*	*aacA4*	128	16	>128	>128	1	0.25	>128	>128/4	32	<0.06
M6	KPN	Stool	*NDM-1*	–	*CTX-M-15*	*SHV-1*	–	–	–	–	64	16	>128	>128	2	0.25	>128	>128/4	4	<0.06
M7	KPN	Blood	*NDM-1*	–	*CTX-M-15*	*SHV-1*	–	–	–	–	64	16	>128	>128	1	0.25	>128	>128/4	8	0.25
M8	KPN	Blood	*NDM-1*	*IMP-4*	*CTX-M-15*	*SHV-1*	–	–	*qnrS1*	–	64	16	>128	>128	1	0.25	>128	>128/4	16	<0.06
M9	KPN	Sputum	*NDM-1*	*IMP-4*	*CTX-M-15*	*SHV-1*	–	–	*qnrS1*	*aacA4*	64	32	>128	>128	1	0.25	>128	>128/4	8	<0.06
M10	KPN	Stool	*NDM-1*	–	*CTX-M-15*	*SHV-1*	–	–	–	–	64	32	>128	>128	1	0.25	>128	>128/4	4	<0.06
M11	KPN	Stool	*NDM-1*	–	*CTX-M-15*	*SHV-1*	–	–	*qnrS1*	*aacA4*	32	4	>128	>128	1	0.5	>128	>128/4	4	<0.06
M12	KPN	Stool	*NDM-1*	–	*CTX-M-15*	*SHV-1*	–	*qnrB4*	*qnrS1*	–	64	16	>128	>128	1	0.5	>128	>128/4	64	<0.06
M13	KPN	Stool	*NDM-1*	–	*CTX-M-15*	*SHV-1*	–	*qnrB4*	*qnrS1*	–	64	128	>128	>128	1	1	>128	>128/4	32	<0.06
M14	KPN	Blood	*NDM-1*	–	*CTX-M-15*	*SHV-1*	–	*qnrB4*	–	–	64	32	>128	>128	1	0.25	>128	>128/4	16	<0.06
M15	KPN	Blood	*NDM-1*	–	*CTX-M-15*	*SHV-1*	–	*qnrB4*	–	–	64	32	>128	>128	1	0.25	>128	>128/4	4	<0.06
M16	KPN	Stool	*NDM-1*	–	*CTX-M-15*	*SHV-1*	–	*qnrB4*	–	*aacA4*	64	>128	>128	>128	8	0.5	>128	>128/4	16	8
M17	KPN	Sputum	*NDM-1*	*IMP-4*	*CTX-M-15*	*SHV-1*	–	*qnrB4*	*qnrS1*	*aacA4*	128	16	>128	>128	1	0.5	>128	>128/4	32	<0.06
M18	KPN	Sputum	*NDM-1*	*IMP-4*	*CTX-M-15*	*SHV-1*	–	*qnrB4*	*qnrS1*	*aacA4*	64	16	>128	>128	1	0.5	>128	>128/4	32	<0.06
M19	KPN	iw	*NDM-1*	*IMP-4*	*CTX-M-15*	*SHV-1*	–	*qnrB4*	*qnrS1*	*aacA4*	64	32	>128	>128	1	0.5	>128	>128/4	16	<0.06

KPN Klebsiella pneumoniae, *ECO Escherichia coli*, *MEM* meropenem, *IPM* imipenem, *CAZ* ceftazidime, *FOX* cefoxitin, *AMK* amikacin, *TIG* tigecycline, *PIP* piperacillin, *PIP/TZB* piperacillin/tazobactam, *ATM* aztreonam, *LEV* levofloxacin, *iw* incubator water

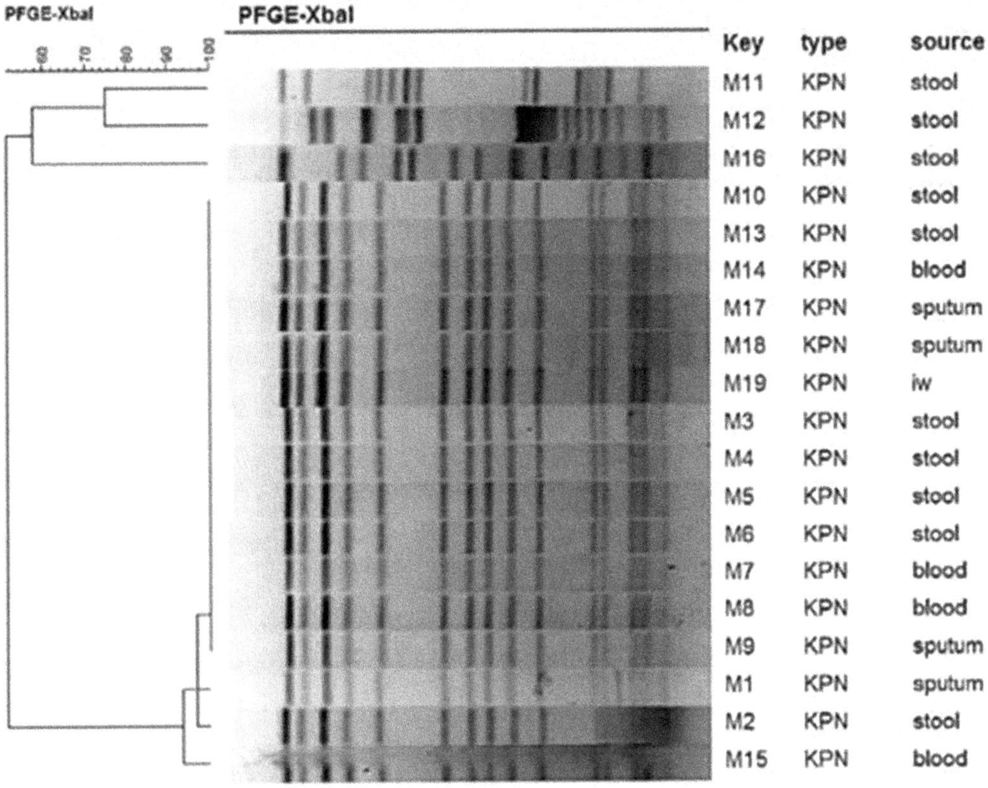

Fig. 1 Dendrogram of PFGE patterns of chromosomal DNA restriction fragments from 19 *K. pneumoniae* isolates in present study. *KPN Klebsiella pneumoniae*, *iw* incubator water

Shandong province, the size and Inc-type of the plasmids harbouring *bla*$_{NDM-1}$ were vary from ~50 to ~336 kb including InX3, IncL/M, IncA/C, and IncN incompatibility group [11, 21–23]. In present study, the plasmid harbouring the *bla*$_{NDM-1}$ belonged to the IncFI-type, which were different from previously replicon type reported in China before. Plasmid replicon types were related to the dissemination of resistance genes [22]. Due to its presence in all the 19 CREs in this study, this IncFI plasmid may be responsible for the dissemination of the *bla*$_{NDM-1}$ in this area.

Moreover, dissemination of *bla*$_{NDM-1}$ is associated with MLST type [24]. NDM-1-producing *K. pneumoniae* have been reported in different countries, and belonged to various kinds of MLST types, including ST11, ST14, ST17, ST25, ST147, ST149, ST231, ST340, and ST1043 [24–29]. Our datas indicated that all 19 NDM-1-producing *K. pneumoniae* strains belong to the same type, viz., ST105, which was different from previous types reported before. PFGE analysis showed 4 clusters for 19 ST105 strains. Among them, one cluster of 16 closely related isolates was found that exhibited ≥90 % similarities including the strains detected in incubator water. Thoese results suggested that 19 NDM-1-producing *K. pneumoniaee* strains were clonally related and easily spread to different patients in NICU ward, environmental reservoirs such as incubator water may contribute to the spread of these organisms within hospital. A previous research showed that *bla*$_{NDM-1}$ gene had disseminated in the NICU via different Gram Negative Bacilli (*E. coli*, *A. baumannii*, *S. maltophilia* and/or *K. pneumoniae*) harbouring *bla*$_{NDM-1}$ [30]. However, it is unclear how the *bla*$_{NDM-1}$ was introduced into the NICU ward in Kunming City Maternal and Child health Hospital. We suspect that isolates in this study represent a novel ST and that autochthonous clones are locally acquiring plasmids carrying the *bla*$_{NDM-1}$, as has been reported previously [27], more research would be needed to uncover it.

In addition, the average days for hospitalization in Kunming City Maternal and Child health Hospital is 6.06 days at present. However, the average hospital stay of the 17 patients including in this study was 18.9 days (more than trebled of average days of hospitalization in this hospital), prolonged hospitalization may contribute to spreading of the ST105 strains in NICU ward.

The *bla*$_{IMP-4}$ carbapenemase-encoding genes have also been detected in the part of NDM-1-producing strains (7/19). *Klebsiella pneumoniae* strains co-harbouring

Table 2 The results of antibiotic susceptibility testing of transconjugants in present study

Strains	MEM	IPM	CAZ	FOX	AMK	TIG	PIP	PIP/TZP	ATM	LEV
M1-J53	32	4	64	64	1	<0.125	>128	>128/4	0.5	<0.06
M2-J53	32	4	64	64	1	<0.125	>128	>128/4	0.5	<0.06
M3-J53	16	4	128	64	1	<0.125	>128	>128/4	0.5	<0.06
M4-J53	32	16	128	64	1	<0.125	>128	>128/4	0.5	<0.06
M5-J53	32	4	64	64	1	<0.125	>128	>128/4	0.5	<0.06
M6-J53	32	4	64	64	1	<0.125	>128	>128/4	0.5	<0.06
M7-J53	32	8	64	64	1	<0.125	>128	>128/4	0.5	<0.06
M8-J53	32	4	64	64	1	<0.125	>128	>128/4	0.5	<0.06
M9-J53	32	4	128	64	1	<0.125	>128	>128/4	0.5	<0.06
M10-J53	32	4	64	64	1	<0.125	>128	>128/4	0.5	<0.06
M11-J53	16	4	>128	64	1	<0.125	>128	>128/4	0.5	<0.06
M12-J53	32	8	64	64	1	<0.125	>128	>128/4	0.5	<0.06
M13-J53	32	4	64	64	1	<0.125	>128	>128/4	4	<0.06
M14-J53	32	4	64	64	1	<0.125	>128	>128/4	2	<0.06
M15-J53	32	8	64	64	1	<0.125	>128	>128/4	0.5	<0.06
M16-J53	32	4	64	64	1	<0.125	>128	>128/4	0.5	<0.06
M17-J53	32	4	32	64	1	<0.125	>128	>128/4	0.5	<0.06
M18-J53	32	16	64	64	1	<0.125	>128	>128/4	4	<0.06
M19-J53	32	4	64	64	1	<0.125	>128	>128/4	4	<0.06
E. coli J53	<0.125	<0.125	<0.125	8	1	<0.125	4	2/4	0.5	<0.06

MEM meropenem, *IPM* imipenem, *CAZ* ceftazidime, *FOX* cefoxitin, *AMK* amikacin, *TIG* tigecycline, *PIP* piperacillin, *PIP/TZB* piperacillin/tazobactam, *ATM* aztreonam, *LEV* levofloxacin

bla_{NDM-1} and bla_{IMP-4} have been identified in China previously, when they were found to be colocalized on a ca. 300-kb plasmid [31]. Plasmid analysis in this study showed that transconjugants acquired a ca. 50-kb plasmid. We analyzed the genomic DNA and plasmid DNA of 19 transconjugants by PCR, and confirmed only the presence of the bla_{NDM-1} and bla_{SHV-1}. This suggested that bla_{IMP-4} was not on the ca. 50-kb IncFI plasmid along with bla_{NDM-1}. We speculate that the bla_{IMP-4} gene may lie on the chromosome or a high molecular weight non-conjugative plasmid of which was not detected by the methodology used, further research was needed to uncover it. $Bla_{CTX-M-15}$ and bla_{NDM-1} have a common origin in the Indian subcontinent [25] and $bla_{CTX-M-15}$ had been identified in the NDM-1-producing strains, irrespective of whether the genes were located on the same plasmid [32, 33] or not [34]. Our study showed the presence of $bla_{CTX-M-15}$ along with bla_{NDM-1} in all strains, but none of the 17 patients or their family had any epidemiological link to the Indian subcontinent. AmpCs always been detected with NMD-1 producers [28], but bla_{ACT-1}, bla_{CMY}, and bla_{DHA-1} were not been found in this study. Although *qnrB4*, *qnrS1* and *aacA4* were detected in some strains, levofloxacin and amikacin maintained a good antibacterial activity in vitro.

Nineteen transconjugants showed increased MIC values for the tested carbapenems as compared with *E. coli* J53 (Az^R). The MIC values of 19 transconjugants for meropenem and imipenem ranged from 16 to 32 μg/mL and 4 to 16 μg/mL respectively, which was more than fourfold higher than those of *E. coli* J53. Due to the transconjugants only acquired bla_{NDM-1} and bla_{SHV-1}, we concluded that bla_{NDM-1} was primarily responsible for the high MIC values of carbapenems. In comprehensive consideration of both the MIC values of clinical isolates (M1–M18) and their transconjugants, bla_{IMP-4} and $bla_{CTX-M-15}$ also played a role in conferring resistance to the carbapenems.

Conclusions

Hospital environment such as incubator water may be the diffusion reservoirs of NDM-1-producing bacteria. Personal contact between the caregivers and the patients hospitalized in the same ward is the most likely transmission route. However, it can not determine how this clone was introduced into the hospital, ST105 *K. pneumoniae* may have been spreading in hospitals in the region and their prevalence may be increasing. Therefore, nosocomial surveillance system should play a more important role in the infection control to limit the spread of NDM-1-producing pathogens.

Abbreviations

CLSI: Clinical and Laboratory Standards Institute; CPE: carbapenemase-producing *Enterobacteriaceae*; CRE: carbapenem-resistant *Enterobacteriaceae*; ESBL: extended-spectrum β-lactamase; MDR: multidrug-resistant; MLST: multilocus-sequence typing; NICU: neonatal intensive care unit; PFGE: pulsed field gel electrophoresis.

Authors' contributions

XX designed the study; RZ drafted the first version of this manuscript; QZ collected the isolates and clinical informations; YG performed the PFGE; RZ and QZ preformed the antimicrobial susceptibility test and conjugation experiment; RZ, YF, LL, AZ, YZ, and XY carried out the molecular biology experiments. All authors read and approved the final manuscript.

Author details

[1] Faculty of Environmental Science and Engineering, Kunming University of Science and Technology, Kunming, Yunnan, China. [2] Faculty of Life Science and Technology, Kunming University of Science and Technology, No. 727 Jing Ming Road, Chenggong District, Kunming, Yunnan, China. [3] Department of Clinical Laboratory, First People's Hospital of Yunnan province, Kunming, Yunnan, China. [4] Department of Clinical Laboratory, Kunming City Maternal and Child health Hospital, Kunming, Yunnan, China. [5] Yunnan Center for Disease Control and Prevention, Kunming, Yunnan, China.

Acknowledgements

Escherchia coli J53 was a kind gift from Prof. Yang Qing, the First Affiliated Hospital of Zhejiang University. This work was supported by Yunnan Science and Technology Commission (2013FB205, 2015BC001) from Yunnan provincial Science and Technology Department and Kunming Medical University.

Competing interests

The authors declare that they have no competing interests.

References

1. Gaynes R, Edwards JR, National Nosocomial Infections Surveillance S. Overview of nosocomial infections caused by gram-negative bacilli. Clin Infect Dis. 2005;41(6):848–54. doi:10.1086/432803.
2. Walsh TR, Toleman MA. The emergence of pan-resistant Gram-negative pathogens merits a rapid global political response. J Antimicrob Chemother. 2012;67(1):1–3. doi:10.1093/jac/dkr378.
3. Li H, Zhang J, Liu Y, Zheng R, Chen H, Wang X, et al. Molecular characteristics of carbapenemase-producing *Enterobacteriaceae* in China from 2008 to 2011: predominance of KPC-2 enzyme. Diagn Microbiol Infect Dis. 2014;78(1):63–5. doi:10.1016/j.diagmicrobio.2013.10.002.
4. Dortet L, Poirel L, Nordmann P. Worldwide dissemination of the NDM-type carbapenemases in gram-negative bacteria. BioMed Res Int. 2014;2014:249856. doi:10.1155/2014/249856.
5. Yong D, Toleman MA, Giske CG, Cho HS, Sundman K, Lee K, et al. Characterization of a new metallo-β-lactamase gene, blaNDM-1, and a novel erythromycin esterase gene carried on a unique genetic structure in Klebsiella pneumoniae sequence type 14 from India. Antimicrob Agents Chemother. 2009;53(12):5046–54.
6. Tzouvelekis LS, Markogiannakis A, Psichogiou M, Tassios PT, Daikos GL. Carbapenemases in *Klebsiella pneumoniae* and other Enterobacteriaceae: an evolving crisis of global dimensions. Clin Microbiol Rev. 2012;25(4):682–707. doi:10.1128/CMR.05035-11.
7. Barman S, Chatterjee S, Chowdhury G, Ramamurthy T, Niyogi SK, Kumar R, et al. Plasmid-mediated streptomycin and sulfamethoxazole resistance in Shigella flexneri 3a. Int J Antimicrob Agents. 2010;36(4):348–51. doi:10.1016/j.ijantimicag.2010.06.037.
8. Coque TM, Novais A, Carattoli A, Poirel L, Pitout J, Peixe L, et al. Dissemination of clonally related *Escherichia coli* strains expressing extended-spectrum beta-lactamase CTX-M-15. Emerg Infect Dis. 2008;14(2):195–200. doi:10.3201/eid1402.070350.
9. Kumarasamy KK, Toleman MA, Walsh TR, Bagaria J, Butt F, Balakrishnan R, et al. Emergence of a new antibiotic resistance mechanism in India, Pakistan, and the UK: a molecular, biological, and epidemiological study. Lancet Infect Dis. 2010;10(9):597–602.
10. Jarvis WR, Munn VP, Highsmith AK, Culver DH, Hughes JM. The epidemiology of nosocomial infections caused by *Klebsiella pneumoniae*. Infect Control. 1985;6(2):68–74.
11. Jin Y, Shao C, Li J, Fan H, Bai Y, Wang Y. Outbreak of multidrug resistant NDM-1-producing *Klebsiella pneumoniae* from a neonatal unit in Shandong Province, China. PLoS One. 2015;10(3):e0119571. doi:10.1371/journal.pone.0119571.
12. Wang X, Xu X, Li Z, Chen H, Wang Q, Yang P, et al. An outbreak of a nosocomial NDM-1-producing *Klebsiella pneumoniae* ST147 at a teaching hospital in mainland China. Microbial Drug Res. 2014;20(2):144–9. doi:10.1089/mdr.2013.0100.
13. CLSI. Performance standards for antimicrobial susceptibility testing; 23rd informational supplement. M100-S23: Clinical and Laboratory Standards Institute, Wayne, PA. 2013.
14. Nordmann P, Poirel L, Dortet L. Rapid detection of carbapenemase-producing *Enterobacteriaceae*. Emerg Infect Dis. 2012;18(9):1503.
15. CLSI. Methods for dilution antimicrobial susceptibility tests for bacteria that grow aerobically, 9th ed. Approved standard M07-A9: Clinical and Laboratory Standards Institute, Wayne, PA. 2012.
16. Yang Q, Wang H, Sun H, Chen H, Xu Y, Chen M. Phenotypic and genotypic characterization of *Enterobacteriaceae* with decreased susceptibility to carbapenems: results from large hospital-based surveillance studies in China. Antimicrob Agents Chemother. 2010;54(1):573–7. doi:10.1128/AAC.01099-09.
17. Institut pasteur MLST databases. http://bigsdb.web.pasteur.fr/klebsiella/klebsiella.html. Accessed 19 Sep 2014.
18. Centers for Disease Control and Prevention. http://www.cdc.gov/pulsenet/protocols.htm. Accessed 20 May 2008.
19. Tenover FC, Arbeit RD, Goering RV, Mickelsen PA, Murray BE, Persing DH, et al. Interpreting chromosomal DNA restriction patterns produced by pulsed-field gel electrophoresis: criteria for bacterial strain typing. J Clin Microbiol. 1995;33(9):2233–9.
20. Carattoli A, Bertini A, Villa L, Falbo V, Hopkins KL, Threlfall EJ. Identification of plasmids by PCR-based replicon typing. J Microbiol Methods. 2005;63(3):219–28. doi:10.1016/j.mimet.2005.03.018.
21. Ho PL, Lo WU, Yeung MK, Lin CH, Chow KH, Ang I, et al. Complete sequencing of pNDM-HK encoding NDM-1 carbapenemase from a multidrug-resistant *Escherichia coli* strain isolated in Hong Kong. PLoS ONE. 2011;6(3):e17989.
22. Qu H, Wang X, Ni Y, Liu J, Tan R, Huang J, et al. NDM-1-producing *Enterobacteriaceae* in a teaching hospital in Shanghai, China: IncX3-type plasmids may contribute to the dissemination of bla. Int J Infect Dis. 2015;34:8–13. doi:10.1016/j.ijid.2015.02.020.
23. Zhou G, Guo S, Luo Y, Ye L, Song Y, Sun G, et al. NDM-1–producing Strains, Family *Enterobacteriaceae*, in Hospital, Beijing, China. Emerg Infect Dis. 2014;20(2):340.
24. Giske CG, Froding I, Hasan CM, Turlej-Rogacka A, Toleman M, Livermore D, et al. Diverse sequence types of *Klebsiella pneumoniae* contribute to the dissemination of blaNDM-1 in India, Sweden, and the United Kingdom. Antimicrob Agents Chemother. 2012;56(5):2735–8. doi:10.1128/AAC.06142-11.
25. Oteo J, Domingo-Garcia D, Fernandez-Romero S, Saez D, Guiu A, Cuevas O, et al. Abdominal abscess due to NDM-1-producing *Klebsiella pneumoniae* in Spain. J Med Microbiol. 2012;61(Pt 6):864–7. doi:10.1099/jmm.0.043190-0.
26. Voulgari E, Gartzonika C, Vrioni G, Politi L, Priavali E, Levidiotou-Stefanou S, et al. The Balkan region: NDM-1-producing *Klebsiella pneumoniae* ST11 clonal strain causing outbreaks in Greece. The Journal of antimicrobial chemotherapy. 2014;69(8):2091–7. doi:10.1093/jac/dku105.
27. Escobar Perez JA, Olarte Escobar NM, Castro-Cardozo B, Valderrama Marquez IA, Garzon Aguilar MI, Martinez de la Barrera L, et al. Outbreak of NDM-1-producing *Klebsiella pneumoniae* in a neonatal unit in Colombia. Antimicrob Agents Chemother. 2013;57(4):1957–60. doi:10.1128/AAC.01447-12.
28. Poirel L, Dortet L, Bernabeu S, Nordmann P. Genetic features of blaNDM-1-positive *Enterobacteriaceae*. Antimicrob Agents Chemother. 2011;55(11):5403–7. doi:10.1128/AAC.00585-11.

29. Pasteran F, Albornoz E, Faccone D, Gomez S, Valenzuela C, Morales M, et al. Emergence of NDM-1-producing *Klebsiella pneumoniae* in Guatemala. J Antimicrob Chemother. 2012;67(7):1795–7. doi:10.1093/jac/dks101.
30. Roy S, Singh AK, Viswanathan R, Nandy RK, Basu S. Transmission of imipenem resistance determinants during the course of an outbreak of NDM-1 Escherichia coli in a sick newborn care unit. J Antimicrob Chemother. 2011;66(12):2773–80. doi:10.1093/jac/dkr376.
31. Chen Z, Wang Y, Tian L, Zhu X, Li L, Zhang B, et al. First Report in China of *Enterobacteriaceae* clinical isolates coharboring blaNDM-1 and blaIMP-4 drug resistance genes. Microbial Drug Res. 2014. doi:10.1089/mdr.2014.0087.
32. Yoo JS, Kim HM, Koo HS, Yang JW, Yoo JI, Kim HS, et al. Nosocomial transmission of NDM-1-producing *Escherichia coli* ST101 in a Korean hospital. J Antimicrob Chemother. 2013;68(9):2170–2. doi:10.1093/jac/dkt126.
33. Solé M, Pitart C, Roca I, Fàbrega A, Salvador P, Muñoz L, et al. First description of an *Escherichia coli* strain producing NDM-1 carbapenemase in Spain. Antimicrob Agents Chemother. 2011;55(9):4402.
34. Poirel L, Revathi G, Bernabeu S, Nordmann P. Detection of NDM-1-producing *Klebsiella pneumoniae* in Kenya. Antimicrob Agents Chemother. 2011;55(2):934–6.

4

Characterization of clinical extensively drug-resistant *Pseudomonas aeruginosa* in the Hunan province of China

Jun Li[1], Mingxiang Zou[1*], Qingya Dou[2], Yongmei Hu[1], Haichen Wang[1], Qun Yan[1] and Wen'en Liu[1]

Abstract

Background: *Pseudomonas aeruginosa* strains that are classed as extensively drug resistant (XDR-PA) are resistant to all antibiotics except for one or two classes and are frequently the cause of hard-to-treat infections worldwide. Our study aimed to characterize clinical XDR-PA isolates recovered during 2011–2012 at nine hospitals in the Hunan province of China.

Methods: Thirty-seven non-repetitive XDR-PA strains from 37 patients were investigated for genes encoding antimicrobial resistance determinants, efflux pumps, outer membrane proteins, and movable genetic elements using polymerase chain reaction (PCR). The expression of genes encoding the efflux pump component MexA and the outer membrane protein OprD was measured using real-time PCR. In addition, clonal relatedness of these XDR-PA isolates was analyzed by pulsed-field gel electrophoresis (PFGE).

Results: Various genes encoding antimicrobial resistance determinants were found in all isolates. In particular, the bla_{TEM-1}, bla_{CARB}, *armA*, bla_{IMP-4}, bla_{VIM-2}, and *rmtB*, were found in 100, 37.8, 22, 22, 19 and 5 % of the isolates, respectively. Remarkably, two isolates coharbored bla_{IMP-4}, bla_{VIM-2}, and *armA*. In all 37 antibiotic-resistant strains, the relative expression of *oprD* was decreased while *mexA* was increased compared to the expression of these genes in antibiotic-susceptible *P. aeruginosa* strains. All of the XDR-PA isolates harbored class I integrons as well as multiple other mobile genetic elements, such as *tnpU*, *tnp513*, *tnpA* (Tn*21*), and *merA*. A high genotypic diversity among the strains was detected by PFGE.

Conclusions: Multiple antibiotic-resistance mechanisms contributed to the drug resistance of the XDR-PA isolates investigated in this study. Thus, the XDR-PA isolates in this area were not clonally related. Instead, multiple types of movable genetic elements were coharbored within each XDR-PA isolate, which may have aided the rapid development of these XDR-PA strains. This is the first report of XDR-PA strains that coharbor bla_{IMP-4}, bla_{VIM-2}, and *armA*.

Keywords: Extensively drug-resistant *Pseudomonas aeruginosa*, Resistance mechanism, Movable genetic elements, Molecular epidemiology, PFGE

Background

Pseudomonas aeruginosa, a rod-shaped, non-fermenting gram-negative bacterium, causes nosocomial infections that can lead to sepsis, pneumonia, endocarditis, and urinary tract infections. The emergence of extensively drug-resistant *P. aeruginosa* (XDR-PA) strains showing resistant to all antimicrobial agents except for one or two classes is becoming a major public health concern [1–5].

That was found by previous studies the mechanisms of antibiotic resistance associated with clinical XDR-PA isolates are complex [6, 7]. The prevailing hypothesis is that XDR-PA isolates acquire numerous drug-resistance determinants through horizontal gene transfer that is mediated by mobile genetic elements [8–10]. In addition, genes encoding the antibiotic-inactivating enzymes

*Correspondence: zoumingxiang@126.com
[1] Department of Clinical Laboratory, Xiangya Hospital, Central South University, No. 87, Xiangya Road; Kaifu District, Changsha 410008, Hunan, China
Full list of author information is available at the end of the article

β-lactamases, aminoglycoside-modifying enzymes (AMEs), and 16S rRNA methylases (16S-RMTases) are frequently associated with antibiotic resistance in XDR-PA strains. In recent studies, an over-expression of drug-efflux pumps and diminished expression of outer membrane proteins are suggested to play a role in drug resistance [11–14].

Although the prevalence of drug-resistance determinants in XDR-PA strains isolated in other countries has been determined [15, 16], few studies have investigated the resistance mechanisms and the epidemiological profiles of clinical XDR-PA isolates found in China. Before 2011, XDR-PA strains were rarely found in China; thereafter, a gradual emergence has occurred in some hospitals. Therefore, the purpose of this study was to analyze the resistance mechanisms and molecular epidemiology of clinical XDR-PA strains isolated earlier in our region recovered from 2011 to 2012.

Methods

Bacterial isolates

Thirty-seven out of 482 (7.7 %) *P. aeruginosa* isolates that were screened were XDR-PA strains displaying resistance to all antimicrobial agents except colistin. The *P. aeruginosa* strains were isolated from September 1, 2011 to June 30, 2012 from nine of fifteen different hospitals in the Hunan province of China. Drug susceptibility of XDR-PA isolates was determined by the Kirby-Bauer (K-B) disk diffusion method and two quality control strains (*Escherichia coli* ATCC25922 and *P. aeruginosa* ATCC27853) were included in the analyses. The results were analyzed and interpreted according to the guidelines of Clinical and Laboratory Standards Institute (CLSI) [17]. To prevent analysis of redundant strains, only the first strain was collected when duplicate strains were from the same patient.

Phenotypic tests for carbapenemase production

The modified Hodge test (MHT) was used to detect the production of carbapenemase using an imipenem disc (10 μg) as described by CLSI [17]. A combined-disc test was carried out to detect the production of metallo-β-lactamase (MBL). Two discs [One disc contained imipenem (10 μg) and 5 μL of 0.5 M EDTA (Sigma Chemicals), and the other disc contained only imipenem (10 μg)] were placed 20 mm apart on a Mueller–Hinton agar plate inoculated with each test strain. A strain was considered positive for metallo-β-lactamase production when the zone diameter around the imipenem-EDTA disc was more than 4 mm of the imipenem-only disc [18].

Detection of genes encoding antimicrobial resistance determinants and genes associated with movable genetic elements

The DNA templates used in polymerase chain reactions (PCR) to amplify genes encoding antimicrobial resistance determinants were obtained as follows: bacterial suspensions were incubated for 10 min at 95 °C followed by centrifugation at 10,000×*g* for 10 min to remove cellular debris. Genes coding for carbapenem β-lactamases (bla_{KPC}, bla_{SME}, bla_{GES}, bla_{IMI}/bla_{NMC}, bla_{NDM-1}, bla_{VIM-2}, bla_{IMP-4}, bla_{SIM-1}, bla_{GIM}, bla_{SPM}, bla_{OXA-23}, and bla_{OXA-51}), extended-spectrum β-lactamases (ESBLs) (bla_{TEM-1}, bla_{CTX-M}, bla_{SHV}, bla_{OXA-1}, bla_{OXA-2}, bla_{OXA-10}, bla_{VEB}, and bla_{PER}), and AmpC β-lactamases (bla_{MOX}, bla_{FOX}, bla_{DHA}, bla_{CIT}, and bla_{EBC}) were performed by PCR with previously described primers [18–20]. In addition, the isolates were screened by PCR for AME genes (*aac(3)-IIa* and *ant(2″)-Ia*) [21], 16S-RMTases (*armA, npmA, rmtA, rmtB, rmtC, rmtD*, and *rmtE*) [22], a drug-efflux pump component (*mexA*), and an outer membrane protein (*oprD*). The PCR primers used to screen for these genes are listed in Table 1. To detect genes associated with the movable genetic elements, *intI, traA, traF, trbC, tnp513,* IS*pa7*, IS*Ecp1*, *tnpU*, *tnpA* (Tn*21*), *tnsA*, and *merA*, PCR was performed with primers shown in Table 1. All amplified DNA fragments were sequenced and then analyzed using the BLAST program (http://www.ncbi.nlm.nih.gov/BLAST).

Quantifying expression of *mexA* and *oprD*

The expression of *mexA* and *oprD* in the XDR-PA isolates was determined by real-time PCR (RT-PCR). The experimental group consisted of the 37 XDR-PA isolates and the control group was made up of 31 *P. aeruginosa* isolates that were collected at the same time as the XDR-PA strains but were shown to be sensitive to all antimicrobial agents tested. The primers used for quantifying *mexA* and *oprD* expression are listed in Table 1. The RT-PCR reactions were carried out by a QuantiFast SYBR Green RT-PCR Kit from Qiagen and a Real-Time PCR System of LightCycler 2.0 from Roche, Burgess Hill, UK, according to the manufacturer protocols. All reactions were repeated three times using 10 ng of RNA template that was prepared using the RNeasy Mini Kit from Qiagen, Crawley, UK and treated with Dnase. Gene expression was normalized relative to that of the *16S rRNA* gene using the $2^{-\triangle\triangle CT}$ method [23]. The expression of *16S rRNA* gene was determined by the primers shown in Table 1.

Table 1 Primers used in this study for PCR and RT-PCR analyses

Gene	Sequence (5′–3′)	Fragment length (bp)
intI	F:CCGAGGATGCGAACCACTTC R:CCGCCACTGCGCCGTTACCA	789
traA	F:AAGTGTTCAGGGTGCTTCTGCGC R:GTCATGTACATGATGACCATTT	272
traF	F:CGGTGATGATTTGCGAACGA R:AGCATTCCGGTCGGCCTGTA	400
trbC	F:CGGYATWCCGSCSACRCTGCG R:GCCACCTGYSBGCAGTCMCC	255
tnp513	F:ATGTCGCTGGCAAGGAACGC R:GGGTTCGCTGCGAGGATTGT	240
IS*pa7*	F:TCAGGCCTTCATCGCTGCCATCAGG R:TAGGCGTACAGTGCTCTTTCAACGCA	300
IS*Ecp1*	F:CTTCATTGGCATTGATAAGTTAG R:TGTAGCATCGGTTTCCCAGTTTC	299
tnpU	F:CCAACTGATGGCGGTGCCTT R:CGGTATGGTGGCTTTCGC	403
tnpA (Tn*21*)	F:ATGCCACGTCGTTCCATCCTGTCC R:CCGGGTCTGCTCCCGCTGGCC	300
tnsA	F:GCAGCAGCCTTACAAGACGAG R:GCCACATAGCGCAACTCCTCC	416
merA	F:GACCAGCCGCAGTTCGTCTA R:GCAGCASGAAAGCT GCTTCA	462
mexA	F:CGACCAGGCCGTGAGCAAGCAGC R:GGAGACCTTCGCCGCGTTGTCGC	275
oprD	F:ATGAAAGTGATGAAGTGGAGCG R:TTACAGGATCGACAGCGGATAG	949
mexA in RT-PCR	F:GGCGACAACGCGGCGAAGG R:CCTTCTGCTTGACGCCTTCCTGC	202
oprD in RT-PCR	F:CGGCGACATCAGCAACACC R:GGGCCGTTGAAGTCGGAGTA	195
16S rRNA in RT-PCR	F:CCTACGGGAGGCAGCAG R:ATTACCGCGGCTGCTGG	194

Pulsed-field gel electrophoresis (PFGE)

Clonal relatedness of the XDR-PA isolates was analyzed by PFGE. Preparation of genomic DNA was done in agarose blocks. The DNA was then digested by the restriction enzyme *Xba*I from Promega, USA, followed by embedding into 1 % PFGE agarose gel. PFGE was performed for 24 h using the GenePath System from Bio-Rad with the follow conditions: 5.5 V/cm, 12 °C, 120°, and a switch time from 4 to 40 s. The molecular size marker, *Salmonella enterica* strain H9812, was obtained from the respiratory laboratory of infectious diseases, CDC, China. The gel was stained for 30 min with ethidium bromide and the gel image was documented using the gel documentation system Gel Doc 2000 from Bio-Rad. Finally, analyses of the results were performed by the BioNumerics software platform (Applied Math, Sint-Maten-Latem, Belgium) and visual inspection with the criteria of relatedness proposed by Tenover et al. [24].

Statistical analysis

WHONET software (version 5.4, WHO) was used to analyze the patient demographic information and the antibiotic resistance data using the 2014 CLSI criteria for breakpoints for *P. aeruginosa*. Comparisons of different groups were analyzed by a two-sided Chi square (χ^2) test with the SPSS13.0 software (SPSS Inc., USA). A $P < 0.05$ was regarded as statistically significant.

Results

Phenotypic screening and resistance determinants

Of the 37 XDR-PA isolates, 13 (35.1 %) isolates were positive for MTH and MBL, while all other isolates were negative (Fig. 1).

Diverse types of genes encoding antibiotic-inactivating enzymes were detected. Specifically, the genes $bla_{\text{TEM-1}}$, bla_{CARB}, *armA*, $bla_{\text{IMP-4}}$, $bla_{\text{VIM-2}}$, and *rmtB* were found in 100, 37.8, 22, 22, 19 and 5 % of the XDR-PA isolates, respectively. The ESBL gene $bla_{\text{TEM-1}}$ was found in all

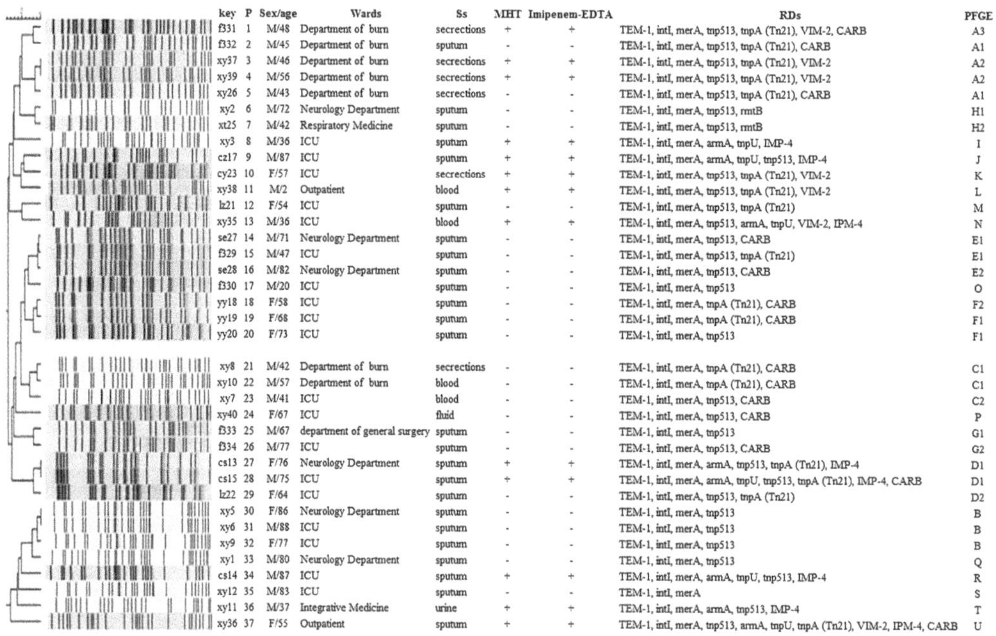

Fig. 1 Clinical features, molecular characterization, and dendrogram based on PFGE of 37 XDR-PA isolates. The dendrogram was developed using the BioNumerics software platform. *P* patients, *Ss* specimens, *RDs* resistance determinants, *xy* Xiangya Hospital, f_3 the Third Xiangya Hospital, *yy* People's Hospital of Liuyang, *cs* the Third Hospital of Changsha, *se* the Second People's Hospital of Hunan province, *xt* Xiangtan Central Hospital, *lz* Chinese Medicine Hospital of Liuyang, *cz* People's Hospital of Chenzhou, *cy* the First Hospital of Changsha, and *A–U* PFGE types

isolates, while the other ESBL genes that were tested were not found in any of the isolates. Among the 37 XDR-PA isolates, 13 (35.1 %) isolates were positive for MBLs genes, 8 contained bla_{IMP-4}, and 7 contained bla_{VIM-2}. Two types of 16S-RMTases genes were detected. Eight isolates contained *armA*, while two isolates contained *rmtB*. Eight isolates coharbored bla_{IMP-4} and *armA* and two isolates coharbored bla_{IMP-4}, bla_{VIM-2}, and *armA*. No isolates harbored genes encoding AmpC β-lactamases or AMEs.

The efflux-pump gene *mexA* and the outer membrane protein gene *oprD* were detected in all 37 XDR-PA isolates. However, no mutations were detected in any of the *oprD* genes. Figure 1 lists the antibiotic resistance genes detected in each isolate.

Expression of *mexA* and *oprD*

The expression of *mexA* was significantly higher in the 37 XDR-PA isolates than in the control group consisting of 31 antibiotic-sensitive isolates (1.95 ± 0.48 and 0.70 ± 0.13, $P = 0.018$, respectively), while expression of *oprD* in the XDR-PA strains was significantly lower than the control group (3.18 ± 0.60 and 0.94 ± 0.08; $P = 0.002$, respectively; Fig. 2).

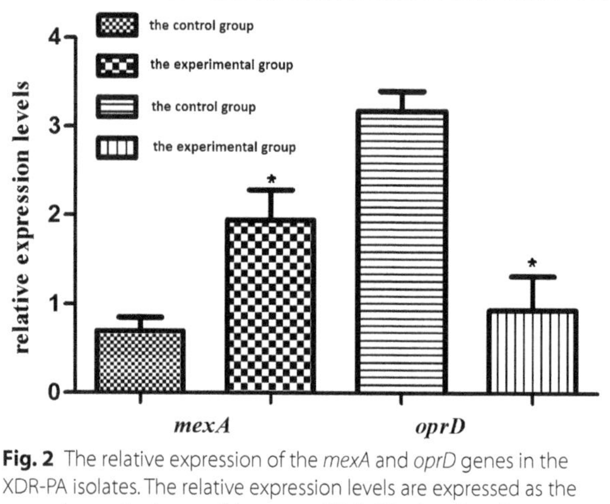

Fig. 2 The relative expression of the *mexA* and *oprD* genes in the XDR-PA isolates. The relative expression levels are expressed as the mean ± standard error of the mean (SEM). **P* values less than 0.05 are considered significant and are indicated by an *asterisk*

Distribution of genes associated with movable genetic elements

Of the movable genetic element genes tested, *intI, merA, tnp513, tnpA* (Tn*21*), and *tnpU* were detected in 100, 100, 81, 49, and 16 % of the isolates, respectively. Moreover, most of the 37 XDR-PA isolates coharbored three or more genes associated with movable genetic elements. For instance, isolates xy36 coharbored five types of movable genetic element genes (Fig. 1).

Clonal relatedness of the XDR-PA isolates

Using PFGE, the 37 XDR-PA isolates were divided into 21 PFGE types (Fig. 1). The main PFGE type found was

A (five strains), including three strains from Xiangya Hospital and two strains from the Third Xiangya Hospital. In addition, an A1 subtype was found in both hospitals. The B- and C-type isolates were found in the Xiangya Hospital, while the D-type isolates were found in the Third Hospital of Changsha as well as Chinese Medicine Hospital of Liuyang. The E-type strains were isolated from the Second People's Hospital of Hunan province and the Third Xiangya Hospital, and an E1 subtype was found in both hospitals. The F-type strains were isolated from the People's Hospital of Liuyang; the G-type strains were isolated from the Third Xiangya Hospital; and the H-type isolates were found at Xiangya Hospital and Xiangtan Central Hospital. The remaining 13 types, from I to U, were collected from the Xiangya Hospital (eight strains), the People's Hospital of Chenzhou (one strain), the First Hospital of Changsha (one strain), the Chinese Medicine Hospital of Liuyang (one strain), the Third Xiangya Hospital (one strain), and the Third Hospital of Changsha (one strain).

Discussion

Pseudomonas aeruginosa is considered one of the primary causes of hospital-acquired infections. An increase in the prevalence of clinical XDR-PA isolates correlates with a rise in mortality and morbidity rates. Consequently, XDR-PA strains pose a considerable threat to public health worldwide. In our study, 37 out of 482 (7.7 %) *P. aeruginosa* strains were found to be XDR-PA strains. The XDR-PA strains were isolated from nine of fifteen teaching hospitals detected in our region, suggesting that the occurrence of XDR-PA isolates in our region is low. To aid the prevention of the spread of XDR-PA strains, we have analyzed the resistance mechanisms and the molecular epidemiology of the XDR-PA strains.

Carbapenems are one of the most effective drugs against severe infections caused by gram-negative bacilli. Unfortunately, pathogens displaying resistance to carbapenems are increasing due to the following three main causes: production of carbapenemases, the over-expression of efflux pumps, and the diminished expression of the outer membrane porin OprD [15]. In *P. aeruginosa*, production of carbapenemases, especially MBLs, is an important antibiotic resistance mechanisms [25]. In this study, 13 (35.1 %) strains produced the metallo-enzymes IMP-4 and VIM-2, indicating that production of carbapenemases played role in carbapenem-resistant in the XDR-PA isolates. Notably, the prevalence of carbapenemases in the 37 XDR-PA isolates in our study were higher than that of other countries in the world [26, 27] and from other regions in China [28]. One isolate that coharbored two MBL genes was reported in previous studies [29]. This observation led to the emergence of a new drug-resistant model for *P. aeruginosa*. In our study, two isolates (xy35 and xy36) coharbored $bla_{\text{IMP-4}}$ and $bla_{\text{VIM-2}}$. To our knowledge, this is the first report of the co-existence of $bla_{\text{IMP-4}}$ and $bla_{\text{VIM-2}}$ in a *P. aeruginosa* strain.

Drug-efflux pumps have been correlated with bacterial resistance since the 1980s [30]. The first efflux pump found in *P. aeruginosa* is the MexAB-OprM pump, which has a broad range of substrates, including carbapenems, quinolones, aminoglycosides, tetracyclines, and macrolides. Therefore, the presence of this efflux pump in bacteria may lead to multi-drug resistance. In our study, the *mexA* gene, encoding a component of MexAB-OprM efflux pump, was found in all 37 XDR-PA isolates. Furthermore, a significant over-expression of *mexA* in the XDR-PA isolates was seen compared with the *mexA* levels in antibiotic-susceptible strains. Thus, over-expression of an efflux pump, especially MexAB-OprM, may play a key role in the antibiotic resistance of these XDR-PA isolates.

Decreased expression of OprD can significantly reduce the susceptibility of *P. aeruginosa* to carbapenems. Previous studies showed that decreased expression of *oprD* is primarily due to mutations in the OprD-encoding genes [31]. In our study, the expression of *oprD* in the 37 XDR-PA isolates was significantly lower than that in susceptible strains confirming that a decreased level of this porin plays a key role in carbapenem-resistance. However, no mutations or deletions were detected for the *oprD* gene in the 37 XDR-PA isolates. This finding was not consistent with previous studies [32, 33], suggesting that decreased expression of *oprD* in the 37 XDR-PA isolates might be due to regulation by small bioactive molecules, amino acids, or efflux pump expression [34]. Therefore, in-depth studies on the role of outer membrane proteins in bacterial drug resistance are needed in the future.

Production of AMEs and 16S-RMTases is the main cause of bacterial resistance to aminoglycoside agents [35, 36]. In contrast to these reports, none of the 37 XDR-PA isolates, which were resistant to aminoglycoside antibiotics, harbored genes encoding AMEs and only 27.0 % ($n = 10$) harbored either *armA* or *rmtB* 16S-RMTases genes. These data suggest that 16S-RMTases play an important role in aminoglycoside resistance in the XDR-PA isolates but also that some of these isolates may utilize an alternative, unknown resistance mechanism, such as new drug efflux pumps, new 16S-RMTases, or mutational activation of the AmgRS two-component system [37].

Movable genetic elements, including integrons, plasmids, transposons, and insertion sequences, play a key role in the horizontal transfer of resistance genes [38]. In this study, most of the XDR-PA isolates coharbored three or more genes associated with movable genetic elements. The most frequently detected genes were *intI*, *merA tnp513*, *tnpA* (Tn*21*), and *tnpU*, and their distribution percentage among the XDR-PA isolates was 100, 100, 81, 49, and 16 %, respectively. Furthermore, two isolates, cs15 and xy36, coharbored 5 types of genes associated with movable genetic elements.

The XDR-PA strains previously isolated in other countries were shown to be clonally related [1]. In contrast, the XDR-PA strains isolated from hospitals within the Hunan province of China were shown to be genetically diverse. The 37 XDR-PA isolates were divided into 21 different PFGE types and no one type predominated amongst the isolates suggesting that none of the XDR-PA isolates are considered to be an epidemic clone. Interestingly, the A-type, D-type, E-type, and H-type were detected in two different hospitals and the B-type, C-type, and F-type were found in two different wards of the same hospital during the same time period. Although prevalence of the XDR-PA isolates in this area was sporadic, dissemination of the same isolate was detected inter- and intra-hospital. The high heterogeneity of the PFGE types suggests that the mobile genetic elements may play a role in the emergence of clinical XDR-PA strains.

Conclusions

In conclusion, this study shows that the extreme antibiotic resistance of the clinical XDR-PA isolates is due to strains coharboring multiple antibiotic resistance genes, over-expressing drug-efflux pumps, and decreasing expression of *oprD*, which encodes an outer membrane porin. Moreover, this study has identified for the first time a *P. aeruginosa* isolate that coharbors the $bla_{\text{IMP-4}}$, $bla_{\text{VIM-2}}$, and *armA* antibiotic resistance genes. Although the XDR-PA isolates were not clonally related, the strains were shown to carry multiple genes encoding different types of movable genetic elements, which may aid the rapid development of XDR-PA isolates.

Authors' contributions

MZ contributed to the conception of the study. JL contributed significantly to analysis and manuscript preparation; QD and YH performed the data analyses and wrote the manuscript; HW, QY and WL helped perform the analysis with constructive discussions. All authors read and approved the final manuscript.

Author details

[1] Department of Clinical Laboratory, Xiangya Hospital, Central South University, No. 87, Xiangya Road; Kaifu District, Changsha 410008, Hunan, China.
[2] Department of Infection Control Center, Xiangya Hospital, Central South University, Changsha 410008, Hunan, China.

Acknowledgements

We are thankful to the staff in the Laboratory of Xiangya Hospital of Central South University who helped us in the collection and identification of these XDR-PA isolates. In particular, we thank Xin Xia, a teacher at the Center for Disease Control (CDC) in the Hunan Province of China, for helping us with the PFGE experiments.

Competing interests

The authors declare that they have no competing interests.

Funding

This work was supported by the Hunan Development and Reform Investment [2012] No. 1493 from the Development and Reform Commission of the Hunan Province, a Grant (14JJ7003) from the Natural Science Foundation of the Hunan Province, and the Hunan Development and Reform Investment [2014] No. 658 from Development and Reform Commission of the Hunan Province.

Informed consent

A signed, informed consent was given by all participants included in the study.

References

1. Ciofi Degli Atti M, Bernaschi P, Carletti M, Luzzi I, Garcia-Fernandez A, Bertaina A, Sisto A, Locatelli F, Raponi M. An outbreak of extremely drug-resistant *Pseudomonas aeruginosa* in a tertiary care pediatric hospital in Italy. BMC Infect Dis. 2014;14:494. doi:10.1186/1471-2334-14-494.
2. Fonseca EL, Freitas Fdos S, Vicente AC. The colistin-only-sensitive Brazilian *Pseudomonas aeruginosa* clone SP (sequence type 277) is spread worldwide. Antimicrob Agents Chemother. 2010;54(6):2743. doi:10.1128/aac.00012-10.
3. Jin JS, Kwon KT, Moon DC, Lee JC. Emergence of *16S rRNA* methylase rmtA in colistin-only-sensitive *Pseudomonas aeruginosa* in South Korea. Int J Antimicrob Agents. 2009;33(5):490–1. doi:10.1016/j.ijantimicag.2008.10.024.
4. Lee YC, Ahn BJ, Jin JS, Kim JU, Lee SH, do Song Y, Lee WK, Lee JC. Molecular characterization of *Pseudomonas aeruginosa* isolates resistant to all antimicrobial agents, but susceptible to colistin, in Daegu, Korea. J Microbiology (Seoul, Korea). 2007;45(4):358–63.
5. Viedma E, Juan C, Acosta J, Zamorano L, Otero JR, Sanz F, Chaves F, Oliver A. Nosocomial spread of colistin-only-sensitive sequence type 235 Pseudomonas aeruginosa isolates producing the extended-spectrum beta-lactamases GES-1 and GES-5 in Spain. Antimicrob Agents Chemother. 2009;53(11):4930–3. doi:10.1128/aac.00900-09.
6. Livermore DM. Multiple mechanisms of antimicrobial resistance in, *Pseudomonas aeruginosa*: our worst nightmare? Clin Infect Dis. 2002;34(5):634–40. doi:10.1086/338782.
7. Poole K. *Pseudomonas aeruginosa*: resistance to the max. Front Microbiol. 2011;2:65. doi:10.3389/fmicb.2011.00065.
8. Beige F, Baseri Salehi M, Bahador N, Mobasherzadeh S. Plasmid mediated antibiotic resistance in isolated bacteria from burned patients. Jundishapur J Microbiol. 2015;8(1):e13567. doi:10.5812/jjm.13567.
9. Kiddee A, Henghiranyawong K, Yimsabai J, Tiloklurs M, Niumsup PR. Nosocomial spread of class 1 integron-carrying extensively drug-resistant Pseudomonas aeruginosa isolates in a Thai hospital. Int J Antimicrob Agents. 2013;42(4):301–6. doi:10.1016/j.ijantimicag.2013.05.009.
10. Stalder T, Barraud O, Casellas M, Dagot C, Ploy MC. Integron involvement in environmental spread of antibiotic resistance. Front Microbiol. 2012;3:119. doi:10.3389/fmicb.2012.00119.
11. Aghazadeh M, Hojabri Z, Mahdian R, Nahaei MR, Rahmati M, Hojabri T, Pirzadeh T, Pajand O. Role of efflux pumps: MexAB-OprM and MexXY(-OprA), AmpC cephalosporinase and OprD porin in non-metallo-beta-lactamase producing Pseudomonas aeruginosa isolated from cystic fibrosis and burn patients. Infect Genet Evol. 2014;24:187–92. doi:10.1016/j.meegid.2014.03.018.
12. Lee JY, KO KS. OprD mutations and inactivation, expression of efflux pumps and AmpC, and metallo-beta-lactamases in carbapenem-resistant Pseudomonas aeruginosa isolates from South Korea. Int J Antimicrob Agents. 2012;40(2):168–72. doi:10.1016/j.ijantimicag.2012.04.004.
13. Quale J, Bratu S, Gupta J, Landman D. Interplay of efflux system, ampC, and oprD expression in carbapenem resistance of Pseudomonas aeruginosa clinical isolates. Antimicrob Agents Chemother. 2006;50(5):1633–41. doi:10.1128/AAC.50.5.1633-1641.2006.
14. Xavier DE, Picao RC, Girardello R, Fehlberg LC, Gales AC. Efflux pumps expression and its association with porin down-regulation and beta-lactamase production among Pseudomonas aeruginosa causing bloodstream infections in Brazil. BMC Microbiol. 2010;10:217. doi:10.1186/1471-2180-10-217.
15. Castanheira M, Deshpande LM, Costello A, Davies TA, Jones RN. Epidemiology and carbapenem resistance mechanisms of carbapenem-non-susceptible Pseudomonas aeruginosa collected during 2009–11

in 14 European and Mediterranean countries. J Antimicrob Chemother. 2014;69(7):1804–14. doi:10.1093/jac/dku048.

16. Polotto M, Casella T, de Lucca Oliveira MG, Rubio FG, Nogueira ML, de Almeida MT, Nogueira MC. Detection of *P. aeruginosa* harboring bla CTX-M-2, bla GES-1 and bla GES-5, bla IMP-1 and bla SPM-1 causing infections in Brazilian tertiary-care hospital. BMC Infect Dis. 2012;12:176. doi:10.1186/1471-2334-12-176.
17. Clinical and Laboratory Standards Institute. Performance standards for antimicrobial susceptibility testing, 24th informational supplement. M100-S24. Wayne: Clinical and Laboratory Standards Institute; 2014.
18. Fang H, Ataker F, Hedin G, Dornbusch K. Molecular epidemiology of extended-spectrum beta-lactamases among Escherichia coli isolates collected in a Swedish hospital and its associated health care facilities from 2001 to 2006. J Clin Microbiol. 2008;46(2):707–12. doi:10.1128/jcm.01943-07.
19. Perez-Perez FJ, Hanson ND. Detection of plasmid-mediated AmpC beta-lactamase genes in clinical isolates by using multiplex PCR. J Clin Microbiol. 2002;40(6):2153–62.
20. Queenan AM, Bush K. Carbapenemases: the versatile beta-lactamases. Clin Microbiol Rev. 2007;20(3):440–58. doi:10.1128/CMR.00001-07 **(table of contents)**.
21. Soleimani N, Aganj M, Ali L, Shokoohizadeh L, Sakinc T. Frequency distribution of genes encoding aminoglycoside modifying enzymes in uropathogenic *E. coli* isolated from Iranian hospital. BMC Res Notes. 2014;7:842. doi:10.1186/1756-0500-7-842.
22. Doi Y, Arakawa Y. Ribosomal RNA methylation: emerging resistance mechanism against aminoglycosides. Clin Infect Dis. 2007;45(1):88–94. doi:10.1086/518605.
23. Arabestani MR, Rajabpour M, Yousefi Mashouf R, Alikhani MY, Mousavi SM. Expression of efflux pump MexAB-OprM and OprD of Pseudomonas aeruginosa strains isolated from clinical samples using qRT-PCR. Arch Iranian Med. 2015;18(2):102–8. doi:015182/AIM.008.
24. Tenover FC, Arbeit RD, Goering RV, Mickelsen PA, Murray BE, Persing DH, Swaminathan B. Interpreting chromosomal DNA restriction patterns produced by pulsed-field gel electrophoresis: criteria for bacterial strain typing. J Clin Microbiol. 1995;33(9):2233–9.
25. Hong DJ, Bae IK, Jang IH, Jeong SH, Kang HK, Lee K. Epidemiology and Characteristics of Metallo-β-Lactamase-Producing *Pseudomonas aeruginosa*. Infect Chemother. 2015;47(2):81–97. doi:10.3947/ic.2015.47.2.81.
26. Kalantar E, Torabi V, Salimizand H, Soheili F, Beiranvand S, Soltan Dallal MM. First survey of metallo-β-lactamase producers in clinical isolates of *Pseudomonas aeruginosa* from a referral burn center in Kurdistan Province. Jundishapur J Nat Pharm Prod. 2012;7(1):23–6. doi:10.17795/jjnpp-3546.
27. Hong JS, Kim JO, Lee H, Bae IK, Jeong SH, Lee K. Characteristics of metallo-β-lactamase-producing *Pseudomonas aeruginosa* in Korea. Infect Chemother. 2015;47(1):33–40. doi:10.3947/ic.2015.47.1.33.
28. Zhang X, Gu B, Mei Y, Wen Y, Xia W. Increasing resistance rate to carbapenem among blood culture isolates of *Klebsiella pneumoniae, Acinetobacter baumannii* and *Pseudomonas aeruginosa* in a university-affiliated hospital in China, 2004–2011. J Antibiot (Tokyo). 2015;68(2):115–20. doi:10.1038/ja.2014.119.
29. Toval F, Guzmán-Marte A, Madriz V, Somogyi T, Rodríguez C, García F. Predominance of carbapenem-resistant *Pseudomonas aeruginosa* isolates carrying bla_{IMP} and bla_{VIM} metallo-β-lactamases in a major hospital in Costa Rica. J Med Microbiol. 2015;64(Pt 1):37–43. doi:10.1099/jmm.0.081802-0.
30. George AM, Levy SB. Amplifiable resistance to tetracycline, chloramphenicol, and other antibiotics in *Escherichia coli*: involvement of a non-plasmid-determined efflux of tetracycline. J Bacteriol. 1983;155(2):531–40.
31. Shu JC, Chia JH, Siu LK, Kuo AJ, Huang SH, Su LH, Wu TL. Interplay between mutational and horizontally acquired resistance mechanisms and its association with carbapenem resistance amongst extensively drug-resistant *Pseudomonas aeruginosa* (XDR-PA). Int J Antimicrob Agents. 2012;39(3):217–22. doi:10.1016/j.ijantimicag.2011.09.023.
32. Shen J, Pan Y, Fang Y. Role of the outer membrane protein OprD2 in carbapenem-resistance mechanisms of *Pseudomonas aeruginosa*. PLoS One. 2015;10(10):e0139995. doi:10.1371/journal.pone.0139995.
33. Rojo-Bezares B, Estepa V, Cebollada R, de Toro M, Somalo S, Seral C, Castillo FJ, Torres C, Sáenz Y. Carbapenem-resistant *Pseudomonas aeruginosa* strains from a Spanish hospital: characterization of metallo-beta-lactamases, porin OprD and integrons. Int J Med Microbiol. 2014;304(3–4):405–14. doi:10.1016/j.ijmm.2014.01.001.
34. Li H, Luo YF, Williams BJ, Blackwell TS, Xie CM. Structure and function of OprD protein in *Pseudomonas aeruginosa*: from antibiotic resistance to novel therapies. Int J Med Microbiol. 2012;302(2):63–8. doi:10.1016/j.ijmm.2011.10.001.
35. Ashenafi M, Ammosova T, Nekhai S, Byrnes WM. Purification and characterization of aminoglycoside phosphotransferase APH(6)-Id, a streptomycin-inactivating enzyme. Mol Cell Biochem. 2014;387(1–2):207–16. doi:10.1007/s11010-013-1886-1.
36. Galani I, Souli M, Panagea T, Poulakou G, Kanellakopoulou K, Giamarellou H. Prevalence of 16S rRNA methylase genes in *Enterobacteriaceae* isolates from a Greek university hospital. Clin Microbiol Infect. 2012;18(3):E52–4. doi:10.1111/j.1469-0691.2011.03738.x.
37. Lau CH, Fraud S, Jones M, Peterson SN, Poole K. Mutational activation of the AmgRS two-component system in aminoglycoside-resistant *Pseudomonas aeruginosa*. Antimicrob Agents Chemother. 2013;57(5):2243–51. doi:10.1128/AAC.00170-13.
38. Ibrahim ME, Magzoub MA, Bilal NE, Hamid ME. Distribution of Class I integrons and their effect on the prevalence of multi-drug resistant *Escherichia coli* clinical isolates from Sudan. Saudi Med J. 2013;34 (3):240–7.

5

Performance evaluation of a rapid whole-blood immunoassay for the detection of IgG antibodies against *Helicobacter pylori* in daily clinical practice

Dietmar Enko[1*], Gabriele Halwachs-Baumann[1], Robert Stolba[1], Ortrun Rössler[2] and Gernot Kriegshäuser[1]

Abstract

Background: A growing number of rapid *Helicobacter pylori* antibody tests are commercially available now, however, some of these tests are often used without sufficient evaluation. The aim of this study was to evaluate the performance of a commercially available rapid whole-blood immunoassay (gabControl® *H. pylori*; gabmed GmbH, Köln, Germany), for the qualitative detection of IgG antibodies against *H. pylori* with the ^{13}C-urea breath test (^{13}C-UBT) serving as a reference method.

Methods: A total of 108 consecutive outpatients, who were referred for ^{13}C-UBT by general practitioners and specialists, were also tested for *H. pylori* infection by the gabControl® *H. pylori* immunoassay. The clinical performance of this rapid whole-blood test was evaluated by determining the sensitivity, specificity, positive predictive value (PPV), and negative predictive value (NPV) compared to the ^{13}C-UBT. The agreement between the two tests was calculated using Cohen's Kappa (κ) with 95 % confidence intervals (CI).

Results: The agreement between the gabControl® *H. pylori* assay and the ^{13}C-UBT was 0.62 [95 % confidence intervals (CIs) 0.47–0.76; $P < 0.001$]. With the ^{13}C-UBT serving as the non-invasive gold standard method of *H. pylori* diagnosis, the gabControl® *H. pylori* assay demonstrated a sensitivity and specificity of 91.4 and 76.7 %, respectively, with a PPV of 65.3 % and a NPV of 94.9 %. Seventeen (15.7 %) individuals with a positive *H. pylori* anamnesis showed a negative ^{13}C-UBT and were typed positive by the gabControl® *H. pylori* assay. Of these, 13 (76.5 %) and 3 individuals (17.6 %) had completed one and two eradication therapies, respectively.

Conclusions: The gabControl® *H. pylori* immunoassay is a rapid and easy to use first line screening tool for *H. pylori* IgG antibody detection in daily clinical practice. However, this assay should not be used for confirmation of the successful *H. pylori* eradication after antibiotic treatment.

Keywords: *Helicobacter pylori*, Immunoassay, Laboratory diagnosis

Background

Helicobacter pylori infection is still a common condition worldwide. In North Europe and North America, about one-third of adults are infected, whereas in South-East Europe, South America, and in Asia, the *H. pylori* prevalence is reported to be higher than 50 % [1].

Since the *H. pylori* infection was recognized as a causative agent of chronic active gastritis and a risk factor for ulcer disease, gastric cancer and the mucosa-associated lymphoid tissue (MALT) lymphoma, numerous invasive and non-invasive methods for the accurate detection of this bacterium have been developed. Invasive techniques include biopsy-based histological methods, culture of the bacterium, the rapid urease test, and molecular tests (e.g. real-time PCR). Non-invasive methods encompass the ^{13}C-urea breath test (^{13}C-UBT), the stool antigen test,

*Correspondence: dietmar.enko@gespag.at
[1] Institute of Clinical Chemistry and Laboratory Medicine, General Hospital Steyr, Sierningerstraße 170, 4400 Steyr, Austria
Full list of author information is available at the end of the article

and the *H. pylori* antibody detection by serological tests [2–4].

The ^{13}C-UBT is considered the non-invasive gold standard method of *H. pylori* diagnosis [5–7]. It is a simple and safe test, which is easily repeated and provides excellent accuracy for the initial diagnosis of *H. pylori* infection, as well as the confirmation of its eradication after treatment [7, 8]. In the presence of the *H. pylori* produced enzyme urease, the ingested labeled urea (^{13}C-urea) is metabolized into labeled carbon dioxide ($^{13}CO_2$) and ammonia (NH_3). The produced $^{13}CO_2$ diffuses into the blood vessels and is eliminated via the lungs. The expired air is collected in order to measure the activity of labeled carbon so as to detect individuals with *H. pylori* infection [5, 9, 10].

Since individuals infected with *H. pylori* develop a local and systematic immune response [11, 12], specific *H. pylori* antibodies can be detected by rapid serological assays. These tests are easy to perform, inexpensive, and enable immediate patient testing for *H. pylori* antibodies in general practice surgeries [13]. A previous study, which evaluated a rapid whole-blood test, demonstrated, that there was no difference in diagnostic accuracy between capillary (fingerstick) and venous blood (venipuncture) collection [14]. A growing number of rapid *H. pylori* antibody tests are commercially available now, however, some of these tests are often used without sufficient evaluation.

The aim of this study was to evaluate the performance of a commercially available rapid whole blood immunoassay (gabControl® *H. pylori*; gabmed GmbH, Köln, Germany), for the qualitative detection of IgG antibodies against *H. pylori* with the ^{13}C-UBT serving as a reference method.

Methods

Patients

In total, 108 patients, who were consecutively referred for ^{13}C-UBT by general practitioners and specialists to our outpatient clinic, were also tested for *H. pylori* infection by the gabControl® *H. pylori* immunoassay (gabmed GmbH, Köln, Germany). The study period was from January to December 2015. The inclusion criteria were a minimum age of >15 years, an overnight fasting state and a non-smoking period >12 h before the ^{13}C-UBT. Patients with antibiotic-based therapy at least 4 weeks before and/or proton pump inhibitor (PPI) therapy at least 2 weeks before the ^{13}C-UBT were excluded from the study. An anamnesis was carried out about the history of *H. pylori* infections, completed eradication therapies, and intake of medication. Written informed consent was provided from all the patients. The ethical approval for this study was obtained from the Ethical Committee of Upper Austria, Linz, Austria. The study was carried out in accordance with the latest version of the Declaration of Helsinki.

^{13}C-UBT

Isotope ratio mass spectrometry was employed using the IRIS®-^{13}C-Infrared Isotope Analyzer System (Wagner Analysen Technik GmbH, Bremen, Germany). The ^{13}C-UBT was performed according to the manufacturer's instructions. Briefly: after a 12 h fasting period, breath samples were obtained before (baseline) and 30 min after the test drink intake (75 mg ^{13}C-urea from the capsule dissolved in 200 mL fruit juice) early in the morning (8:00–10.00 a. m.). ^{13}C/^{12}C-isotope ratio differences between the value at 30 min and the baseline value were determined and expressed in delta over baseline (DOB, ‰). A sample was considered positive if the 30 min value was above a 4 ‰ cut-off level [15]. Eating, drinking and/or smoking were not allowed until the ^{13}C-UBT was completed.

GabControl® *H. pylori*

This commercially available test is a qualitative membrane based immunoassay for the qualitative detection of *H. pylori* IgG antibodies in whole-blood, serum or plasma. The test was performed in accordance with the manufacturer's instructions. Approximately 50 µL of fingerstick whole-blood was sampled in a glass capillary tube and transferred to the specimen well (S) on the test device (Fig. 1a–c). One drop (approximately 40 µL) of dilution buffer containing *H. pylori* antigen-coated particles was added and allowed to migrate along a lateral-flow membrane thereby interacting with anti-human IgG antibodies immobilized as parallel lines. The test results were read after 10 min: a red control (C) line signal together with a red test (T) line signal (intense or faint) indicated the presence of *H. pylori* IgG antibody (Fig. 1a, b); showing a single red C line signal only, the assay was interpreted as negative (Fig. 1c). Assay read-out was performed independently by two physicians (i.e. four eyes principle), which were both blinded to the respective ^{13}C-UBT result.

Statistical analysis

The agreement between the ^{13}C-UBT and the gabControl® *H. pylori* assay was calculated using Cohen's Kappa (κ) with 95 % confidence intervals (CIs) [16]. Sensitivity, specificity, positive predictive value (PPV) and negative predictive value (NPV) of the gabControl® *H. pylori* assay were calculated compared to the ^{13}C-UBT. No adjustment for type I error was made. Therefore the concerning P values are only descriptive. Analyse-it® software version 2.30 (Analyse-it Software, Ltd, Leeds, United Kingdom) was used for statistical analysis.

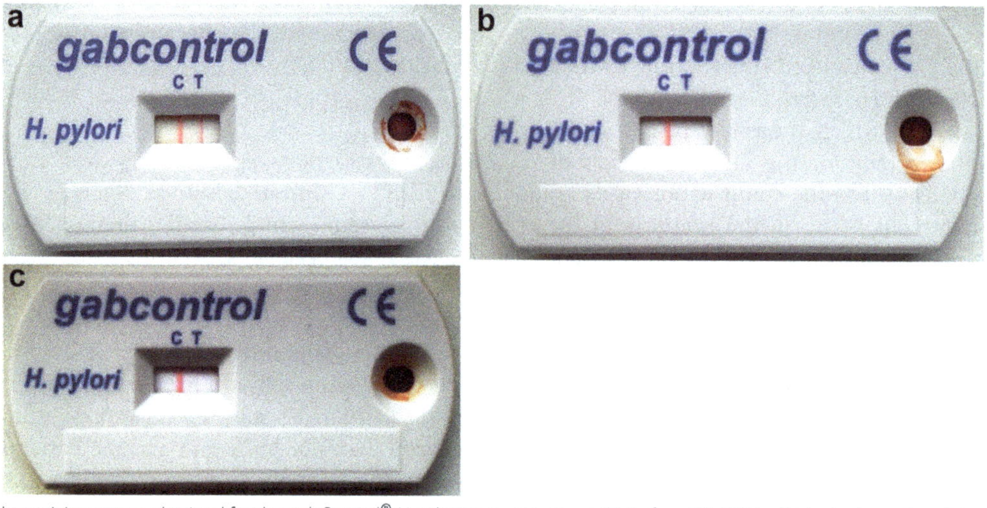

Fig. 1 Typical reactivity patters obtained for the gabControl® *H. pylori* immunoassay: **a** thirty-four (31.5 %) individuals showed an intense T line signal, **b** 15 (13.9 %) individuals were observed with faint to faintest T line signals, **c** 59 (54.6 %) patients demonstrated a C line signal only. *C* control line; *T* test line

Results

Study population characteristics

Of 108 consecutively enrolled patients, 36 (33.3 %) were male and 72 (66.7 %) were female. The median age was 44.0 (range: 15–88) years. The main demographic and clinical characteristics of the study population are provided in Table 1. Fifty-eight (53.7 %) individuals had a positive history of previous *H. pylori* infections.

Performance of the gabControl® *H. pylori* assay

The gabControl® *H. pylori* assay was found positive and negative in 49/108 (45.4 %) and 59/108 (54.6 %) patients, respectively (Table 2). Of those patients with a positive result, fifteen (30.6 %) individuals showed faint red colored changes in the test line region (T) only (Fig. 1b).

The agreement between the gabControl® *H. pylori* assay and the ^{13}C-UBT was 0.62 (95 % CI 0.47–0.76; $P < 0.001$). With the ^{13}C-UBT serving as the non-invasive gold standard method of *H. pylori* diagnosis [5–7], the gabControl® *H. pylori* assay demonstrated a sensitivity and specificity of 91.4 and 76.7 %, respectively, with a PPV of 65.3 % and a NPV of 94.9 % (Table 2).

Thirty-five (32.4 %) individuals had a positive ^{13}C-UBT. Twenty-seven (77.1 %) of these patients had a positive *H. pylori* anamnesis, whereas in 8 patients (22.9 %) *H. pylori* infection was detected for the first time. Seventeen (15.7 %) individuals with a positive *H. pylori* anamnesis showed a negative ^{13}C-UBT and were typed positive by the gabControl® *H. pylori* assay. Of these, 13 (76.5 %) and 3 individuals (17.6 %) had completed one and two eradication therapies, respectively. One patient (5.9 %), however, did not undergo any kind of antibiotic treatment.

Table 1 Basic characteristics of the study population

	Study population
Patients	n = 108
Gender	
Male	n = 36 (33.3 %)
Female	n = 72 (66.7 %)
Median age (years)	44 (range: 15–88)
History of previous H. pylori infections	
Negative history	n = 50 (46.3 %)
Positive history	n = 58 (53.7 %)
Completed eradication therapies (one or more)	n = 54 (50 %)

Discussion

This study aimed to compare the performance of the gabControl® *H. pylori* rapid immunoassay with the ^{13}C-UBT in 108 patients, who were referred by general practitioners and specialists to our outpatient clinic. As the ^{13}C-UBT

Table 2 GabControl® *H. pylori* versus ^{13}C-UBT

	n = 108	
	GabControl® *H. pylori* [a] +	GabControl® *H. pylori* [a] −
^{13}C-UBT +	32 (29.6 %)	3 (2.8 %)
^{13}C-UBT −	17 (15.7 %)	56 (51.9 %)

[a] The gabControl® *H. pylori* immunoassay showed a sensitivity of 91.4 % and a specificity of 76.7 % with the ^{13}C-UBT serving as a reference method

was considered the non-invasive gold standard method of *H. pylori* diagnosis [5–7], the gabControl® *H. pylori* assay demonstrated a sensitivity and specificity of 91.4 and 76.7 %, respectively, with a PPV of 65.3 % and a NPV of 94.9 %.

Several previous studies have evaluated other rapid whole blood test kits for *H. pylori* antibody detection, reporting sensitivities and specificities of 80.3–89.5 % and 78.0–93.5 %, and PPVs and NPVs of 83–92.9 % and 57.4–93.5 %, respectively [13, 17–19].

Herein, seventeen patients (15.7 %), who had a negative ^{13}C-UBT result were found positive for *H. pylori* antibody by the gabControl® *H. pylori* testing. Of these, 16 (94.1 %) individuals had a positive *H. pylori* anamnesis with one or two completed eradication therapies most likely responsible for the relatively low specificity of 76.7 % observed for the gabControl® *H. pylori* assay as well as the substantial agreement of 0.62 (95 % CI 0.47–0.76; $P < 0.001$) between the two methodologies investigated here. Patients with previous eradication therapy might recently have overcome their infection and the ^{13}C-UBT, as an indicator of current active infection, might be negative [20, 21]. Furthermore, it is known that it may take more than 1 year for *H. pylori* antibody to disappear after successful eradication [22]. Moreover, post-treatment circulating *H. pylori* antibodies are considered to remain positive for a significant period or perhaps indefinitely in some patients [3, 4, 20].

The intake of proton pump inhibitors (PPIs) may be another possible explanation of discrepant test results between the ^{13}C-UBT and the gabControl® *H. pylori* assay. While PPI intake at least 2 weeks before the ^{13}C-UBT was an exclusion criterion of this study, the authors cannot guarantee, that all individuals strictly followed this instruction. Individuals with PPI intake within 2 weeks before the ^{13}C-UBT may have false-negative breath test results, whereas *H. pylori* antibodies are serologically detectable [23–25].

Previous studies, which were performed in various populations with different geographical and socio-economic status, demonstrated, that the prevalence of antibodies against *H. pylori* increases with age [26–28]. A cross-sectional population study in Germany comprising 1797 individuals showed a *H. pylori* antibody prevalence of 48 % [29]. These seroprevalence data are in agreement with our study that found IgG antibodies against *H. pylori* in 49/108 (45.4 %) individuals.

In clinical practice, it should be considered, that a positive IgG serology does not necessarily indicate an ongoing infection [30]. As a consequence the ^{13}C-UBT may not be replaced through rapid whole-blood IgG antibody screening tests for confirmation of the successful *H. pylori* eradication after antibiotic treatment.

Using finger-stick blood samples the gabControl® *H. pylori* assay is rapid and easy to perform as centrifugation is no necessary and results are available within 10 min. However, low antibody titers resulting in faintest signal intensities may lead to false negative read-outs as interpretation becomes highly subjective and should therefore be based on the four eyes principle.

The major limitation of this study is the lack of invasive biopsy-based methods (e.g. histology, bacterial culture and real-time PCR) for *H. pylori* detection.

In conclusion, the gabControl® *H. pylori* immunoassay is a rapid and easy to use first-line screening tool for *H. pylori* IgG antibody detection in daily clinical practice. However, it should not be used for confirmation of the successful *H. pylori* eradication after antibiotic treatment.

Abbreviations

H: Helicobacter; MALT: Mucosa-associated lymphoid tissue; ^{13}C-UBT: ^{13}C-urea breath test; CO_2: Carbon dioxide; NH_3: Ammonia; DOB: Delta over baseline; κ: Kappa; PPV: Positive predictive value; NPV: Negative predictive value; PPI: proton pump inhibitor.

Authors' contributions

All authors contributed to the design of the study. DE and GK collected the data. DE analyzed the data and wrote the first draft of the manuscript. GK revised the paper critically. All authors read and approved the final manuscript.

Author details

[1] Institute of Clinical Chemistry and Laboratory Medicine, General Hospital Steyr, Sierningerstraße 170, 4400 Steyr, Austria. [2] Institute of Pathology, General Hospital Steyr, Sierningerstraße 170, 4400 Steyr, Austria.

Competing interests

The authors declare that they have no competing interests.

References

1. Eusebi LH, Zagari RM, Bazzoli F. Epidemiology of *Helicobacter pylori* infection. Helicobacter. 2014;19(Suppl 1):1–5.
2. Mentis A, Lehours P, Mégraud F. Epidemiology and diagnosis of *Helicobacter pylori* infection. Helicobacter. 2015;20(Suppl 1):1–7.
3. Cutler AF, Prasad VM. Long-term follow-up of *Helicobacter pylori* serology after successful eradication. Am J Gastroenterol. 1996;91(1):85–8.
4. Sharma TK, Young EL, Miller S, Cutler AF. Evaluation of a rapid, new method for detecting serum IgG antibodies to *Helicobacter pylori*. Clin Chem. 1997;43(5):832–6.
5. Patel SK, Pratap CB, Jain AK, Gulati AK, Nath G. Diagnosis of *Helicobacter pylori*: what should be the gold standard? World J Gastroenterol. 2014;20(36):12847–59.
6. Parente F, Bianchi Porro G. The (13)C-urea breath test for non-invasive diagnosis of *Helicobacter pylori* infection: which procedure and which measuring equipment? Eur J Gastroenterol Hepatol. 2001;13(7):803–6.
7. Savarino V, Vigneri S, Celle G. The 13C urea breath test in the diagnosis of *Helicobacter pylori* infection. Gut. 1999;45(Suppl 1):I18–22.
8. Lopes AI, Vale FF, Oleastro M. *Helicobacter pylori* infection—recent developments in diagnosis. World J Gastroenterol. 2014;20(28):9299–313.
9. Epple HJ, Kirstein FW, Bojarski C, Frege J, Fromm M, Riecken EO, Schulzke JD. 13C-urea breath test in *Helicobacter pylori* diagnosis and eradication. Correlation to histology, origin of "false" results, and influence of food intake. Scand J Gastroenterol. 1997;32(4):308–14.
10. Kawakami E, Machado RS, Reber M, Patrício FR. 13 C-urea breath test with infrared spectroscopy for diagnosing *Helicobacter pylori* infection in children and adolescents. J Pediatr Gastroenterol Nutr. 2002;35(1):39–43.

11. Blanchard TG, Nedrud JG, Czinn SJ. Local and systematic antibody responses in humans with *Helicobacter pylori* infection. Can J Gastroenterol. 1999;13(7):591–4.
12. Rathbone BJ, Wyatt JI, Worsley BW, Shires SE, Trejdosiewicz LK, Heatley RV, Losowsky MS. Systemic and local antibody responses to gastric *Campylobacter pyloridis* in non-ulcer dyspepsia. Gut. 1986;27(6):642–7.
13. Hackelsberger A, Schultze V, Peitz U, Günther T, Nilius M, Diete U, Schumacher M, Roessner A, Malfertheiner P. Performance of a rapid whole blood test for *Helicobacter pylori* in primary care: a German multicenter study. Helicobacter. 1998;3(3):179–83.
14. Chen TS, Chang FY, Lee SD. No difference of accuracy between capillary and venous blood in rapid whole blood test for diagnosis of *Helicobacter pylori* infection. Dig Dis Sci. 2002;47(11):2519–22.
15. Burucoa C, Delchier JC, Courillon-Mallet A, de Korwin JD, Mégraud F, Zerbib F, Raymond J, Fauchère JL. Comparative evaluation of 29 commercial *Helicobacter pylori* serological kits. Helicobacter. 2013;18(3):169–79.
16. Viera AJ, Garrett JM. Understanding interobserver agreement: the kappa statistic. Fam Med. 2005;37(5):360–3.
17. Jones R, Phillips I, Felix G, Tait C. An evaluation of near-patient testing for *Helicobacter pylori* in general practice. Aliment Pharmacol Ther. 1997;11(1):101–5.
18. Harrison JR, Bevan J, Furth EE, Metz DC. AccuStat whole blood fingerstick test for *Helicobacter pylori* infection: a reliable screening method. J Clin Gastroenterol. 1998;27(1):50–3.
19. Laine L, Knigge K, Faigel D, Margaret N, Marquis SP, Vartan G, Fennerty MB. Fingerstick *Helicobacter pylori* antibody test: better than laboratory serological testing? Am J Gastroenterol. 1999;94(12):3464–7.
20. Newell DG, Hawtin PR, Stacey AR, MacDougall MH, Ruddle AC. Estimation of prevalence of *Helicobacter pylori* infection in an asymptomatic elderly population comparing [14C] urea breath test and serology. J Clin Pathol. 1991;44(5):385–7.
21. Domínguez-Muñoz JE, Leodolter A, Sauerbruch T, Malfertheiner P. A citric acid solution is an optimal test drink in the 13C-urea breath test for the diagnosis of *Helicobacter pylori* infection. Gut. 1997;40(4):459–62.
22. Kim SG, Jung HK, Lee HL, Jang JY, Lee H, Kim CG, Shin WG, Shin ES, Lee YC, Korean College of Helicobacter and Upper Gastrointestinal Research. Guidelines for the diagnosis and treatment of *Helicobacter pylori* infection in Korea, 2013 revised edition. J Gastroenterol Hepatol. 2014;29(7):1371–86.
23. Laine L, Estrada R, Trujillo M, Knigge K, Fennerty MB. Effect of proton-pump inhibitor therapy on diagnostic testing for *Helicobacter pylori*. Ann Intern Med. 1998;129(7):547–50.
24. Graham DY, Opekun AR, Hammoud F, Yamaoka Y, Reddy R, Osato MS, El-Zimaity HM. Studies regarding the mechanism of false negative urea breath tests with proton pump inhibitors. Am J Gastroenterol. 2003;98(5):1005–9.
25. Mana F, Van Laer W, Bossuyt A, Urbain D. The early effect of proton pump inhibitor therapy on the accuracy of the 13C-urea breath test. Dig Liver Dis. 2005;37(1):28–32.
26. Jones DM, Eldridge J, Fox AJ, Sethi P, Whorwell PJ. Antibody to the gastric campylobacter-like organism (*"Campylobacter pyloridis"*)—clinical correlations and distribution in the normal population. J Med Microbiol. 1986;22(1):57–62.
27. Mégraud F, Brassens-Rabbé MP, Denis F, Belbouri A, Hoa DQ. Seroepidemiology of *Campylobacter pylori* infection in various populations. J Clin Microbiol. 1989;27(8):1870–3.
28. Veldhuyzen van Zanten SJ, Pollak PT, Best LM, Bezanson GS, Marrie T. Increasing prevalence of Helicobacter pylori infection with age: continuous risk of infection in adults rather than cohort effect. J Infect Dis. 1994;169(2):434–7.
29. Michel A, Pawlita M, Boeing H, Gissmann L, Waterboer T. *Helicobacter pylori* antibody patterns in Germany: a cross-sectional population study. Gut Pathog. 2014;6:10. doi:10.1186/1757-4749-6-10.
30. Zagari RM, Romano M, Ojetti V, Stockbrugger R, Gullini S, Annibale B, Farinati F, Ierardi E, Maconi G, Rugge M, Calabrese C, Di Mario F, Luzza F, Pretolani S, Savio A, Gasbarrini G, Caselli M. Guidelines for the management of *Helicobacter pylori* infection in Italy: The III Working Group Consensus Report 2015. Dig Liver Dis. 2015;47(11):903–12.

6

Characteristics of multidrug-resistant *Acinetobacter baumannii* strains isolated in Geneva during colonization or infection

Abdessalam Cherkaoui[1*], Stéphane Emonet[1], Gesuele Renzi[1] and Jacques Schrenzel[1,2]

Abstract

This study determined the antibiotic susceptibility profile and genetic mechanisms of β-lactam resistance in 27 clinical strains of *Acinetobacter baumannii* isolated at the University Hospitals of Geneva, Switzerland. The antimicrobial susceptibility testing was performed using Etest and the disc diffusion method in accordance with CLSI guidelines. All of the strains were defined as multi-drug resistant (MDR) and were susceptible to colistin and moderately susceptible to tigecycline. Uniplex PCR assays were used to detect the following β-lactamase genes: four class D carbapenem-hydrolysing oxacillinases (*bla*OXA-51, *bla*OXA-23, *bla*OXA-24 and *bla*OXA-58), four class B metallo-β-lactamases genes (*bla*IMP, *bla*VIM, *bla*SPM and *bla*NDM) and two class A carbapenemases (*bla*KPC and *bla*GES). All of the strains were positive for *bla*OXA-51 (intrinsic resistance), 14/27 strains carried *bla*OXA-23, 2/27 strains carried a *bla*OXA-24-like gene, and 4/27 strains had a *bla*OXA-58 gene. *bla*GES-11 was found in three strains, and NDM-1-harbouring strains were identified in three patients. All of the *A. baumannii* isolates were typed by rep-PCR (DiversiLab) and excluded any clonality. Altogether, this analysis suggests a very high genetic diversity of imported MDR *A. baumannii*.

Keywords: Multi-drug resistant, *Acinetobacter baumannii*, β-lactamase genes, PCR, DiversiLab, rep-PCR

Background

Acinetobacter baumannii, a Gram-negative opportunistic coccobacilli, has emerged globally in healthcare institutions because it is hard to eradicate, most likely because it is resistant to desiccation and to ultraviolet and chemical sanitizers [1]. *A. baumannii* displays numerous intrinsic and acquired drug-resistance mechanisms. Of the multidrug-resistant organisms, the highly resistant *Acinetobacter* spp. isolates deserve special mention. These organisms can be resistant to all of the currently available antimicrobial agents or remain susceptible only to older, potentially more toxic agents, such as polymyxins, leaving limited and suboptimal options for treatment [2]. Carbapenem- and colistin-resistant *A. baumannii* infections were recently reported in two Sicilian hospitals [3]. *Acinetobacter* spp. may develop resistance to carbapenems through various mechanisms, including class B and D carbapenemase production, decreased permeability, altered penicillin-binding proteins, and even in some cases the overexpression of efflux pumps [4, 5]. Carbapenem resistance in *Acinetobacter* species is most commonly caused by the production of OXA-type carbapenemases and metallo-β-lactamases (MBLs) [6, 7]. The OXA-type carbapenemases comprise four broad groups: *bla*OXA-23-like, *bla*OXA-40-like, *bla*OXA-58-like and an intrinsic *bla*OXA-51-like [8–10]. The OXA-51-like β-lactamases are intrinsic to *A. baumannii* and have therefore been used as a method of species identification [8, 11]. The MBLs require a zinc ion for their activity, which is inhibited by metal chelators, such as EDTA, and thiol-based compounds but not by sulbactam, tazobactam or clavulanic acid. Among the multiple types of MBL genes described throughout the world, the *bla*IMP and *bla*VIM types are the most common [9]. The genes responsible for MBL production may be chromosomal or plasmidic, and the latter pose a threat of horizontal transfer among Gram-negative bacteria [12]. To

*Correspondence: abdessalam.cherkaoui@hcuge.ch
[1] Bacteriology Lab, Division of Laboratory Medicine, Department of Genetics and Laboratory Medicine, Geneva University Hospitals, 4 rue Gabrielle-Perret-Gentil, 1205 Geneva, Switzerland
Full list of author information is available at the end of the article

date, infections associated with *A. baumannii* New Delhi metallo-β-lactamase-1 (NDM-1)-positive strains have been reported in several countries, including Switzerland [13, 14]. The genes encoding NDM-1 are carried on a plasmid, thus promoting the spread of resistance among Gram-negative organisms, most likely by horizontal gene transfer [15, 16]. An NDM-2 variant (Pro-to-Ala substitution at position 28) was recently described [17]. This allele was first found in a multidrug-resistant *A. baumannii* strain isolated from a German patient previously hospitalised in Egypt and subsequently isolated in Israel [12, 17, 18].

Despite the implementation of infection control measures, *A. baumannii* remains an important problem in many healthcare institutions around the world. Several studies have reported high rates of faecal carriage of *Acinetobacter*, making the digestive tract a potential reservoir for nosocomial infections and outbreaks caused by multidrug-resistant *Acinetobacter* strains [19, 20]. To control the dissemination of these organisms, rectal swabs are routinely collected from admitted patients based on their recent travel history or hospitalization in foreign countries. The infection control policies that are implemented at the institution where this study was performed request the screening of admitted patients based on their recent travel history or hospitalization in foreign countries. Rectal swab specimens (e-Swab, Copan, Brescia, Italy) from patients fulfilling these criteria were screened for multi-resistant *A. baumannii* using CHROMagar ESBL (Becton, Dickinson, Allschwil, Switzerland) and MacConkey plates (bioMérieux, Geneva, Switzerland) with imipenem, meropenem, and ertapenem disks (MacD) [21]. Suspected colonies were sub-cultured on sheep blood agar for identification (MALDI Biotyper 3.0, Bruker Daltonics, Bremen, Germany) and full antimicrobial susceptibility testing according to CLSI criteria. Multidrug resistance is defined as resistance to at least two different classes of antibiotics [22].

The aim of the present study was to investigate the β-lactam resistance mechanisms involved in a collection of multidrug-resistant *A. baumannii* strains isolated at Geneva University Hospitals, Switzerland.

Methods

Strains and growth conditions

The study included 27 non-duplicate multidrug-resistant *A. baumannii* strains recovered from clinical specimens. Most of the isolates were obtained from rectal swabs of colonised patients during routine screening, whereas a minority of the clinical specimens comprised samples of urine, exudative skin specimens, and lower respiratory tract secretions (Table 1). All of the strains were stored at −80 °C in skim milk with 15 % glycerol. The *A. baumannii* strains were grown on Columbia blood agar at 37 °C with 5 % CO_2, and their identification was confirmed by MALDI-TOF/MS [23].

Antimicrobial susceptibility testing

The susceptibility to various classes of antibiotics was determined by Etest (bioMérieux SA, Geneva, Switzerland) and the disc diffusion method in accordance with CLSI guidelines. The antibiotics tested were amikacin (30 μg), ciprofloxacin (5 μg), ceftazidime (30 μg) and piperacillin-tazobactam (100/10 μg). The minimum inhibitory concentrations (MICs) of imipenem, meropenem, tigecycline, and colistin were determined using the Etest method. The interpretation breakpoints were based on published data from the Clinical Laboratory Standards Institute (CLSI). The colistin and tigecycline MICs were interpreted using the European Clinical Antimicrobial Susceptibility Testing (EUCAST) guidelines (*Acinetobacter* breakpoints for colistin and *Enterobacteriaceae* breakpoints for tigecycline).

Detection of carbapenem resistance genes by polymerase chain reaction (PCR)

The DNA from an overnight culture on Columbia blood agar was extracted using a MagNA Pure LC instrument (Roche, Rotkreuz, Switzerland) according to the manufacturer's instructions. The final elution volume was 100 μl, and 5 μl of the DNA extract was used for each PCR analysis. Uniplex PCR assays were used to detect the following β-lactamase genes: four carbapenem-hydrolysing oxacillinases (*bla*OXA-51, *bla*OXA-23, *bla*OXA-24 and *bla*OXA-58), four metallo-β-lactamases genes (*bla*IMP, *bla*VIM, *bla*SPM and *bla*NDM), *bla*KPC, and *bla*GES. The primers used for PCR amplification of the carbapenemase genes are listed in Table 2.

Molecular typing methods

The DNA was extracted as described above and amplified using the DiversiLab *Acinetobacter* kit (bioMérieux, La Balme-les-Grottes, France) for DNA fingerprinting according to the manufacturer's instructions. PCR was run on a preheated thermal cycler using the parameters recommended by the manufacturer. The kit-specific positive and negative controls were run with each reaction set to validate the amplification. The rep-PCR products were detected, and the amplicons were separated using microfluidics lab-on-a-chip technology and analysed using the DiversiLab system. Further analysis was performed with the web-based DiversiLab software (version 3.4) using the band-based modified Kullback–Leibler distance for the calculation of the percent similarities. The manufacturer provides guidelines for strain-level discrimination: strains with greater than 97 % similarity are considered

Table 1 Antimicrobial susceptibility of multidrug-resistant *Acinetobacter baumannii* isolates collected at Geneva University, Switzerland (n = 27)

Strain ID	Age, years	Gender	Origin	Sample type	E-test / MIC (mg/L)				Carbapenemase				
					IMI	MER	TIG	COL	NDM-1	GES-11	OXA-23	OXA-24	OXA-58
1	66	male	Switzerland	skin swab	128	64	6	0.19			+		
2	50	male	Pakistan	rectal swab	48	48	3	0.094			+		
3	35	male	Libya	rectal swab	64	48	4	0.19		+	+		
4	76	male	Switzerland	urine	64	64	1.5	0.094			+		
5	66	male	Switzerland	rectal swab	64	48	4	0.19	+		+		
6	40	female	Sudan	rectal swab	128	64	3	0.19				+	
7	72	male	Switzerland	rectal swab	192	64	3	0.064			+		
8	2	male	ND	rectal swab	64	64	6	0.19			+		
9	78	male	Thailand	wound swab	128	192	3	0.125			+		
10	72	male	ND	urine	32	12	3	0.094					+
11	68	male	Switzerland	rectal swab	64	192	6	0.25					
12	20	male	Syria	rectal swab	128	256	2	0.19				+	
13	79	male	Switzerland	rectal swab	192	192	4	0.19			+		
14	27	female	Egypt	rectal swab	64	48	3	0.19			+		
15	62	male	Roumania	rectal swab	64	48	3	0.19					+
16	35	male	Libya	blood	48	64	16	0.19			+		
17	27	male	Switzerland	respiratory sample	24	3	4	0.19					+
18	41	male	Kosovo	skin swab	192	24	3	0.19					+
19	80	male	Switzerland	wound swab	64	192	3	0.094			+		
20	ND	male	Libya	wound swab	12	64	1	0.25					
21	64	male	Libya	rectal swab	12	24	0.25	0.094		+			
22	77	female	Switzerland	rectal swab	192	192	3	0.38					
23	62	male	Switzerland	wound swab	256	256	3	0.25					
24	48	male	Switzerland	rectal swab	256	256	4	0.25			+		
25	71	male	England	skin swab	6	32	4	0.25		+			
26	43	male	Egypt	rectal swab	24	32	3	0.5	+		+		
27	24	male	Egypt	rectal swab	256	64	4	0.38	+				
				MIC 50	64	64	3	0.19					
				MIC 90	192	192	6	0.25					

ND, not determined; IMI, imipenem; MER, meropenem; TIG, tigecycline; COL, colistin

indistinguishable (no differences in fingerprints), strains with greater than 95 % similarity are considered similar (1- to 2-band differences in fingerprints), and strains with less than 95 % similarity are considered different. In this study, the optimal cut-off for clustering was 95 %.

Results and discussion

Antimicrobial susceptibility

All of the isolates analysed in this study were resistant to amikacin, ciprofloxacin, ceftazidime, and piperacillin-tazobactam. The MIC of imipenem ranged from 6 to 256 mg/L, and the MIC of meropenem ranged from 3 to 256 mg/L. The MIC50 and MIC90 values for imipenem and meropenem were 64 and 192 mg/L, respectively. All of the tested isolates were susceptible to colistin. The MIC of colistin ranged from 0.064 to 0.5 mg/L, and the MIC50 and MIC90 values for colistin were 0.19 and 0.25 mg/L, respectively. The MIC of tigecycline ranged from 0.25 to 16 mg/L, whereas the MIC50 and MIC90 values for tigecycline were 3 and 6 mg/L, respectively. Susceptibility to tigecycline was observed in two (7.4 %) of the 27 *A. baumannii* isolates.

Bacterial isolates, species identification and molecular analysis

Carbapenem resistance in *A. baumannii* is most often associated with class D β-lactamases (OXA-23-like, OXA-40-like and OXA-58-like) and MBLs. OXA-type carbapenemases are predominant in *A. baumannii*, particularly in worldwide outbreaks of OXA-23 [24]. The molecular analysis of the isolates tested in this study revealed that 14 strains (51.8 %) carried the *bla*OXA-23-like gene and that two strains carried a *bla*OXA-24-like gene. All of the strains had a *bla*OXA-51-like gene, and four strains had a *bla*OXA-58

Table 2 Primers used in the amplification of selected carbapenemase genes

Name	Nucleotide sequence (5′ → 3′)	Product size (bp)	Location	References
OXA-23-like	F- GATCGGATTGGAGAACCAGA R- ATTTCTGACCGCATTTCCAT	501	*bla*OXA-23	[31]
OXA-24-like	F- GGTTAGTTGGCCCCCTTAAA R- AGTTGAGCGAAAAGGGGATT	246	*bla*OXA-24	[31]
OXA-51-like	F- TAATGCTTTGATCGGCCTTG R- TGGATTGCACTTCATCTTGG	353	*bla*OXA-51	[31]
OXA-58-like	F- AAGTATTGGGGCTTGTGCTG R- CCCCTCTGCGCTCTACATAC	599	*bla*OXA-58	[31]
IMP[a]	F- GGAATAGAGTGGCTTAA**Y**TCTC R- GGTTTAA**Y**AAAACAACCACC	232	*bla*IMP	[32]
VIM	F- GATGGTGTTTGGTCGCATA R- CGAATGCGCAGCACCAG	390	*bla*VIM	[32]
SPM	F- AAAATCTGGGTACGCAAACG R- ACATTATCCGCTGGAACAGG	271	*bla*SPM	[32]
NDM	F- GGTTTGGCGATCTGGTTTTC R- CGGAATGGCTCATCACGATC	621	*bla*NDM	[32]
GES	F-ATGCGCTTCATTCACGCAC R-CTATTTGTCCGTGCTCAGGA	863	*bla*GES	[33]
GES	F- CGGTTTCTAGCATCGGGACACAT R- CCGCCATAGAGGACTTTAGCMACAG *Probe*: Quasar 705-CGACCTCAGAGATACAACTACGCCTATTGC-BHQ2	263	*bla*GES	[34]
NDM-1	F- ATTAGCCGCTGCATTGAT R- CATGTCGAGATAGGAAGTG ***Probe***: FAM-CTG[+ C]CA [+ G]AC [+ A]TT [+ C]GG TGC-TAMRA	154	*bla*NDM	[35]
KPC	F- GATACCACGTTCCGTCTGG R- GCAGGTTCCGGTTTTGTCTC ***Probe***: FAM-AGCGGCAGCAGTTTGTTGATTG-3′–BHQ1	246	*bla*KPC	[36]

[a] Y = C or T

gene. In this study, the OXA-58 isolates presented lower MIC values for meropenem than OXA-23-like-positive isolates, which systematically exhibited higher MIC values (Table 1). The isolates with non-acquired OXA genes displayed a marked variation and included some carbapenem-resistant genes. Naturally occurring OXA carbapenemases, such as OXA-51-like enzymes (e.g., OXA 64-66, OXA 68-71, OXA 78-80, OXA-82, OXA-86, OXA-92 and OXA104-112), have been identified in *A. baumannii* isolates worldwide. In addition, strains producing OXA-58 derivatives have been found in isolates recovered from Italy, Belgium, France, Greece, Iran, the United States and Argentina [25]. OXA-23, OXA-58 and OXA-51 have been reported in Turkey [25, 26]. All of the strains investigated in this study had an intrinsic blaOXA-51-like gene, supporting the use of this resistance gene as a surrogate for the identification of a strain as *A. baumannii* [27]. Recently, the presence of Ambler class A GES (Guiana extended-spectrum) β-lactamases has also been reported in *A. baumannii* and can confer a high level of resistance to carbapenems [8]. *bla*GES genes have been reported in several countries in Europe, Asia, South America and South Africa [8]. In addition, several GES-1 mutants, such as GES-11, GES-12, GES-14, and GES-22, have been detected in *A. baumannii* [8]. In the present study, *bla*GES-11 was detected in three strains, one of which also carried a *bla*OXA-23-like gene (Table 1). The most important characteristic of the GES family of enzymes is their ability to evolve into carbapenemases. GES and OXA-type enzymes are jointly responsible for the high carbapenem-resistance levels observed in the tested strains. The emergence of NDM-1-producing *Acinetobacter* spp. has been recently reported in many countries, such as India, Israel, Egypt, Germany, Spain, Switzerland, the United Arab Emirates and China [13, 28, 29]. Interestingly, *bla*NDM-1 has been shown to be a chimeric gene constructed by the fusion of the aminoglycoside-resistance gene *aphA6* with a mannose-binding lectin (MBL) gene, an event that most likely occurred in *Acinetobacter* spp., indicating that *Acinetobacter* spp. are the likely origin of this gene [30]. *A. baumannii* is the most common NDM-1-producing *Acinetobacter* spp., and the *bla*NDM-1 gene is mostly chromosomal [13, 16]. In this study, NDM-1-harbouring strains were identified in three patients, and two of these originated from Egypt. These isolates have been found to carry mixed carbapenemase genes (*bla*OXA-23 with *bla*NDM-1), yielding very broad-spectrum antibiotic resistance profiles. These isolates are susceptible only to colistin. Taking into account the relationship between North African countries and many European countries, it is possible that the spread of NDM-1 carbapenemases may occur rapidly, mostly through *A. baumannii* rather than *Enterobacteriaceae* because *A. baumannii* may become markedly more difficult to eradicate [28]. *bla*KPC was not detected in any of the 27 isolates. The emergence and coexistence of these major resistance mechanisms seriously limit therapeutic options, raising concerns regarding their transmission to other organisms. It is important to highlight the fact that most of the multidrug-resistant isolates analysed in this study were derived from intestinal colonization and that this—mostly unrecognized—carriage in hospitalized patients may constitute a reservoir of *A. baumannii* strains that are not susceptible to carbapenem.

The genomic pattern of all of the isolates revealed a high degree of variability. Neither a dendrogram nor a computer-generated image of rep-PCR banding patterns showed clustering between the three oxacillinase genes (OXA-23-like, OXA-24-like and OXA-58; Fig. 1).

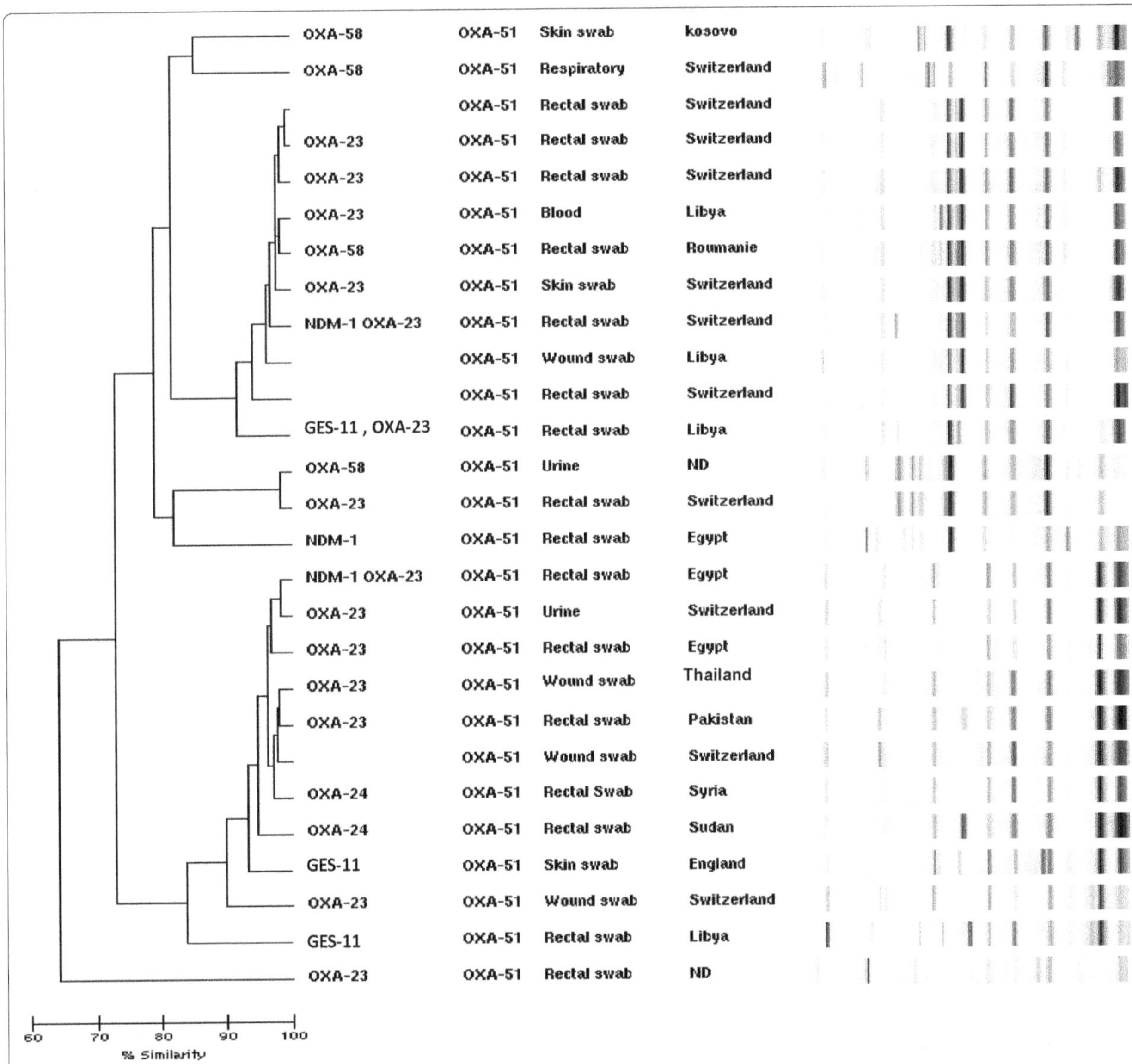

Fig. 1 Results of the DiversiLab typing analysis of isolates from patients infected/colonised with multidrug-resistant *Acinetobacter baumannii* strains from Geneva University Hospitals, Switzerland (n = 27)

Conclusion

In recent years, *A. baumannii* has emerged as one of the most challenging pathogens responsible for healthcare-associated infections. Despite being less frequently identified in *A. baumannii* than OXA-type carbapenemases, MBLs exhibit significantly more potent hydrolytic activities against carbapenems. Interestingly, the results of this study provide evidence that NDM-encoding genes may be widespread in *A. baumannii* and that further molecular surveys will be necessary to more carefully evaluate their distribution in this species. The routine implementation of simple and inexpensive screening methods to detect carbapenemase production in microbiology laboratories is therefore crucial for the optimal treatment of patients infected with carbapenemase-producing pathogens and for controlling the spread of resistance.

Authors' contribution

AC: performed the disk diffusion and Etest assays, carried out the molecular genetic studies, sequence alignment and drafted the manuscript. SE: participated in drafting the manuscript. GR: carried out the molecular genetic studies and participated in the sequence alignment. JS: supervised the research and participated in drafting the manuscript. All authors read and approved the final manuscript.

Author details

[1] Bacteriology Lab, Division of Laboratory Medicine, Department of Genetics and Laboratory Medicine, Geneva University Hospitals, 4 rue Gabrielle-Perret-Gentil, 1205 Geneva, Switzerland. [2] Genomic Research Laboratory, Service of Infectious Diseases, Geneva University Hospitals, 4 rue Gabrielle-Perret-Gentil, 1205 Geneva, Switzerland.

Competing interests

The authors declare that they have no competing interests.

References

1. Yamamoto M, Nagao M, Matsumura Y, Matsushima A, Ito Y, Takakura S, Ichiyama S. Interspecies dissemination of a novel class 1 integron carrying blaIMP-19 among Acinetobacter species in Japan. J Antimicrob Chemother. 2011;66(11):2480–3.
2. Villalon P, Valdezate S, Medina-Pascual MJ, Carrasco G, Vindel A, Saez-Nieto JA. Epidemiology of the Acinetobacter-derived cephalosporinase, carbapenem-hydrolysing oxacillinase and metallo-beta-lactamase genes, and of common insertion sequences, in epidemic clones of Acinetobacter baumannii from Spain. J Antimicrob Chemother. 2013;68(3):550–3.
3. Agodi A, Voulgari E, Barchitta M, Quattrocchi A, Bellocchi P, Poulou A, Santangelo C, Castiglione G, Giaquinta L, Romeo MA, Vrioni G, Tsakris A. Spread of a carbapenem- and colistin-resistant Acinetobacter baumannii ST2 clonal strain causing outbreaks in two Sicilian hospitals. J Hosp Infect. 2014;86(4):260–6.
4. Heritier C, Poirel L, Lambert T, Nordmann P. Contribution of acquired carbapenem-hydrolyzing oxacillinases to carbapenem resistance in Acinetobacter baumannii. Antimicrob Agents Chemother. 2005;49(8):3198–202.
5. Quale J, Bratu S, Landman D, Heddurshetti R. Molecular epidemiology and mechanisms of carbapenem resistance in Acinetobacter baumannii endemic in New York City. Clin Infect Dis Off Publ Infect Dis Soc Am. 2003;37(2):214–20.
6. Amudhan MS, Sekar U, Kamalanathan A, Balaraman S. bla(IMP) and bla(VIM) mediated carbapenem resistance in Pseudomonas and Acinetobacter species in India. J Infect Develop Ctries. 2012;6(11):757–62.
7. Thomson JM, Bonomo RA. The threat of antibiotic resistance in Gram-negative pathogenic bacteria: beta-lactams in peril! Curr Opin Microbiol. 2005;8(5):518–24.
8. Cicek AC, Saral A, Iraz M, Ceylan A, Duzgun AO, Peleg AY, Sandalli C. OXA- and GES-type beta-lactamases predominate in extensively drug-resistant Acinetobacter baumannii isolates from a Turkish University Hospital. Clin Microbiol Infect. 2014;20(5):410–5.
9. Tsakris A, Ikonomidis A, Pournaras S, Tzouvelekis LS, Sofianou D, Legakis NJ, Maniatis AN. VIM-1 metallo-beta-lactamase in Acinetobacter baumannii. Emerg Infect Dis. 2006;12(6):981–3.
10. Kusradze I, Diene SM, Goderdzishvili M, Rolain JM. Molecular detection of OXA carbapenemase genes in multidrug-resistant Acinetobacter baumannii isolates from Iraq and Georgia. Int J Antimicrob Agents. 2011;38(2):164–8.
11. Lee YT, Kuo SC, Chiang MC, Yang SP, Chen CP, Chen TL, Fung CP. Emergence of carbapenem-resistant non-baumannii species of Acinetobacter harboring a blaOXA-51-like gene that is intrinsic to A. baumannii. Antimicrob Agents Chemother. 2012;56(2):1124–7.
12. Ghazawi A, Sonnevend A, Bonnin RA, Poirel L, Nordmann P, Hashmey R, Rizvi TA, Bh M, Pal T. NDM-2 carbapenemase-producing Acinetobacter baumannii in the United Arab Emirates. Clin Microbiol Infect Off Publ Eur Soc Clin Microbiol Infect Dis. 2012;18(2):E34–6.
13. Poirel L, Bonnin RA, Boulanger A, Schrenzel J, Kaase M, Nordmann P. Tn125-related acquisition of blaNDM-like genes in Acinetobacter baumannii. Antimicrob Agents Chemother. 2012;56(2):1087–9.
14. Abbas M, Cherkaoui A, Fankhauser C, Schrenzel J, Harbarth S. Epidemiology and clinical implications of carbapenemase-producing bacteria in Switzerland. Revue Medicale Suisse. 2012;8(338):882–4.
15. Chen Y, Zhou Z, Jiang Y, Yu Y. Emergence of NDM-1-producing Acinetobacter baumannii in China. J Antimicrob Chemother. 2011;66(6):1255–9.
16. Pfeifer Y, Wilharm G, Zander E, Wichelhaus TA, Gottig S, Hunfeld KP, Seifert H, Witte W, Higgins PG. Molecular characterization of blaNDM-1 in an Acinetobacter baumannii strain isolated in Germany in 2007. J Antimicrob Chemother. 2011;66(9):1998–2001.
17. Kaase M, Nordmann P, Wichelhaus TA, Gatermann SG, Bonnin RA, Poirel L. NDM-2 carbapenemase in Acinetobacter baumannii from Egypt. J Antimicrob Chemother. 2011;66(6):1260–2.
18. Espinal P, Fugazza G, Lopez Y, Kasma M, Lerman Y, Malhotra-Kumar S, Goossens H, Carmeli Y, Vila J. Dissemination of an NDM-2-producing Acinetobacter baumannii clone in an Israeli rehabilitation center. Antimicrob Agents Chemother. 2011;55(11):5396–8.
19. Doi Y, Onuoha EO, Adams-Haduch JM, Pakstis DL, McGaha TL, Werner CA, Parker BN, Brooks MM, Shutt KA, Pasculle AW, Muto CA, Harrison LH. Screening for Acinetobacter baumannii colonization by use of sponges. J Clin Microbiol. 2011;49(1):154–8.
20. Corbella X, Pujol M, Ayats J, Sendra M, Ardanuy C, Dominguez MA, Linares J, Ariza J, Gudiol F. Relevance of digestive tract colonization in the epidemiology of nosocomial infections due to multiresistant Acinetobacter baumannii. Clin Infect Dis Off Publ Infect Dis Soc Am. 1996;23(2):329–34.
21. Adler A, Navon-Venezia S, Moran-Gilad J, Marcos E, Schwartz D, Carmeli Y. Laboratory and clinical evaluation of screening agar plates for detection of carbapenem-resistant Enterobacteriaceae from surveillance rectal swabs. J Clin Microbiol. 2011;49(6):2239–42.
22. Magiorakos AP, Srinivasan A, Carey RB, Carmeli Y, Falagas ME, Giske CG, Harbarth S, Hindler JF, Kahlmeter G, Olsson-Liljequist B, Paterson DL, Rice LB, Stelling J, Struelens MJ, Vatopoulos A, Weber JT, Monnet DL. Multidrug-resistant, extensively drug-resistant and pandrug-resistant bacteria: an international expert proposal for interim standard definitions for acquired resistance. Clin Infect Dis Off Publ Infect Dis Soc Am. 2012;18(3):268–81.
23. Cherkaoui A, Hibbs J, Emonet S, Tangomo M, Girard M, Francois P, Schrenzel J. Comparison of two matrix-assisted laser desorption ionization-time of flight mass spectrometry methods with conventional phenotypic identification for routine identification of bacteria to the species level. J Clin Microbiol. 2010;48(4):1169–75.
24. Adams-Haduch JM, Paterson DL, Sidjabat HE, Pasculle AW, Potoski BA, Muto CA, Harrison LH, Doi Y. Genetic basis of multidrug resistance in

Acinetobacter baumannii clinical isolates at a tertiary medical center in Pennsylvania. Antimicrob Agents Chemother. 2008;52(11):3837–43.
25. Nowak P, Paluchowska P, Budak A. Distribution of blaOXA genes among carbapenem-resistant Acinetobacter baumannii nosocomial strains in Poland. New Microbiol. 2012;35(3):317–25.
26. Peleg AY, Seifert H, Paterson DL. Acinetobacter baumannii: emergence of a successful pathogen. Clin Microbiol Rev. 2008;21(3):538–82.
27. Turton JF, Woodford N, Glover J, Yarde S, Kaufmann ME, Pitt TL. Identification of Acinetobacter baumannii by detection of the blaOXA-51-like carbapenemase gene intrinsic to this species. J Clin Microbiol. 2006;44(8):2974–6.
28. Decousser JW, Jansen C, Nordmann P, Emirian A, Bonnin RA, Anais L, Merle JC, Poirel L. Outbreak of NDM-1-producing Acinetobacter baumannii in France, January to May 2013. Eurosurveillance. 2013;18(31). doi:10.2807/1560-7917.ES2013.18.31.20547
29. Yang J, Chen Y, Jia X, Luo Y, Song Q, Zhao W, Wang Y, Liu H, Zheng D, Xia Y, Yu R, Han X, Jiang G, Zhou Y, Zhou W, Hu X, Liang L, Han L. Dissemination and characterization of NDM-1-producing Acinetobacter pittii in an intensive care unit in China. Clin Microbiol Infect Off Publ Eur Soc Clin Microbiol Infect Dis. 2012;18(12):E506–13.
30. Toleman MA, Spencer J, Jones L, Walsh TR. blaNDM-1 is a chimera likely constructed in Acinetobacter baumannii. Antimicrob Agents Chemother. 2012;56(5):2773–6.
31. Woodford N, Ellington MJ, Coelho JM, Turton JF, Ward ME, Brown S, Amyes SG, Livermore DM. Multiplex PCR for genes encoding prevalent OXA carbapenemases in Acinetobacter spp. Int J Antimicrob Agents. 2006;27(4):351–3.
32. Poirel L, Walsh TR, Cuvillier V, Nordmann P. Multiplex PCR for detection of acquired carbapenemase genes. Diagn Microbiol Infect Dis. 2011;70(1):119–23.
33. Cicek AC, Saral A, Iraz M, Ceylan A, Duzgun AO, Peleg AY, Sandalli C. OXA- and GES-type beta-lactamases predominate in extensively drug-resistant Acinetobacter baumannii isolates from a Turkish University Hospital. Clin Microbiol Infect Off Publ Eur Soc Clin Microbiol Infect Dis. 2014;20(5):410–5.
34. Swayne RL, Ludlam HA, Shet VG, Woodford N, Curran MD. Real-time TaqMan PCR for rapid detection of genes encoding five types of non-metallo- (class A and D) carbapenemases in Enterobacteriaceae. Int J Antimicrob Agents. 2011;38(1):35–8.
35. Naas T, Ergani A, Carrer A, Nordmann P. Real-time PCR for detection of NDM-1 carbapenemase genes from spiked stool samples. Antimicrob Agents Chemother. 2011;55(9):4038–43.
36. Hindiyeh M, Smollen G, Grossman Z, Ram D, Davidson Y, Mileguir F, Vax M, Ben David D, Tal I, Rahav G, Shamiss A, Mendelson E, Keller N. Rapid detection of blaKPC carbapenemase genes by real-time PCR. J Clin Microbiol. 2008;46(9):2879–83.

Detection of a CTX-M group 2 beta-lactamase gene in a *Klebsiella pneumoniae* isolate from a tertiary care hospital, Trinidad and Tobago

Paul Cheddie[1*], Francis Dziva[2^] and Patrick Eberechi Akpaka[3]

Abstract

Background: Identification of the prevalence and spread of ESBL-mediated antibiotic resistance is essential especially in the hospital setting. It is for this reason, more and more studies are highlighting the importance of complementing phenotypic ESBL-detection techniques with molecular techniques in order to understand the basis and extent of this form of resistance among clinically evolved bacterial populations, especially those belonging to the *Enterobacteriaceae* family. However, in Trinidad and Tobago and other Caribbean countries, very little is known regarding ESBL detection rates and/or the prevalence of genes conferring ESBL resistance.

Methodology: Sixty-six *Klebsiella pneumoniae* isolates from clinical specimens phenotypically identified by the Microscan Walkaway-96 System as potential ESBL-producers were analysed in this study. Screening and confirmation of these isolates as ESBL producers was done by the Clinical and Laboratory Standards Institute (CLSI) approved methods. Polymerase chain reaction amplification of beta-lactamase genes bla_{TEM}, bla_{SHV}, $bla_{CTX\text{-}M1}$, $bla_{CTX\text{-}M2}$ and bla_{AmpC} was performed to identify mechanisms of β-lactam resistance.

Results: ESBL-producing *K. pneumoniae* was confirmed in 78.8% (41/52) from isolates collected from a variety of sources during the period, April–July 2015. bla_{SHV} (84.8%) and $bla_{CTX\text{-}M}$ (46.9%) were the predominant β-lactamase genes identified. A single *K. pneumoniae* isolate possessed a $bla_{CTX\text{-}M}$ group 2 beta-lactamase gene. RAPD analysis identified a number of epidemiologically related isolates. However, current isolates were unrelated to isolates from previous years.

Conclusion: This study revealed that among *K. pneumoniae* isolates exhibiting extended spectrum β-lactam resistance, there was a high prevalence of bla_{SHV} and $bla_{CTX\text{-}M}$ genes. This result highlights the need for a reliable epidemiological apparatus that involves the molecular characterisation of ESBL resistance.

Keywords: Extended-spectrum beta-lactamase, Polymerase chain reaction, Random amplification of polymorphic DNA, Trinidad and Tobago

Background

Organisms harbouring genes for extended spectrum β-lactamase (ESBL) production are a major public health concern especially given their association with cephalosporin therapy failure, and the burden they place on infection control practices. Since the first reported case in *Klebsiella* isolates in Germany in the late twentieth century [1], they have increasingly been described worldwide, including in the Caribbean [2–4]. ESBLs are β-lactam hydrolysing enzymes capable of conferring bacterial resistance to the penicillins, 1st-, 2nd-, and 3rd-generation cephalosporins, and azetronam (but not the cephamycins or carbapenems), and which are inhibited

*Correspondence: paul.cheddie@gmail.com
^ Deceased
[1] Department of Medical Technology, University of Guyana, Georgetown, Guyana
Full list of author information is available at the end of the article

by β-lactamase inhibitors such as clavulanic acid [5, 6]. The clinical significance of these enzymes is underpinned by the fact that often times in vitro activity of antimicrobial drugs against ESBL-producing organisms does not always translate into clinical efficacy in patients [7].

Most *Klebsiella pneumoniae* ESBLs are plasmid-encoded enzymes derived classically from the TEM- and SHV- type β-lactamases [1] which belong to molecular class A, according to the classification scheme of Ambler, and Bush–Jacoby–Medeiros 2be group of β-lactamases [5]. TEM and SHV ESBLs are functionally similar to another group of rapidly proliferating β-lactamase enzymes, the CTX-M enzymes, that are related to chromosomally determined β-lactamases in species of *Kluyvera* [8, 9].

Due to the complex epidemiology of ESBL-producing *K. pneumoniae*, the frequency of isolation varies among institutions [10]. Exploring the population diversity of ESBL-harbouring *K. pneumoniae* in a single institution is essential to understanding the role of the genes, plasmids, and clones, involved in ESBL-production, and therapy failure with cephalosporins (and to some extent carbapenems) as well as providing useful information for infection prevention and control initiatives.

The presence and characterization of ESBL-producing genes in clinical isolates of *K. pneumoniae* and other *Enterobacteriaceae* have previously been described in Trinidad and Tobago [2, 3, 11]. However, this study sought to determine the evolving nature of these genes, specifically in the hospital setting, in order to provide data that could be useful in improving infection control measures and guide antimicrobial stewardship programmes.

Methods

Setting

The Eric Williams Medical Sciences Complex (EWMSC), a tertiary ambulatory regional hospital in Trinidad and Tobago that provides general healthcare for both paediatric and adult populations.

Clinical isolates

Seventy-two *K. pneumoniae* isolates were used in this study. This comprised 52 non-duplicate *K. pneumoniae* isolates recovered from the microbiology laboratory during the study period, April–July 2015, and identified as resistant to extended-spectrum β-lactam agents. Additionally, 20 isolates representing a subset recovered in 2008, 2009 and 2010—which were stored at −70 °C in BHI and 5% glycerol and were identified as β-lactamase producers—were also included in this study. Preliminary identification and susceptibility testing of the isolates collected in the current study was determined using the Microscan WalkAway-96 (Beckman Coulter, Inc.). The procedures were performed in accordance with the manufacturer's recommendations. The breakpoints were interpreted in accordance with Clinical and Laboratory Standards Institute (CLSI) guidelines [12].

Antimicrobial susceptibility

Extended-spectrum β-lactamase production were confirmed according to the CLSI confirmatory testing guidelines [12]. Briefly, confirmatory testing was performed on Mueller–Hinton agar (BD) using cefotaxime 30 μg, ceftazidime 30 μg, cefotaxime/clavulanic acid 30/10 μg and ceftazidime 30/10 μg (Oxoid, Remel Inc, USA) (Additional file 1). Quality control of the test procedures was performed with *K. pneumoniae* ATCC 700603 and *Escherichia coli* ATCC 25922.

PCR amplification

From the sum total of isolates analysed (n = 72), 66 (consisting of 57 phenotypically confirmed ESBL producers and 9 non-ESBL producers randomly selected from the pool) were subjected to polymerase chain reaction (PCR) analysis. The non-ESBL producers were included to detect AmpC beta-lactamase production. The PCR amplification of *bla* genes, including bla_{TEM}, bla_{SHV}, $bla_{CTX\text{-}M\text{-}1}$, $bla_{CTX\text{-}M\text{-}2}$ and bla_{AmpC} were carried out with GoTaq® Green Master Mix (Promega, Madison, Wisconsin) using primers listed in Table 1. All PCR amplicons were separated by gel electrophoresis on a 1.5% (wt/vol) agarose gel. Staining of the gel was conducted with 0.5 μg/ml GelRed™ (Biotium, Hayward, CA).

Random amplification of polymorphic DNA (RAPD) typing

Bacteria were grown overnight on MacConkey agar (Hardy Diagnostics) at 37 °C. Genomic DNA was then extracted using the ChargeSwitch® gDNA Mini Bacteria Kit (Invirogen, Carlsbad, CA) following the specific manufacturer's instructions. Samples were initially screened for RAPD typing using five different primers:

Table 1 Primers used for PCR amplification of *bla* genes

Target	Primer name	Primer sequence (5′–3′)
bla_{TEM}	TEM-F	GCGGAACCCCTATTTG
	TEM-R	ACCAATGCTTAATCAGTGAG
bla_{SHV}	SHV-F	TTATCTCCCTGTTAGCCACC
	SHV-R	GATTTGCTGATTTCGCTCGG
$bla_{CTX\text{-}M\text{-}1}$	CTX-M1-F	GGTTAAAAAATCACTGCGTC
	CTX-M1-R	TTGGTGACGATTTTAGCCGC
$bla_{CTX\text{-}M\text{-}2}$	CTX-M2-F	GATGAGACCTTCCGTCTGGA
	CTX-M2-R	CAGAAACCGTGGGTTACGAT
bla_{AmpC}	AmpC-F	ATGATGGGGGGGTCGTTATGC
	AmpC-R	TTGCAGCTTTTCAAGAATGCGC

All primers were obtained from Sigma-Aldrich (St. Louis, MO, USA)

RAPD1 (5′-CGTGGGCCT), RAPD2 (5′-TCGTCG-GCGT), RAPD3 (5′-GTGACGTAGG), RAPD4 (5′-CTTGAGTGGA), RAPD5 (5′-GAGATGACGA) (Sigma-Aldrich). RAPD–PCR was conducted under reaction conditions described by Ashayeri-panah et al. [13]. The amplified products were separated by electrophoresis in a 2.0% agarose gel containing GelRed™ run in 1 × TAE buffer at 65 V for 3 h 30 min until amplified fragments are separated. RAPD1 was chosen because it gave the best banding pattern. RAPD typing was then performed using selected isolates (Additional file 1). The resulting gel was photographed under UV light. RAPD fingerprints were analysed with PyElph version 1.4 gel analysis software [14], and a dendrogram generated using the unweighted pair group method with arithmetic averages (UPGMA).

Results

Description of isolates and CLSI confirmatory test results

Following initial testing, 52 *K. pneumoniae* isolates were identified during the study period, (April 2015–July 2015), by the Microscan Walkaway-96 as potential ESBL producers. Phenotypic AST confirmatory testing indicated that 41 (78.8%) of these isolates were indeed extended-spectrum β-lactamase producing. Additionally, of the subset of 20 *K. pneumoniae* isolates tested from previous years, 16 (80%) were identified as ESBL-producers after confirmatory testing. Four were *K. pneumoniae* isolated in 2008, nine were isolated in 2009, and three were isolated in 2010.

Detection and characterisation of *K. pneumoniae* isolates expressing extended-spectrum β-lactamase resistance

Of the 72 *K. pneumoniae* isolates, 66 were examined by PCR to detect the presence of bla_{TEM}, bla_{SHV}, $bla_{CTX\text{-}M1}$, $bla_{CTX\text{-}M2}$ and bla_{AmpC}. This comprised the 41 ESBL-confirmed *K. pneumoniae* isolates collected during the study period along with the 16 ESBL-confirmed *K. pneumoniae* isolates collected between 2008 and 2010. Additionally, nine *K. pneumoniae* isolates identified as non-ESBL-producers were chosen randomly and added to the pool. 65 of the 66 isolates possessed a gene that may contribute to β-lactamase production (Table 2). bla_{TEM} was detected in 39 of the isolates tested, comprising n = 30 (2015), n = 2 (2008), n = 6 (2009) and n = 1 (2010) *K. pneumoniae* isolates respectively. bla_{SHV} was identified in n = 3 (2008), n = 9 (2009), n = 3 (2010), and n = 41(2015) of *K. pneumoniae* isolates respectively. $bla_{CTX\text{-}M1}$ genes were detected in 30 of the isolates collected in 2015 as well as n = 2 (2008), n = 6 (2009) and n = 2 (2010). Interestingly, 88.9% (8/9) isolates, representing non-ESBL producing isolates that were tested with PCR, were positive for a

Table 2 Correlation between ESBL confirmatory results and PCR results

PCR result	Phenotypic confirmatory testing result (Not-confirmed isolates)		Phenotypic confirmatory testing result (Confirmed isolates)	
	Negative (9)	% Total	Positive (57)	% Total
Negative				
bla_{TEM}	8	88.8	18	31.6
bla_{SHV}	1	11.1	1	1.7
$bla_{CTX\text{-}M1}$	8	88.9	17	29.8
$bla_{CTX\text{-}M2}$	9	100	56	98.2
bla_{AmpC}	9	100	57	100
Positive				
bla_{TEM}	1	11.1	39	68.4
bla_{SHV}	8	88.9	56	98.2
$bla_{CTX\text{-}M1}$	1	11.1	40	70.2
$bla_{CTX\text{-}M2}$	0	0	1	1.7
bla_{AmpC}	0	100	0	100

bla_{SHV} gene. Only one *K. pneumoniae* isolate, recovered in 2015, tested positive for a $bla_{CTX\text{-}M2}$ gene.

Twenty five isolates were positive for bla_{TEM}, bla_{SHV}, and $bla_{CTX\text{-}M1}$ β-lactamase genes representing 21 of the *K. pneumoniae* isolates collected in 2015 in addition to 1 isolate from 2008 and 3 isolates from 2009. Notably, a single isolate collected in 2015 was positive for bla_{TEM}, bla_{SHV}, $bla_{CTX\text{-}M1}$ and $bla_{CTX\text{-}M2}$ genes.

The majority of the isolates, 80.5% (33/41), that were identified in 2015 as ESBL-producing were retrieved from urine specimens, whilst the remainder were recovered from blood, sputum, wound and genital sources. Records were not available for the 16 ESBL-positive isolates from previous years.

For the generation of DNA fingerprints using RAPD-PCR analysis, 18 isolates were used representing *K. pneumoniae* strains from 2008 to 2010 as well as isolates recovered during the duration of this study (Fig. 1). Banding patterns revealed DNA weights between 250 and 2000 bp (Fig. 1). RAPD analysis revealed that six *K. pneumoniae* isolates had the same banding patterns and these were placed into four genotypic groups. While there were similarities in some of the band positions of the remaining 12 *K. pneumoniae* isolates, their overall RAPD profiles were not similar. Therefore, the conclusion was that these isolates belonged to distinct genotypic groups.

The results from cluster analysis using UPGMA (Fig. 2) showed diversity between strains isolated from 2008 to 2010 and those isolated in 2015. However, relatedness was noted for one *K. pneumoniae* strain isolated in 2008 and another isolated in 2009. Also, two strains isolated in 2010 were also similar in their RAPD profiles. Finally, three separate pairs of *K. pneumoniae* strains isolated in

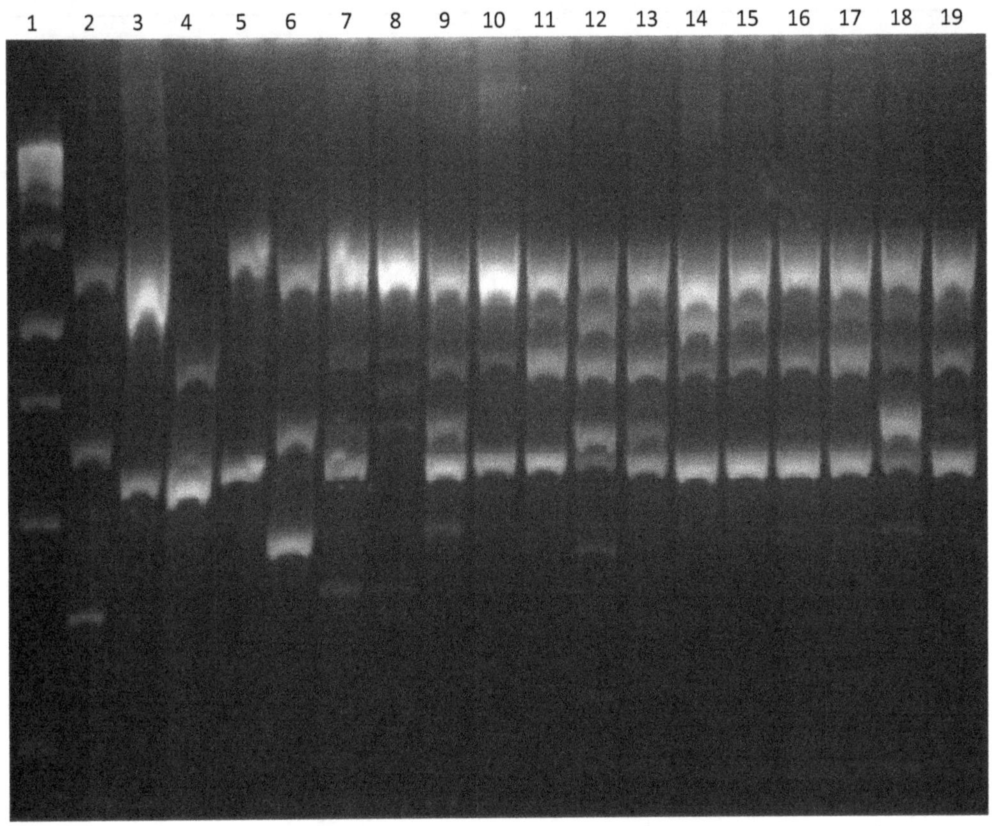

Fig. 1 RAPD profiles for a fraction of ESBL-producing *Klebsiella pneumoniae* isolates amplified by RAPD1 primers. From *left* to *right*: GeneRuler 1 kb ladder followed by isolates from 2008 (*lanes 2* and *3*), 2009 (*lanes 4* and *5*), 2010 (*lanes 6–8*) and 2015 (*lanes 9–19*)

2015 were found to be closely related based on their genotypic profiles.

Discussion

The CLSI disk diffusion ESBL confirmatory test proved suitable for the identification of *K. pneumoniae* isolates included in this study, correctly identifying 41 (78.85%) isolates as possessing β-lactamases capable of hydrolysing oximino-cephalosporins. Although it was not the intention of this study to evaluate the effectiveness of the Microscan WalkAway-96 System, the sensitivity being reported here is much less than that reported by Wiegand et al. [15] of 84 and 87% by Vespero et al. [16]. However, this 21.15% (11/52) "false positive" rate should be interpreted with caution as well as interest. In a SENTRY report authored by Bell et al. [17], they found that 20.3% of screen-positive isolates failed to show clavulanate synergy, and, subsequently, 75% of these nonconforming results were due to the presence of a plasmid-borne AmpC enzyme of the CIT or DHA type. Munier et al. [18] also found that 70% of ESBL screen-positive isolates (which were characterised by *E. coli*, *K. pneumoniae*, *K. oxytoca*, and *Proteus mirabilis*) were actually producing an AmpC β-lactamase, while only 13% represented true ESBL producers. Although this study did assess whether isolates that produced negative confirmatory results possessed a gene that coded for an AmpC β-lactamase (data not shown), all of the isolates returned negative results. However, this finding does not rule out the possibility of these isolates harbouring other AmpC varieties, and further investigation is warranted.

Another possible reason that may be posited for the "high" number of false positives involves the influence of the inoculum effect. In their clinical update paper, Patterson and Bonomo highlight that in vitro, MICs of cephalosporins may rise as the inoculum of ESBL-producing organism increases [5]. This was further substantiated by Thauvin-Eliopoulos et al. [19] who showed that the cefotaxime MIC for a *K. pneumoniae* strain harbouring TEM-26 increased from 0.25 μg/ml at an inoculum of 10^5 CFU/ml to 64 μg/ml at an inoculum of 10^7 CFU/ml. Similarly, Bedenic et al. [20] found that SHV harbouring *klebsiellae* were more resistant to cephalosporin agents when the inoculum size was higher. This reason may certainly be applicable in the case of this study especially given that eight of nine negative confirmatory test isolates were

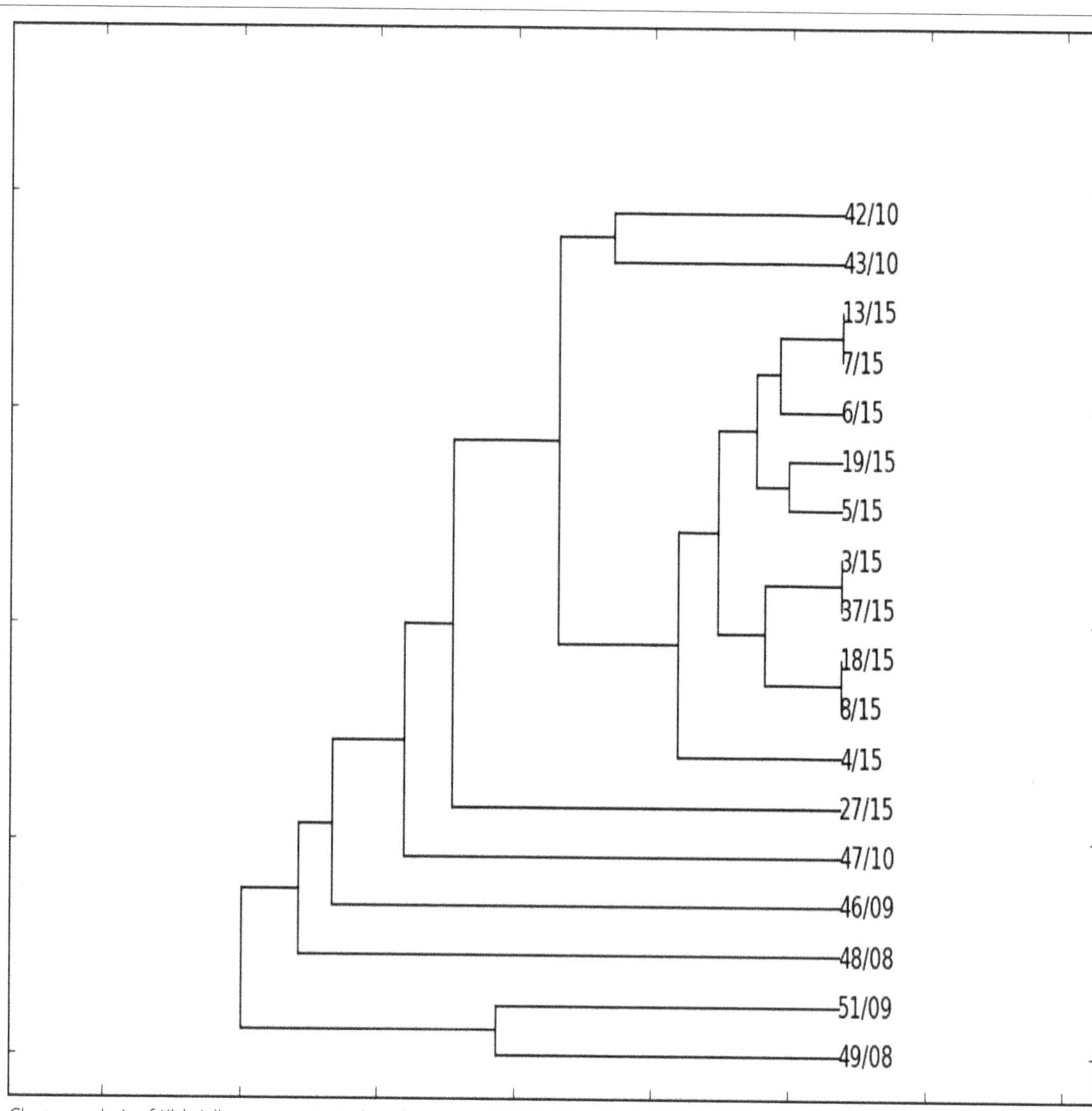

Fig. 2 Cluster analysis of *Klebsiella pneumoniae* isolates based on RAPD-PCR typing with the RAPD1 primer

identified as possessing a SHV-type β-lactamase gene when examined with a molecular assay.

It is also worth noting that even though there was PCR amplification of TEM and SHV genes in most of the isolates, without sequencing it cannot be determined whether these genes contributed to mediating extended spectrum beta-lactam resistance. Sequencing allows for the differentiation of the non-ESBL genes (e.g., TEM-1, -2, and SHV-1) from the ESBL variants (e.g., TEM-3 and SHV-2) [21].

The distribution of the three groups of ESBL-genes for *K. pneumoniae* identified in this study was different from what was reported at this institution by Akpaka et al. [2]. That study reported that there were 84.3% bla_{TEM}, 34.5% bla_{SHV} and 58.8% $bla_{\text{CTX-M}}$ of the ESBL genes present in *K. pneumoniae* isolates recovered at the institution (EWMSC) over a 3-year period. In comparison, this study found lower rates for bla_{TEM} (59%; 39/66) and $bla_{\text{CTX-M}}$ (46.9%; 31/66, $bla_{\text{CTX-M1}}$ plus $bla_{\text{CTX-M2}}$), and a higher rate for bla_{SHV} (84.8%; 56/66). Most noteworthy is that 37.8% (25/66) of the *K. pneumoniae* isolates possessed all three β-lactamase genes. This suggests that one or more of these β-lactamase genes may have been acquired from transferrable plasmids, however, a conjugative assay was not performed at the time the study was conducted to confirm this. Moreover, this finding increases the likelihood that other genes such as plasmid-mediated fluoroquinolone and aminoglycoside resistance genes may also be co-transferred, thereby contributing to the dissemination of multidrug resistance mechanisms [22].

The emergence and spread of CTX-M continues to be well documented and reported across Latin America and the Caribbean [2, 9, 23, 24]. In this study there was widespread distribution of β-lactamases belonging to the CTX-M-1 group, and one instance of an isolate with a β-lactamase from the CTX-M-2 group- the first such account of this particular enzyme in *K. pneumoniae* from a Caribbean territory. This simultaneous production of both cefotaximase and ceftazidimase poses a serious problem to the characterization of resistance by clinical laboratories since these enzymes confer a higher level of resistance to oxyimino-cephalosporinases [25].

For RAPD typing, isolates that possessed two or more β-lactamase genes were chosen with the majority of isolates being those recovered in 2015. RAPD-PCR was chosen because it is a rapid and simple method which when optimized has proven competitive with the gold standard of pulse field gel electrophoresis [26, 27]. RAPD1, also referred to as Primer 640 by other authors [13, 26], proved to be optimal for DNA fingerprinting since it allowed the clear distinction of DNA banding patterns for all of the isolates tested. The resulting RAPD profiles for this select group of isolates showed that there was diversity among those isolated during 2008–2010 and those recovered in 2015. However, it was found that *K. pneumoniae* isolates with the same genotype possessed three or more extended-spectrum β-lactamase genes. This seems to suggest that these strains may have been epidemic in the hospital environment, but due to the lack of patient information this fact could not be proven with certainty.

This study was not without some limitations. The loss of transferrable genetic elements, i.e. plasmids, in stored *K. pneumoniae* isolates from 2008 to 2010 could not be accounted for, and, therefore, genes contributing to resistance might have been lost as has been highlighted by previous authors [5]. Secondly, RAPD-PCR was only conducted on a small subset of the isolates recovered due to inadequate resources for DNA extraction and purification.

Conclusion

This study serves as an important update on the ESBL genes conferring β-lactam antimicrobial resistance among clinical isolates of *K. pneumoniae* isolated from patients being treated at the EWMSC, Trinidad. Along with identifying the traditional bla_{TEM}, bla_{SHV}, and $bla_{CTX\text{-}M1}$ genes, it also identified a previously uncharacterised gene belonging to the $bla_{CTX\text{-}M2}$ group. These findings suggest that both phenotypic and genotypic methods are required to determine and describe the genes responsible for resistance in *K. pneumoniae*, and thus, better guide infection control and antimicrobial stewardship measures directed at preventing the heterogeneous spread of plasmid-mediated resistance genes. Improving the results of studies, conducted at the EWMSC, similar to ours would require conducting plasmid conjugation transfer experiments and sequencing in order to determine: (1) the extent to which the resistance genes amplified by PCR are chromosomally-mediated or plasmid-mediated, and (2) what ESBL genotypes are prevalent among *K. pneumoniae* and other gram negative bacteria within the hospital setting.

Abbreviations

ATCC: American Type Culture; AST: antimicrobial sensitivity testing; *Bla*: used to designate "beta-lactamase" gene; CLSI: Clinical Laboratory Standards Institute; DNA: deoxyribonucleic acid; EWMSC: Eric Williams Medical Sciences Complex; ESBL: extended-spectrum beta (β)-lactamase; ID: identification; MIC: minimum inhibitory concentration; PCR: polymerase chain reaction; RAPD: random amplification of polymorphic DNA; UPGMA: unweighted pair group method with arithmetic averages.

Authors' contributions

PC was the principal investigator, participated in the planning and execution of the study, performed data entry and data analysis, laboratory work and was the main responsible author. FD and PEA coordinated the study, participated in planning, data analysis and writing. All authors read and approved the final manuscript.

Author details

[1] Department of Medical Technology, University of Guyana, Georgetown, Guyana. [2] Faculty of Medical Sciences, The University of the West Indies, St. Augustine, Trinidad and Tobago. [3] Department of Para-Clinical Sciences, Faculty of Medical Sciences, The University of the West Indies, St. Augustine, Trinidad and Tobago.

Acknowledgements

PC would like to acknowledge Ms. C. Dacron and others working in the Vet Laboratory, Eric Williams Medical Sciences Complex for use of the facilities during the different phases of laboratory testing as well as providing guidance about troubleshooting during the molecular-based testing phase of this research.

Competing interests

The authors declare that they have no competing interests

Funding

Funding was not provided for the completion of this research.

References

1. Philippon A, Arlet G, Lagrange PH. Origin and impact of plasmid-mediated extended spectrum beta-lactamases. Eur J Clin Microbiol Infect Dis. 1994;13(Suppl 1):S17–29.
2. Akpaka PE, Legall B, Padman J. Molecular detection and epidemiology of extended-spectrum beta-lactamase genes prevalent in clinical isolates of *Klebsiella pneumoniae* and *E. coli* from Trinidad and Tobago. West Indian Med J. 2010;59(6):591–6.
3. Nicholson AM, Gayle P, Roye-Green K. Extended spectrum beta-lactamase producing organisms at the University Hospital of the West Indies. West Indian Med J. 2004;53(2):104–8.

4. Akpaka PE, Swanston WH. Phenotypic detection and occurrence of extended-spectru beta-lactamases in clinical isolated of *Klebsiella pneumoniae* and *Escherichia coli* at a tertiary hospital in Trinidad and Tobago. Braz J Infect Dis. 2008;12(6):516–20.
5. Paterson DL, Bonomo RA. Extended-spectrum beta-lactamases: clinical update. Clin Microbiol Rev. 2005;18(4):657–86.
6. Lee JH, Bae IK, Lee SH. New definitions of extended-spectrum beta-lactamases conferring worldwide emerging antibiotic resistance. Med Res Rev. 2012;32(1):216–32.
7. Pitout JDD, Laupland KB. Extended-spectrum beta-lactamases-producing *Enterobacteriaceae*: an emerging public-health concern. Lancet. 2008;8:159–66.
8. Bush K, Jacoby GA. Updated functional classification of beta-lactamases. Antimicrob Agents Chemother. 2010;54(3):969–76.
9. Bonnet R. Growing group of extended-spectrum beta-lactamases: the CTX-M enzymes. Antimicrob Agents Chemother. 2004;48:1–14.
10. Coque TM, Oliver A, Perez-Diaz JC, Baquero F, Canton R. Genes encoding TEM-4, SHV-2, and CTX-M-10 extended-spectrum beta-lactamases are carried by multiple *Klebsiella pneumoniae* clones in a single hospital (Madrid 1989 to 2000). Antimicrob Agents Chemother. 2002;46(2):500–10.
11. Cherian BP, Singh N, Charles W, Prabhakar P. Extended spectrum beta-lactamase producing *Salmonella enteritidis* in Trinidad and Tobago. Emerg Infect Dis. 1999;5:181–2.
12. Clinical and Laboratory Standard Institute. M100-S24 Performance standards for antimicrobial susceptibility testing: twenty-fourth informational supplement. Performance standards for antimicrobial susceptibility testing. Pennsylvania: Clinical and Laboratory Institute; 2014. Report No.: M100-S24.
13. Ashayeri-panah M, Eftekhar F, Feizabadi M. Development of an optimized random amplified polymorphic DNA protocol for fingerprinting of *Klebsiella pneumoniae*. Lett Appl Microbiol. 2012;54(2):272–9.
14. Pavel AB, Vasile CL. PyElph- a software tool for gel images analysis and phylogenetics. BMC Bioinform. 2012;13(9):1–6.
15. Wiegand I, Geiss HK, Mack D, Sturenburg E, Seifert H. Detection of extended-spectrum beta-lactamases among *Enterobacteriaceae* by use of semiautomated microbiology systems and manual detection procedures. J Clin Microbiol. 2007;45(4):1167–74.
16. Vespero E, Perugini M, Saridakis H. Screening and confirmatory assays for detection of ESBLs (extended spectrum beta-lactamases) production by *Klebsiella pneumoniae* isolates. Semina Ciênc Biol e da Saúde Londrina. 2007;28(1):33–8.
17. Bell JM, Chitsaz M, Turnidge JD, Barton M, Walters LJ, Jones RN. Prevalence and significance of a negative extended-spectrum beta-lactamase (ESBL) confirmation test result after a positive ESBL screening test result for isolates of *Escherichia coli* and *Klebsiella pneumoniae*: results from the SENTRY Asia-Pacific surveillance program. J Clin Microbiol. 2007;45(5):1478–82.
18. Munier GK, Johnson CL, Snyder JW, Moland ES, Hanson ND, Thomson KS. Positive extended-spectrum-beta-lactamase (ESBL) screening results may be due to AmpC beta-lactamases more often than ESBLs. J Clin Microbiol. 2010;48(2):673–4.
19. Thauvin-Eliopoulos C, Tripodi MF, Moellering RC Jr, Eliopoulos GM. Efficacies of piperacillin–tazobactam and cefepime in rats with experimental intra-abdominal abscesses due to an extended-spectrum beta-lactamase-producing strain of *Klebsiella pneumoniae*. Antimicrob Agents Chemother. 1997;41:1053–7.
20. Bedenic B, Beader N, Zagar Z. Effect of inoculum size on the antibacterial activity of cefpirome and cefepime against *Klebsiella pneumoniae* producing SHV extended-spectrum beta-lactamases. Clin Microbiol Infect. 2001;7(11):626–35.
21. Shaikh S, Fatima J, Shakil S, Rizvi SM, Kamal MA. Antibiotic resistance and extended spectrum beta-lactamases: types, epidemiology and treatment. Saudi J Biol Sci. 2015;22(1):90–101.
22. Poulou A, Grivakou E, Vrioni G, et al. Modified CLSI extended-spectrum β-lactamase (ESBL) confirmatory test for phenotypic detection of ESBLs among *Enterobacteriaceae* producing various β-lactamases. Bourbeau P, ed. J Clin Microbiol. 2014;52(5):1483–9.
23. Espinal P, Garza-Ramos U, Reyna F, Rojas-Moreno T, Sanchez-Perez A, Carrillo B, et al. Identification of SHV-type and CTX-M-12 extended-spectrum beta-lactamases (ESBLs) in multiresistant *Enterobacteriaceae* from Colombian Caribbean hospitals. J Chemother. 2010;22(3):160–4.
24. Pallecchi L, Bartoloni A, Fiorelli C, Mantella A, Di Maggio T, Gamboa H, et al. Rapid dissemination and diversity of CTX-M extended-spectrum beta-lactamase genes in commensal *Escherichia coli* isolates from healthy children from low-resource settings in Latin America. Antimicrob Agents Chemother. 2007;51(8):2720–5.
25. Ryoo NH, Kim EC, Hong SG, Park YJ, Lee K, Bae IK, et al. Dissemination of SHV-12 and CTX-M-type extended-spectrum beta-lactamases among clinical isolates of *Escherichia coli* and *Klebsiella pneumoniae* and emergence of GES-3 in Korea. J Antimicrob Chemother. 2005;56(4):698–702.
26. Ashayeri-Panah MM, Eftekhar F, Ghamsari MM, Parvin M. Genetic profiling of *Klebsiella pneumoniae*: comparison of pulsed field gel electrophoresis and random amplified polymorphic DNA. Braz J Microbiol. 2013;7:823–8.
27. Eftekhar F, Nouri P. Correlation of RAPD-PCR profiles with ESBL production in clinical isolates of *Klebsiella pneumoniae* in Tehran. J Clin Diagn Res. 2015;9(1):DC01–3.

8

Phenotypic and genetic changes in the life cycle of small colony variants of *Salmonella enterica* serotype *Typhimurium* induced by streptomycin

Wanli Li[1], Yinghui Li[2], Yarong Wu[3], Yujun Cui[3], Yao Liu[1], Xiaolu Shi[2], Qian Zhang[2], Qiongcheng Chen[2], Qun Sun[1*] and Qinghua Hu[2*]

Abstract

Background: Small colony variants (SCVs), constituting a slow-growing subpopulation of bacteria that facilitates persistence in lethal environmental conditions, are able to revert to the phenotype of rapid growth for further proliferation and transmission. *Salmonella enterica* serotype *Typhimurium* is one of the most important foodborne pathogens. This study investigated the genetic mechanisms how SCVs induced by streptomycin reverted to the fast-growing phenotype and the phenotypic changes of SCVs among their complete life cycle in *S. Typhimurium*.

Methods: *Salmonella Typhimurium* SCVs were obtained by streptomycin treatment and their revertants were collected in the absence of antibiotics. The fitness, antimicrobial susceptibility, biofilm formation, and the biofilm-related genes expression were analyzed in comparison to their wild type strain, and the whole genome sequencing was performed to identify the genetic changes in the life cycle of *S. Typhimurium* SCVs.

Results: Small colony variants were characterized by an increased antimicrobial resistance to streptomycin (64-fold), imipenem (twofold), and gentamicin (fourfold). A significant increase in biofilm production with higher expression of *csgB* was observed in SCVs ($P < 0.01$). The genetic alterations of all SCVs occurred in *ubiE* gene (coenzyme Q_8 and menaquinone synthesis) with frameshift mutations. However, all fast-growing revertants again lost the trait of increased biofilm production ($P > 0.05$), in which two modes of the genetic changes for reversing to the rapidly growing form were observed: four revertants harbored a secondary mutation in *ubiE*, which reinstated most of the amino acid sequence of the *ubiE*, and other four revertants harbored a mutation in *prfB*.

Conclusions: *Salmonella Typhimurium* could switch to the phenotype of SCVs under the treatment of streptomycin by a mutation in *ubiE*, partially combined with increased production of biofilm, and these SCVs could escape from growth restriction by a compensatory mutation in *prfB* or a new mutation in *ubiE*. These findings may contribute to establishing phenotype-directed treatments against SCVs of *S. Typhimurium*.

Keywords: Small colony variants, *Salmonella*, Biofilm, *ubiE*, *prfB*

*Correspondence: qunsun@scu.edu.cn; huqinghua03@163.com
[1] Key Laboratory of Bio-resources and Eco-environment of the Ministry of Education, College of Life Sciences, Sichuan University, 29# Wangjiang Rd., Chengdu, Sichuan 610064, P. R. China
[2] Shenzhen Major Infectious Disease Control Key Laboratory, Shenzhen Centre for Disease Control and Prevention, Shenzhen, Guangdong 518055, P. R. China
Full list of author information is available at the end of the article

Background

Small colony variants (SCVs), an aberrant form of bacterial phonotype, constitute a slow-growing subpopulation typically characterized with reduced metabolic activity and increased resistance to antibiotics [1, 2], thereby protecting bacterial cells against some non-optimal and lethal environmental conditions [3]. Incidences of SCVs have been reported in clinical specimens [4], livestock and even in foods [5].

Bacterial SCVs can be induced by cold stress [6], triclosan and living inside eukaryotic cells [1]. Additionally, exposure to antibiotics, like quinolones and aminoglycosides, has been shown to be able to induce bacterial SCVs [7, 8], resulting in an increased bacterial survival and ability to further proliferate. For example, streptomycin (STR), one of the aminoglycoside antibiotics, has been reported to induce SCVs of *S. aureus* [9]. STR, which was first used in plant agriculture in the 1950's, remains to be an important antibiotic for bacterial disease control in both animals and plants, especially in developing countries [10, 11]. However, agricultural products, such as fruits, vegetables, livestock and poultry meats were found to be the most common sources of *Salmonella enterica* infections [12–14]. Therefore, *Salmonella* spp. SCVs may be induced by exposure to STR in agricultural products in these countries.

Salmonella spp. is a major causative agent of foodborne disease outbreaks, with *Typhimurium* as the most important serotype in outpatients with acute diarrhea [15]. Currently, SCV has been widely recognized to be part of the bacterial natural life cycle, including in *Salmonella* spp. [16]. Only a few literatures elucidated the genetic mechanisms for the development of *S. Typhimurium* SCVs by exposure to protamine or in the intracellular environment of fibroblasts. For example, mutations in the genes *lpd, hemL, aroD, hemA* and *ubiA* were reported to be responsible for the occurrence of *S. Typhimurium* SCVs [16, 17]. The SCVs have a slow growth rate; however, these mutants are unstable that can revert to a phenotype of rapid growth at high frequency [18]. In *S. enterica*, only one genetic basis for SCV reversion was described by Maria et al. [19]. There can be multiple pathways involved in SCV reversion, and so far for a number of *S. enterica* revertants, the mechanism of reversion is still a speculation. Accordingly, it is of importance to disclose the full lifestyles of *S. Typhimurium*, its survival strategy, and to identify the genetic changes underlying the life cycle of *S. Typhimurium* SCVs.

In addition, some bacterial SCVs, such as *Pseudomonas aeruginosa* and *S. aureus* [18, 20], showed increased biofilm formation compared to their wild-type (WT) strains. The ability to form biofilms, which contributes to antibiotic resistance and protects bacteria against suboptimal environments, makes the pathogen extremely difficult to be eradicated [21, 22]. Several studies have demonstrated biofilm formation of *S. enterica* in abiotic surfaces, plant surfaces and animal epithelial cells [23]. However, the ability of biofilm formation in the life cycle of SCVs in *S. Typhimurium* is still poorly understood.

In order to disclose the mode of *S. Typhimurium* survival after treated with STR and identify the genetic changes underlying the complete life cycle of *S. Typhimurium* SCVs, the fitness, antimicrobial susceptibility, biofilm formation, and the biofilm-related genes expression during the life cycle of SCVs were analyzed in comparison with their parent strains. Then whole genome sequencing of WT strain, SCVs, and revertants in *S. Typhimurium* was performed to analyze the genetic changes in SCVs.

Methods

Bacterial strains

Selection of resistant mutants was performed as described previously [24] with some modifications. Briefly, WT strain 5, a susceptible clinical isolate obtained from stool sample from an infant with acute diarrhea in Shenzhen, China, was cultured at 37 °C on Mueller–Hinton agar (MHA) added with STR (Sigma-Aldrich, St. Louis, MO) to allow cells to undergo a multistep selection process to obtain SCV strains. STR was only present in the agar during the selection, starting at 16 μg/mL and increasing twofold each step to a maximum concentration of 1024 μg/mL. A total of five *S. Typhimurium* SCVs (mutation rate: 5×10^{-8}) were obtained in vitro. Based on the results of biofilm formation analysis, two representative SCVs (1024-4 and 1024-5) were selected for further studies. In addition, one class of fast-growing strains (approximately 10 %) was observed on antibiotic-free MHA agar after 5-day incubation at room temperature, and eight revertants reverted from strain 1024-4 or 1024-5 were collected. Two representative strains 4V1 and 5V1, which reverted respectively from 1024-4 and 1024-5, were randomly selected for further studies. All the mutants were serially passaged on *Salmonella* chromogenic agar plates (CHROMagar, France) in the absence of STR for 7 days. The stock cultures were stored at −80 °C in tryptone soy broth (TSB; Oxoid Ltd., Cambridge, UK) supplemented with 20 % glycerol until use.

Molecular subtyping of mutants

The homology of all the mutants, including WT strain, SCVs and revertants, were identified by pulsed-field gel electrophoresis (PFGE; using XbaI) and multiple-locus variable-number tandem-repeat analysis (MLVA) following standard PulseNet protocols (http://www.cdc.gov/pulsenet/pathogens/). Dendrograms of MLVA and PFGE patterns were then analyzed using Bionumerics software (Version No. 6.0; Applied Maths, Sint-Martens-Latem, Belgium).

Transmission electron microscopy (TEM)

Transmission electron microscopy was performed to assess the phenotypic characteristics at single cell level and the distribution of flagella, as described previously [25] with some modifications. In brief, 400-mesh carbon-coated Cu/Rh grids were incubated on 10 μL of fresh culture grown overnight for 1 min. After which, the excess media were removed by blotting off with filter paper. Each grid was dipped in 20-μL 2 % (w/v) phosphotungstic acid for 3 min. Then the grids were air-dried. To count the flagella manually, grids were examined in a TEM (Hitachi HT7700) operated at 80.0 kV and at a magnification of 10,000×.

Fitness

In order to determine the growth of bacteria, WT strain, SCVs and revertants were incubated overnight in Luria–Bertani broth (LB) at 37 °C and adjusted to obtain the same optical density at 595 nm by fresh LB. Then, bacteria were cultured in LB medium at 37 °C for 15 h with shaking (200 r/min). The growth of bacteria in 96-well microplate was measured by Multiskan FC (Thermo Fisher Scientific Inc., USA) at 595 nm every 30 min. Each isolate was conducted with eight replicates. The broth without inoculation was used as the blank control.

Antimicrobial susceptibility tests

Minimal inhibitory concentration (MIC) for 15 antimicrobial agents, including streptomycin (STR), imipenem (IMI), chloramphenicol (CHL), gentamicin (GEN), ciprofloxacin (CIP), trimethoprim/sulfamethoxazole (SXT), ceftriaxone (AXO), amoxicillin/clavulanic acid 2:1 ratio (AUG2), ampicillin (AMP), nalidixic acid (NAL), tetracycline (TET), cefoxitin (FOX), doxycycline (DOX), cefepime (FEP), and azithromycin (AZI), were determined by broth microdilution method using Thermo Scientific™ Sensititre™ susceptibility MIC plates (Thermo Scientific Inc., USA) following the manufacturer's instructions. Breakpoints for sensitive, intermediate and resistant were defined by the Clinical and Laboratory Standards Institute, 2012. The *Escherichia coli* ATCC 25922 was used as quality control.

Biofilm formation assay

Biofilm production was analyzed using crystal violet assay [26]. In passing, bacterial cultures grown at 37 °C with shaking (200 r/min) overnight were adjusted to the optical density (OD_{595}) of 0.01 by diluting with TSB (1:10). Then, 100 μL of the diluted bacterial suspension was added to each well and incubated at 28 °C for 48 h without shaking. The medium was then discarded, and each well was washed with distilled water and stained with 100 μL of crystal violet for 15 min. Finally, the wells were again washed for five times with distilled water, and the biofilm formation was assayed with addition of 100 μL of 95 % ethanol to determine the OD at 570 nm by Multiskan FC (Thermo Fisher Scientific Inc., USA). The TSB (1:10) was used as the negative control. Each isolate was conducted with eight replicates.

Confocal laser scanning microscopy (CLSM) was used to study biofilm structure in mutants with the ability to form biofilm as described by Bridier et al. [27] with some modifications. Overnight bacterial cultures were adjusted to an OD_{595} of 0.01 by diluting with TSB (1:10) before being suspended in a 35-mm glass-bottom dish and incubated at 28 °C for 48 h without shaking. After the formation of biofilm, the dishes were washed five times with distilled water and refilled with diluted (1:10) TSB containing 5 μM Syto9 (1: 1000 dilution from a Syto9 stock solution at 5 mM in DMSO; Invitrogen, USA). The dishes were then incubated in the dark at 28 °C for 20 min to enable the fluorescent labeling of the bacteria. Images were acquired by CLSM (Leica microsystems Inc., Germany). Stack images were captured with a z-step of 1 μm and then biofilm images were reconstructed into three-dimensional images (3D) by IMARIS 8.0 software. The number of pixels of green fluorescent in images was determined for substratum coverage of biofilm.

Congo red phenotype

The "rdar" (red, dry and rough) morphotype related to biofilm formation is indicative of curli fimbriae and cellulose production on Congo red plate. WT strain and all mutants were cultured overnight in TSB at 37 °C before being normalized to the same OD at 595 nm. Then, 10 μL of each culture was spotted onto an LB plate (without NaCl) containing 40 μg/mL Congo red, and further incubated for 48 h at 28 °C.

RNA extraction and real-time PCR

RNA were extracted from WT strain, SCVs and revertants bacterial cultures grown at 28 °C for 48 h using the RNeasy Mini Kit (Qiagen; Germany), which was later used to synthesize complementary DNA (PrimeScript™ cDNA Synthesis Kit; TaKara, China). The expression levels of biofilm-related genes *csgB*, *csgD*, *adrA* and *bapA* were determined by real-time PCR following standard protocols coupled with primers described by Fa`brega et al. [24]. Relative gene expression was evaluated using the $2^{-\triangle\triangle CT}$ method, and the 16S rRNA gene was used as reference gene. Each strain was tested in triplicate.

Whole-genome resequencing and identification of genetic variations

Genomic DNA of WT (strain 5), SCVs (strain 1024-4 and 1024-5) and revertants (4V1 and 5V1) was extracted from overnight cultures using a TIANamp bacteria DNA Kit (TIANGEN, China). Nucleic materials were sent to Beijing Genomics Institute (BGI) for whole genome sequencing using Illumina Hiseq 2000™ platform with an average of 100× coverage per bacterial genome. Quality-filtered reads for each strain were separately aligned to the assembled contigs of WT to determine variations using SOAPaligner (v 2.21) and BWA (v 0.6.2-r126). Then the reads with indels and SNPs were mapped back to the reference genome of *S. Typhimurium* LT2 (RefSeq NC_003197.1). The indels and SNPs were further verified by PCR and Sanger sequencing method (Invitrogen, China). Also, the genetic alterations in the other revertants (strain 4V2, 4V3, 4V4, 5V2, 5V3 and 5V4) were further identified by PCR and Sanger sequencing method.

Statistical analysis

All statistical analyses were performed using the software SPSS 13.0 for Windows as P value <0.05 considered to be significant.

Results

Phenotypic characterization of *S. Typhimurium* SCVs and revertants

One clinical isolate of *S. Typhimurium* was selected as wild-type strain, and two SCV mutants induced by STR were successfully obtained in vitro. Moreover, two fast-growing strains that reverted back from their corresponding SCVs were also obtained (Fig. 1a). WT strain and all the mutants showed identical PFGE and MLVA profiles (Additional file 1: Figure S1).

In order to study the phenotypic characteristics in the different life stages of *S. Typhimurium* SCV, the morphologies of colonies, the distribution of the number of flagella and the fitness were analyzed. The SCV colonies on *Salmonella* chromogenic agar plates appeared to be small compared with the wild-type parental strain and revertants (Representative data were shown in Fig. 1b). Based on TEM images, both strains 4V1 and 5V1 showed significantly more flagella compared to their SCV mutants (ANOVA, $P < 0.05$; Additional file 1: Figure S2). Moreover, strain 4V1 had significantly more flagella than the WT strain ($P < 0.05$). The SCVs of *S. Typhimurium* displayed slower growth rate in comparison with the WT strain, while the revertants and WT strain growing in LB obtained similar growth rate (Fig. 1c).

Antimicrobial susceptibility test

As resistance to a variety of antibiotics is one of the typical characteristics of SCVs, we determined the MICs of several antibiotics for WT strain, SCVs and revertants (Table 1). SCVs showed two- to fourfold increments of MICs for IMI and GEN, and a drastic 64-fold increase in STR when compared with the wild-type parental strain. The revertants also showed an increase of two- to fourfold in the MICs of STR and decrease of two- to fourfold in the MICs of AMP and AZI when compared with the wild-type parental strain.

Biofilm formation

Biofilm production was analyzed in WT strain, SCVs, and revertants (Fig. 2) and the biofilm structures of SCVs were presented in Fig. 2a. Substratum coverage of biofilm in SCVs (strain 1024-4 and 1024-5) was significantly bigger than WT strain ($P < 0.01$; Fig. 2b). Consistent with this, SCVs of strain 1024-4 and 1024-5 also exhibited significantly increased production of biofilm according to crystal violet assay ($P < 0.01$; Fig. 2c). However, this characteristic lost in all eight fast growing strains when SCVs reverted back to the normal phenotype ($P > 0.05$; Additional file 1: Figure S3).

Expression of biofilm-related genes in SCVs

The relative expression of biofilm-related genes was analyzed in mutants with the ability to form biofilm by the RT-PCR. For strain 1024-4, expression of the gene *csgB* ($P < 0.01$) was 32 times higher (Fig. 3), while a fourfold increase was observed in both *adrA* and *bapA* genes ($P < 0.05$), and no significant change was found in *csgD* in comparison with WT strain ($P > 0.05$). For strain 1024-5, a significant increase was found in *csgB* (eightfold; $P < 0.01$), but no significant change in *adrA*, *csgD* and *bapA* ($P > 0.05$). Based on the Congo red staining, SCV strain (1024-4) showed rdar morphology which is indicative of curli and cellulose production.

Genetic alterations

To explore the genetic changes in the life cycle of SCVs, whole-genome sequences of the SCVs (strain 1024-4 and 1024-5) and revertants (strain 4V1 and 5V1) were compared to the WT strain (strain 5). Only five mutations were identified in four mutants by analyzing the data of whole genome sequencing, and notably, three of them were associated with the gene *ubiE* (Fig. 4a and Table 2). A four bp length deletion occurred in *ubiE* of SCV strain 1024-5, which might de-activate the gene through

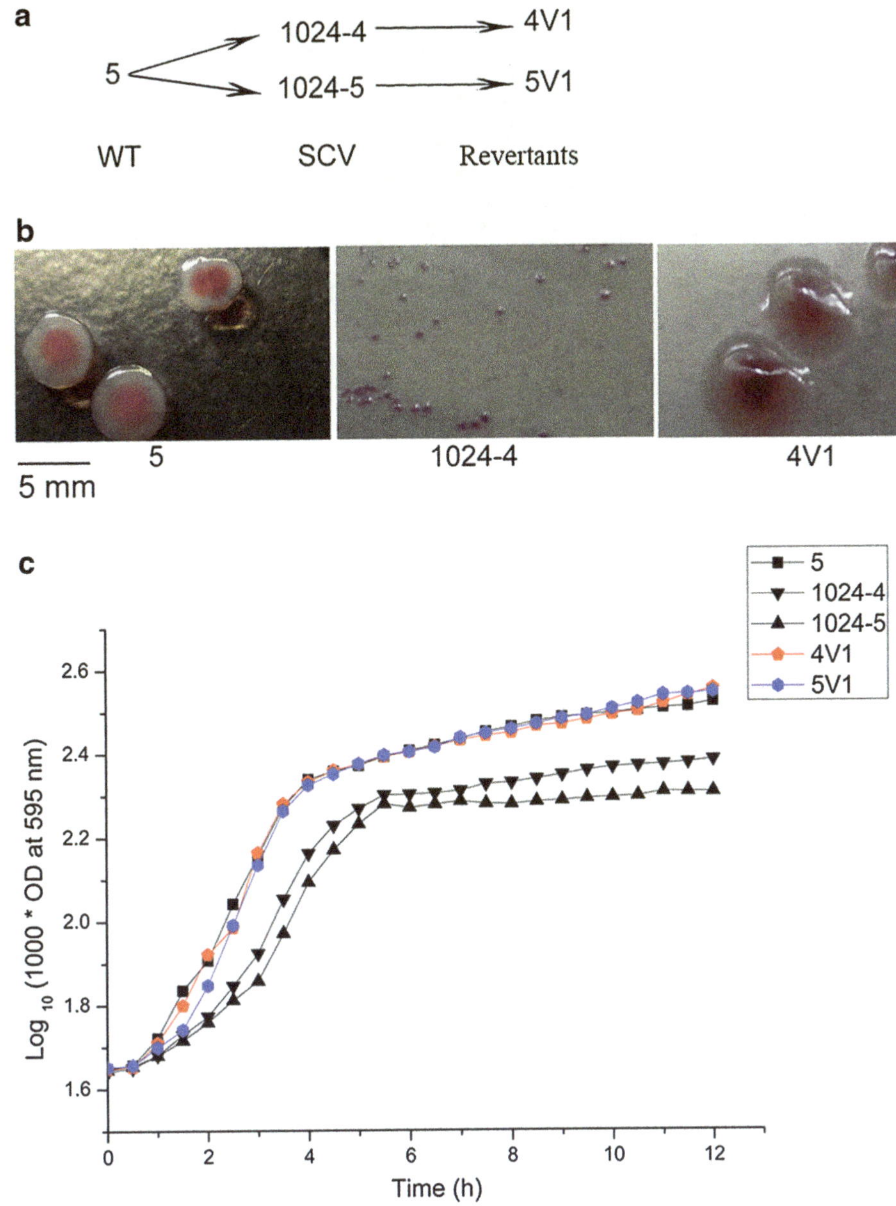

Fig. 1 Phenotypic characterization of WT, SCVs and revertants of *S. Typhimurium*. **a** The relationship between WT (wide-type; strain 5), SCVs (strain 1024-4 and 1024-5) and revertants (strain 4V1 and 5V1). **b** Representative data on the colony morphologies of strains on chromogenic agar plate. **c** Bacterial fitness evaluated by growth curves, and strains were incubated in Luria–Bertani broth (LB) at 37 °C with shaking

Table 1 MIC determination in wide-type strain (WT), small colony variants (SCV), and revertants

Strain	MIC (μg/mL)														
	STR	IMI	CHL	GEN	CIP	SXT	AXO	AUG2	AMP	NAL	TET	FOX	DOX	FEP	AZI
5 (WT)	16	<0.5	<2	<1	<0.03	<0.12/2.38	<0.25	<1/0.5	2	4	<2	4	4	<1	8
1024-4 (SCV)	>1024	1	<2	4	<0.03	0.25/4.75	<0.25	2/1	2	4	<2	4	4	<1	<2
1024-5 (SCV)	>1024	1	<2	4	<0.03	<0.12/2.38	<0.25	<1/0.5	<1	4	<2	4	4	<1	<2
4V1 (revertant)	32	<0.5	4	<1	<0.03	<0.12/2.38	<0.25	<1/0.5	<1	4	<2	4	4	<1	4
5V1 (revertant)	64	<0.5	4	2	<0.03	<0.12/2.38	<0.25	<1/0.5	<1	4	<2	4	4	<1	4

STR streptomycin; *IMI* imipenem; *CHL* chloramphenicol; *GEN* gentamicin; *CIP* ciprofloxacin; *SXT* trimethoprim/sulfamethoxazole; *AXO* ceftriaxone; *AUG2* amoxicillin/clavulanic acid 2:1 ratio; *AMP* ampicillin; *NAL* nalidixic acid; *TET* tetracycline; *FOX* cefoxitin; *DOX* doxycycline; *FEP* cefepime; *AZI* azithromycin

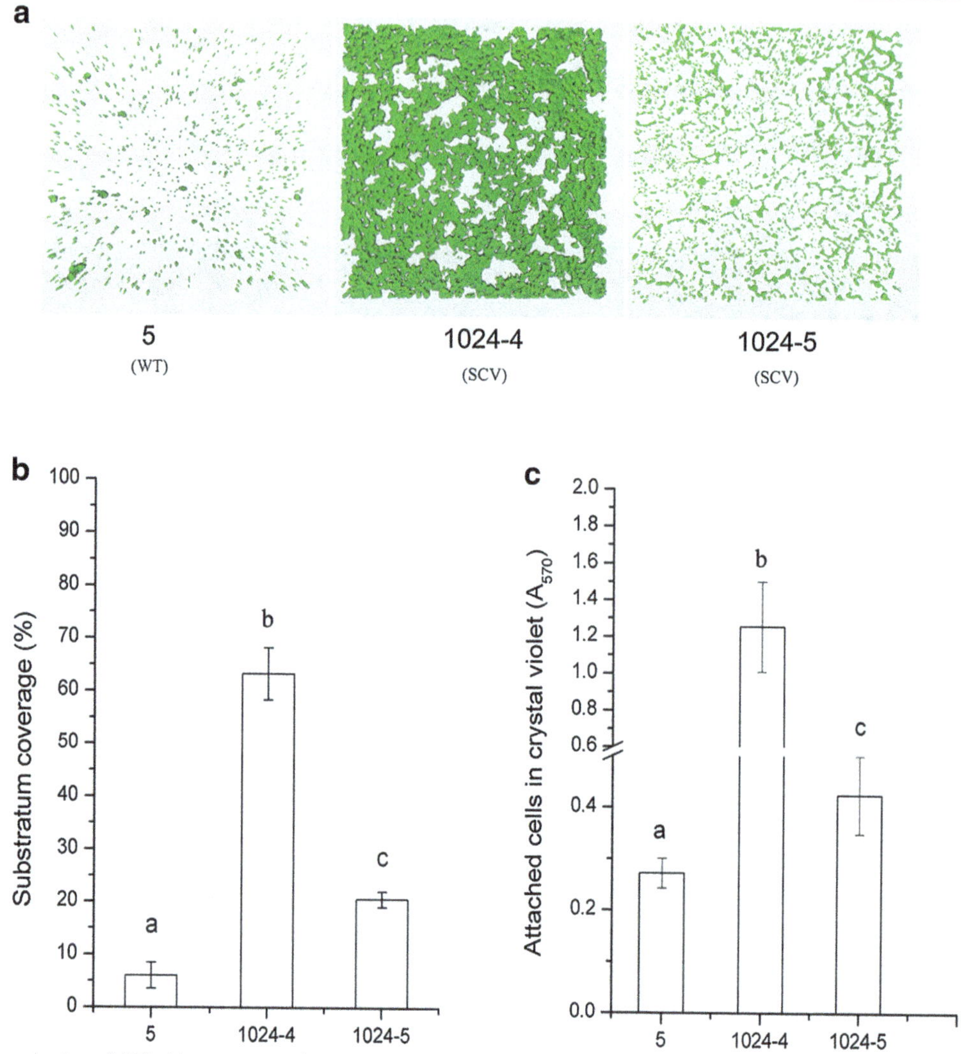

Fig. 2 Biofilm production of WT (wide-type; strain 5) and SCVs (strain 1024-4 and 1024-5). **a** A 3D projection of a biofilm structure of SCVs obtained by CLSM. **b** Ability of biofilm formation by using substratum coverage. **c** Ability of biofilm formation based on crystal violet assay. Data are presented as mean ± SD. *Different letters* on the *error bars* indicate statistically significant differences between strains in each group based on ANOVA ($P < 0.01$)

frameshift and premature termination (Fig. 4b). Interestingly, in its revertant strain, 5V1, the second mutation in *ubiE* (a one base pair insertion) recovered most of the amino acid sequence of the *ubiE* and hence might re-activate this gene (Fig. 4b). A frameshift mutation in *ubiE* was also observed in another SCV strain, 1024-4, suggesting a close association between the activity of the *ubiE* and the SCV phenotype (Table 2).

For strain 4V1, the revertant of 1024-4, carried two SNPs beside in addition to the defective *ubiE* (Fig. 4a). One SNP occurred in a putative gene that encodes for an inner membrane protein (Table 2). However, this SNP did not change the amino acid sequence of the product, and could then just be a neutral mutation. Another SNP in the gene *prfB* led to a substitution of serine by leucine (S271L). This non-synonymous mutation could compensate the functional deficiency of mutated *ubiE*, resulting in the recovery of the phenotype (Fig. 4c).

Based on the results of PCR amplification and sequencing of mutated genes in the other revertants (5V2, 5V3, 5V4, 4V2, 4V3 and 4V4), a total of two modes of genetic change for reversion to a rapidly growing form were observed. The revertants (strain 5V2, 5V3 and 5V4) that reverted back from strain 1024-5, also harbored a secondary mutation in *ubiE* (Fig. 4b), which reinstated most of the amino acid sequence of the *ubiE*. In addition, revertants (strain 4V2, 4V3, 4V4) from 1024-4 harbored a mutation in *prfB* (Fig. 4c).

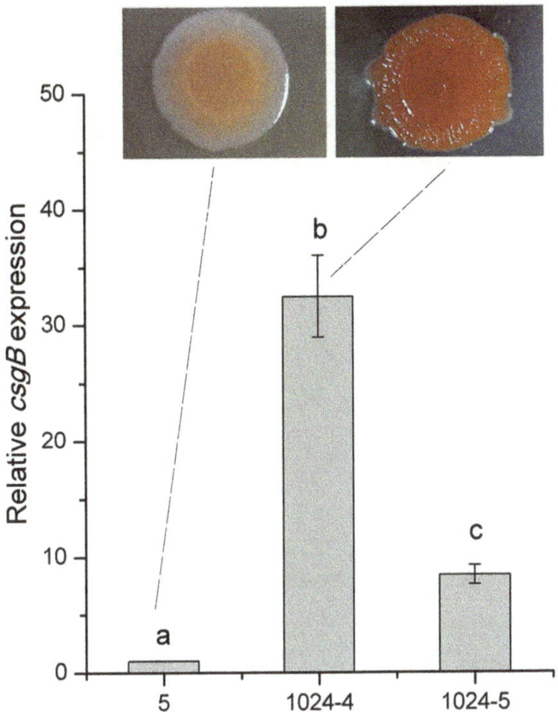

Fig. 3 Relative expression of *csgB* gene in correlation with the rdar morphotype in SCVs (strain 1024-4 and 1024-5). Data are presented as mean ± SD. Measurement of relative expression was normalized to the WT (wide-type; strain 5). *Different letters* on the *error bars* indicate statistically significant differences between strains in each group ($P < 0.01$)

Discussion

Slower growth, reduced metabolic activity and increased antimicrobial resistance are typical characteristics for bacterial SCVs [28], which have been most extensively studied for *S. aureus*. In this study, *S. Typhimurium* SCVs obtained by the treatment of STR also displayed slower growth rate and increased antimicrobial resistance, additionally, with partially increased production of biofilm in comparison to the WT strain.

From the perspectives of food industry, the occurrence of *S. Typhimurium* SCV may increase the potential infection risks. Since STR is still widely used in farm industry in developing countries, exposure to STR could result in the occurrence of *S. Typhimurium* SCVs. Slower growth and reduced metabolic activity are typical characteristics for SCVs of many bacteria. Conventional identification tests (i.e. biochemical tests) are hampered or modified by the decreased metabolism of these SCVs giving no reaction or false negative results [1, 29], which may complicate the routine isolation and identification of bacteria for laboratory-based surveillance of contamination in food. In this way, the risk of *Salmonella* infection might become increased.

Clinically, the phenotypes of SCVs are associated with persistent and recurrent infections in *S. aureus* and *P. aeruginosa* due to their increased ability to persist in mammalian cells and increased antimicrobial resistance [2]. In *S. aureus*, Long et al. have demonstrated that the minimum bacteriocidal concentration was two- to four-fold higher than the parental strain, which may correlate to the bacterial persister cells, however, there was very little change in MIC for SCVs [30]. Consistently, a slightly increase in MIC of IMI and GEN was observed in *S. Typhimurium* SCV mutants. In addition, these SCVs remained susceptible to critical antimicrobials, such as AUG2, AMP and CIP. These data confirm that switching to the SCVs phenotype does not bring a great change in MIC. Additionally, there was a great increase in STR resistance as these SCVs were selected by STR.

In most bacteria, the ability to form biofilm contributes to conferring tolerance and firm adhesion, which helps the bacteria to survive in suboptimal environments, making it extremely difficult to be eradicated. Therefore, the food borne pathogenic bacteria with the ability to form biofilm may threaten the safety of food industry [31]. In this study, a total of five *S. Typhimurium* SCVs were obtained, among which two mutants (strain 1024-4 and 1024-5) displayed a significantly increased biofilm formation in comparison to their wild type strain (ANOVA, $P < 0.05$; data not shown). Consistent with this, approximately 30 % of *P. aeruginosa* SCVs was observed to exhibit increased attachment to glass by Drenkard et al. [32]. Several genes, including *csgD, adrA, csgB* and *bapA*, have been identified to be associated with biofilm formation in *S. enterica* and they were quantified by RT-PCR in this study. *csgD*, a transcriptional regulator, decides whether *S. enterica* strains would form biofilms [33]. On the other hand, the gene *adrA*, which controls the levels of cyclic di-GMP, is related to cellulose production, and *csgB* is the nucleator of the curli fimbriae [34]. In addition, BapA is a large secreted protein required for biofilm formation in *S.* Enteritidis [35]. In our study, *csgB* expressed at a much higher level in SCVs, compared with the WT strain. Particularly, the relative expression of *csgB* reached a maximum of 32-fold in strain 1024-4, suggesting that "rdar" morphotype and biofilm production observed in this strain were possibly attributable to an increased expression of this gene. The associated production of cellulose and curli fimbriae have been well characterized as the "rdar" morphotype which is related to biofilm formation in *S. enterica* [36].

Coenzyme Q is a redox lipid that functions in the respiratory electron transport chain, and also plays a critical role in energy generating processes [37]. Biosynthesis of coenzyme Q in *E. coli* depends on the *ubi* genes [38]. The *ubiE* gene encodes ubiquinone/menaquinone

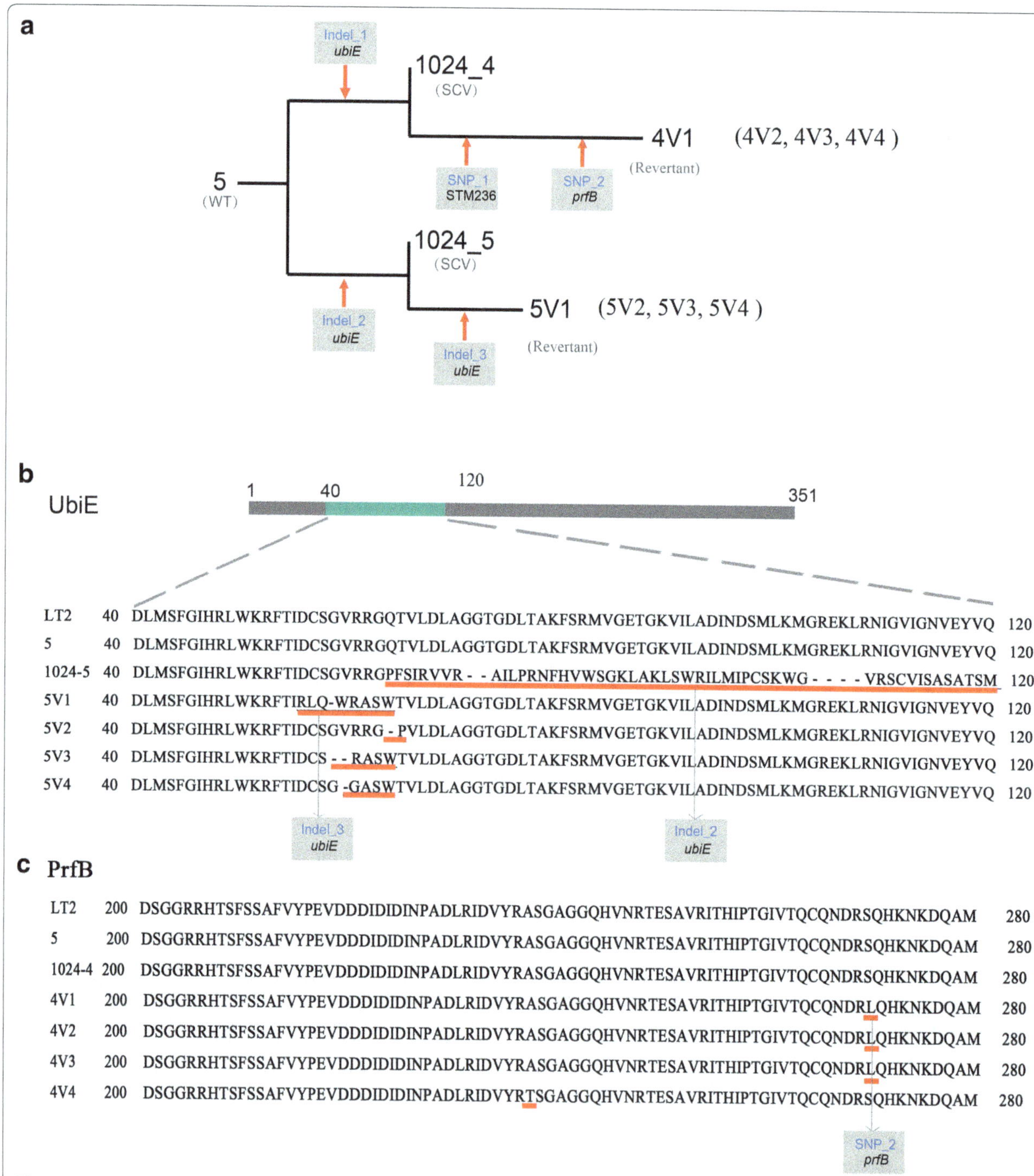

Fig. 4 Two modes of genetic change for reversion to a rapidly growing form in SCVs. **a** Whole-genome resequencing was performed in wide-type strain (WT, strain 5), SCVs (strain 1024-4 and 1024-5) and revertants (strain 4V1 and 5V1) and the genetic alterations in the other revertants (strain 4V2, 4V3, 4V4, 5V2, 5V3 and 5V4) were further identified by PCR and Sanger sequencing method. **b** Amino acid sequence alignment of UbiE for reference strain (*S. Typhimurium* LT2), WT, SCVs and revertants. **c** Amino acid sequence alignment of PrfB for reference strain (*S. Typhimurium* LT2), WT, SCVs and revertants

biosynthesis methyltransferase, which is required for C-methylation reactions in both coenzyme Q_8 and menaquinone biosynthesis [39]. In this study, a frameshift mutation in *ubiE* was observed in all SCVs, which possibly led to the deficiency of electron-transport and the formation of SCV phenotype. As previously reported,

Table 2 List of genetic changes in *S. Typhimurium* SCVs and revertants

Mutation[a]	LT2 Position[b]	Mutant strain	Mutant type	Amino acid change	Gene name	Gene product
Indel_1	4,177,676	1024_4, 4V1	Insertion: T	Frame shift	*ubiE* (STM3970)	Ubiquinone/menaquinone Biosynthesis C-methyltransferase UbiE
Indel_2	4,177,484:4,177,487	1024_5, 5V1	Deletion: GTTT	Frame shift	*ubiE* (STM3970)	Ubiquinone/menaquinone biosynthesis C-methyltransferase UbiE
Indel_3	4,177,459	5V1	Insertion: T	Frame shift	*ubiE* (STM3970)	Ubiquinone/menaquinone biosynthesis C-methyltransferase UbiE
SNP_1	2,480,126	4V1	SNP: G to A	F125F	STM2367	Inner membrane protein
SNP_2	3,201,008	4V1	SNP: G to A	S271L	*prfB* (STM3041c)	Peptide chain release factor 2

[a] The genetic changes in SCVs and revertants were compared to the wild-type parental strain by analyzing the data of whole genome sequencing

[b] Corresponding position in the reference genome of *S. Typhimurium*, LT2 (Accession number: NC_003197.1)

the biogenesis of flagella would be inhibited in the strains bearing deletion mutation of *ubiE* due to the lack of energy source [40]. However, complete deletion of *ubiE* is not naturally occurring in any life stages of bacteria. In this study, SCVs displayed less flagella with a mutation that naturally occurred in *ubiE*, which may be due to the reduced energy generating for flagellar biogenesis [41].

Fitness costs can be offset by compensatory mutations. In this study, two modes of the genetic changes for reversion to the rapidly growing form were observed. All the four revertants that reverted back from strain 1024-5, harbored secondary mutations in *ubiE*. It was possible that the secondary changes in the protein-coding domain led to recovery on the electron-transport compared with SCV strain (strain 1024-5). Moreover, another mode of genetic change for reversion to a rapidly growing form was observed in the revertants reverting back from 1024-4 (strain 4V1, 4V2, 4V3, 4V4). All the revertants harbored a mutation in *prfB* (encoding for peptide chain release factor 2), suggesting that the deficiency in electron-transport could be compensated by the mutation of *prfB* gene. Peptide chain release factor 2 gene, *prfB*, was catalyzes translational termination at UGA or UAA codons [42], but how the mutation in *prfB* compensated the growth cost of SCVs needs to be further investigated.

Conclusion

To conclude, this study disclosed the specific genetic changes that involved in the life cycle of SCVs in *S. Typhimurium*, which helps to get a better understanding of the genetic basis for the ability of SCVs to revert to the phenotype of rapid growth. *S. Typhimurium* could switch to the phenotype of SCV by a mutation in *ubiE* under the treatment of STR. Moreover, the available biofilm formation of *S. Typhimurium* SCVs may be a strategy for survival. Therefore, the rational use of STR in agriculture or farm industry should be considered to reduce the potential risk of *S. Typhimurium* infection. Under a favorable environmental condition, these SCVs can escape from the growth restriction by a second-site compensatory mutation in *prfB* or a new mutation in *ubiE*. These genetic changes (SNPs and indels) that occurred in the life cycle of *S. Typhimurium* SCVs were different to those previously reported in the literature. And these findings may contribute to developing phenotype-directed treatments against *S. Typhimurium* SCVs.

Abbreviations

S. Typhimurium: *Salmonella enterica* serotype *Typhimurium*; SCVs: small colony variants; STR: streptomycin; WT: wild-type strains; MHA: Mueller–Hinton agar; TSB: tryptone soy broth; PFGE: pulse field gel electrophoresis; MLVA: multilocus variable number tandem repeat analysis; CDC: center for disease control and prevention; TEM: transmission electron microscopy; PCR: polymerase chain reaction; SNP: single-nucleotide polymorphism; LB: Luria–Bertani broth; MIC: minimal inhibitory concentration; IMI: imipenem; CHL: chloramphenicol; GEN: gentamicin; CIP: ciprofloxacin; SXT: trimethoprim/sulfamethoxazole; AXO: ceftriaxone; AUG2: amoxicillin/clavulanic acid 2:1 ratio; AMP: ampicillin; NAL: nalidixic acid; TET: tetracycline; FOX: cefoxitin; DOX: doxycycline; FEP: cefepime; AZI: azithromycin; CLSM: confocal laser scanning microscopy; cDNA: complementary DNA; rdar: red, dry and rough.

Authors' contributions

All authors contributed to this work. All authors read and approved the final manuscript.

Author details

[1] Key Laboratory of Bio-resources and Eco-environment of the Ministry of Education, College of Life Sciences, Sichuan University, 29# Wangjiang Rd., Chengdu, Sichuan 610064, P. R. China. [2] Shenzhen Major Infectious Disease Control Key Laboratory, Shenzhen Centre for Disease Control and Prevention, Shenzhen, Guangdong 518055, P. R. China. [3] State Key Laboratory of Pathogen and Biosecurity, Beijing Institute of Microbiology and Epidemiology, Beijing 100071, P. R. China.

Acknowledgements

This research was supported by the China National Science and Technology Major Projects Foundation (2012ZX10004215-003-005), the Department of Science and Technology of Sichuan Province of China (2016NZ005, 2016SZ0068).

Competing interests

The authors declare that they have no competing interests.

References

1. Kahl BC. Small colony variants (SCVs) of *Staphylococcus aureus*—a bacterial survival strategy. Infect Genet Evol. 2014;21:515–22.
2. Proctor RA, von Eiff C, Kahl BC, Becker K, McNamara P, Herrmann M, Peters G. Small colony variants: a pathogenic form of bacteria that facilitates persistent and recurrent infections. Nat Rev Microbiol. 2006;4(4):295–305.
3. Yagci S, Hascelik G, Dogru D, Ozcelik U, Sener B. Prevalence and genetic diversity of *Staphylococcus aureus* small-colony variants in cystic fibrosis patients. Clin Microbiol Infec. 2013;19(1):77–84.
4. Anderson SW, Stapp JR, Burns JL, Xuan Q. Characterization of small-colony-variant *Stenotrophomonas maltophilia* isolated from the sputum specimens of five patients with cystic fibrosis. J Clin Microbiol. 2007;45(2):529–35.
5. Atalla H. Characterization of a *Staphylococcus aureus* small colony variant (SCV) associated with persistent bovine mastitis. Foodborne Pathog Dis. 2008;5(6):785–99.
6. Onyango LA, Dunstan RH, Gottfries J, Von EC, Roberts Tk. Effect of low temperature on growth and ultra-structure of *Staphylococcus spp*. PLoS One. 2012;7(1):339.
7. Xiao-Su P, Hamlyn PJ, Raquel TV, Alovero FL, Manzo RH, L Mark F. Small-colony mutants of *Staphylococcus aureus* allow selection of gyrase-mediated resistance to dual-target fluoroquinolones. Antimicrob Agents Ch. 2002;46(8):2498–506.
8. Schaaff F, Bierbaum G, Baumert N, Bartmann P, Sahl HG. Mutations are involved in emergence of aminoglycoside-induced small colony variants of *Staphylococcus aureus*. Int J Med Microbiol. 2004;293(6):427–35.
9. Massey RC, Buckling A, Peacock SJ. Phenotypic switching of antibiotic resistance circumvents permanent costs in *Staphylococcus aureus*. Curr Biol. 2001;11(22):1810–4.
10. Wen-Hong LI, Cheng Y, Jin JX, Feng-Liang LI. History and research advance of streptomycin for controlling plant bacterial diseases. Hubei Agricultural Sciences 2013. (**In Chinese**).
11. Door APDL, Chacón AR, Muñiz CA. Detection of streptomycin resistance in *Erwinia amylovora* strains isolated from apple orchards in Chihuahua, Mexico. Eur J Plant Pathol. 2013;137(2):223–9.
12. Patel J, Sharma M. Differences in attachment of *Salmonella enterica* serovars to cabbage and lettuce leaves. Int J Food Microbiol. 2010;139(1–2):41–7.
13. Bolton DJ, Ivory C, McDowell D. A study of *Salmonella* in pigs from birth to carcass: serotypes, genotypes, antibiotic resistance and virulence profiles. Int J Food Microbiol. 2013;160(3):298–303.
14. Singh R, Yadav AS, Tripathi V, Singh RP. Antimicrobial resistance profile of *Salmonella* present in poultry and poultry environment in north India. Food Control. 2013;33(2):545–8.
15. Liang Z, Ke B, Deng X, Liang J, Ran L, Lu L, He D, Huang Q, Ke C, Li Z, et al. Serotypes, seasonal trends, and antibiotic resistance of non-typhoidal *Salmonella* from human patients in Guangdong Province, China, 2009–2012. BMC Infect Dis. 2015;15:53.
16. Cano DA, Pucciarelli MG, Martinez-Moya M, Casadesus J, Garcia-del Portillo F. Selection of small-colony variants of *Salmonella enterica* serovar *typhimurium* in nonphagocytic eucaryotic cells. Infect Immun. 2003;71(7):3690–8.
17. Koskiniemi S, Pränting M, Gullberg E, Näsvall J, Andersson DI. Activation of cryptic aminoglycoside resistance in *Salmonella enterica*. Mol Microbiol. 2011;80(6):1464–78.
18. Eliana N, Ausubel FM. *Pseudomonas* biofilm formation and antibiotic resistance are linked to phenotypic variation. Nature. 2002;416(6882):740–3.
19. Pränting M, Andersson DI. Escape from growth restriction in small colony variants of *Salmonella typhimurium* by gene amplification and mutation. Mol Microbiol. 2011;79(2):305–15.
20. Singh R, Ray P, Das A, Sharma M. Enhanced production of exopolysaccharide matrix and biofilm by a menadione-auxotrophic *Staphylococcus aureus* small-colony variant. J Med Microbiol. 2010;59(5):521–7.
21. Nguyen HDN, Yuk H-G. Changes in resistance of *Salmonella typhimurium* biofilms formed under various conditions to industrial sanitizers. Food Control. 2013;29(1):236–40.
22. Vázquez-Sánchez D, Cabo ML, Ibusquiza PS, Rodríguez-Herrera JJ. Biofilm-forming ability and resistance to industrial disinfectants of *Staphylococcus aureus* isolated from fishery products. Food Control. 2014;39:8–16.
23. Steenackers H, Hermans K, Vanderleyden J, De Keersmaecker SCJ. *Salmonella* biofilms: an overview on occurrence, structure, regulation and eradication. Food Res Int. 2012;45(2):502–31.
24. Fabrega A, Soto SM, Balleste-Delpierre C, Fernandez-Orth D, Jimenez de Anta MT, Vila J. Impact of quinolone-resistance acquisition on biofilm production and fitness in *Salmonella* enterica. J Antimicrob Chemoth. 2014;69(7):1815–24.
25. van Ditmarsch D, Boyle Kerry E, Sakhtah H, Oyler Jennifer E, Nadell Carey D, Déziel É, Dietrich Lars EP, Xavier Joao B. Convergent evolution of hyper-swarming leads to impaired biofilm formation in pathogenic bacteria. Cell Rep. 2013;4(4):697–708.
26. Ben-Jacob E, Bogino P, Abod An, Nievas F, Giordano W. Water-limiting Conditions alter the structure and biofilm-forming ability of bacterial multispecies communities in the alfalfa rhizosphere. PLoS One. 2013;8(11):e79614.
27. Bridier A, Dubois-Brissonnet F, Boubetra A, Thomas V, Briandet R. The biofilm architecture of sixty opportunistic pathogens deciphered using a high throughput CLSM method. J Microbiol Meth. 2010;82(1):64–70.
28. Eiff CV, Peters G, Becker K. The small colony variant (SCV) concept—the role of staphylococcal SCVs in persistent infections. Injury. 2006;37(2):S26–33.
29. Von EC, Mcnamara PK, Bates D, Lei XH, Ziman M, Bochner BR, Peters G, Proctor RA. Phenotype microarray profiling of *Staphylococcus aureus* menD and hemB mutants with the small-colony-variant phenotype. J Bacteriol. 2006;188(2):687–93.
30. Bui LMG, Kidd SP. A full genomic characterization of the development of a stable small colony variant cell-type by a clinical *Staphylococcus aureus* strain. Infect Genet Evol. 2015;36:345–55.
31. Srey S, Jahid IK, Ha SD. Biofilm formation in food industries: a food safety concern. Food Control. 2013;31(31):572–85.
32. Drenkard E, Ausubel FM. *Pseudomonas* biofilm formation and antibiotic resistance are linked to phenotypic variation. Nature. 2002;416(6882):740–3.
33. Chambers JR, Sauer K. Small RNAs and their role in biofilm formation. Trends Microbiol. 2013;21(1):39–49.
34. Grantcharova N, Peters V, Monteiro C, Zakikhany K, Romling U. Bistable expression of CsgD in biofilm development of *Salmonella enterica* serovar *typhimurium*. J Bacteriol. 2009;192(2):456–66.
35. Latasa C, Roux A, Toledo-Arana A, Ghigo JM, Gamazo C, Penadés JR, Lasa I. BapA, a large secreted protein required for biofilm formation and host colonization of *Salmonella enterica* serovar Enteritidis. Mol Microbiol. 2005;58(5):1322–39.
36. Römling U, Bokranz W, Rabsch W, Zogaj X, Nimtz M, Tschäpe H. Occurrence and regulation of the multicellular morphotype in *Salmonella* serovars important in human disease. Int J Med Microbiol. 2003;293(4):273–85.
37. Laurent A, Laurent L, Mahmoud HC, Bérengère P, Marc F, Fabien P, Frédéric B. ubiJ, a new gene required for aerobic growth and proliferation in macrophage, is involved in coenzyme Q biosynthesis in *Escherichia coli* and *Salmonella enterica* Serovar *typhimurium*. J Bacteriol. 2014;196(1):70–9.
38. Gulmezian M, Hyman KR, Marbois BN, Clarke CF, Javor GT. The role of UbiX in *Escherichia coli* coenzyme Q biosynthesis. Arch Biochem Bioph. 2007;467(2):144–53.
39. Aussel L, Loiseau L, Hajj Chehade M, Pocachard B, Fontecave M, Pierrel F, Barras F. ubiJ, a new gene required for aerobic growth and proliferation in macrophage, is involved in coenzyme Q biosynthesis in *Escherichia coli* and *Salmonella enterica* serovar *typhimurium*. J Bacteriol. 2013;196(1):70–9.
40. Barker CS, Meshcheryakova IV, Sasaki T, Roy MC, Sinha PK, Yagi T, Samatey FA: Randomly selected suppressor mutations in genes for NADH : quinone oxidoreductase-1, which rescue motility of a *Salmonella* ubiquinone-biosynthesis mutant strain. Microbiology. 2014; 160(Pt_6):1075–86.

9

Determinants of felt demand for dengue vaccines in the North Caribbean region of Colombia

Yalil T. Bracho-Churio[1], Ruth A. Martínez-Vega[1], Alfonso J. Rodriguez-Morales[1,2], Ronald G. Díaz-Quijano[1], María L. Luna-González[1] and Fredi A. Diaz-Quijano[3*]

Abstract

Background: The increasing burden associated with dengue in Latin America makes it essential to understand the community's interest in acquiring vaccines, as an input to plan its introduction in endemic regions. The objective of this study is to learn the felt demand for dengue vaccines by estimating the willingness to pay and its associated factors in endemic communities of the North Caribbean region of Colombia.

Methods: A population survey was administered from October to December 2015, including 1037 families in 11 municipalities in Colombia. One adult per family was interviewed on their perception and history of dengue. Participants received a description of four hypothetical scenarios of dengue vaccines, administered in a single dose or in 3 doses, with an effectiveness of 70% for 5 years or 95% for 30 years. The willingness to pay for each one of these vaccines was inquired vs. 5 hypothetical prices in Colombian pesos.

Results: Most participants recognized dengue as a serious disease in children (99.3%) and adults (98.6%). 33 (3.2%) of the total respondents reported having suffered dengue and 19 (57.6%) of them required hospitalization. The price of the vaccine was inversely related to the willingness to pay. In addition, single dose vaccines (compared to 3 doses) and one with a protection of 95% for 30 years (compared to an effectiveness of 70% for 5 years), were associated with greater willingness to pay. Greater willingness to pay was observed among the respondents who considered it likely to get the disease, either themselves (OR 1.56; CI 95% 1.08–2.26) or their children (OR 1.89; CI 95% 1.28–2.81), in the next 5 years. The participants who have been diagnosed with dengue also showed greater willingness to pay (OR 1.89; CI 95% 1.01–3.54) compared to those who did not have this history.

Conclusion: Factors such as price, number of doses and effectiveness can independently influence the decision to purchase a vaccine against an endemic disease, such as dengue. Additionally, this study reveals that background and perceptions of the disease can affect individuals' interest in acquiring this type of preventive interventions.

Background

Dengue continues to be the viral disease with the highest incidence transmitted by arthropods [1]. Recent estimates suggest that the annual incidence of dengue infections is 390 million, worldwide [1, 2]. In the Americas, dengue is a growing cause of morbidity and mortality, especially in the Caribbean region [3–5], representing a high burden in terms of disability-adjusted life years (DALYs) and associated costs [6]. In Colombia, dengue is a priority in public health, which in 2016 caused more than 100,000 reported cases with 195 associated deaths [7]. The Colombian Caribbean region has shown a tendency to rise and its departments, such as La Guajira, exhibit since 2011 incidence rates that exceed the country's average [4].

Unfortunately, there is still no specific antiviral therapy and the current vector control seems to be insufficient to reduce the burden caused by dengue. Therefore, different

*Correspondence: frediazq@msn.com
[3] Department of Epidemiology, Faculdade de Saúde Pública, Universidade de São Paulo, Av. Dr. Arnaldo, 715, São Paulo, SP CEP-01246-904, Brazil
Full list of author information is available at the end of the article

vaccines are being developed with different levels of effectiveness and dosage schedules [8–11]. For example, CYD-TDC (Dengvaxia®) was the first vaccine to gain regulatory approval in some endemic countries. However, this vaccine requires a 3 dose regimen and showed only moderate efficacy (60%) in children and adolescents [12]. Other vaccines under evaluation would be potential alternatives with less dose schedules [13, 14]. Therefore, it is feasible that aspects such as the number of doses and the effectiveness of the vaccine are issues pertinent to the choice of a vaccine against dengue.

Given the increasing burden associated with dengue in the Americas [3], it is relevant to learn the felt demand of this intervention in the community, which serves as an input for the governments that must make decisions regarding prioritization of interventions for prevention and control. In addition, it is essential to understand the potential economic returns that the introduction of any vaccine would have [5]. Previous studies have been conducted in other populations evaluating the demand for vaccines through the estimation of willingness to pay [5, 15–19]. These studies have shown important differences among countries but few of them have evaluated the determinants of felt demand for dengue vaccines [17].

On the other hand, only one of the previous studies was developed in Colombia [5], specifically in Medellín, a city where only 0.1% of the population is self-recognized as indigenous and 6.2% as afro-descendant [20]. However, this demographic structure is very different from that observed in the Colombian Caribbean, where in addition to the ethnic differences there is a high socio-economic vulnerability.

Accordingly, the objective of this study is to learn the felt demand for dengue vaccines by estimating the willingness to pay and its associated factors in endemic communities of the North Caribbean region of Colombia.

Methods

Study setting

This research is part of a population-based cohort study (4). A population survey was administered from October to December 2015, including 1037 families selected through probabilistic sampling by conglomerates in eleven municipalities of three departments in Colombia. One adult from each family was interviewed on their perception and history of dengue. In addition, participants received a description of four scenarios of dengue vaccines, changing the effectiveness or the number of doses required in each scenario. The willingness to pay for each one of these vaccines was inquired vs. five hypothetical prices in Colombian pesos (COP).

Study population and sampling technique

For this study, a sample was planned of at least 1000 families selected in 11 municipalities in the Colombian Caribbean. The municipalities included nine in the department of La Guajira (Riohacha, Albania, Fonseca, San Juan del Cesar, Distracción, Maicao, Villanueva, Uribia and Manaure) one in Cesar (Valledupar) and one in Magdalena (El Retén) (Fig. 1). Together these municipalities are estimated to have a total population of 1.3 million inhabitants [21]. Most of the surveys were administered in the Department of La Guajira (89.2%), in which approximately 42.4% of the population is self-recognized as indigenous and nearly 14% as afro-descendant [20].

The number of homes per municipality was assigned considering the size of the population, ranging from 20 families in El Retén (Magdalena) to 203 in Riohacha (La Guajira). Sampling by conglomerates was carried out for the selection of participants. Thus, blocks were selected in each municipality and on each block, following a mapping and population analysis, the number of homes was selected. Both selections were carried out at random. In each of the homes, residents were invited to participate and the questionnaire of this study was administered to the responsible adult who was at home at the time of the visit.

Only people in charge of the house at the time of the visit, who were at least 16 years old, were considered eligible to respond to the survey. People planning to change their place of residence in the next 6 months were excluded [4]. The respondents had not a dengue diagnosis at the time of the interview, but they may or may not have had the disease in the past [22]. In that sense, only 3.2% of the respondents reported a diagnosis of dengue in the past.

Study procedure

Interviews were conducted by previously trained professional nurses, who carried out the informed consent process and the interview using a standardized questionnaire. This questionnaire was developed seeking to include the variables previously evaluated in a multi-country study for hypothetical vaccines with a 3 dose regimen [5]. In addition, we incorporated analogous scenarios for single-dose vaccines.

This questionnaire included questions on participants' perception and experience regarding dengue. This was followed by a process of presentation of a scenario in which there is a vaccine with an effectiveness of 70% for 5 years, administered in 3 doses. This process included a graphical presentation of the concept of effectiveness as proposed by other authors for the respondent's appropriate capacity to respond [5].

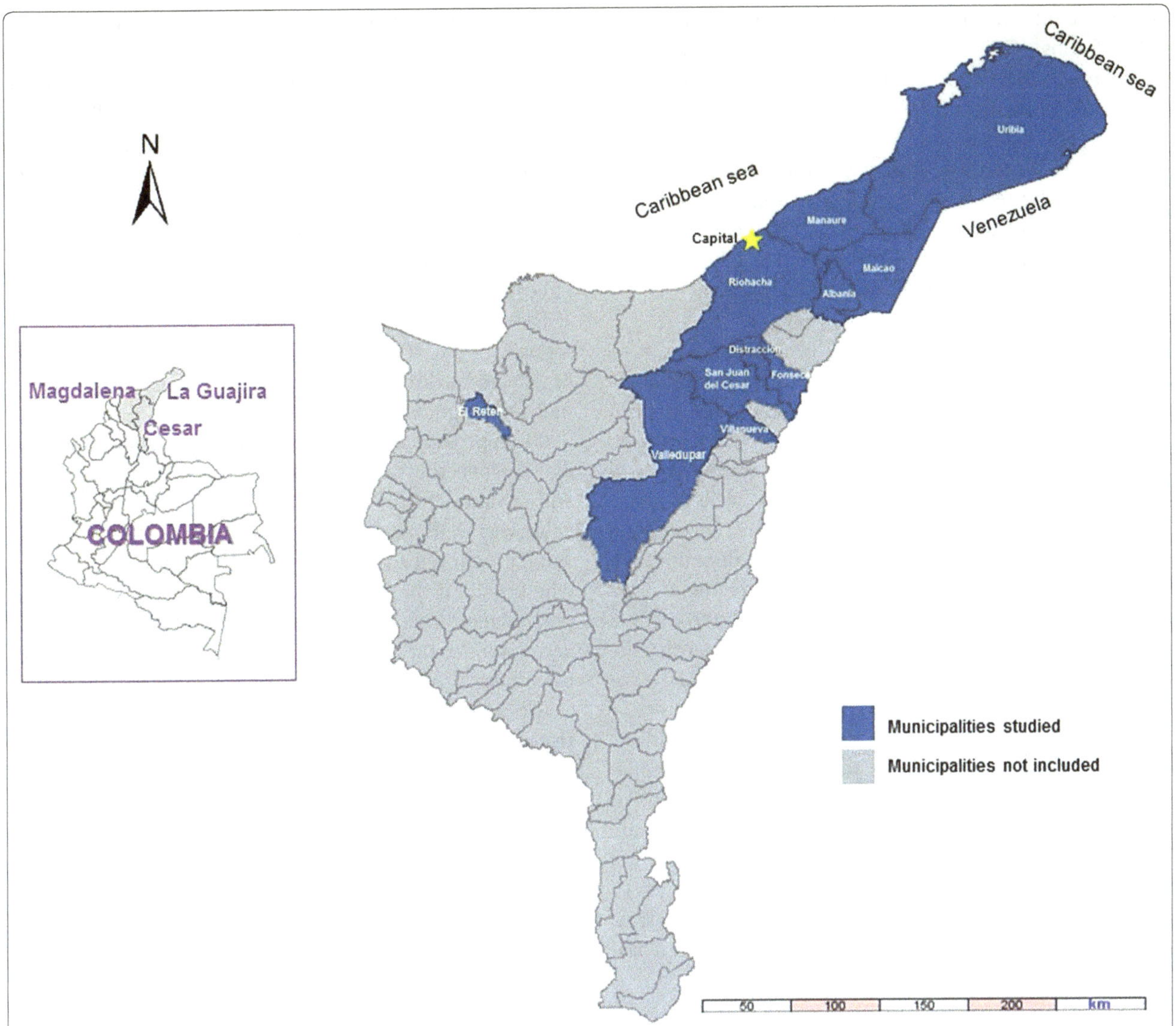

Fig. 1 Relative location of the study sites in the North Caribbean region of Colombia

After that, participants were questioned on their willingness to pay for a vaccine for themselves with these characteristics, based on the following hypothetical prices: COP 3000, COP 60,000, COP 150,000, COP 300,000 and COP 900,000. These values are close to the following values in US dollars (USD) respectively (at the exchange rate of June 15, 2016): USD 1, USD 20, USD 50, USD 100 and USD 300. Subsequently, participants were asked if they would accept the same vaccine as provided freely. Then, the questionnaire of willingness to pay was repeated but presenting a scenario in which the vaccine would have an effectiveness of 95% for 30 years, administered in 3 doses. Then, these procedures were repeated for single-dose vaccines. Finally, the interviewers asked with a single question what is the average monthly income in the participant's home. The value referred was recorded in COP.

Statistical analysis

The analysis focused on modeling the willingness to pay as a binary variable. Number of doses, effectiveness and hypothetical price were considered as independent variables. Since the same person was providing information for a number of scenarios, logistic regression with the cluster option was used (applied to the participant) for the estimation of standard errors. The resulting model was evaluated in relation to goodness of fit using the Pearson and Hosmer–Lemeshow tests, with a confidence level of 95%.

This was followed by an exploratory analysis of the sociodemographic variables, perceptions and experiences of participants in relation to their intention to pay. The Odds Ratios (OR) were estimated for these analyses with 95% confidence intervals (CI 95%) for each of the responses, adjusting these estimates by the characteristics of the hypothetical vaccines. Variables with few data, for example those that were not applicable to the majority of the respondents or those categories with ten observations or less, were not considered for the multiple analysis. The Stata program (Version 11, 2009; College Station, TX) was used for the statistical analysis.

Results

A total of 1037 individuals answered the survey and were included in the analysis, most of which were women (85%). Median age of participants was 42 years with an interquartile interval from 32 to 54. Regarding level of educational, 30.4% of participants had a basic primary level or lower, 43.9% had high school (either incomplete or graduated) and 25.7% had any superior education. On the other hand, referred income ranged between none and approximately COP 9 million (USD 3000) with a median of COP 600.000 (USD 200) and an interquartile interval from COP 300.000 to COP 800.000 (USD 100 to USD 267).

Almost all participants recognized dengue as a serious disease in children (99.3%), as well as in adults (98.6%). In addition, the majority of respondents considered it was likely they would get dengue in the next few years (Table 1). In turn, 33 respondents (3.2%) reported having previously had dengue (diagnosed by a physician) and 19 (1.84%) of them required hospitalization due to the virus. It is interesting that 15 respondents (1.45%) reported that a family member has died of dengue and 55 (5.33%) mentioned the death of a neighbor caused by dengue.

In relation to vaccines, the majority of respondents (85.3%) claim to have received a dose of the yellow fever vaccine. Only 60 (5.81%) individuals claim to have paid for any vaccine. Other background information is presented in Table 1. According to the criteria of the interviewer, 92.2% (955/1036) of participants answered the questions related to effectiveness and duration of the effect of the vaccine adequately.

The price of the vaccine was inversely related to the willingness to pay (Fig. 2). The vaccine with an effectiveness of 70% and a duration of 5 years, administered in 3 doses, had a willingness to pay of 88.6% when its value was COP 3000 (approximately USD 1); this percentage dropped to 51.8% when the value was COP 60,000 (≈USD 20); 29% with a value of COP 150,000 (≈USD 50); 22.1% when the value was COP 300,000 (≈USD 100); and, 18.9% when the value amounted to COP 900,000 (≈USD 300). However, when asked if they would accept the vaccine for free, the percentage of acceptance was 98.1%. This proportion of acceptance of the vaccine for free was similar for the other hypothetical vaccines (Fig. 2).

The willingness to pay for a vaccine with an effectiveness of 95% and a duration of 30 years, as well as a single-dose vaccine, showed a very similar tendency in relation to the price of the vaccine (Figs. 2a, b). However, the logistic regression model showed that, in addition to price, effectiveness and number of doses also had an impact on the willingness to pay (Table 2). Specifically, the vaccine with an effectiveness of 95% and a duration of 30 years had an odds 19% higher in the willingness to pay,

Table 1 Perceptions and experiences regarding dengue

Questions about dengue	(n)	Responses		
		Yes	No	Does not know/does not remember
Is dengue is a serious disease for children?	(1037)	1030 (99.3%)	4 (0.4%)	3 (0.3%)
Is dengue is a serious disease for adults?	(1037)	1022 (98.6%)	10 (1%)	5 (0.5%)
Are you likely to get dengue in the next 5 years?	(1034)	836 (80.9%)	88 (8.5%)	110 (10.6%)
Are your children likely to get dengue in the next 5 years?	(1032)	785 (76.1%)	78 (7.6%)	169 (16.4%)
Has a doctor ever diagnosed you with dengue?	(1037)	33 (3.2%)	998 (96.2%)	6 (0.6%)
Did you require hospitalization due to dengue?	(33)	19 (57.6%)	14 (42.4%)	
Has a doctor ever diagnosed anyone in your family with dengue?	(1035)	236 (22.8%)	798 (77.1%)	1 (0.1%)
Did the family member require hospitalization due to dengue?	(236)	206 (87.3%)	27 (11.4%)	3 (1.3%)
Has a family member ever died from dengue?	(1025)	15 (1.5%)	1003 (97.9%)	7 (0.7%)
Has a doctor ever diagnosed anyone in your neighborhood with dengue?	(1036)	238 (23%)	459 (44.3%)	339 (32.7%)
Has anyone in your neighborhood been hospitalized due to dengue?	(1037)	232 (22.4%)	437 (42.1%)	368 (35.5%)
Has anyone in your neighborhood died from dengue?	(1035)	55 (5.3%)	594 (57.4%)	386 (37.3%)
Have you ever been vaccinated against yellow fever?	(1037)	885 (85.3%)	81 (7.8%)	71 (6.8%)
Have you ever paid for a vaccine to prevent a disease?	(1033)	60 (5.8%)	960 (92.9%)	13 (1.3%)

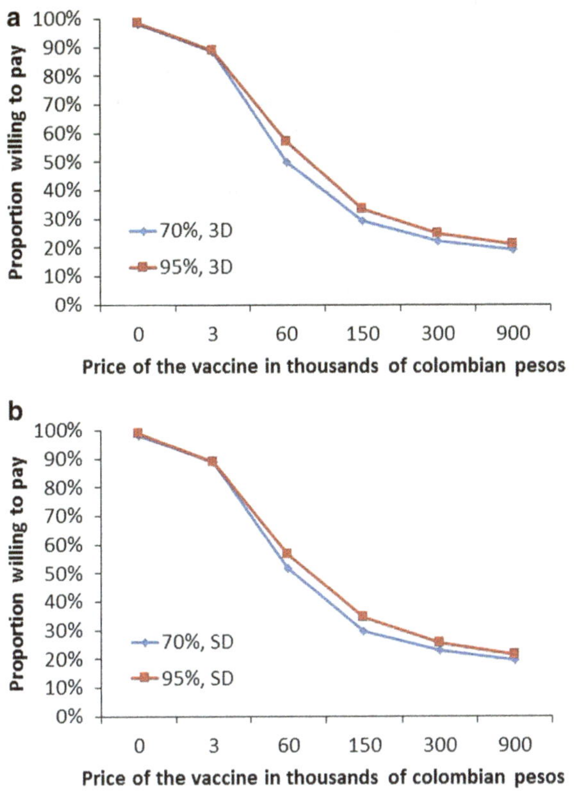

Fig. 2 Willingness to pay for a vaccine against dengue, depending on the price of the vaccine and its effectiveness. **a** Vaccine administered in 3 doses (3D). **b** Vaccine administered in a single dose (SD). *Blue* shows the willingness to pay for a vaccine with an effectiveness of 70% and a duration of 5 years. *Red* shows the willingness to pay for a vaccine with an effectiveness of 95% and a duration of 30 years

Table 2 Association between the characteristics of the hypothetical dengue vaccine and the intention to pay for it

Characteristic	OR (CI 95%)	p value
Effectiveness of 95%[a]	1.19 (1.14–1.24)	<0.001
Value of the vaccine in COP[b]	1	
3000 (USD 1)	0.13 (0.09–0.2)	<0.001
60,000 (USD 20)	0.02 (0.013–0.03)	<0.001
150,000 (USD 50)	0.008 (0.005–0.012)	<0.001
300,000 (USD 100)	0.005 (0.003–0.008)	<0.001
900,000 (USD 300)	0.004 (0.003–0.007)	<0.001
3 dose (vs. single dose)	0.97 (0.95–0.99)	0.001

The values predicted by this model were similar to those observed according to the Pearson (p = 0.98) and Hosmer–Lemeshow (p = 0.99)

[a] In reference to an effectiveness of 95% for 30 years, compared to an effectiveness of 70% for 5 years

[b] The free category was used as the reference. Value in US dollars for 15 June 2016

compared with that of a 70% effectiveness and a duration of 5 years (OR 1.19; CI 95% 1.14–1.24).

In turn, the vaccine that requires 3 doses, would have an odds 3% lower of willingness to pay, compared to single-dose vaccines (OR 0.97; CI 95% 0.95–0.99). The model made up of the above variables presented a high goodness of fit, considering that the predicted values were similar to those observed according to the Pearson (p = 0.98) and Hosmer–Lemeshow (p = 0.99) tests. In addition, associations of this model were maintained when they were adjusted by municipality (data not shown).

Regarding sociodemographic variables, sex and age were not associated with the willingness to pay for a dengue vaccine. However, independently of the characteristics of vaccine (price, number of doses and effectiveness), willingness to pay was positively associated with level of education (Table 3). In relation to the monthly income mentioned by the respondent, we observed a positive association between this variable and the willingness to pay. Specifically, each increase of COP 300,000 (≈USD 100) in monthly income was associated with an 11% increase in the odds of paying for a dengue vaccine (Table 3).

On the other hand,, greater willingness to pay was observed among the respondents who considered it likely to get the disease, either themselves (OR 1.56; CI 95% 1.08–2.26) or their children (OR 1.89; CI 95% 1.28–2.81), in the next 5 years (Table 3). The participants who have been diagnosed with dengue also showed greater willingness to pay (OR 1.89; CI 95% 1.01–3.54) compared to those who did not have this history. In addition, participants who have been vaccinated against yellow fever also indicated greater willingness to pay for a dengue vaccine (OR 1.82; CI 95% 1.22–2.73).

Moreover, the responses indicated that the lack of knowledge of background information related to dengue were associated with lower odds to pay. Specifically, participants who mentioned they did not know whether they were diagnosed as having dengue (OR 0.17; CI 95% 0.05–0.54), or whether anyone in the neighborhood had been diagnosed (OR 0.64; CI 95% 0.5–0.82) or died from dengue (OR 0.54; CI 95% 0.43–0.68), showed a significantly lower odds of paying for the vaccine (Table 3). Finally, the individuals who said they did not know or could not remember having paid for any vaccines, also showed less willingness to pay, compared to those who responded negatively to the same question (OR 0.18; CI 95% 0.1–0.32).

Table 3 Sociodemographic factors, perceptions and experiences associated with the willingness to pay for a vaccine against dengue

Variable	OR[a] (CI 95%)	p value
Sociodemographic		
Sex (female compared with men)	1.01 (0.76–1.34)	0.94
Age (years)	1 (0.99–1.01)	0.96
Level of education		
Basic primary or lower	1	
High school (graduated or incomplete)	1.56 (1.21–2.03)	0.001
Any superior education	2.05 (1.53–2.75)	<0.001
Income (every COP 300,000 ≈ USD 100)	1.11 (1.05–1.17)	<0.001
Perceptions		
Are you likely to get dengue in the next 5 years?		
No	1.0	
Yes	1.56 (1.08–2.26)	0.02
Does not know	1.27 (0.81–1.99)	0.30
Are your children likely to get dengue in the next 5 years?		
No	1.0	
Yes	1.89 (1.28–2.81)	0.001
Does not know	1.2 (0.78–1.86)	0.41
Experiences		
Has a doctor ever diagnosed you with dengue? (yes vs. no)	1.89 (1.01–3.54)	0.05
Has a doctor ever diagnosed anyone in your family with dengue? (yes vs. no)	1.16 (0.9–1.51)	0.25
Has a family member ever died from dengue? (yes vs. no)	1.26 (0.61–2.63)	0.53
Has a doctor ever diagnosed anyone in your neighborhood with dengue?		
No	1.0	
Yes	1.04 (0.79–1.37)	0.78
Does not know	0.64 (0.5–0.82)	<0.001
Has anyone in your neighborhood been hospitalized due to dengue?		
No	1.0	
Yes	0.96 (0.72–1.26)	0.75
Does not know	0.6 (0.47–0.77)	<0.001
Has anyone in your neighborhood died from dengue?		
No	1.0	
Yes	0.71 (0.44–1.15)	0.17
Does not know	0.54 (0.43–0.68)	<0.001
Have you ever been vaccinated against yellow fever?		
No	1.0	
Yes	1.82 (1.22–2.73)	0.003
Does not know	1.66 (0.95–2.89)	0.08
Have you ever paid for a vaccine to prevent a disease?		
No	1.0	
Yes	0.93 (0.6–1.45)	0.75
Does not know	0.18 (0.1–0.32)	<0.001

[a] Each OR is adjusted by the vaccine characteristics (price, number of doses and effectiveness)

Discussion

Dengue continues to be a major global public health problem. In the study of the global burden of disease, an average of 9221 deaths from dengue per year was estimated between 1990 and 2013 [6]. The incidence increased significantly between 1990 and 2013, with a number of cases that multiplies each decade, from 8.3 million in 1990, to 58.4 million cases in 2013 [6]. Considering the fatal and non-fatal results as a whole, dengue was responsible for 1.14 million DALYs in 2013 [6]. In Colombia, it is a widely distributed disease that has caused epidemics over the past three decades (3), especially in the Colombian Caribbean, where the municipalities assessed in this paper are located [4].

For all the above reasons, there was therefore a marked interest in having dengue vaccines, both in endemic areas, as well as for travelers going to these regions, in order to reduce the impact of this burden. Decisions about introduction of a vaccine require careful assessment at the country level, including consideration of local priorities, dengue epidemiology, affordability and budget impact [23], as well as, the cost-effectiveness of dengue vaccination compared with other potential strategies [24].

In that sense, vaccine introduction must consider the felt demand in order to involve the community in the prioritization of specific interventions. In this context, economic evaluations, including the willingness to pay for vaccines, take on great importance and are related to the potential vaccination coverage, especially for those that will not be included in the national immunization programs but may be purchased by the population concerned [11].

The results of this study reveal aspects, such as the fact that the number of doses and the effectiveness of the vaccine are associated with the community's willingness to pay. These associations suggest that the population studied could be less interested in the CYD-TDC (Dengvaxia®) because this vaccine, besides requiring 3 doses, have exhibited only a 60% of effectiveness [12], which is lower than those hypothetical scenarios evaluated in our study.

Regarding the price, this study shows that the median willingness to pay is about COP 60,000 (approximately USD 20). Higher values would make more than half of the population decline the immunization (Fig. 2). In similar studies, the median willingness to pay in Vietnam was USD 26, USD 70 in Thailand and USD 23 in a district of Medellin, Colombia, where 400 families were evaluated [5], which is very similar to our results and consistent for the country.

On the other hand, the median willingness to pay in our study was higher than that observed in Indonesia for an hypothetically safe and fully protective dengue vaccine, which was about USD 4 [17]; but it was lower than that reported in Brazil for the CYD-TDC (Dengvaxia®), which was about USD 33 [15]. This indicates that the estimates of this study are within the range observed in the literature.

These results, as in previous studies [5], suggest that respondents took the hypothetical scenario of buying a dengue vaccine seriously. They also suggest the possibility that there is a market for dengue vaccines and that sales can be robust if prices are lower than the estimated median of our study, which in the case of Colombia included a greater number of households assessed than the previous study [5]. However, it is important to mention that despite the willingness to pay, similar to that reported in other dengue studies, less than 6% of subjects evaluated claimed to have paid for some vaccine in their life.

Our study identified several associations between willingness to pay and factors such as the educational level, income, perceptions and previous experiences of the interviewee. Although evaluated, these associations were not statistically significant in a recent study in Indonesia [17]. This was probably due to that study having a smaller sample size. However, the aforementioned study found that the willingness to pay is associated with good attitudes and preventive practices of the population. The joint evidence from these studies indicates that the felt demand for a dengue vaccine will be conditioned by multiple factors of the population, including the educational level, the economic situation, the experience with the disease, and the way in which people are currently facing this arbovirosis.

This type of willingness-to-pay studies may have significant limitations. For example, to identify the maximum amount of money that a respondent would be willing to pay, the interviewers went through a list of vaccine prices in an ascending manner starting from a cheapest vaccine bid. This might have caused an anchoring effect bias and therefore a risk of underestimating the price which participants would pay [17]. In the present study, the risk of this bias could be reduced because the free vaccine scenario was offered at the end for each type of vaccine.

On the other hand, it is possible that other types of bias affect respondents' responses. For example, desirability bias in which participants might tend to give favorable answers; and/or, the "hypothetical bias", in which participants misstate their actual preferences in a hypothetical survey compared to a real-life situation [17]. Indeed, it is difficult to know the direction of the joint effect of all potential biases on estimation. However, we consider that possible biases would not invalidate the associations found between the willingness to pay and the determinants identified.

As another limitation, this study does not refer to any particular available vaccine. In fact, it could be considered that the scenarios raised exclude vaccines with effectiveness lower than 70% or those designed to apply in two doses [8, 11]. However, the purpose of this study was to understand vaccine demand, which was performed in an objective way in a country where there is no supply of any dengue vaccine. Thus, this study allowed us to identify determinants of the demand for vaccines that could even be extrapolated by analogy to other diseases. These determinants included characteristics of vaccines (dose, effectiveness and price), as well as, epidemiological factors such as previous exposure to the disease and the perception of risk.

For example, participants who believe that they are likely to get the disease and those who have been diagnosed as having it, showed greater willingness to pay. In another sense, patients who are unaware that there has been morbidity or mortality from dengue in their environment, showed less interest in buying a vaccine. Therefore, it is feasible that education in dengue and its epidemiology can raise community awareness and increase the demand for preventive interventions.

All this suggests that the intention to pay can be considered a good indicator of the felt demand for vaccines, since it is closely related to the perception of risk and personal experiences. So it is expected that the felt demand for vaccines is greater in areas with higher morbidity and mortality rates. Therefore, it could be expected that other endemic municipalities, not specifically included in this evaluation, have similar values based on the epidemiological importance of dengue therein.

In addition, aspects such as having been vaccinated for yellow fever was associated with a greater willingness to pay, suggesting greater awareness of the benefit of immunization, which may be associated with positive reinforcement, low frequency of adverse effects and access to health services, among other factors. In addition, the relationship between monthly income and the dependent variable is consistent and validates the consistency of the questionnaire, as was to be expected because individuals with better incomes tend to be more willing to pay for a vaccine.

Another relevant aspect in the region is the co-circulation of other viruses transmitted by the same vector, such as Chikungunya and Zika, which have taken on great importance over the last year [25, 26]. This epidemiological phenomenon can reinforce community awareness of the arboviruses [27, 28] in general and, thus, positively reinforce the willingness to pay for dengue vaccines [16].

Secondly, this study also showed an apparent coverage of self-referenced vaccination for yellow fever in the region of study of more than 85%. This is particularly important at a time when yellow fever is the subject of global concern due to epidemics in Africa and other regions of the world [29, 30].

The increase in the number of dengue cases and the lack of vaccines against arboviruses leads governments to take into account several types of effective means to control the disease [31]. Similar to previous studies [5, 15, 17], this paper provides important information on the number of individuals in endemic areas who are willing to pay for a dengue vaccine to avoid the risk of getting the infection, perhaps especially those who have only had a previous infection by one serotype and want to avoid further infection by other serotypes.

The results of this study can be used in a cost-benefit analysis to plan an appropriate introduction of dengue vaccines. Some studies have already used information generated in this regard [32], where with a theoretical efficiency of 70%, a potential effect of herd immunity can even be reached with a vaccination coverage of 82%. At these values, the dengue vaccine could be cost-effective for costs of vaccination of up to USD 534 per individual vaccinated, saving up to USD 204. It is suggested that even at lower effectiveness rates, they are still cost-effective [32].

These estimates, which are consistent with those of previous studies in Colombia and in Asia [5, 16, 18], present an approach that can be associated with the impact that they can also have on the reduction of the disease. The results can be incorporated in the analysis of prioritization of different health interventions on the national level [5]. Moreover, studies such as the one carried out could be suggested to health authorities to be conducted at the national level in municipalities prioritized by their epidemiological characteristics in the country.

The study can also help decision makers understand how a large part of the population in endemic areas, can be covered by the subsidy of dengue vaccines in the implementation of campaigns on the national level and contribute to the design of public vaccination policies, which should definitely be integrated with other preventive strategies to control dengue in the country [10], and even more so since new vaccines show a better effectiveness and safety profile [33]. On the other hand, knowledge about contextual factors determining willingness to pay are essential to design vaccine introduction programs [34].

In conclusion, this study shows evidence, for the first time for the Colombian Caribbean region, of how factors such as price, number of doses and effectiveness can independently influence the decision to purchase a vaccine against an endemic disease, such as dengue. Additionally, this study reveals how community background and perceptions of the disease can affect individuals' interest in acquiring this type of preventive interventions.

Abbreviations

COP: Colombian pesos; USD: US dollars; OR: odds ratio; CI 95%: confidence intervals of 95%; 3D: 3 doses; SD: single-dose.

Authors' contributions

YTBC participated in the preparation of the questionnaire and coordination of the study and carried out a review of the manuscript; RAMV participated in the preparation of manuals and instruments and contributed to the discussion of the results; AJRM participated in the coordination of the study, assisted in drafting the manuscript and the design of illustrations; RGDQ participated in the design and management of the study and contributed to the discussion of the results; MLLG participated in the design of instruments to collect and store information, data management and carried out critical reviews of the manuscript; and FADQ conceived the study, participated in the design and coordination thereof, analyzed the data and prepared the first draft of the manuscript. All authors read and approved the final manuscript.

Author details

[1] Organización Latinoamericana para el Fomento de la Investigación en Salud, Bucaramanga, Santander, Colombia. [2] Public Health and Infection Research Group, Faculty of Health Sciences, Universidad Tecnológica de Pereira, Pereira, Risaralda, Colombia. [3] Department of Epidemiology, Faculdade de Saúde Pública, Universidade de São Paulo, Av. Dr. Arnaldo, 715, São Paulo, SP CEP-01246-904, Brazil.

Acknowledgements

The authors would like to thank Dr. Alexander Rojas Calero and Diana Martínez Vega, Engineer, for their invaluable support in administrative activities of the project. In addition, we would like to acknowledge the outstanding participation of the following professionals who collaborated in the collection of information: Dallys Almazo, Sorangel Brito, Greys C. Rios, Jacinta Arrieta, Heidist Bermúdez, Maripaz Vergara, Stephanie Arévalo, Yulibeth Gutierrez, Karen Kammerer, Maria A. Sierra, Milli Brito, Dainis Nieves, Johanna Perez, Rubys Oyola, Adriana Miranda, Jennifer Brito, Maria M. Kammerer, Eivis Morales.

This study was previously presented in part at the 10th National Meeting of Research in Infectious Diseases, Colombian Association of Infectious Diseases (ACIN), Medellin, Antioquia, Colombia, 17–19 November 2016 (Oral presentation #52, Virology Section).

Competing interests

The authors declare that they have no competing interests. However, RAMV wanted to state that she is participating in a research project of the Public Health Institute of Mexico that received funding from Sanofi-Pasteur.

Consent for publication

It is not applicable because the manuscript does not contain anyone's individual data.

Funding

The project was funded by the Department of La Guajira in an agreement with Organización Latinoamericana para el Fomento de la Investigación en Salud [Latin American Organization for the Promotion of Research in Health] (OLFIS). Convention 019/2014.

References

1. Gubler DJ. Dengue, urbanization and globalization: the unholy trinity of the 21st century. Trop Med Health. BioMed Central. 2011;39:3–11. http://www.ncbi.nlm.nih.gov/pubmed/22500131. Accessed 2 May 2017.
2. Bhatt S, Gething PW, Brady OJ, Messina JP, Farlow AW, Moyes CL, et al. The global distribution and burden of dengue. Nature. 2013;496:504–7. http://www.ncbi.nlm.nih.gov/pubmed/23563266. Accessed 2 May 2017.
3. Díaz-Quijano FA, Waldman EA. Factors associated with dengue mortality in Latin America and the Caribbean, 1995–2009: an ecological study. Am J Trop Med Hyg. 2012;86:328–34.
4. Martínez-Vega RA, Rodriguez-Morales AJ, Bracho-Churio YT, Castro-Salas ME, Galvis-Ovallos F, Díaz-Quijano RG, et al. A prospective cohort study to assess seroprevalence, incidence, knowledge, attitudes and practices, willingness to pay for vaccine and related risk factors in dengue in a high incidence setting. BMC Infect Dis. 2016;16:705.
5. Lee J-S, Mogasale V, Lim JK, Carabali M, Sirivichayakul C, Anh DD, et al. A multi-country study of the household willingness-to-pay for dengue vaccines: household surveys in Vietnam, Thailand, and Colombia. PLoS Negl. Trop Dis. Public Library of Science; 2015;9:e0003810. http://www.ncbi.nlm.nih.gov/pubmed/26030922. Accessed 2 May 2017.
6. Stanaway JD, Shepard DS, Undurraga EA, Halasa YA, Coffeng LE, Brady OJ, et al. The global burden of dengue: an analysis from the Global Burden of Disease Study 2013. Lancet Infect Dis. Europe PMC Funders; 2016;16:712–23. http://www.ncbi.nlm.nih.gov/pubmed/26874619. Accessed 2 May 2017.
7. PAHO. Number of reported cases of dengue and severe dengue (SD) in the americas, by country: figure for 2016. 2017. http://www2.paho.org/hq/index.php?option=com_topics&view=rdmore&cid=6290&Itemid=40734. Accessed 4 May 2017.
8. Hadinegoro SR, Arredondo-García JL, Capeding MR, Deseda C, Chotpitayasunondh T, Dietze R, et al. Efficacy and long-term safety of a dengue vaccine in regions of endemic disease. N Engl J Med. Massachusetts Medical Society; 2015;373:1195–206. http://www.nejm.org/doi/abs/10.1056/NEJMoa1506223. Accessed 2 May 2017.
9. Villabona-Arenas CJ, Ocazionez Jimenez RE, Jimenez Silva CL. Dengue vaccine: considerations before rollout in Colombia. PLoS Negl. Trop Dis. Public Library of Science; 2016;10:e0004653. http://www.ncbi.nlm.nih.gov/pubmed/27280803. Accessed 2 May 2017.
10. Pitisuttithum P, Bouckenooghe A. The first licensed dengue vaccine: an important tool for integrated preventive strategies against dengue virus infection. Expert Rev. Vaccines. Taylor & Francis; 2016;15:795–8. http://www.tandfonline.com/doi/full/10.1080/14760584.2016.1189331. Accessed 2 May 2017.
11. Halstead SB, Aguiar M. Dengue vaccines: are they safe for travelers? Travel Med Infect Dis. 2016. http://www.sciencedirect.com/science/article/pii/S1477893916300710. Accessed 4 May 2017.
12. Godói IP, Lemos LLP, de Araújo VE, Bonoto BC, Godman B, Guerra Júnior AA. CYD-TDV dengue vaccine: systematic review and meta-analysis of efficacy, immunogenicity and safety. J Comp Eff Res. 2017;6:165–80. http://www.ncbi.nlm.nih.gov/pubmed/28084784. Accessed 14 Apr 2017.
13. Precioso AR, Palacios R, Thomé B, Mondini G, Braga P, Kalil J. Clinical evaluation strategies for a live attenuated tetravalent dengue vaccine. Vaccine. 2015;33:7121–5. http://www.sciencedirect.com/science/article/pii/S0264410X1501395X. Accessed 2 May 2017.
14. Torresi J, Ebert G, Pellegrini M. Vaccines licensed and in clinical trials for the prevention of dengue. Hum Vaccin Immunother. Taylor & Francis; 2017;1–14. https://www.tandfonline.com/doi/full/10.1080/21645515.2016.1261770. Accessed 2 May 2017.
15. Godói IP, Santos AS, Reis EA, Lemos LLP, Brandão CMR, Alvares J, et al. Consumer willingness to pay for dengue vaccine (CYD-TDV, Dengvaxia(®)) in Brazil; implications for future pricing considerations. Front Pharmacol. Frontiers Media SA; 2017;8:41. http://www.ncbi.nlm.nih.gov/pubmed/28210223. Accessed 14 Apr 14.
16. Hadisoemarto PF, Castro MC, Sirivichayakul C, Limkittikul K, Chanthavanich P. Public Acceptance and willingness-to-pay for a future dengue vaccine: a community-based survey in Bandung, Indonesia. Ribeiro GS, editor. PLoS Negl. Trop Dis. Public Library of Science; 2013;7:e2427. http://dx.plos.org/10.1371/journal.pntd.0002427. Accessed 3 May 2017.
17. Harapan H, Anwar S, Bustamam A, Radiansyah A, Angraini P, Fasli R, et al. Willingness to pay for a dengue vaccine and its associated determinants in Indonesia: a community-based, cross-sectional survey in Aceh. Acta Trop.2017;166:249–56. http://www.sciencedirect.com/science/article/pii/S0001706X16305149. Accessed 3 May 2017.
18. Palanca-Tan R. The demand for a dengue vaccine: a contingent valuation survey in Metro Manila. Vaccine. 2008;26:914–23. http://www.sciencedirect.com/science/article/pii/S0264410X07014600. Accessed 3 May 2017.
19. Harapan H, Anwar S, Setiawan AM, Sasmono RT. Dengue vaccine acceptance and associated factors in Indonesia: a community-based cross-sectional survey in Aceh. Vaccine. 2016;34:3670–5. http://www.sciencedirect.com/science/article/pii/S0264410X16303164. Accessed 3 May 2017.
20. DANE. Geoportal DANE—Censo General 2005. https://geoportal.dane.gov.co/v2/?page=elementoCNPV. Accessed 3 May 2017.
21. DANE. Proyecciones de población. https://www.dane.gov.co/index.php/estadisticas-por-tema/demografia-y-poblacion/proyecciones-de-poblacion. Accessed 4 May 2017.
22. Timothy C. Haab, Kenneth E McConnell. Valuing environmental and natural resources. Massachusetts: Edward Elgar Publishing, Inc.; 2002. http://s1.downloadmienphi.net/file/downloadfile8/200/1375235.pdf. Accessed 2 May 2017.
23. World Health Organization. Dengue vaccine: WHO position paper, July 2016—recommendations. Vaccine. 2017. p. 1200–1. http://www.sciencedirect.com/science/article/pii/S0264410X16310192. Accessed 4 May 2017.
24. Webster DP, Farrar J, Rowland-jones S. Progress towards a dengue vaccine. Lancet Infect Dis. Elsevier Ltd; 2009;9:678–87. 10.1016/S1473-3099(09)70254-3. Accessed 4 May 2017.
25. Rodriguez-Morales AJ, García-Loaiza CJ, Galindo-Marquez ML, Sabogal-Roman JA, Marin-Loaiza S, Lozada-Riascos CO, et al. Zika infection GIS-based mapping suggest high transmission activity in the border area of la Guajira, Colombia, a northeastern coast Caribbean department, 2015–2016: implications for public health, migration and travel. Travel Med Infect Dis. 2016;14:286–8.
26. Rodriguez-Morales AJ, Villamil-Gómez WE, Franco-Paredes C. The arboviral burden of disease caused by co-circulation and co-infection of dengue, chikungunya and Zika in the Americas. Travel Med Infect Dis. 2016;14:177–9. http://linkinghub.elsevier.com/retrieve/pii/S1477893916300370. Accessed 4 May 2017.
27. Siddiqui TR, Ghazal S, Bibi S, Ahmed W, Sajjad SF, Stuyft P Van der. Use of the health belief model for the assessment of public knowledge and household preventive practices in Karachi, Pakistan, a dengue-endemic city. Rabaa MA, editor. PLoS Negl. Trop Dis. John Wiley & Sons; 2016;10:e0005129. http://dx.plos.org/10.1371/journal.pntd.0005129. Accessed 4 May 2017.
28. Fritzell C, Raude J, Adde A, Dusfour I, Quenel P, Flamand C. Knowledge, Attitude and Practices of Vector-Borne Disease Prevention during the Emergence of a New Arbovirus: implications for the control of chikungunya virus in French Guiana. Akogun OB, editor. PLoS Negl. Trop Dis. Harwood Academic Publishers; 2016;10:e0005081. http://dx.plos.org/10.1371/journal.pntd.0005081. Accessed 4 May 2017.
29. Vasconcelos PFC, Monath TP. Yellow fever remains a potential threat to public health. Vector-Borne Zoonotic Dis. Mary Ann Liebert, Inc. 140 Huguenot Street, 3rd Floor New Rochelle, NY 10801 USA; 2016;16:566–7. http://online.liebertpub.com/doi/10.1089/vbz.2016.2031. Accessed 4 May 2017.
30. Woodall JP, Yuill TM. Why is the yellow fever outbreak in Angola a "threat to the entire world"? Int J Infect Dis. 2016;48:96–7. http://linkinghub.elsevier.com/retrieve/pii/S120197121631044X. Accessed 4 May 2017.
31. Dickinson KL, Hayden MH, Haenchen S, Monaghan AJ, Walker KR, Ernst KC. Willingness to pay for mosquito control in key west, Florida and Tucson, Arizona. Am J Trop Med Hyg. The American Society of Tropical Medicine and Hygiene; 2016;94:775–9. http://www.ncbi.nlm.nih.gov/pubmed/26903603. Accessed 4 May 2017.
32. Durham DP, Ndeffo Mbah ML, Medlock J, Luz PM, Meyers LA, Paltiel AD, et al. Dengue dynamics and vaccine cost-effectiveness in Brazil. Vaccine. 2013;31:3957–61. http://www.ncbi.nlm.nih.gov/pubmed/23791696. Accessed 4 May 2017.

10

Genetic characterization of TEM-type ESBL-associated antibacterial resistance in *Enterobacteriaceae* in a tertiary hospital in Ghana

Daniel Oduro-Mensah[1,5*], Noah Obeng-Nkrumah[2], Evelyn Yayra Bonney[3], Ebenezer Oduro-Mensah[4], Kingsley Twum-Danso[2], Yaa Difie Osei[1] and Sammy Tawiah Sackey[1]

Abstract

Background: Antibiotic resistance due to the presence of extended-spectrum beta-lactamases (ESBLs) among *Enterobacteriaceae* is a worldwide problem. Data from Ghana regarding this resistance mechanism is limited. This study was designed to investigate the presence of TEM-type ESBL genes, their locations and their conjugabilities in clinical isolates of enterobacteria collected from the Korle-Bu Teaching Hospital in Ghana.

Methods: Study isolates were characterized with respect to ESBL phenotype, TEM-type ESBL gene detection, location of the ESBL gene(s) and conjugability of the ESBL phenotype using nalidixic acid-resistant *Escherichia coli* K-12 as recipient. Phenotyping was by Kirby Bauer disk diffusion using cefpodoxime, ceftazidime, cefotaxime and their combinations with clavulanate. Gene detections were by PCR using *bla*TEM primers.

Results: Overall, 37.96 % of 137 clinical isolates showed ESBL phenotype. The ESBLs occurred mostly in *Klebsiella* spp. (42.3 %) and then *Escherichia coli* (34.6 %). The TEM gene was detected in 48.1 % of ESBL-positive isolates and was determined to be plasmid-borne in 24 of 25 *bla*TEM detections. Overall, 62.7 % of TEM-producing isolates transferred the ESBL phenotype by conjugation.

Conclusions: The results highlight the presence of TEM-type ESBLs in the Korle-Bu Teaching Hospital and show considerable risk of environmental contamination through the urine of infected persons. An inhibition zone chart was generated which indicates the possible presence of complex beta-lactamase types. The data points to the fact that the ESBL-producing bacteria may disseminate this resistance mechanism via conjugation.

Keywords: Beta-lactamase, Inhibition zone chart, Conjugation, Reamplification

Background

The *Enterobacteriaceae* comprise a large family of clinically significant Gram-negative bacteria. They cause over 30 % of the morbidity and mortality associated with bacterial infections [1, 2] [CDC 2015, unpublished observation]. Resistance to β-lactam antimicrobials in *Enterobacteriaceae* has been due to largely the presence of β-lactamase enzymes [3, 4]. β-lactamase genes (*bla*) were originally found to be chromosomal [5]. Since the emergence of the first reports on plasmid-borne *blaTEM-1* in the 1960s, many more which appear to be mutants of the classic *TEM* genes, as well as novel types including SHV, CTX-M and OXA, have been found [6–8]. β-lactamase-mediated resistance may develop in vivo during chemotherapy, lending support to the prevalent view that ESBL plasmids are conjugative, may be borne on transposons, and that the genes may have high mutation frequencies [9, 10]. Also of concern is the increasing

*Correspondence: danomensah@gmail.com

[1] Department of Biochemistry, Cell and Molecular Biology, School of Biological Sciences, University of Ghana, Legon, Accra, Ghana

Full list of author information is available at the end of the article

dissemination of ESBLs across hitherto wildtype species [11].

ESBL-producing bacterial isolates have been reported across Africa, even in isolated remote communities [11–16]. Beyond detection, data on specific identification of ESBLs are needed for deciding local therapy options, control strategies and recognition of unusual cases. In Ghana, investigations into mechanisms of *β*-lactam resistance have often been limited to phenotypic characterizations. This study reports the presence of TEM-type *β*-lactamase genes, their location(s) and their transferability by conjugation in clinical enterobacteria isolates collected at the Korle-Bu Teaching Hospital (KBTH).

Methods

Study isolates

Bacteria were isolated from clinical specimen (sputum, blood, feces, urine, cerebrospinal fluid, high vaginal swabs, wound swabs, pus) submitted to the Microbiology Laboratory of Korle-Bu Teaching Hospital (KBTH). A total of 137 isolates were included in the study. The isolates comprised only those recovered as members of the family *Enterobacteriaceae* [17] and identified as being responsible for patients' clinical conditions. Conclusive identification of isolates was done with API 20E rapid test strips (bioMerieux SA, Marcy l'Etoile, France). Isolates were stocked in Luria–Bertani (LB)-ampicillin (60 μg/ml) broth containing 15 % glycerol and kept at −20 °C. All stocks were routinely plated to check for purity. Four National Collection of Typed Cultures (NCTC) isolates were included in the study as controls; NCTC 10418 (*β*-lactamase negative), NCTC 13352 (TEM 10 positive), NCTC 13353 (CTX-M-15 positive), NCTC 165032 (SHV-3).

Detection of ESBL phenotype

Isolates were examined for ESBL phenotype by the Kirby-Bauer disk diffusion method of susceptibility testing and according to United Kingdom Health Protection Agency (HPA) guidelines (QSOP 51i2.2, 2008). Screening and confirmatory tests were done simultaneously on the same plate. Briefly, each test isolate was plated on Mueller–Hinton agar (Oxoid, UK). After incubating overnight at 37 °C, a 0.5 McFarland suspension in peptone broth (MAST, UK) of each was prepared. This suspension was then swabbed onto a cation-balanced Mueller–Hinton agar plate (MAST, UK) and left to dry completely. Antibiotic discs from a D52C ESBL detection kit (MAST, UK) were applied onto the plate and the setup was incubated at 37 °C for 18 h. Discs used were cefpodoxime (10 μg), ceftazidime (30 μg), cefotaxime (30 μg) and combination discs of cefotaxime/clavulanate (30/10 μg) and ceftazidime/clavulanate (30/10 μg). After incubation, inhibition zone diameters were measured and interpreted. A zone difference of ≥5 mm between the single and the combination disks for any of the antibiotics was regarded positive for ESBL production. *Klebsiella pneumoniae* ATCC 700603 was used as positive control for ESBL production.

Assessment of antibiotics for ESBL phenotyping

The diagnostic performance of each antibiotic used for ESBL phenotyping was assessed on the following criteria: sensitivity, specificity, positive predictive value (PPV) and negative predictive value (NPV).

Conjugation study

Only isolates confirmed as ESBL-producers were included in subsequent experiments. Conjugations were done using nalidixic acid^R *E. coli* K-12 as the recipient strain. Three of the study isolates that had shown resistance to nalidixic acid were excluded from this stage of the study. Donor isolates were grown in LB-ampicillin (60 μg/ml) broth overnight. An aliquot of a pure stock of the recipient strain was also grown overnight in LB broth but with no antibiotic. For conjugation, aliquots of each donor and the recipient (1 ml each) were transferred into fresh LB broth and incubated for 2 h. Volumes of 500 μl of each donor culture were each taken and mixed with an equal volume of the recipient culture. The mixed cultures were incubated for 6 h at 37 °C. Selection for transconjugants was carried out on MacConkey agar (MAST, UK) supplemented with 32 μg/ml nalidixic acid and 100 μg/ml ampicillin [16]. Transconjugants were confirmed for ESBL production as previously described.

Plasmid DNA extraction

Plasmid DNA was extracted from both ESBL-producing donor isolates and transconjugants according to previously described methods [18, 19]. For electrophoresis, 10 μl of each extract was mixed with 2 μl of 6X gel loading dye and electrophoresed on 0.7 % agarose gel stained with ethidium bromide (1 μg/ml). Electrophoresis was carried out in 1X Tris–acetate-EDTA (TAE) buffer at 10 V/cm for 1 h and visualized under UV transillumination [20]. The plasmid DNA samples obtained were used in subsequent PCRs.

Total DNA extraction

Total DNA was also extracted from ESBL-producing donor isolates according to the method described by [21]. The DNA samples obtained by this procedure were used in subsequent PCR procedures.

PCR for ESBL Genes

PCR amplifications of bla_{TEM}, bla_{SHV} and $bla_{CTX\text{-}M}$ genes were performed in 25 μl reaction mixes containing

25 units/ml of *Taq* DNA polymerase, 200 µM each of dATP, dGTP, dTTP and dCTP, 0.2 µM of each primer, 1.5 mM $MgCl_2$ and 5 µl of plasmid or total DNA template. Amplifications were carried out with the following thermal cycling profile: initial denaturation for 10 min at 94 °C followed by 35 cycles of amplification consisting of 30 s at 94 °C, 1 min at the appropriate annealing temperature for the specific primer and 1 min at 72 °C for primer extension, and then 10 min at 72 °C for the final extension with a soaking step at 4 °C.

In cases where reamplifications of the previous PCR product were necessary, the reagent concentrations were modified to use only half the primer concentration used in the previous reaction and 1.0 µl of the previous product as template. Primers used and their corresponding annealing temperatures are shown in Table 1. For electrophoresis, 10 µl of each PCR product were prepared and run as already described.

Results

A total of 137 clinical isolates belonging to *E. coli*, *Klebsiella* spp., *Citrobacter* spp., *Enterobacter* spp. and *Proteus* spp. were collected for this study. Table 2 shows the species distribution and clinical specimens from which isolates were recovered.

Detection of ESBL-producing isolates

Figure 1 shows the setup for the disc diffusion assays for ESBL phenotype detection. Sensitivity values were 100 % for cefpodoxime (CPD), 100 % for cefotaxime (CTX) and 97.06 % for ceftazidime (CAZ). Cefpodoxime had highest specificity of 95.24 %, followed by CTX (94.64 %) and CAZ (92.98 %). Similarly, CPD recorded the highest PPD (92.98 %), then CTX (93.02 %) and CAZ (89.19 %).

Table 1 Sequences, annealing temperatures and expected product sizes of primer sequences targeting the specified ESBL genes

Gene	Primer	Annealing temp. (°C)	Expected product size (bp)
bla$_{TEM}$	*f*: 5′-AAA CGC TGG TGA AAG TA-3′ *r*: 5′-AGC GAT CTG TCT AT-3′	45	720
bla$_{SHV}$	*f*: 5′-ATG CGT TAT ATT CGC CTG TG-3′ *r*: 5′-TGC TTT GTT ATT CGG GCC AA-3′	60	726
bla$_{CTX-M}$	*f*: 5′-GAC GAT GTC ACT GGC TGA GC-3′ *r*: 5′-AGC CGC CGA CGC TAA TAC A-3′	55	499

Sources Bonomo et al. [22] (*bla*$_{TEM}$), Hanson et al. [23] (*bla*$_{CTX-M}$), Bonomo et al. [24] (*bla*$_{SHV}$)

For NPV, CPD and CTX showed 100 %. Inhibition-zone size differences for *Klebsiella* spp. and *E. coli* isolates for all three antibiotics are presented in Fig. 2. Overall, 52 (37.96 %) of the 132 isolates included in this study expressed ESBLs (Table 3). The ESBL phenotype was most predominant in *Enterobacter* spp. (62.5 %) followed by *Citrobacter* spp. (60 %). Meanwhile, *Klebsiella* species comprised the majority of ESBL-producing isolates (42.3 %). Table 4 shows distribution of ESBL-producing isolates across clinical samples.

Conjugation studies

Results from the conjugation study indicated 64 % overall conjugability of ESBL genes amongst the ESBL-producing isolates (Table 5).

ESBL genotyping

The TEM gene was found in 25 (19.6 %) of the 127 isolates with ESBL-producing phenotype. None of the ESBL-positive isolates had SHV- or CTX-M-type genes (Fig. 3). Of the 25 strains with TEM-type genes, 12 (48 %) transferred their ESBL phenotype in conjugation assays (Table 6). In 24 (0.96 %) of the 25 TEM-gene positive strains, the gene was detected in both plasmid and total-DNA extracts.

Discussion

Over the last decade, many studies have demonstrated the presence of ESBL-mediated resistance in bacteria causing infections in patients [25–28]. Despite several reports of ESBL presence in Ghana, the characterization of ESBL genotypes in relation to chromosomal or plasmid locations—and their transferability by conjugation—are not described.

ESBLs in study isolates

The study revealed a moderate [37.96 % (n = 52/137)] prevalence of ESBL phenotype among the study isolates. In Table 3, the column for those that were not confirmed positive included all the bacteria that failed the screening tests as well as those that may have passed a screening test but failed all three confirmatory tests. The ESBL-producing isolates were found among every genus tested.

Two observations merit attention. First, the level of ESBLs is comparable to that reported by other ESBL-affected institutions in Ghana [29, 30] but higher than figures reported in many other reviews spanning across several regions [25–27]. In the African context however, the situation in KBTH appears to be rather moderate [13, 14, 30]. If current trends of lack of routine ESBL-monitoring and lack of ESBL-control strategies continue however, it can be expected that the prevalence will rapidly increase. This will lead to increased treatment expenses,

Table 2 Distribution of study isolates according to clinical sources

Isolate	Clinical source						Number of species	
	Urine	Blood	Sputum	CSF	HVS	Other[a]	Total	%
Citrobacter spp.	2	1	6	0	1	0	10	7.3
Enterobacter spp.	2	5	1	0	0	0	8	5.8
Escherichia coli	42	9	7	1	3	7	69	50.4
Klebsiella spp.	23	6	8	0	4	3	44	32.1
Proteus spp.	1	0	4	0	1	0	6	4.4
Total	70 (51.1 %)	21 (15.3 %)	26 (19.0 %)	1 (0.7 %)	9 (6.6 %)	10 (7.3 %)	137	100

Though only one instance of infection was observed from three CSF samples tested, it was separated due to the clinical significance of infection in the normally sterile cerebrospinal region

CSF cerebrospinal fluid, *HVS* high vaginal swab

[a] Refers to miscellaneous clinical sources (wound swabs, pus, aspirates, ear swabs)

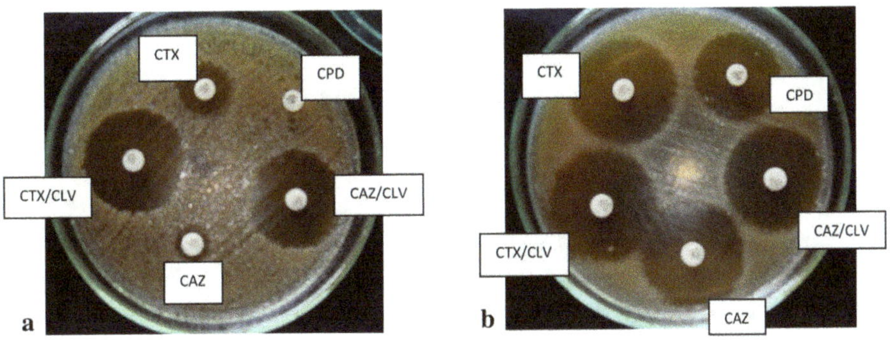

Fig. 1 Appearance after over-night incubation for ESBL phenotyping of (**a**) an ESBL-positive strain and **b** an ESBL-negative strain. *Plate* **a** shows an example of what was taken as a positive ESBL test result. *Plate* **b** shows an example of a negative ESBL test result. In both cases, cefpodoxime was used only to screen and not in confirmation. Cefotaxime and ceftazidime were used in both screening and confirmation. *CPD* cefpodoxime 10 µg, *CPD/CLV* cefpodoxime 10 µg + clavulanate 10 µg, *CTX* cefotaxime 30 µg, *CTX/CLV* cefotaxime 30 µg + clavulanate 10 µg, *CAZ* ceftazidime 30 µg, *CAZ/CLV* ceftazidime 30 µg + clavulanate 10 µg

longer hospital stays and possibly, mortality. Second, our results point to ESBL-producing isolates as being present among various members of the family *Enterobacteriaceae* and not just *Escherichia coli* and *Klebsiella* spp. In contrast to the attention paid mostly to ESBLs in *Escherichia coli* and *Klebsiella* spp. [25–28], the study showed that although a minority of the isolates were non-*Escherichia coli* and non-*Klebsiella* species, >40 % of these were ESBL-producers.

It is also noteworthy that ESBL detection was considerably high among *Citrobacter freundii* (>50 %) and *Enterobacter cloacae* (>60 %). Though only six *Proteus* spp. isolates were included in the study, their producer prevalence of 16.7 % cannot be over-looked. Therefore, the practice of not investigating ESBL presence in these pathogens may have an adverse impact on patients who are treated with extended-spectrum cephalosporins. With their hypermotility and ability to easily dominate biofilms, ESBL-producing *Proteus* spp. is a very uncomfortable prospect.

ESBL-producing strains appeared to be most common amongst isolates cultured from urine samples. Considering the fact that some bacteria will certainly be expelled in situ when urine is excreted, this has rather significant implications for risk of environmental contamination and cross-infections.

Performance of detection agents

Extent of reliability of phenotypic screening and confirmatory agents is needed to confidently rule out isolates that do not pass screening and/or confirmatory tests. Both cefpodoxime and cefotaxime had 100 % sensitivity scores and 100 % negative predictive value (NPV) scores. After comparing specificity and positive predictive value (PPV) scores however, it was evident that cefotaxime had a lesser likelihood of refusing a possible-positive than cefpodxime. It is generally accepted that cefpodoxime is the best single agent for ESBL detection [31]. From these results however, cefotaxime, with its slightly lower

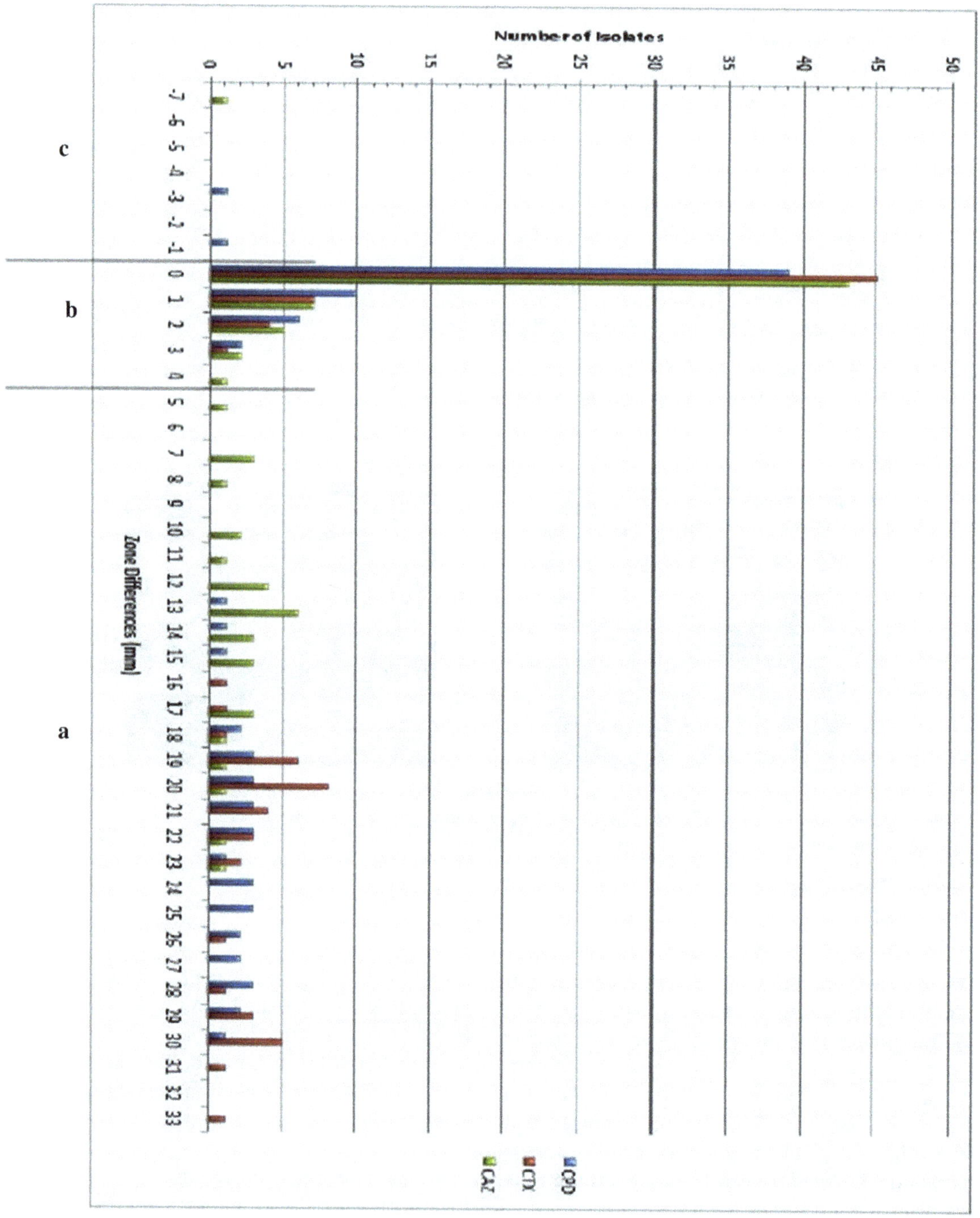

Fig. 2 Inhibition zone chart for *Klebsiella* spp. and *E. coli* isolates. Zone differences observed between screening and confirmatory tests using each of the screening antibiotics alone and in its appropriate combination with clavulanate for confirmation. *CPD* cefpodoxime, *CTX* cefotaxime, *CAZ* ceftazidime. *Region* **a** zone differences for ESBL-positive phenotype. *Region* **b** zone-differences for ESBL-negative phenotype. *Region* (**c**) unusual zone differences

specificity score but higher positive predictive value score, performed just as well as, if not better than, cefpodoxime. Data of this nature are very important since for a given study involving large numbers of samples, one cannot screen all collected isolates by genotypic methods which are the gold standard in ESBL detection.

Unusual inhibition zone patterns should however be treated on a case-by-case basis.

Table 3 ESBL prevalence amongst study isolates

Isolate	Not confirmed ESBL-positive[a]	ESBL prevalence	
		Confirmed ESBL-positive	% of overall prevalence
Citrobacter spp.	4	6 (60 %)	11.5
Enterobacter spp.	3	5 (62.5 %)	9.6
Escherichia coli	51	18 (26.1 %)	34.6
Klebsiella spp.	22	22 (50.0 %)	42.3
Proteus spp.	5	1 (16.7 %)	1.9
Total	85	52 (37.9 %)	100

ESBL prevalence was determined using MAST D52C combined discs by the Kirby-Bauer method of antibiotic susceptibility testing

[a] The column for "not confirmed ESBL-positive" includes isolates that failed screening tests as well as those isolates that may have passed the screening test(s) but failed confirmatory tests

Table 4 Distribution of ESBL-producing strains according to clinical sources

Clinical source	Sample size	ESBL phenotype present	
		Number	% of total number of ESBL-producers
Urine	70	31 (44.3 %)	59.6
Blood	21	9 (42.9 %)	17.3
CSF	1	0 (0)	0
HVS	9	3 (33.3 %)	5.8
Sputum	26	5 (19.2 %)	9.6
Other[a]	10	4 (40 %)	7.7
Total	137	52	100

HVS high vaginal swab, *CSF* cerebrospinal fluid

[a] Refers to miscellaneous clinical sources (wound swabs, pus, aspirates, and ear swabs)

Table 5 Conjugabilities of ESBL-producer phenotype from isolates confirmed for ESBL production

Donor isolate	Total	Conjugation successful	Percent conjugability (%)
Klebsiella pneumoniae	22	19	86.4
Escherichia coli	18	9	50.0
Enterobacter spp.	5	2	40.0
Citrobacter spp.	4	1	25.0
Proteus spp.	1	1	100
Total	50	32	64

ESBL-positive study isolates were conjugated to nalidixic acid-resistant *E. coli* K-12. Selection of transconjugants was done on MacConkey agar (MAST, UK) supplemented with ampicillin and nalidixic acid

Inferences from inhibition zones

Comparing the cefpodoxime zone size differences represented in Fig. 2 to data from the British society for antimicrobial chemotherapy [32], certain implications were realised. It was seen that the patterns of size differences represented in both figures were quite different. In the reference data, zone differences of the majority of ESBL-producer isolates fell between the ranges of 6–26 mm whereas from this study, zone differences fell between 13–30 mm with the majority ranging from 18 to 30 mm. The relatively higher zone sizes realized from this data may be indicative of differences in plasmid copy numbers and activity profiles of the enzymes as well as differences in permeability characteristics of the isolates from the two different localities.

Two *Klebsiella* isolates had cefpodoxime zone size differences that were in the negatives; −1 and −3 (Fig. 2). The lack of synergistic effect with the addition of clavulanate might suggest that they produce AmpC enzymes. However, they both tested screen-negative with each antibiotic used, uncharacteristic of AmpC-producing strains. Comparing to the reference data, those isolates were likely to produce K1 β-lactamases. The K1 enzymes are a family of β-lactamses, encoded by chromosomal genes, and which are presently thought to be unique to *Klebsiella oxytoca*. The two isolates however had corresponding ceftazidime zone-size differences of −7 and 1 mm. This implies that any K1 presence in them is unlikely since ceftazidime is notably susceptible to K1 enzymes. Also, the activity of K1 enzymes on ceftazidime is greatly diminished with the addition of clavulanate [33, 34]. Both isolates were amongst those most susceptible to the screening agents used, including ceftazidime, but were obviously not affected by clavulanate synergy. Currently, the only β-lactamase class that fits this profile of decreased affinity for β-lactam substrates and non-inhibition by clavulanate is the mutants of the inhibitor-resistant TEMs (IRTs) which belong to class A, subgroup 2br. The 2br subgroup contains the inhibitor-resistant TEM-type enzymes that evolved from the classical TEMs by acquiring the substitutions M69 V and N276D [29]. Derivatives of these enzymes are the complex TEM mutants (CTMs) that combine inhibitor-resistance with decreased affinity for cephalosporins [35].

A few isolates (4 for cefpodoxime, 3 for cefotaxime and 5 for ceftazidime) were screen-positive but failed the confirmatory tests, with 2 strains common to cefpodoxime and cefotaxime and 1 strain being common to all three antibiotics. This kind of phenotype, though typical of ampC-producers, may also be expressed by strains with CTMs, high levels of the TEM-1 enzyme and OXA-type ESBLs.

An interesting observation was one *Klebsiella* isolate which was clearly screen-positive with cefpodoxime, tested screen-negative for ceftazidime but was affected by clavulanate synergy with ceftazidime. Screening by

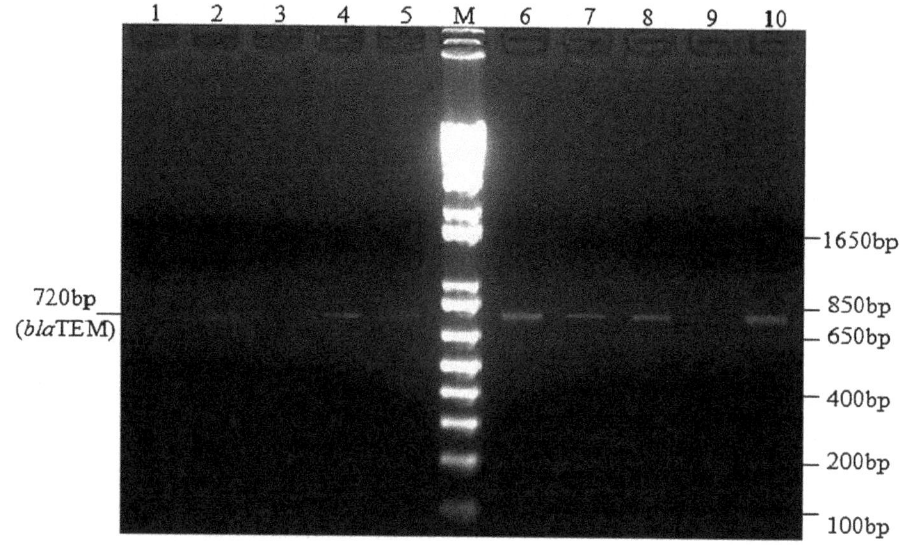

Fig. 3 Bands observed after reamplification of previous PCR product with the TEM family-specific primers. PCR products were resolved on 2 % agarose gel stained with 1 μg/ml ethidium bromide at 100 V for 30 min. The gel was photographed under UV illumination. *Lane M* 1 kb plus DNA ladder, *Lanes 2, 4, 5, 7, 8, 10* PCR product from showing amplified *TEM* gene with band position at 720 bp, *Lane 6* TEM-3-producing *E. coli* NCTC 13351, *Lanes 1, 3, 9* PCR product with no amplification

Table 6 Numbers of detected conjugative TEM genes

Isolate	TEM	Number that had transferred by conjugation
Citrobacter spp.	0	0
Enterobacter spp.	1	0
Escherichia coli	11	3
Klebsiella spp.	12	8
Proteus spp.	1	1

The TEM primer produced PCR amplification product in DNA extracts from 25 of the ESBL-positive isolates. Verification of which of these genes had been transferred by conjugation was obtained by comparing this data to results of PCR on plasmid-DNA extracts from the transconjugants

ceftazidime alone would have led to the isolate being ruled as an ESBL non-producing strain. However, the observed synergy upon addition of clavulanate suggests, besides the possibility of AmpC-production, the presence of other β-lactamase types that are susceptible to the inhibitor.

It is seen from Fig. 2 that from 5 to 15 mm in region (a), inhibition of cefotaxime hydrolysis by clavulanate is not shown. This is a likely indication of the presence of CTX-M enzymes which preferentially hydrolyse cefotaxime relative to cefpodoxime and ceftazidime. Like all other ESBLs, CTX-M enzymes are susceptible to inhibition by clavulanate. The effect of clavulanate synergy with cefpodoxime and ceftazidime is seen but since CTX-M's normally hydrolyse these with relatively lower turn-over rates, the zone size differences there are not as large as for cefotaxime which the enzymes would hydrolyse with greater efficiency in the absence of clavulanate.

Conjugation study

In the present study, about 63 % conjugability was observed, higher than the 38.7 % reported in Cameroon by [36]. In contrast to the report by [37] where *E. coli* showed higher ESBL conjugability than *Klebsiella* spp., *Klebsiella* had the highest rate of 86.4 % followed by *E. coli's* 50 % (Table 5). This pattern of results may stem from the fact that *Klebsiellae* have been found to frequently harbor plasmids bearing bla_{SHV} -type genes, and considering the usual sizes of bla_{TEM}—(less than 80 kb) and bla_{SHV}—(from about 80 kb to up to 350 kb in some *Klebsiella* isolates) bearing plasmids, the latter are probably more likely to be conjugable.

DNA extraction and PCR

All isolates positive for ESBL-production were selected for DNA extraction. Attempts at linearization of plasmids using *Pst*I, *Hind*III and *Eco*RI restriction enzymes always failed. A plasmid which consistently appeared in the 22 kb position (data not shown) was found to be present in some of the plasmid extracts in which TEM genes were detected. Further resolution of the 22 kb band showed that it consisted of two clearly distinct bands placed closely together. All the plasmid extracts had the lower band. Plasmid preparations from a few of the transconjugants showed only the lower band, suggesting that the higher band may have been a non-conjugable plasmid species.

DNA extracted by a Promega Plus SV Miniprep DNA kit and [20] were used for PCR with *bla*TEM, *bla*SHV and *bla*CTX-M primers. Initial PCR rounds on control isolates showed amplification products for *bla*TEM but none for *bla*SHV and *bla*CTX-M positive controls (data not shown). Generally, the bla_{TEM} products required re-amplification to be clearly visible (Fig. 3). A total DNA extract belonging to an *Enterobacter* spp. isolate produced amplification product but nothing was observed with its corresponding plasmid extract. This suggested that the detected gene may have been chromosomal. With the *Klebsiella* spp. and *E. coli* isolates that produced amplicons with both DNA extracts, there is at least a plasmid-borne bla_{TEM} gene present even if there may be others that are chromosomal. Particularly with the *Proteus* spp. DNA sample, the detection made with the total-DNA extract was notably very faint relative to that from its plasmid extract. Due to the fact that any plasmid template present would be very dilute in the total-DNA preparation, this strongly suggested again that the gene detected by PCR may have been plasmid-borne in the *Proteus* isolate.

Plasmid mediation and conjugability

TEM-producing isolates that did not have the 22 kb plasmid included 2 *E. coli*, 1 *Enterobacter* and 1 *Proteus* isolate. This may have been a TEM-bearing plasmid since it was common to 84 % of the isolates in which TEM was detected. Judging from its size however, it was unlikely to be conjugative and this had been demonstrated by its absence in the plasmid extracts from the transconjugants. It was unlikely also to be mobilisable since it was not observed in any of the transconjugants tested. [38] has however previously reported the successful conjugation of a 10 kb ESBL-associated resistance determinant. The *Proteus* isolate had transferred its phenotype during the conjugation study (Table 6), suggesting that the gene it carried was on a mobilisable plasmid. The proportion of ESBL conjugability reported here also suggests that precautions should be taken to minimise the possibility of horizontal transfer of ESBL genes as well as clonal spread as reported by [39].

Conclusions

Detection level of ESBL-producing strains amongst the isolates studied was 37.96 % (n = 137). It is important that subsequent work carried out on ESBL-producing strains should take ampC β-lactamase detection as well as influence from other types of β-lactamases that may be present into account. This is because as more and more isolates begin to concomitantly produce these enzymes, interactions between them will make antibiograms of the isolates rather difficult to interpret. In the majority of cases, ESBL-producing bacteria in the hospital could transfer the phenotype by conjugation. Interpretative reading of the inhibition-zone chart suggests that other types of β-lactamases such as inhibitor-resistant TEMs (IRTs) and ampCs might have been present amongst the isolates. These need to be investigated.

Abbreviations

AmpC: ampicillin-hydrolyzing cephalosporinase; bla: beta-lactamase gene; ESBL: extended spectrum β-lactamase; M: methionine; V: valine; N: asparagine; D: aspartate.

Authors' contributions

DO-M, NO-N and EYB carried out the laboratory work for the study. KT-D supervised the microbiological aspects of laboratory work. YDO and STS supervised the laboratory work in molecular biology. DO-M, EO-M and STS prepared the manuscript. EO-M and NO-N reviewed the manuscript. All authors read and approved the final manuscript.

Author details

[1] Department of Biochemistry, Cell and Molecular Biology, School of Biological Sciences, University of Ghana, Legon, Accra, Ghana. [2] Department of Microbiology, University of Ghana Medical School, Korle-Bu, Accra, Ghana. [3] Department of Virology, Noguchi Memorial Institute for Medical Research, University of Ghana, Legon, Accra, Ghana. [4] Adabraka Polyclinic, Ghana Health Service, Accra, Ghana. [5] Department of Applied Chemistry and Biochemistry, University for Development Studies, Navrongo Campus, Navrongo, Ghana.

Acknowledgements

The authors are grateful to the Virology Department of Noguchi Memorial Instiitute for Medical Research and the technicians of the Microbiology Unit, Central Laboratory, Korle-Bu Teaching Hospital for the use of their facilities and for their assistance in various ways.

Competing interests

The authors declare that they have no competing interests.

References

1. Kocsis B. Antibiotic resistance mechanisms in *Enterobacteriaceae*. In: Mendez-Vilas A, editor. Microbial pathogens and strategies for combating them: science, technology and education. Badajoz: Formatex; 2013. p. 251–7.
2. Rossolini GM, Mantengoli E, Docquier J-D, Musmanno RA, Coratza G. Epidemiology of infections caused by multiresistant Gram-negatives: ESBLs, MBLs, panresistant strains. New Microbiol. 2007;30:332–9.
3. Shaikh S, Fatima J, Shakil S, Mohd S, Rizvi D, Kamal MA. Antibiotic resistance and extended spectrum beta-lactamases: Types, epidemiology and treatment. Saudi J Biol Sci. 2015;22(1):90–101.
4. Jacoby GA, Munoz-Price LS. Mechanisms of disease: the new β-lactamases. N Engl J Med. 2005;352:380–91.
5. Araj GF, Samaha-Kfoury JN. Recent developments in β-Lactamases and extended-spectrum β-lactamases. BMJ. 2003;327:1209–13.
6. Moya B, Beceiro A, Cabot G, Juan C, Zamorano L, Alberti S, Oliver A. Pan-beta-lactam resistance development in *Pseudomonas aeruginosa* clinical srains: molecular mechanisms, penicillin-binding protein profiles and binding affinities. Antimicrob Agents Chemother. 2012;56(9):4771–8.
7. Elliot E, Brink AJ, van Greune J, Els Z, Woodford N, Turton J, Warner M, Livermore DM. *In vivo* development of ertapenem resistance in a patient with pneumonia caused by *Klebsiella peneumoniae* with an extended-spectrum beta-lactamase. Clin Infect Dis. 2006;42(11):e95–8.
8. Bayer AS, Peters J, Parr TR, Chan L, Hancock RE. Role of beta-lactamase in in vivo development of ceftazidime resistance in experimental

Pseudomonas aeruginosa endocarditis. Antimicrob Agents Cemother. 1987;31(2):253–8.

9. Bush K. New β-Lactamases in Gram-negative bacteria: diversity and impact on the selection of antimicrobial therapy. Clin Infect Dis. 2001;32:1085–9.
10. Bradford P, Cherubin CE, Idemyor V. Multiply resistant *Klebsiella pneumoniae* from two Chicago hospitals: identification of the extended spectrum TEM-12 and TEM-10 ceftazidime-hydrolyzing β-lactamases in a single isolate. Antimicrob Agents Chemother. 1994;38:761–6.
11. Obeng-Nkrumah N, Twum-Danso K, Krogfelt KA, Newman MJ. High levels of extended-spectrum beta-lactamases in a major teaching hospital in Ghana: the need for regular monitoring and evaluation of antibiotic resistance. Am J Trop Med Hyg. 2013;89(5):960–4.
12. Fegloa P, Adu-Sarkodie Y, Jain R, Spurbeck RR, Springman AC, Englebergb NC, Newton DW, Xi C, Walk ST. Emergence of a Novel Extended-Spectrum-β-Lactamase (ESBL)-producing, fluoroquinolone-resistant clone of extraintestinal pathogenic *Escherichia coli* in Kumasi, Ghana. J Clin Microbiol. 2014;51(2):728–30.
13. Maningi NE, Ehlers MM, Hoosen AA, Makgothlo E, Omar S, Kock MM. Prevalence of ESBL and MBL antibiotic resistance genes in *Klebsiella pneumoniae* in pretoria academic hospital. Health sciences faculty day posters. 2008. http://hdl.handle.net/2263/8293. Accessed on 10 Nov 2015.
14. Iroha RI, Oji AE, Afiukwa TN, Nwuzo AC, Ejikeugwu PC. Extended spectrum β-lactamase (ESBL) mediated resistance to antibiotics among *Klebsiella pneumoniae* in Enugu metropolis. Macedonian J. Med. Sci. 2009;2(3):196–9.
15. Blomberg B, Jureen R, Manji KP, Tamim BS, Mwakagile DSM, Urassa WK, Fataki M, Msangi V, Tellevik MG, Maselle SY, Langeland N. High rate of fatal cases of pediatric septicemia caused by gram-negative bacteria with extended-spectrum β-lactamases in Dar es Salaam. Tanzania J Clin Microbiol. 2005;43:745–9.
16. Kariuki S, Corkill JE, Revathi G, Musoke R, Hart CA. Molecular characterization of a novel plasmid-encoded cefotaximase (CTXM-12) found in clinical *Klebsiella pneumoniae* isolates from Kenya. Antimicrob Agents Chemother. 2001;45:2141–3.
17. Cowan ST, Steel KJ. Characteristics of gram negative bacteria. In: Barrow GI, Feltham RKA, editors. Cowan's and Steel's manual for identification of medical bacteria. London: Cambridge University Press; 1993. p. 94–150.
18. Birnboim HC, Doly J. A rapid alkaline extraction procedure for screening recombinant plasmid DNA. Nucl Acid Res. 1979;7(6):1513–23.
19. Takahashi S, Nagano Y. Rapid procedure for isolation of plasmid DNA and application to epidemiological analysis. J Clin Microbiol. 1984;20(4):608–13.
20. Maniatis T, Fritsch EF, Sambrook J. Molecular cloning: a laboratory manual. New York: Cold Spring Harbor Laboratory Press; 1982.
21. Ruiz-Barba JL, Maldonado A, Jimenez-Diaz R. Small-scale total DNA extraction from bacteria and yeast for PCR applications. J Anal Biochem. 2005;347:333–5.
22. Bonomo RA, Paterson DL, Jacobs MR, Ewell AJ, Fishbain JT, Craft DW, Rather PN, Thomson JD, Sampath R, Eshoo MW, Massire C, Ecker DJ, Donskey CJ, Adams JM, Bajaksouzain S, Hulten EA, Hujer AM, Hujer KM. Multi-drug resistant Acinetobacter spp. isolates from military and civilian patients treated at the Walter Reed Army Medical Center: analysis of antibiotic resistance genes. Antimicrob Agents Chemother. 2006;50(12):4114–23.
23. Hanson, ND, Hossain A and Pitout JDD. Phenotypic and molecular detection of CTX-M-β-lactamases produced by *Escherichia coli* and *Klebsiella* spp. J Clin Microbiol. 2004;42(12):5715–21.
24. Bonomo RA, Paterson DL, Yeiser B, Hujer KM, Hujer AM, Bonomo MD, Rice LB; International Klebsiella Study Group. Extended-spectrum β-lactamases in Klebsiella pneumonia bloodstream isolates from seven countries: dominance and widespread prevalence of SHV- and CTX-M-type β-lactamases. Antimicrob Agents Chemother. 2003;47(11):3554–60.
25. Tansarli GS, Poulikakos P, Kapaskelis A, Falagas ME. Proportion of extended-spectrum β-lactamase (ESBL)-producing isolates among Enterobacteriaceae in Africa: evaluation of the evidence-systematic review. J Antimicrob Chemother. 2014;69:1177–84.
26. Hoban DJ, Lascols C, Nicolle LE, Badal R, Bouchillon S, Hackel M, Hawser S. Antimicrobial susceptibility of enterobacteriaceae, including molecular characterization of extended-spectrum beta-lactamase-producing species, in urinary tract isolates from hospitalized patients in North America and Europe: results from the SMART study. Diagn Microbiol Infect Dis. 2012;74:62–7.
27. Sharma M, Pathak S, Srivastava P. Prevalence and antibiogram of extended spectrum β-lactamase (ESBL) producing Gram negative bacilli and further molecular characterization of ESBL producing *Escherichia coli* and *Klebsiella* spp. J Clin Diagn Res. 2013;7:2173–7.
28. Cantón R, Novais A, Valverde A, Machado E, Peixe L, Baquero F, Coque TM. Prevalence and spread of extended-spectrum beta-lactamase-producing enterobacteriaceae in Europe. Clin Microbiol Infect. 2008;4(Suppl 1):144–53.
29. Hackman HK, Brown C, Twum-Danso K. Antibiotic Resistance Profile of Non-Extended Spectrum Beta-Lactamase-producing *Escherichia coli* and *Klebsiella pneumoniae* in Accra, Ghana. J Biol Agric Healthc. 2014;4:12–6.
30. Aibinu IE, Ogunsola FT, Ohaegbulam VC, Adenipekun EA, Odugbemi TO, Mee BJ. Extended-spectrum β-lactamase enzymes in clinical isolates of *Enterobacter* species from Lagos, Nigeria. J Clin Microbiol. 2003;41(5):2197–8.
31. Jacoby GA, Walsh KE, Walker VJ. Identification of extended-spectrum, ampC and carbapenem-hydrolyzing β-Lactamases in *Escherichia coli* and *Klebsiella pneumoniae* by Disk Tests. J Clin Microbiol. 2006;44(6):1971–6.
32. Livermore DM. Detection of ESBLs and AmpC. The british society for antimicrobial chemotherapy. 2008. www.bsac.org.uk/wp-content/uploads/.../Detecting_AmpC__ESBL_pruned.ppt. Accessed 28 June 2014.
33. Livermore DM, Hall LMC, Yuan M, Gheorghui R. Bases of variation in resistance to β-lactams in *Klebsiella oxytoca* isolates hyperproducing K1 β-lactamase. J Antimicrob Chemother. 1997;40:533–41.
34. Livermore DM. Determinants of the activity of β-lactamase inhibitor combinations. J Antimicrob Chemother. 1993;31(Suppl A):9–21.
35. Robin F, Delmas J, Schweitzer C, Tournilhac O, Lesens O, Chanal C, Bonnet R. Evolution of TEM-type enzymes: biochemical and genetic characterization of two new complex mutant TEM enzymes, TEM-151 and TEM-152, from a single patient. Antimicrob Agents Chemother. 2007;51(4):1304–9.
36. Gangoue-Pieboji J, Bedenic B, Koulla-Shiro S, Randegger C, Adiogo D, Ngassam P, Ndumbe P, Hachler H. Extended-spectrum beta-lcatamase-producing *Enterobacteriaceae* in Yaounde. J Clin Microbiol. 2005;43(7):3273–7.
37. Rao SPN, Rama PS, Gurushanthappa V, Manipura R, Srinivasan K. Extended-spectrum beta-lactamase producing *Escherichia coli* and *Klebsiella pneumoiae*: a multi-centric study across Karnataka. J Lab Physicians. 2014;6(1):7–13.
38. AitMhanda R, Soukrib A, Moustaouia N, Amarouchb H, Elmdaghria N, Sirotc D, Benbachira M. Plasmid-mediated TEM-3 extended-spectrum beta-lactamase production in Salmonella typhimurium in Casablanca. J Antimicrob Chemother. 2002;49(1):169–72.
39. Agyekum A, Fajardo-Lubiána A, Ansong D, Partridge SR, Agbenyega T, Iredell JR. *bla*CTX-M-15 carried by IncF-type plasmids is the dominant ESBL gene in *Escherichia coli* and *Klebsiella pneumoniae* at a hospital in Ghana. Diagn Microbiol Infect Dis. 2015;. doi:10.1016/j.diagmicrobio.2015.12.010.

11

Phenotypic and molecular characterization of clinical isolates of *Acinetobacter baumannii* isolated from Delhi, India

Dabet Rynga[1,3], Malini Shariff[1*] and Monorama Deb[2]

Abstract

Background: Acinetobacter has gained importance as a multi-drug resistant and hence a difficult to treat pathogen. This study was done to characterize our isolates with respect to drug resistance and presence of beta-lactamases which is a major mechanism of resistance and to type using RAPD and MLST so that comparison of our clones can be made with the existing international clones.

Methods: 100 isolates recovered from clinical samples from two hospitals in Delhi were tested for their susceptibility against major groups of antimicrobials. The resistant isolates were screened and confirmed phenotypically for presence of ESBL, MBL and AmpC and MBLs also by PCR. The isolates were typed by RAPD and MLST.

Results: Out of the 100 isolates, 91, 78 and 2 % were MDR, XDR and PDR respectively. 97, 100 and 85 were screen positive for ESBL, AmpC and MBL respectively. Of these, 38.1 % were confirmed phenotypically to produce ESBL, 99 % produced AmpC and 29.4 % produced MBL comprising of GIM, VIM, SIM and IMP. MLST showed known STs 110, 188, 146, 69, 103, 108 and 194. Eight new STs were encountered. The RAPD showed a high degree of genetic variability among the isolates.

Conclusion: Majority of our isolates were MDR, producing one or more types of beta-lactamases. We encountered drug resistant international clones by MLST which are found in other continents there by confirming their spread to Indian sub continent. No data on ST types of other Indian isolates is available in the MLST database and hence comparison is not possible.

Keywords: *Acinetobacter baumannii*, Molecular characterization, MLST, RAPD, Beta-lactamases

Background

Acinetobacter species, once considered as opportunistic, low virulence pathogens have now emerged as important nosocomial pathogens due to their increase in antimicrobial resistance. The resistance is due to various mechanisms including production of different types of beta-lactamases including oxacillinases. They are responsible for a number of hospital acquired infections. To control the spread of *Acinetobacter baumannii* (*A. baumannii*) in the hospital, it is necessary to distinguish the outbreak strain from epidemiologically unrelated *Acinetobacter*. This requires the comparison of isolates at the subspecies level which is done by epidemiological typing methods. Phenotypic typing systems based on biochemical profiles (biotyping), antibiotic susceptibility patterns, serological reactions (serotyping), phage typing and protein profiles have mostly been replaced by molecular typing systems like ribotyping, Pulsed-field gel electrophoresis (PFGE), Amplified fragment length polymorphisim (AFLP) analysis, Random amplification of polymorphic DNA (RAPD) and many more. PFGE is

*Correspondence: malini.shariff@gmail.com
[1] Department of Microbiology, Vallabhbhai Patel Chest Institute, University of Delhi, Delhi 110007, India
Full list of author information is available at the end of the article

more sensitive in analysis of *Acinetobacter* epidemiology but it is cumbersome as well as expensive, so RAPD is preferred. However, reproducibility and inter-laboratory exchange of data for global epidemiological analysis have been problematic which is solved by MLST by offering the possibility to transfer typing data from laboratory to laboratory or compare results via the internet [1].

The present study was undertaken to identify and characterize clinical isolates of *A. baumannii* with reference to its antibiotic susceptibility, presence of the different types of β-lactamases in the resistant isolates and molecular typing of the isolates using RAPD and MLST and compare them with international clones.

Methods

Institutional ethics committee clearance was taken before the start of the project. A total of one hundred (100) non repetitive isolates of *A. baumannii* were collected from various clinical specimens from patients attending two hospitals in New Delhi after taking patient's consent. The species identification of the isolates was done using the API 20NE strips (Biomerieux, Cat No. 20 050) and it was further confirmed using Amplified ribosomal DNA restriction analysis (ARDRA) [2, 3].

Susceptibility of the isolates to various antibiotics was tested by using the Kirby Bauer's Disk diffusion method. The antibiotics used included cefoxitin (30 μg), ceftazidime (30 μg), cefotaxime (30 μg), cefpodoxime (30 μg), aztreonam (30 μg), cefepime (30 μg), imipenem (10 μg), amikacin (30 μg), ciprofloxacin (30 μg), gentamicin (10 μg), ampicillin/sulbactam (20/10 μg), piperacillin/tazobactam (100/10 μg), tigecycline (15 μg) and colistin(10 μg) discs (Becton–Dickinson). The diameters of the zones of inhibition were recorded and interpreted as sensitive, intermediate sensitive or resistant, according to the CLSI guidelines 2013 [4] except colistin and tigecycline where in CLSI guidelines for *Acinetobacter* is not available. Keeping the breakpoints of ≤ 2 as sensitive and ≥ 4 as resistant [5] the zone sizes of colistin in disk diffusion test was taken as ≥ 11 as susceptible and ≤ 10 as resistant [6, authors unpublished data]. The interpretation for tigecycline was ≥ 16 mm as sensitive and ≤ 12 as resistant according to Jones et al. [7]. *A. baumannii* isolates were labelled as Multi-drug resistant (MDR) if the isolate was resistant to at least three classes of antimicrobial agents—all Penicillins and Cephalosporins (including inhibitor combinations), Fluroquinolones, and Aminoglycosides, Extensive drug resistant (XDR) when they were MDR and also resistant to Carbapenems and finally, Pan-drug resistant (PDR), those that are XDR and also resistant to polymyxins and tigecycline [8].

The isolates were screened for ESBL production by checking their susceptibility against ceftazidime, cefotaxime, cefpodoxime and aztreonam (each disk of 30 μg) and the screen positive isolates were confirmed phenotypically by the Modified combined disc test in which AmpC inhibitory substances, like cloxacillin (200 μg/ml) is added into the Mueller–Hinton Agar as the coexistence of AmpC β-lactamases along with ESBL have been shown to mask the production of ESBL. If the zone of inhibition around cefotaxime-clavulanate is larger than the zone around the cefotaxime disc then the isolate is ESBL positive [9].

Isolates resistant to imipenem and ceftazidime were further confirmed for MBL production by Combined disc test. An organism was considered to be MBL positive if there was an increase of ≥ 7 mm in the zone of inhibition around the imipenem + EDTA disc as compared to imipenem disc alone [10]. They were further confirmed for the presence of MBL genes, VIM, IMP, GIM, SPM and SIM, using multiplex PCR [11].

Similarly, isolates resistant to cefoxitin were confirmed phenotypically for the presence of AmpC β-lactamase by the AmpC disc test. Briefly, a lawn culture of cefoxitin sensitive *E.coli* (ATCC 25922) was prepared on Muller Hinton Agar plate and a cefoxitin disk (30 μg) was placed on it. A sterile plain disk was placed next (almost touching) to the cefoxitin disk, moistened with 20 μl of sterile saline and inoculated with several colonies of the test organism. A flattening or indentation of the cefoxitin inhibition zone in the vicinity of the inoculated disc was considered as a positive test [12].

Typing of the isolates was done using RAPD and MLST methods.

RAPD was performed by the method described by Karthika et al. 2009 [13]. Amplification was carried out in a final volume of 10 μl of the amplification mixture containing 1U of *Taq* Polymerase, 1X of PCR buffer (with MgCl2), 50 pmol of primer, 50 μM of deoxynucleotide triphosphate (dNTP) and 1 μl of DNA template. AP6 CCCGTCAGCA was used as a primer. 35 cycles of 94 °C for 30 s, 45 °C for 45 s, 72 °C for 2 min followed by a final extension 72 °C for 5 min. The PCR products were resolved using 1.2 % agarose gel. A low molecular weight DNA ladder (New England Biolabs Inc., Category no. N3233S) was used. The image of the gel was captured and the banding pattern was analyzed using Gelcompar II software (Applied-Maths, Kortrijk, Belgium) and the dendrogram was generated.

For MLST, seven housekeeping genes were amplified using the method described by Bartual et al., [14] with some modifications in the sequence of *gyrB* and *rpoD* primers as given by Park et al. [15]. The PCR products were resolved by 1 % agarose gel electrophoresis. Amplified fragments were sequenced by outsourcing to a commercial company. The sequences obtained were trimmed using the Bio Edit Sequence alignment editor software (Ibis Biosciences, Carlsbad, CA, USA). The assignment of alleles and sequence types was performed by the software available in the Department of Zoology, Oxford University website noted above. The sequence types not present in the database were submitted to the website and assigned new ST types.

Results

Out of the 100 isolates of *A. baumannii* 14 % were isolated from sputum, 31 % from ET aspirate, 28 % from pus, 25 % from wound swab, 1 % from drain fluid and 1 % from high vaginal swab. *A. baumannii* was isolated from ICU (28 %), followed by burns ward and respiratory medicine ward (15 % each), surgery ward (14 %) burns ICU (11 %) gynaecology ward (9 %), orthopaedics ward (5 %), respiratory medicine OPD (2 %). Respiratory samples were from patients suffering from exacerbation of Chronic obstructive pulmonary disease, Asthma, Chronic bronchitis and Ventilator associated pneumonia.

The results for detection of *A. baumannii* by ARDRA (using three enzymes) and API 20 NE strips were identical.

The antibiotic susceptibility of the isolates is as shown in Table 1. High percentage of resistance was seen to most antibiotics except colistin and tigecycline.

Out of the 100 isolates, 91 % were MDR, 78 % were XDR and 2 % were PDR.

Screening tests showed 97 (97 %), 100 (100 %) and 85 (85 %) were positive for ESBL, AmpC and MBL respectively. Out of these screen positive isolates, 37 (38.1 %), 99 (99 %) and 25 (25 %) were confirmed phenotypically to produce ESBL, AmpC and MBL respectively. 18 out of the 25 isolates that were confirmed phenotypically for MBL production, were positive for GIM (n = 6), VIM (n = 9), SIM (n = 2) and IMP (n = 1) by PCR. AmpC was seen to be produced by all but one isolate. It existed in combination with ESBL in 37 isolates and with MBL in 25. Interestingly, 7 isolates showed the production of all three.

Table 1 Antibiotic susceptibility pattern of *A. baumannii* isolates (n = 100)

Antibiotics	Resistant (%)	Intermediate (%)	Susceptible (%)
Ceftazidime	99 (99)	1 (1)	0 (0)
Cefotaxime	100 (100)	0 (0)	0 (0)
Cefpodoxime	100 (100)	0 (0)	0 (0)
Aztreonam	99 (99)	1 (1)	0 (0)
Imipenem	85 (85)	5 (5)	10 (10)
Cefoxitin	100 (100)	0 (0)	0 (0)
Amikacin	97 (97)	0 (0)	3 (3)
Ciprofloxacin	98 (98)	1 (1)	1 (1)
Gentamicin	95 (95)	1 (1)	4 (4)
Piperacillin–tazobactam	85 (85)	8 (8)	7 (7)
Cefepime	100 (100)	0 (0)	0 (0)
Ampicillin–sulbactam	65 (65)	14 (14)	21 (21)
Tigecycline	42 (42)	–	58 (58)
Colistin	3 (3)	–	97 (97)

Total of 100 isolates were typed using RAPD. 86 isolates were from one hospital and 14 from the other. Figure 1 shows the dendrogram of the isolates showing percentage similarity between them. A high degree of genetic variability was observed among the 100 isolates, including 53 distinct RAPD patterns with >20 % difference in UPGMA generated dice coefficients. 18 of these showed 100 % similarity. Majority of the isolates in each clonal type were restricted to the same hospital. However, few clonal types showed isolates from both the hospitals. The discriminatory index of 0.984 was found to be good.

MLST was done on 21 isolates representative of different clones as indicated by RAPD. One isolate each of STs 110, 103, 108, 194 and 14, two isolates each of ST 146 and 69 and three isolates of ST 188 were encountered. Nine isolates were found to have new ST types and were submitted to the PUBMLST site and were assigned the types. The new STs assigned were, ST 386 (n = 1), ST 387 (n = 1), ST 388 (n = 1), ST 389 (n = 1), ST 390 (n = 2) and ST 391 (n = 3) (Table 2).

Discussion

The distribution of the isolates among the specimen and the wards were similar to a recent study done in North India where it was seen that maximum number of *Acinetobacter* were isolated from pus (37.14 %), followed by blood (23 %) and urine (13.6 %). The highest percentage of isolation was from the ICU (22 %), followed by paediatrics (21 %), neurosurgery (16 %) and general surgery ward (13 %) [16].

When compared with other Gram-negative bacilli, the outer membrane of *A. baumannii* is less permeable which might be due to the small number and size of porins and thus it is intrinsically less susceptible to antimicrobial agents [17].

The resistance of *A. baumannii* isolates to Cephalosporins was similar to the findings of studies done in Saudi Arabia and Nigeria where in the resistance was found to range from 70 to 100 % [19] which might be due to the extensive use of Cephalosporins in these hospitals.

The resistance to the Aminoglycosides—amikacin and gentamicin was similar to the results in two studies where it was found to be 78.2–79.5 and 96.2 % respectively [20, 21]. In contrast, a few studies which were carried out in China and Malaysia showed that it was as low as 20.5–57.4 and 66.7 % respectively, which might be due

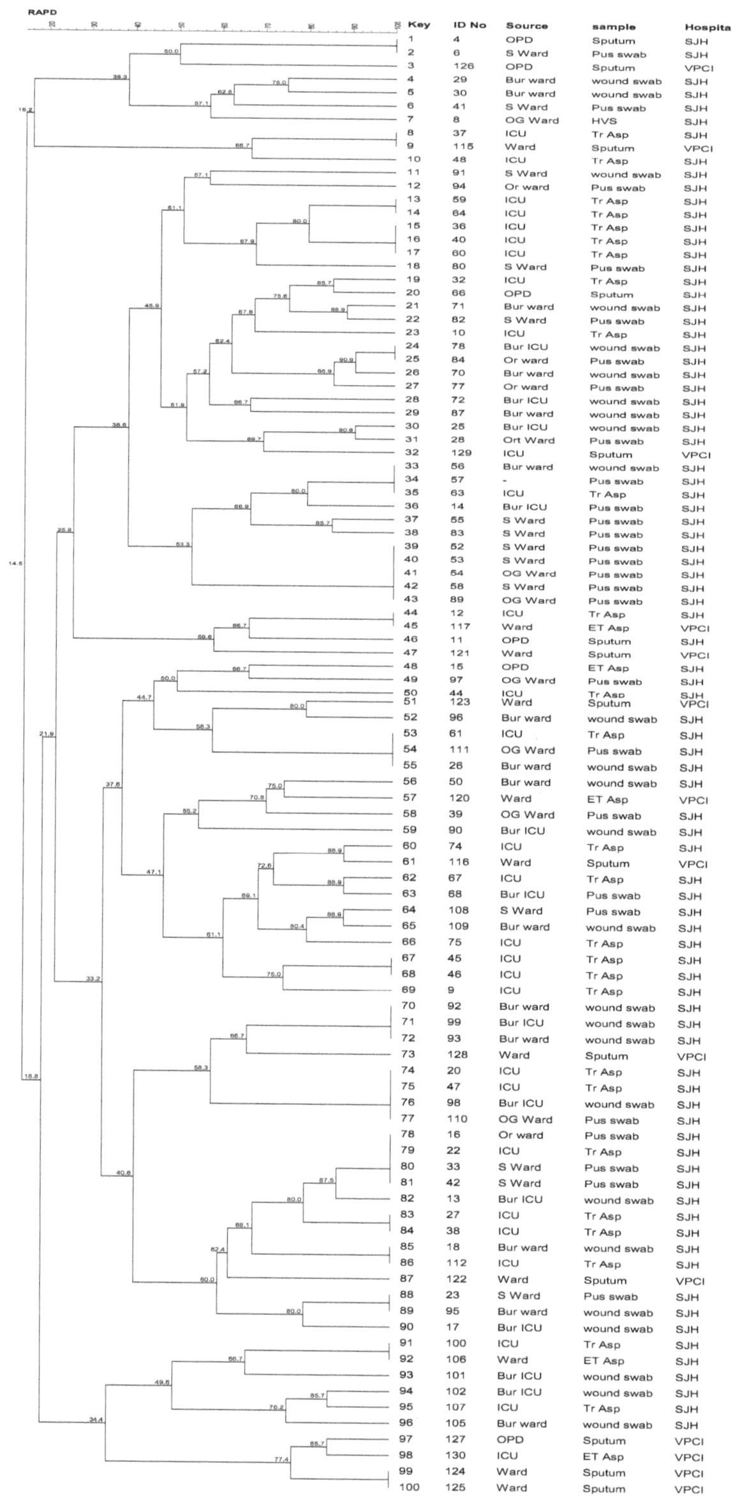

SJH- Safdarjung Hospital VPCI- VP Chest Institute

Fig. 1 UPGMA clustering dendrogram indicating percentage similarity between RAPD patterns of *A. baumannii* isolates from Safdarjung hospital and VPCI

Table 2 Sequence types of *Acinetobacter baumannii* isolates encountered in the study

S. no	ST	gltA	gyrB	gdhB	recA	cpn60	Gpi	rpoD	Strain
1	386*	31	33	67	40	1	102	7	In-S 58938
2	387*	1	15	4	11	4	140	4	In-S 95167
3	388*	1	15	4	11	4	95	4	In-S 91318
4	389*	1	7	8	11	1	4	14	In-S 93192
5	390*	31	33	67	40	1	58	7	In-S 100924
6	391*	1	15	13	12	4	102	2	In-V 1687/11
7	391*	1	15	13	12	4	102	2	In-V 323/05
8	391*	1	15	13	12	4	102	2	In-V 5930/11
9	390*	31	33	67	40	1	58	7	In-V 5290/10
10	14	1	10	8	6	1	4	14	In-S 84570
11	103	12	17	12	1	29	3	39	In-S 90868
12	69	1	46	3	2	2	58	3	In-S 98632
13	69	1	46	3	2	2	58	3	In-S 101149
14	108	10	12	4	6	4	9	5	In-S 101767
15	194	1	15	4	11	4	58	4	In-S 102704
16	110	1	15	2	28	1	52	32	In-V 5290/08
17	188	31	33	67	40	16	58	7	In-V 7362/07
18	188	31	33	67	40	16	58	7	In-V 3507/06
19	188	31	33	67	40	16	58	7	In-S 88877
20	146	1	15	13	12	4	14	2	In-V 8095/10
21	146	1	15	13	12	4	14	2	In-S 92729

S.no. serial number

* New STs found in the study

to the controlled use of Aminoglycosides in these hospitals [22, 23].

The resistance to Fluroquinolone, like ciprofloxacin, was similar to a study from Egypt which showed the resistance to be 85 % [24].

After the development of resistance to Fluoroquonolones, Carbapenem is usually the drug of choice for infections caused by Multi-drug resistant *A. baumannii* but unfortunately, Carbapenem-resistant isolates are constantly on the rise. In the present study, the resistance to imipenem (85 %) was similar to the findings from other parts of the world. [25–27]. In contrast three studies, two from India and one from Saudi Arabia, showed the resistance to be still as low as 0 and 9 % respectively. This might be due to the small number of isolates tested in these studies. [28–30].

With the increase in Carbapenem-resistance, tigecycline and colistin have been used for treatment of the infections caused by Extensive-drug resistant (XDR) *A. baumannii.*

There is no CLSI guidelines for the disk diffusion criteria for *A. baumannii.* United States Food and Drug Administration breakpoint criteria for tigecycline when testing Enterobactericeae (Susceptibility at ≤2 μg/ml, intermediate at 4 μg/ml and resistant at ≥8 μg/ml and the corresponding disc diffusion diameters as ≥19 and ≤14 mm for sensitive and resistant strains respectively) is being followed by various authors. But it was observed by Jones et al., that using these zone sizes many isolates were falsely labelled as resistant [7]. She proposed that by using the zone diameters as ≥16 mm for sensitive and ≤12 mm for resistant isolates reduced the error rate to a minimum. Thus, using these criteria, in the present study, resistance to tigecycline was found to be 42 % which was similar to a study done in Taiwan in which it was 45.5 % [31]. But, it was very high in comparison to a study by Behera et al. [32] in which, in spite of using the FDA breakpoints, the resistance was only 7.6 %. This could be due to the fact that the study was conducted in 2007 when tigecycline was not used as frequently as Carbapenems for the treatment of these infections. Resistance to tigecycline has also increased in the past few years [33].

In this study, the resistance to colistin was similar to that seen in three other studies, one each from India, Egypt and Taiwan which showed a resistance of 3.5, 5 and 10 % respectively [18, 22, 30]. This might be due to the fact that colistin is a reserve drug and used only for multi-drug resistant cases. However, a recent study from the United States showed that 14 out of 28 isolates were colistin resistant [34]. This is because of the rise in

MDR *Acinetobacter* where in, colistin is the only choice available for the treatment. Hence, resistance to it is also emerging. The resistance to antibiotics reflects on the policy of antimicrobial usage and the circulation of drug resistant clones in different countries.

In the present study it was seen that out of the 100 isolates, 91 % were MDR, 78 % were XDR and 2 % were PDR. Similar findings were seen in another study. [35]. However, a study from North India showed lower percentage of isolates to be MDR. [20]. This could be due to the fact that the study was done in 2007–2008 and usage of Carbapenems and hence, resistance to it has increased since then.

The resistance to the various antibiotics is commonly due to the production of β-lactamases out of which the Extended spectrum β-lactamse (ESBL), AmpC β-lactamase and the Metallo β-lactamase (MBL) were studied here. All these three mechanisms have been observed in the present study.

Detection of lower number of MBLs by PCR is due to the fact that MBLs are only one of many mechanisms for Carbapenem resistance. Oxacillanases are important cause of Carbapenem resistance in *Acinetobacter*. Unfortunately we could not test for it.

In the present study, 99 % of the isolates produced AmpC, 37 % in combination with ESBL and 25 % in combination with MBL. Co-production of all the three, ESBL, AmpC and MBL were found in 7 % of our isolates. This could explain the increased rates of MDR in our study.

RAPD was done to detect clones which could be further typed by MLST. In the current study RAPD showed a high degree of genetic variability among the 100 isolates, with 53 distinct RAPD patterns out of which 18 (consisting of 2–5 isolates each) showed 100 % similarity between the isolates. The clonal types were not restricted to specific wards but were spread all over. They seem to be mostly restricted to the same hospital though a few were seen in both hospitals. Interestingly, one clonal type comprising of 5 isolates isolated from tracheal aspirates of different patients in the ICU of SJH, were Extensive-drug resistant, resistant to tigecycline, sensitive to colistin. Another clonal type included 6 isolates from different samples and different wards of SJH but all were Extensive-drug resistant, sensitive to colistin and all but one were sensitive to tigecycline. There were many other clonal types but they did not correlate with the antibiotypes. In a study done in India it was seen that the RAPD results did not correlate with those of antibiotypes since the isolates showed highly divergent resistance profiles. Only a few correlations could be made [13].

PUBMLST database has 2738 *Acinetobacter baumannii* isolates with 920 assigned STs. Analyzing the data by eBURST, 78 groups (each having 6 or more loci in common) were identified. Out of all the STs identified 319 were singletons not belonging to any group. Even among the 78 groups a founder could only be identified in very few suggesting high diversity among the isolates (http://pubmlst.org/abaumannii/). Few of the STs found in the study with clonal complex 92, 104, 109, 110 and 20 belonged to international clones and are distributed in different continents of the world suggesting their spread to India due to frequent travel between the continents. Most of these clones are multidrug resistant and that could explain the increased percentage of MDR in our study. So far, there is no published data on the sequence types of other Indian isolates. MLST database does not contain ST of Indian isolates. Therefore, the prevalence of the ST types in India cannot be commented upon.

In comparison of ST types with the antibiotic resistance pattern it was observed that, ST146 (CC20) clone consisting of 2 isolates which were XDR and sensitive to both tigecycline and colistin, did not produce ESBL or MBL but produced AmpC β-lactamase, were from different clinical samples and different wards. CC20 is an international clone and is known to produce Oxa 51- and 68-variants. This could explain the XDR nature of our isolates though we did not test for oxacillinases. Two other isolates belonged to another clone ST69 and they were both XDR, resistant to tigecycline and sensitive to colistin, producing both ESBL and AmpC β-lactamase but they belonged to different wards. ST110 clone consisted of two isolates which although had different antibiotic susceptibility, they produced the same type of β-lactamase. ST188 clone with three isolates showed similar antibiotic susceptibility but differed in the type of β-lactamase produced. The discordance between the ST types and antibiotic resistance and/or the β-lactamase types could be due to the fact that MLST is based on the house keeping genes but the genes responsible for resistance and virulence could be located on mobile elements and clustered in genomic islands and are not linked to particular sequence types. The new STs encountered in our study were mostly sensitive to colistin and resistant to tigecycline. They were closely related and were either single locus variants or double locus variants of existing clones. For example ST 390 is a SLV and 386 a DLV of known ST 188. These two differed from 188 in that both were resistant to tigecycline. All of these were isolates from respiratory samples. Similarly ST 387 and 388 were SLV and DLV of ST 194 respectively. All these isolates were from burns unit of the same hospital. Two of the three were resistant to tigecycline. These data show that genetic variations have occurred locally in the existing clones to give the new STs.

Conclusion

A high percentage of MDR and XDR *Acinetobacter* obtained in the study is due to acquisition of various kinds of beta lactamases most of these belonging to resistant international clones. Hence, *A. baumannii* has developed into one of the most difficult hospital pathogens to control and treat. As of now colistin is the only drug of choice due to its low resistance. But keeping in mind the nephrotoxicity, patients should be carefully treated giving adequate dosage and proper scheduling. Restrained and careful use of antibiotics as well as strict infection control policy is crucial for preventing the emergence of complete resistance and spread of this pathogen. RAPD with a discriminatory index of 0.984 can be used to type isolates. MLST should be performed for epidemiological surveillance so as to learn about the variability and prevalence of MDR clones in the world.

Authors' contributions

MS proposed and designed the study, analyzed the generated data; DR carried out the experimental part of the manuscript. MD provided with strains from SJH, MS and MD helped to draft the manuscript and in critical revision. All authors read and approved the final manuscript.

Author details

[1] Department of Microbiology, Vallabhbhai Patel Chest Institute, University of Delhi, Delhi 110007, India. [2] Vardhaman Mahavir Medical College and Safdarjung Hospital, New Delhi 110029, India. [3] Present Address: Department of Microbiology, Vardhaman Mahavir Medical College and Safdarjung Hospital, New Delhi, India.

Acknowledgements

It was supported by Vallabhbhai Patel chest Institute through their annual departmental funding.

This work was carried out at Department of Microbiology, Vallabhbhai Patel Chest Institute.

Competing interests

The authors declare that there are no competing interests associated with this work. The authors declare that the research work has been approved by their Institute's ethics committees.

References

1. Peleg AY, Seifert H. Paterson DL *Acinetobacter baumannii*: emergence of a successful pathogen. Clin Microbiol Rev. 2008;21:538–82.
2. Chandra R, Kapil A, Sharma P, Das B. Identification of *Acinetobacter* species isolated from clinical specimens by amplified ribosomal DNA restriction analysis. Indian J Med Res. 2002;116:1–4.
3. Vaneechoutte M, Dijkshoorn L, Tjernberg I, Elaichouni A, de Vos P, Claeys G, Verschraegen G. Identification of *Acinetobacter* genomic species by amplified ribosomal DNA restriction analysis. J Clin Microbiol. 1995;33:11–5.
4. Clinical Laboratory Standards Institute (CLSI). Performance standards for antimicrobial susceptibility testing. Twenty-Third Informational Supplement (M100-S23), Wayne, PA.2013.
5. Wikler MA, editor. Performance standards for antimicrobial susceptibility testing; Eighteenth informational supplement. 18th ed. Wayne (PA): Clinical and Laboratory Standards institute; 2008.
6. Somily AM. Comparison of E-test and disc diffusion methods for the in vitro evaluation of the antimicrobial activity of colistin in multi-drug resistant Gram-negative bacilli. Saudi Med J. 2010;31:507–11.
7. Jones RN, Ferraro MJ, Reller LB, Schreckenberger PC, Swenson JM, Sader HS. Multicenter studies of tigecycline disk diffusion susceptibility results for *Acinetobacter spp*. J Clin Microbiol. 2007;45:227–30.
8. Manchanda V, Sanchaita S, Singh NP. Multidrug resistant *Acinetobacter*. J Global Infect Dis. 2010;2:291–304.
9. Thomson KS. Extended-spectrum-beta-lactamase, AmpC, and carbapenemase issues. J Clln Microbiol. 2010;48:1019–25.
10. Yong D, Lee K, Yum JH, Shin HB, Rossolini GM, Chong Y. Imipenem-EDTA disk method for differentiation of metallo-beta-lactamase-producing clinical isolates of *Pseudomonas* spp. and *Acinetobacter* spp. J Clin Microbiol. 2002;40:3798–801.
11. Ellington MJ, Kistler J, Livermore DM, Woodford N. Multiplex PCR for rapid detection of genes encoding acquired metallo beta-lactamases. J Antimicrob Chemother. 2007;59:321–2.
12. Black JA, Moland ES, Hossain A, Lockhart TJ, Olson LB, Thomson KS (2003) Abstr. 43rd intersci. Conf. Antimicrob. Agents Chemother., abstr C2-2034. Prevalence of plasmid-mediated AmpC β-lactamase in *Klebsiella pneumoniae* (kp), *Klebsiella* spp. and 21 non-ICU sites in the United States.
13. Karthika RU, Rao RS, Sahoo S, Shashikala P, Kanungo R, Jayachandran S. Prashanth K Phenotypic and genotypic assays for detecting the prevalence of metallo-beta-lactamases in clinical isolates of *Acinetobacter baumannii* from a South Indian tertiary care hospital. J Med Microbiol. 2009;58:430–5.
14. Bartual SG, Seifert H, Hippler C. Domı´nguez Luzon MA, Wisplinghoff H, Rodrı´guez-Valera F. Development of a multilocus sequence typing scheme for characterization of clinical isolates of *Acinetobacter baumannii*. J Clin Microbiol. 2005;43:4382–90.
15. Park YK, Jung SI, Park KH, Cheong HS, Peck KR, Song JH, Ko KS. Independent emergence of colistin-resistant *Acinetobacter* spp. isolates from Korea. Diagn Microbiol Infect Dis. 2009;64:43–51.
16. Sinha N, Agarwal J, Srivastava S, Singh M. Analysis of carbapenem resistant *Acinetobacter* from a tertiary care setting in North India. Indian J Med Microbiol. 2013;31:60–3.
17. Vila J, Martí S, Sánchez-Céspedes J. Porins, efflux pumps and multidrug resistance in *Acinetobacter baumannii*. J Antimicrob Chemother. 2007;59:1210–5.
18. El-Ageery SM, Abo-Shadi MA, Alghaithy AA, Ahmad MA, Alsharif NH, Alharbi SA. Epidemiological investigation of nosocomial infection with multidrug-resistant *Acinetobacter baumannii*. Eur Rev Med Pharmacol Sci. 2012;16:1834–9.
19. Nwadike VU, Ojide CK, Kalu EI. Multidrug resistant *Acinetobacter* infection and their antimicrobial susceptibility pattern in a Nigerian tertiary hospital ICU. Afr J Infect Dis. 2014;8:14–8.
20. Taneja N, Singh G, Singh M, Sharma M. Emergence of tigecycline and colistin resistant *Acinetobacter baumannii* in patients with complicated urinary tract infections in North India. Indian J Med Res. 2011;133:681–4.
21. Patwardhan RB, Dhakephalkar PK, Niphadkar KB, Chopade BA. A study on nosocomial pathogens in ICU with special reference to mutiresistant *Acinetobacter baumannii* harboring multiple plasmids. Indian J Med Res. 2008;128:178–87.
22. Ning D, De-zhi L, Ji-chao C, Yu-sheng C, Rong G, Ying-hui HU, Jing-ping Y, Juan D, Cheng-ping H, Wei Z, Jia-shu L, Qin Y, Huan-ying W, Lan M, Xiao-ning Z, Li-ping W, Jian-jun M, Qiu-yue W, Ke H, Gui-zhen T, Shao-xi C, Rui-qin W, Bei H, Si-qin W, Zhan-wei W, Su-rui Z, Zhan-cheng G. Drug-resistant genes carried by *Acinetobacter baumannii* isolated from patients with lower respiratory tract infection. Chin Med J. 2010;123:2571–5.
23. Lean SS, Suhaili Z, Ismail S, Rahman NIA, Othman N, Abdullah FH, Jusoh Z, Yeo CC, Thong KL. Prevalence and Genetic Characterization of Carbapenem- and Polymyxin-Resistant *Acinetobacter baumannii* Isolated from a Tertiary Hospital in Terengganu, Malaysia. ISRN, Microbiology. 2014;1:1–9.
24. Al-Agamy MH, Khalaf NG, Tawfick MM, Shibl AMA, Kholy AE. Molecular characterization of carbapenem-insensitive *Acinetobacter baumannii* in Egypt. Int J Infect Dis. 2014;22:49–54.

25. Denys GA, Callister SM, Dowzicky MJ. Antimicrobial susceptibility among gram-negative isolates collected in the USA between 2005 and 2011 as part of the Tigecycline Evaluation and Surveillance Trial (T.E.S.T.). Ann Clin Microbiol Antimicrob. 2013;12:24–34.
26. Ertürk A, Çiçek AC, Gümüş A, Cüre E, Şen A, Kurt A, Karagöz A, Aydoğan N, Sandall Durmaz R. Molecular characterisation and control of *Acinetobacter baumannii* isolates resistant to multi-drugs emerging in inter-intensive care units. Ann Clin Microbiol Antimicrob. 2014;13:36–43.
27. Dettori M, Piana A, Deriu MG, Curto PL, Cossu A, Musumeci R, Cocuzza C, Astone V, Contu MA, Sotgiu G. Outbreak of multidrug-resistant *Acinetobacter baumannii* in an intensive care unit. New Microbiol. 2014;37:185–91.
28. Shete VB, Ghadage DP, Muley VA, Bhore AV. Multi-drug resistant *Acinetobacter* ventilator-associated pneumonia. Lung India. 2010;27:217–20.
29. Shete VB, Ghadage DP, Muley VA, Bhore AV. *Acinetobacter* septicaemia in neonates admitted to intensive care units. J Lab Phys. 2009;1:73–6.
30. Said KB, Al-Jarbou AN, Alrouji M, Al-Harbi HO. Surveillance of antimicrobial resistance among clinical isolates recovered from a tertiary care hospital in Al Qassim, Saudi Arabia. Int J Health Sci (Qassim). 2014; 8:3–12.
31. Chang KC, Lin MF, Lin NT, Wu WJ, Kuo HY, Lin TY, Yang TL, Chen YC, Liou ML. Clonal spread of multidrug-resistant *Acinetobacter baumannii* in eastern Taiwan. J Microbiol Immunol Infect. 2012;45:37–42.
32. Behera B, Das A, Mathur P, Kapil A, Gadepalli R, Dhawan B. Tigecycline susceptibility report from an Indian tertiary care hospital. Indian J Med Res. 2009;129:446–50.
33. Spiliopoulou A, Jelastopulu E, Vamvakopoulou S, Bartzavali C, Kolonitsiou F, Anastassiou ED, Christofidou M. In vitro activity of tigecycline and colistin against *A. baumannii* clinical bloodstream isolates during an 8-year period. J Chemother. 2014. doi:10.1179/1973947814Y.0000000193 **[Epub ahead of print]**.
34. Lesho E, Yoon EJ, McGann P, Snesrud E, Kwak Y, Milillo, Onmus-Leone F, Preston L, St. Clair K, Nikolich M, Viscount H, Wortmann G, Zapor M, Grillot-Courvalin C, Courvalin P, Clifford R, Waterman PE. Emergence of colistin-resistance in extremely drug-resistant Acinetobacter baumannii containing a novel pmrCAB operon during colistin therapy of wound infections. J Infect Dis. 2013;208:1142–51.
35. Navon-Venezia S, Leavitt A, Carmeli Y. High tigecycline resistance in multidrug-resistant *Acinetobacter baumannii*. J Antimicrob Chemother. 2007;59:772–4.

12

Molecular characterization of clinical IMP-producing *Klebsiella pneumoniae* isolates from a Chinese Tertiary Hospital

Kaisheng Lai†, Yanning Ma†, Ling Guo, Jingna An, Liyan Ye and Jiyong Yang*

Abstract

Background: IMP-producing *Klebsiella pneumoniae* (IMPKpn) exhibits sporadic prevalence in China. The mechanisms related to the spread of IMPKpn remain unclear.

Methods: Carbapenem non-susceptible *K. pneumoniae* isolates were collected from our hospital. The genetic relatedness, antimicrobial susceptibility, as well as sequence types (ST) were analyzed by pulsed-field gel electrophoresis (PFGE), VITEK 2 AST test Kit, and multilocus sequence typing (MLST), respectively. S1-PFGE, Southern blot analysis and multiple PCR amplification were used for plasmid profiling.

Results: Between October 2009 and June 2016, 25 non-repetitive IMPKpn isolates were identified. PFGE results showed that these isolates belonged to 20 genetically unrelated IMPKpn strains. Diverse STs were identified by MLST. Most strains carried $bla_{\text{IMP-4}}$, followed by $bla_{\text{IMP-1}}$. Four incompatibility types of bla_{IMP}-carrying plasmids were identified, which included A/C (n = 2), B/O (n = 2), L/M (n = 1) and N (n = 14), while type of other one plasmid failed to be determined.

Conclusions: The IMPKpn isolates exhibited sporadic prevalence in our hospital. IncN types of plasmids with various sizes have emerged as the main platform mediating the spread of the bla_{IMP} genes in our hospital.

Keywords: IMP, *Klebsiella pneumoniae*, Sequence type

Background

The spread of carbapenemase-producing *Enterobacteriaceae* has been a major challenge both for treatment of individual patients and for policies of infection control [1]. IMP-1 is the first identified metallo-β-lactamase conferring carbapenem resistance and was described in 1988 in a *Pseudomonas aeruginosa* strain in Japan [2]. IMP-type carbapenemases can hydrolyze almost all β-lactams. The popular IMP-type carbapenemases have been widespread in non-fermenting Gram-negative bacilli, including *Pseudomonas aeruginosa*, *Acinetobacter* spp., and members of the *Enterobacteriaceae* family [3]. The bla_{IMP} genes are usually located on large plasmids with different replicon types or incompatibility (Inc) types, such as IncA/C, L/M, N, and HI2, which have been commonly associated with the carriage and transmission of various bla_{IMP} genes [4–7].

Klebsiella pneumoniae is an important pathogen causing various infections. IMP-producing *K. pneumoniae* (IMPKpn) isolates have been identified worldwide and caused a few small-scale outbreaks [3, 5, 6, 8, 9]. Up to now, diverse sequence types (ST) of IMPKpn have been reported, including STs 15, 37, 107, 133, 252, 323, 340, 476, 478, 626, 686, 889, 903, 1114 and 1306 [5–11].

In China, IMP-producing *Enterobacteriaceae* isolates have been found across the country [3, 6, 7, 9–21]. Variants of bla_{IMP} have been identified in *K. pneumoniae*, *Escherichia coli* and *Enterobacter cloacae*. Among IMPKpn, IMP-4 is the most commonly encountered isoform in clinical isolates, followed by IMP-8, IMP-26 and IMP-38 [6, 9–18, 22]. Meanwhile, the IMPKpn isolates exhibit high diversity of sequence type (ST), and IMPKpn STs15,

*Correspondence: yangjy301@hotmail.com
†Kaisheng Lai and Yanning Ma contributed equally to this work
Department of Microbiology, Chinese PLA General Hospital, 301 Hospital, 28# Fuxing Road, Beijing 100853, China

37, 107, 133, 323, 476, 686, 889, 1114 and 1306 have been recovered [6, 7, 10, 11].

In the present study, a retrospective study of clinical carbapenem-non-susceptible *enterobacteriaceae* isolates from our hospital was performed. In total, 25 IMPKpn isolates were identified in this study. Phenotypic and genotypic characteristics of these isolates were further analyzed.

Methods

Bacterial isolates

All clinical *Enterobacteriaceae* isolates were collected from a 4000-bed tertiary-care hospital and were identified by VITEK® MS (bioMérieux SA, Marcy-l'Etoile, France). The isolates exhibiting resistance or intermediate to any one of ertapenem or imipenem or meropenem will be defined as carbapenem non-susceptibility strain, and will be screened for bla_{IMP} by PCR and subsequent amplicon sequencing using the primers IMP-1F: 5′-TGAGCAAGTTATCTGTATTC and IMP-1R: 5′-TTAGTTGCTTGGTTTTGATG [11]. *E. coli* ATCC 25922 was used as a quality control strain for antimicrobial susceptibility testing. The *Salmonella* ser. Braenderup strain H9812 was used as a reference standard for pulsed-field gel electrophoresis (PFGE). No ethical approval was obtained for using the clinical samples, because they were collected during routine bacteriologic analyses in public hospitals, and the data were anonymously analyzed.

Antimicrobial susceptibility testing

The MICs of clinical commonly used antimicrobial agents (listed in Fig. 1) were measured using VITEK 2 AST-GN09 and AST-GN13 test Kit (bioMérieux, Inc.) according to the manufacturer's instructions. All susceptibility results were interpreted according to the 2017 CLSI performance standards [23].

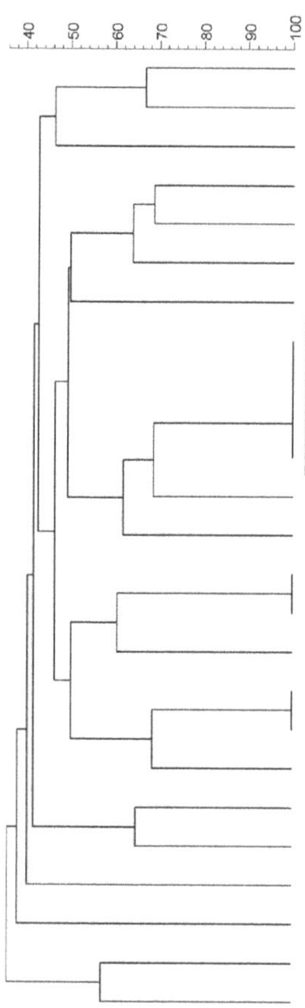

No.	PFGE type	ST	Isolating date	Source	IMP variants	Plasmids size and type	CAZ	FEP	TZP	IMP	MEM	ETP	AK	CIP
IR5010	D	ST147	2011-07-09	Urine	IMP-38	110 kb, N	≥64	≥64	≥128	4	≥16	≥8	≤2	≥4
IR5020	G	ST1326	2012-02-16	Drainage	IMP-4	220 kb, B/O	≥64	≥64	≥128	8	4	≥8	≥64	≥4
IR5068	P	ST1737	2013-07-04	Drainage	IMP-4	60 kb, N	≥64	≥64	≥128	≥16	8	≥8	≤2	1
IR5049	N	ST1405	2012-11-25	Sputum	IMP-4	260 kb, N	≥64	≥64	8	4	1	≥8	≤2	≤0.25
IR5623	T	ST629	2014-11-26	Sputum	IMP-4	55 kb, N	≥64	≥64	64	8	1	≥8	≤2	≥4
IR5005	B	ST629	2010-08-30	Blood	IMP-4	30 kb, N	≥64	≥64	64	4	8	≥8	≥64	≥4
IR5055	O	Novel	2013-01-24	Sputum	IMP-4	50 kb, N	≥64	8	8	8	1	4	≤2	1
IR5015	F	ST11	2011-10-21	Sputum	IMP-1	30 kb, N	≥64	≥64	64	≥16	≥16	≥8	≥64	≥4
IR5016	F	ST11	2011-11-04	Sputum	IMP-1	30 kb, N	≥64	≥64	64	≥16	≥16	≥8	≥64	≥4
IR5017	F	ST11	2011-11-11	Sputum	IMP-1	30 kb, N	≥64	≥64	64	≥16	≥16	≥8	≥64	≥4
IR5018	F	ST11	2011-11-29	Sputum	IMP-1	30 kb, N	≥64	≥64	64	≥16	≥16	≥8	≥64	≥4
IR5038	I	ST11	2012-06-25	Blood	IMP-4	280 kb, N	≥64	≥64	≥128	≥16	≥16	≥8	≤2	≥4
IR5091	R	ST37	2014-03-07	Sputum	IMP-4	90 kb, N	≥64	16	16	2	2	≥8	≤2	≥4
IR5011	E	ST48	2011-07-19	Catheter	IMP-4	55 kb, L/M	≥64	≥64	≥128	≤1	8	≥8	≤2	≥4
IR5012	E	ST48	2011-07-20	Urine	IMP-4	55 kb, L/M	≥64	≥64	≥128	≤1	8	≥8	≤2	≥4
IR5041	J	ST454	2012-07-08	Bile	IMP-4	230 kb, N	≥64	16	8	4	1	≥8	≤2	≤0.25
IR5033	H	Novel	2012-06-15	Drainage	IMP-1	260 kb, N	≥64	16	8	4	1	≥8	≤2	≤0.25
IR5040	H	Novel	2012-07-04	Drainage	IMP-1	260 kb, N	≥64	16	8	4	1	≥8	≤2	≤0.5
IR5044	K	ST873	2012-08-21	Sputum	IMP-4	55 kb, N	≥64	16	64	8	1	≥8	≥64	≥4
IR5047	L	ST1240	2012-08-17	Blood	IMP-4	170 kb, B/O	≥64	≥64	≥128	≥16	8	≥8	≤2	≤0.25
IR5079	Q	ST11	2013-10-20	Drainage	IMP-4	260 kb, N	≥64	≥64	≥128	4	1	4	16	≥4
IR5096	S	ST514	2014-05-18	Sputum	IMP-4	320 kb, UT	≥64	≥64	≥128	4	8	≥8	≤2	1
IR5002	A	Novel	2009-10-23	Sputum	IMP-4	120 kb, A/C	≥64	≥64	≥128	4	4	≥8	≤2	≥4
IR5008	C	ST1697	2011-03-26	Drainage	IMP-26	310 kb, A/C	≥64	≥64	64	≤1	8	≥8	≤2	≥4
IR5048	M	ST761	2012-08-22	Abscess	IMP-1	245 kb, N	≥64	16	8	2	1	≥8	≤2	≤0.25

(Minimum inhibitory concentration (mg/L): CAZ, FEP, TZP, IMP, MEM, ETP, AK, CIP)

Fig. 1 Dendrogram of patterns generated by PFGE of IMP-producing *K. pneumoniae* isolates. The PFGE types, ST, isolating date of the IMPKpn isolates, IMP variants, the size and type of bla_{IMP}-carrying plasmids and the MICs of common-used antimicrobial agents were list in this figure. The frame indicated the characterization of IMP-producing *K. pneumoniae* isolates causing an outbreak. *ST* sequence type, *CAZ* ceftazidime, *FEP* cefepime, *TZP* piperacillin–tazobactam, *IMP* imipenem, *MEM* meropenem, *ETP* ertapenem, *AK* amikacin, *CIP* ciprofloxacin, *UT* unable type

PFGE and MLST analyses

PFGE with *Xba*I was performed for IMPKpn isolates as previously described [24]. MLST was carried out for IMPKpn according to protocols provided on their MLST websites (http://www.pasteur.fr/recherche/genopole/PF8/mlst/Kpneumoniae).

Plasmid and southern blot analyses

A bla_{NDM} probe was generated by labeling the PCR product using the PCR DIG Probe Synthesis Kit (Roche Applied Sciences, Mannheim, Germany). The size and incompatibility types of bla_{IMP}-carrying plasmids were analyzed by the S1-PFGE, Southern blot and multiple PCR as previously described [24, 25]. The whole genomic DNA including the plasmid of the isolates was digested with 20 U of S1 nuclease at 37 °C for 20 min, and separated by PFGE. Then, the DNA fragments were transferred to positively charged nylon membranes (Roche Applied Science). Hybridization was carried out with the DIG Easy Hyb Granules (Roche Applied Sciences), and the detection was performed using the DIG Nucleic Acid Detection Kit (Roche Applied Sciences).

Results

Prevalence and genetic relatedness of IMPKpn

The first IMPKpn isolate in our hospital was identified in October 2009. Since then until June 2016, 25 non-repetitive IMPKpn isolates have been recovered. The source of the IMPKpn isolates included 11 sputum, 6 drainges, 3 bloods, 2 urines, 1 catheter, 1 bile and 1 abscess. The 25 IMPKpn isolates were categorized into 20 PFGE types (type A to T). Type F contained 4 isolates, and types E and H contained 2 isolates, other 16 types contained only 1 isolate (Fig. 1). Isolates with same PFGE type were considered as the same strain. Therefore, a total of 20 IMPKpn strains with no genetic relationship were further analyzed.

Antimicrobial susceptibility

The antimicrobial susceptibility patterns of the isolates were listed in Fig. 1. All isolates presented resistance to ceftazidime, cefepime and piperacillin–tazobactam, and exhibited heterogeneous resistance patterns to carbapenem, amikacin and ciprofloxacin (Fig. 1).

bla_{IMP} variants

PCR and subsequent amplicon sequence alignment revealed that most strains carried bla_{IMP-4}, and several bla_{IMP} gene sequences displayed 100% identity with the published sequence of the bla_{IMP-1} (for 3 strains), bla_{IMP-26} (for 1 strains) and bla_{IMP-38} (for 1 strains) genes, respectively (Fig. 1).

MLST

Among 20 IMPKpn strains, a diversity of STs was identified. Three strains were identified as ST11, two strains were defined as ST629, and 12 strains belonged to independent STs. Three novel STs were identified with the allelic profile 18-71-26-125-115-2-51 (type A strain), 42-22-25-96-115-20-49 (type H strain) and 71-1-1-83-16-121-5 (type O strain), respectively (Fig. 1).

Plasmid analysis

The bla_{IMP} genes were located on plasmids with sizes ranged from approximately 30 to 320 kb (Fig. 1). Four incompatibility types of bla_{IMP}-carrying plasmids including A/C, B/O, L/M and N were identified, whereas type of one plasmid was unable to be determined. In total, 14 IMPKpn strains carried the IncN plasmids with sizes ranging from 30 to 280 kb, while two A/C (120- and 310-kb), two IncB/O (170- and 220-kb) and one IncL/M (55 kb) plasmids were characterized.

Discussion

The worldwide spread of carbapenemase-producing *K. pneumoniae* has been a growing clinical problem and threat to public health [1]. In this study, 25 non-duplicated IMPKpn isolates were collected between October 2009 and June 2016. During this period, 8.5% (537 of 6310) of clinical *K. pneumoniae* isolates exhibited carbapenem-resistant phenotypes, and only 0.19% (25/537) of carbapenem-non-susceptible *K. pneumoniae* strains produced IMP. Further analysis showed that the majority of carbapenemase-producing *K. pneumoniae* was the KPC-2-producing *K. pneumoniae*, followed by OXA-48- and NDM-producing *K. pneumoniae* [24–26]. Therefore, IMPKpn exhibited sporadic prevalence in our hospital. In China, IMPKpn isolates have been identified across the country, and the main variants are IMP-4 and IMP-8 [3, 6, 7, 9–21], while IMP-26 and IMP-38 have also been identified [16, 18]. In this study, besides the scattered emergence of IMP-1, IMP-26 and IMP-38, we found that the majority of IMPKpn isolates produced IPM-4 (Fig. 1) which was different from the prevalence of IMP variants that were reported from other Asian regions, where IMP-1 accounted for the majority [3]. Taken together, the source, evolution and dissemination of IMPKpn may be different in different regions.

In this study, PFGE analysis revealed that the majority of IMPKpn isolates belonged to different types, while an outbreak at small scales (type F strain) that covered only four patients was observed (Fig. 1), suggesting that the majority of IMPKpn isolates analyzed in this study were genetically unrelated strains. Meanwhile, most strains exhibited high ST diversity. Only three and two clones of IMPKpn strains belonged to ST11 and ST629, respectively, while other STs were only identified in single strain. Three strains were identified as new clones with novel STs (Fig. 1). Other reports also showed that the STs of IMPKpn are highly dispersed [5–11], suggesting the clonal diversity of IMPKpn isolates. Thus, the IMPKpn exhibited a significant sporadic prevalence across the world. Under the same medical condition and selective pressure, the KPC-2-producing *K. pneumoniae* spread throughout our hospital [24]. However, the IMPKpn strains only exhibited low prevalence and small scale of outbreaks at the same time. A study revealed that some biological characteristics, such as cell motility, secretion, DNA repair and modification, may contribute to the rapid spread of KPC-producing *K. pneumoniae* ST258 and ST11 [27]. Recent genomic analysis of *K. pneumoniae* has established that the genomic background was closely related to the pathogenicity of *K. pneumoniae* [28]. Therefore, the virulence characteristics, rather than their drug-resistant phenotype, may be the major driving force responsible for the emergence and widely spread of antibiotic-resistant pathogens. The urgent efforts are needed to reveal the genetic background of these pathogens, as well as its relationship with their pathogenic and transmission abilities, which is the essential first step to design intervention strategies preventing their spread.

In this study, most of the clinical isolates exhibited low-level resistance or even sensitivity to imipenem and meropenem, but high-level resistance to ertapenem (Fig. 1). Similar results have also been reported in other studies from China [9, 13, 14, 16, 20]. These studies showed that the effects of IMP hydrolase on different carbapenems may be diverse, and therefore, the carbapenem-sensitive phenotype does not mean negative for carbapenemase. In most laboratories in China, the production of carbapenemases was not usually detected by modified Hodge test [23] in clinical IMPKpn isolates with carbapenem-sensitive phenotype. The weak hydrolytic ability of IMPs to carbapenems may lead to an underestimation of the prevalence of IMPKpn isolates. It was reported that some IMP variants (such IMP-26) exhibited increased carbapenem-hydrolyzing activity [29]. However, the IMP-26-producing IMPKpn were sensitive to imipenem in this study (Fig. 1). Another study also showed that the IMP-26-producing IMPKpn displayed only low-level resistance to imipenem [14]. Therefore, the production of IMPs was not the only factor responsible for high-level carbapenem resistance, other resistance mechanisms may also confer this process, which include hyperexpression of efflux systems, and loss of the outer membrane channel OprD that allows the entry of carbapenems into the cell [30]. For clinical IMPKpn isolates, it is less clear to what extent the different resistant mechanisms have impact on the carbapenem-resistant phenotype.

Plasmid analysis in this study showed that the majority (13 of 20) of bla_{IMP}-carrying plasmids belonged to IncN. Another study in China found the dissemination of IncN bla_{IMP}-coding plasmids among *K. pneumoniae* of different genotypes [7]. These results suggested that IncN plasmids have a unique advantage and fitness in the spread of bla_{IMP} genes. However, because most of the IncN plasmids had different sizes in this study (Fig. 1), it was possible that the dissemination of bla_{IMP} genes in our hospital may not mediated by transfer of plasmids but other mechanisms.

The present study has several limitations. First, because this study was retrospective analysis and only limited patient information was available, thus the study focused on the characterization of phenotype and genotype of clinical IMPKpn isolates. Second, the genetic environment of bla_{IMP} genes remained to be characterized in our future study. Another limitation of the study included the absence of analyzing other resistance-related determinants, the outer-membrane permeabilities, and efflux systems of IMPKpn isolates. Further studies are needed to address these limitations.

Authors' contributions

KL, YM, LG, JA and LY performed the phenotypic and genotypic analysis of clinical isolates. JY designed the study, performed data analysis and drafted the manuscript. All authors read and approved the final manuscript.

Acknowledgements

Not applicable.

Competing interests

The authors declare that they have no competing interests.

Consent for publication

We give our permission for the above material to appear in the print, online, and licensed versions of *Annals of Clinical Microbiology and Antimicrobials*.

Funding

This study was supported by the China Mega-Project on Infectious Disease Prevention (Grant No. 2017ZX10103002-002-002).

References

1. van Duin D. Doi Y. The global epidemiology of carbapenemase-producing Enterobacteriaceae. Virulence. 2016;11:1–10. doi:10.1080/21505594.2016.1222343.
2. Watanabe M, Iyobe S, Inoue M, Mitsuhashi S. Transferable imipenem resistance in *Pseudomonas aeruginosa*. Antimicrob Agents Chemother. 1991;35(1):147–51.

3. Zhao WH, Hu ZQ. IMP-type metallo-beta-lactamases in Gram-negative bacilli: distribution, phylogeny, and association with integrons. Crit Rev Microbiol. 2011;37(3):214–26.
4. Ho PL, Lo WU, Chan J, Cheung YY, Chow KH, Yam WC, Lin CH, Que TL. pIMP-PH114 carrying bla IMP-4 in a *Klebsiella pneumoniae* strain is closely related to other multidrug-resistant IncA/C2 plasmids. Curr Microbiol. 2014;68(2):227–32.
5. Peirano G, Lascols C, Hackel M, Hoban DJ, Pitout JD. Molecular epidemiology of Enterobacteriaceae that produce VIMs and IMPs from the SMART surveillance program. Diagn Microbiol Infect Dis. 2014;78(3):277–81.
6. Wang JT, Wu UI, Lauderdale TL, Chen MC, Li SY, Hsu LY, Chang SC. Carbapenem-nonsusceptible Enterobacteriaceae in Taiwan. PLoS ONE. 2015;10(3):e0121668.
7. Feng W, Zhou D, Wang Q, Luo W, Zhang D, Sun Q, Tong Y, Chen W, Sun F, Xia P. Dissemination of IMP-4-encoding pIMP-HZ1-related plasmids among *Klebsiella pneumoniae* and *Pseudomonas aeruginosa* in a Chinese teaching hospital. Sci Rep. 2016;6:33419.
8. Fukigai S, Alba J, Kimura S, Iida T, Nishikura N, Ishii Y, Yamaguchi K. Nosocomial outbreak of genetically related IMP-1 beta-lactamase-producing *Klebsiella pneumoniae* in a general hospital in Japan. Int J Antimicrob Agents. 2007;29(3):306–10.
9. Yu F, Ying Q, Chen C, Li T, Ding B, Liu Y, Lu Y, Qin Z, Parsons C, Salgado C, et al. Outbreak of pulmonary infection caused by *Klebsiella pneumoniae* isolates harbouring blaIMP-4 and blaDHA-1 in a neonatal intensive care unit in China. J Med Microbiol. 2012;61(Pt 7):984–9.
10. Wang Y, Cao W, Zhu X, Chen Z, Li L, Zhang B, Wang B, Tian L, Wang F, Liu C, et al. Characterization of a novel *Klebsiella pneumoniae* sequence type 476 carrying both bla KPC-2 and bla IMP-4. Eur J Clin Microbiol Infect Dis. 2012;31(8):1867–72.
11. Ho PL, Cheung YY, Wang Y, Lo WU, Lai EL, Chow KH, Cheng VC. Characterization of carbapenem-resistant *Escherichia coli* and *Klebsiella pneumoniae* from a healthcare region in Hong Kong. Eur J Clin Microbiol Infect Dis. 2016;35(3):379–85.
12. Yan JJ, Ko WC, Wu JJ. Identification of a plasmid encoding SHV-12, TEM-1, and a variant of IMP-2 metallo-beta-lactamase, IMP-8, from a clinical isolate of *Klebsiella pneumoniae*. Antimicrob Agents Chemother. 2001;45(8):2368–71.
13. Yang Q, Wang H, Sun H, Chen H, Xu Y, Chen M. Phenotypic and genotypic characterization of Enterobacteriaceae with decreased susceptibility to carbapenems: results from large hospital-based surveillance studies in China. Antimicrob Agents Chemother. 2010;54(1):573–7.
14. Xia Y, Liang Z, Su X, Xiong Y. Characterization of carbapenemase genes in Enterobacteriaceae species exhibiting decreased susceptibility to carbapenems in a university hospital in Chongqing, China. Ann Lab Med. 2012;32(4):270–5.
15. Chen S, Feng W, Chen J, Liao W, He N, Wang Q, Sun F, Xia P. Spread of carbapenemase-producing enterobacteria in a southwest hospital in China. Ann Clin Microbiol Antimicrob. 2014;13:42.
16. Jian Z, Li Y, Liu W, Li H, Zhang Y, Gu X, Peng W. Detection of the novel IMP-38 among carbapenemase-producing Enterobacteriaceae in a university hospital, China. J Infect Dev Ctries. 2014;8(8):1044–8.
17. Li H, Zhang J, Liu Y, Zheng R, Chen H, Wang X, Wang Z, Cao B, Wang H. Molecular characteristics of carbapenemase-producing Enterobacteriaceae in China from 2008 to 2011: predominance of KPC-2 enzyme. Diagn Microbiol Infect Dis. 2014;78(1):63–5.
18. Hu L, Zhong Q, Shang Y, Wang H, Ning C, Li Y, Hang Y, Xiong J, Wang X, Xu Y, et al. The prevalence of carbapenemase genes and plasmid-mediated quinolone resistance determinants in carbapenem-resistant Enterobacteriaceae from five teaching hospitals in central China. Epidemiol Infect. 2014;142(9):1972–7.
19. Wei Z, Yu T, Qi Y, Ji S, Shen P, Yu Y, Chen Y. Coexistence of plasmid-mediated KPC-2 and IMP-4 carbapenemases in isolates of *Klebsiella pneumoniae* from China. J Antimicrob Chemother. 2011;66(11):2670–1.
20. Li B, Xu XH, Zhao ZC, Wang MH, Cao YP. High prevalence of metallo-beta-lactamase among carbapenem-resistant *Klebsiella pneumoniae* in a teaching hospital in China. Can J Microbiol. 2014;60(10):691–5.
21. Lo WU, Cheung YY, Lai E, Lung D, Que TL, Ho PL. Complete sequence of an IncN plasmid, pIMP-HZ1, carrying blaIMP-4 in a *Klebsiella pneumoniae* strain associated with medical travel to China. Antimicrob Agents Chemother. 2013;57(3):1561–2.
22. Cao XL, Cheng L, Zhang ZF, Ning MZ, Zhou WQ, Zhang K, Shen H. Survey of clinical extended-spectrum beta-lactamase-producing enterobacter cloacae isolates in a Chinese Tertiary Hospital, 2012–2014. Microb Drug Resist. 2017;23(1):83–9.
23. CLSI. Performance standards for antimicrobial susceptibility testing. 27th ed. Wayne: Clinical and Laboratory Standards Institute, 950 West Valley Road, Suite 2500; 2017.
24. Yang J, Ye L, Guo L, Zhao Q, Chen R, Luo Y, Chen Y, Tian S, Zhao J, Shen D, et al. A nosocomial outbreak of KPC-2-producing *Klebsiella pneumoniae* in a Chinese hospital: dissemination of ST11 and emergence of ST37, ST392 and ST395. Clin Microbiol Infect. 2013;19(11):E509–15.
25. An J, Guo L, Zhou L, Ma Y, Luo Y, Tao C, Yang J. NDM-producing Enterobacteriaceae in a Chinese hospital, 2014–2015: identification of NDM-producing Citrobacter werkmanii and acquisition of blaNDM-1-carrying plasmid in vivo in a clinical *Escherichia coli* isolate. J Med Microbiol. 2016;65(11):1253–9.
26. Guo L, An J, Ma Y, Ye L, Luo Y, Tao C, Yang J. Nosocomial outbreak of OXA-48-producing *Klebsiella pneumoniae* in a Chinese hospital: clonal transmission of ST147 and ST383. PLoS ONE. 2016;11(8):e0160754.
27. Chmelnitsky I, Shklyar M, Hermesh O, Navon-Venezia S, Edgar R, Carmeli Y. Unique genes identified in the epidemic extremely drug-resistant KPC-producing *Klebsiella pneumoniae* sequence type 258. J Antimicrob Chemother. 2013;68(1):74–83.
28. Brisse S, Fevre C, Passet V, Issenhuth-Jeanjean S, Tournebize R, Diancourt L, Grimont P. Virulent clones of Klebsiella pneumoniae: identification and evolutionary scenario based on genomic and phenotypic characterization. PLoS ONE. 2009;4(3):e4982.
29. Tada T, Nhung PH, Miyoshi-Akiyama T, Shimada K, Tsuchiya M, Phuong DM, Anh NQ, Ohmagari N, Kirikae T. Multidrug-resistant sequence type 235 *Pseudomonas aeruginosa* clinical isolates producing IMP-26 with increased carbapenem-hydrolyzing activities in vietnam. Antimicrob Agents Chemother. 2016;60(11):6853–8.
30. Zavascki AP, Carvalhaes CG, Picao RC, Gales AC. Multidrug-resistant *Pseudomonas aeruginosa* and *Acinetobacter baumannii*: resistance mechanisms and implications for therapy. Expert Rev Anti Infect Ther. 2010;8(1):71–93.

13

Occurrence of co-existing bla_{VIM-2} and bla_{NDM-1} in clinical isolates of *Pseudomonas aeruginosa* from India

Deepjyoti Paul[1], Debadatta Dhar[2], Anand Prakash Maurya[1], Shweta Mishra[3], Gauri Dutt Sharma[4], Atanu Chakravarty[2] and Amitabha Bhattacharjee[1*]

Abstract

Background: bla_{VIM-2} harboring *Pseudomonas aeruginosa* has been reported worldwide and considered as the most prevalent metallo-β-lactamase after NDM which are found horizontally transferable and mostly associated with integron gene cassettes. The present study investigates the genetic background, transmission dynamics as well as stability of bla_{VIM-2} in clinical isolates of *P. aeruginosa* harbor bla_{NDM-1} as well which were collected from October 2012 to September 2013.

Methods: Two *P. aeruginosa* strains harboring bla_{VIM-2} along with bla_{NDM-1} were isolated from Silchar Medical College and Hospital, India. Genetic environment of these resistance determinants was determined and transferability was checked by transformation and conjugation assay which was further confirmed by Southern hybridization. Replicon typing was performed to determine the incompatibility group of the resistant plasmid and their stability was checked by serial passage method. Antimicrobial susceptibility pattern of the isolates was determined and their clonal relatedness was checked by pulsed field gel electrophoresis.

Results: bla_{VIM-2} was found to be horizontally transferable through an Inc F type plasmid of approximately 30 kb in size. bla_{VIM-2} was found to be associated with integron gene cassette and was flanked by two different types of cassette arrays. Both the isolates were co-harboring bla_{NDM-1} which was carried within Inc N type of plasmid with an approximate 24 kb in size and associated with IS*Aba125* in their upstream region. Reduced susceptibility rate as well as high MIC range was observed in case of wild strains and transformants carrying bla_{VIM-2} and bla_{NDM-1}.

Conclusions: The detection of this co-existence of multiple carbapenem resistance genes in this part of world is worrisome and further investigation is required in order to trace the source and to initiate proper treatment option.

Keywords: bla_{VIM-2}, bla_{NDM-1}, Integron, Inc F type, *Pseudomonas aeruginosa*

Background

Carbapenems are considered as the last drug of choice for most of the serious infections caused by Gram negative bacteria, but due to the prevalence of multidrug resistant organisms these lifesaving drugs were compromised in treating the patients with severe illness. Gram negative bacteria have been documented as the most serious threat in the management of acute infections, as of exhibiting resistance to antibiotics due to the production of carbapenemase enzyme especially metallo-β-lactamase [1, 2]. *Pseudomonas aeruginosa* is one of the most common nosocomial pathogen causing acute infections and frequently reported for carbapenem resistance. VIM metallo-β-lactamase, the second most predominant MBL type responsible for antimicrobial resistance, is pandemic and becoming a health hazard. Among the 37 variant of VIM enzymes, bla_{VIM-2} has now been spread as prevalent MBL among *P. aeruginosa* in all European countries [3] whereas bla_{NDM-1} and bla_{VIM-18} has known to be originated from India [4, 5] where irrational use of

*Correspondence: ab0404@gmail.com
[1] Department of Microbiology, Assam University, Silchar, India
Full list of author information is available at the end of the article

antibiotic is a major contributor for their emergence [6]. VIM and NDM type of MBLs are horizontally transferable and found to be associated with mobile genetic elements, however few molecular information and genetic context is available from this part of India. The potential for quick and extensive dissemination rate of these resistance genes make over a great concern. The present study describes genetic background, transmission dynamics as well as stability of *bla*$_{\text{VIM-2}}$ and *bla*$_{\text{NDM-1}}$ in clinical isolates of *P. aeruginosa*.

Methods

Bacterial collection

From October 2012 to September 2013, a total of seventeen *P. aeruginosa* with reduced susceptibility to at least a single carbapenem were collected from Silchar Medical College and Hospital, Silchar. The isolates were then identified by standard biochemical reactions, cytochrome oxidase activity, citrate utilization, pigment production and growth on Cetrimide agar [7].

Characterization of carbapenemases

For detection of carbapenemase production, isolates were subjected to modified Hodge test (MHT) and imipenem-EDTA disc test for metallo-β-lactamase production [4]. MHT uses *Escherichia coli* ATCC 25922 as an indicator organism. The presence of clover leaf like indentation in MHT was interpreted as a positive result for carbapenem hydrolysis.

Molecular characterization of *bla*$_{\text{VIM}}$ and *bla*$_{\text{NDM}}$ gene

PCR assay was performed for detection of *bla*$_{\text{VIM}}$ as described earlier [8] as well as other metallo-β-lactamase gene (*bla*$_{\text{NDM}}$, *bla*$_{\text{IMP}}$, *bla*$_{\text{GIM}}$, *bla*$_{\text{SIM}}$, *bla*$_{\text{SMB}}$) [4] and amplified products were further sequenced to confirm the presence of resistant gene.

Detection of co-existing of ESBL genes

Co-existence of ESBL genes were determined by multiplex PCR targeting *bla*$_{\text{TEM}}$, *bla*$_{\text{PER}}$, *bla*$_{\text{OXA-2}}$, *bla*$_{\text{SHV}}$, *bla*$_{\text{CTX-M}}$, *bla*$_{\text{VEB}}$ and *bla*$_{\text{GES}}$ [9]. Reactions were performed under the following conditions: initial denaturation at 94 °C for 5 min, 33 cycles of 94 °C for 35 s, 51 °C for 1 min, 72 °C for 1 min and final extension at 72 °C for 7 min. The amplified products were further sequenced to confirm the co-existence of ESBL genes.

Detection of genetic context of *bla*$_{\text{VIM-2}}$

Genetic environment of *bla*$_{\text{VIM-2}}$ was determined by performing integrase gene PCR [10] for characterizing the class 1 and class 2 integron. The conserved sequences 5′CS and 3′CS flanking the *bla*$_{\text{VIM}}$ were determined using two sets of primers 5′CS and the reverse primer of *bla*$_{\text{VIM}}$, 3′CS and forward primer of *bla*$_{\text{VIM}}$ as described earlier [10]. Amplified products were sequenced to determine genetic map of *bla*$_{\text{VIM-2}}$. The reaction condition was: initial denaturation at 95 °C for 3 min, 34 cycles at 95 °C for 30 s, 46 °C for 1 min, 72 °C for 3 min and final extension at 72 °C for 7 min. The presence of mobile element like ISCR in each strain was determined by performing PCR using primers ISCR F (5′-RNSBATAGGAADWWNAAHMNV-3′) and ISCR R (5′-BNKDTTNWWHTTCCTATVSNY-3′).

Determination of genetic environment of *bla*$_{\text{NDM-1}}$

Integron carriage was assessed by performing integrase gene PCR for characterizing the class 1 and class 2 integron. PCR reaction conditions followed was described as earlier [10]. The flanking region of *bla*$_{\text{NDM}}$ were determined using two sets of primers 5CS and the reverse primer of *bla*$_{\text{NDM}}$, 3CS and forward primer of *bla*$_{\text{NDM}}$ [10]. The linkage of *bla*$_{\text{NDM-1}}$ with insertion sequence IS*Aba125* was determined by using forward primer of IS*Aba125* (5′GAA ACT GTC GCA CCT CAT GTT TG-3′) and reverse of *bla*$_{\text{NDM-1}}$ (5′-GTA GTG CTC AGT GTC GGC AT-3′) [11].

Plasmid analysis, transformation and conjugation assay

bla$_{\text{VIM}}$ positive bacterial isolates were cultured in Luria–Bertani broth (Hi-Media, India) containing 0.25 μg/ml of imipenem. After overnight incubation, plasmids were extracted by using QIAprep Spin Miniprep Kit (Qiagen, Germany). Isolated plasmids were transformed into recipient strain *Escherichia coli* JM107 by heat shock method and transformants were selected on LB agar with 0.25μg/ml of imipenem. Conjugation experiment was carried out using *bla*$_{\text{VIM-2}}$ and *bla*$_{\text{NDM-1}}$ harboring transformants as donors and a streptomycin resistant *E. coli* recipient strain B (Genei, India), both the donor and reciepient cells were cultured in Luria–Bertani Broth (Hi-Media, India) till it reach an O.D. of 0.8–0.9 at A_{600}. Cells were mixed at 1:5 donor-to-recipient ratios and transconjugants were selected on imipenem (0.25 μg/ml) and streptomycin (400 μg/ml) agar plates. Additionally conjugation experiment was also tried using *P. aeruginosa* harboring *bla*$_{\text{NDM-1}}$ and *bla*$_{\text{VIM-2}}$ as donor and *E. coli* strain B as recipient.

Southern hybridization for detection of transferability

Southern blotting was performed on agarose gel by in-gel hybridization with the *bla*$_{\text{VIM-2}}$ and *bla*$_{\text{NDM-1}}$ probe labelled with DIG HIGH PRIME LABELING MIX (Roche, Germany) detection Kit. The digoxigenin-labeled *bla*$_{\text{VIM-2}}$ and *bla*$_{\text{NDM-1}}$ specific probe was prepared using primers VIM-F, VIM-R, NDM-F and NDM-R. Plasmid DNA from transformants and transconjugants was separated by PFGE (CHEF DR-III System, Bio-Rad; USA) and transferred to nylon membrane (Hybond N, UK) and then hybridised with prepared bla_{VIM} and bla_{NDM} specific probe. Detection was performed by using an NBT color detection Kit (Roche, Germany).

PCR based replicon typing

The incompatibility type of the plasmids encoding $bla_{\text{VIM-2}}$ and $bla_{\text{NDM-1}}$ were characterized by PCR based replicon typing targeting 18 different replicon types such as FIA, FIB, FIC, HI1, HI2, I1/Iγ, L/M, N, P, W, T, A/C, K, B/O, X, Y, F and FIIA [12].

Antibiotic susceptibility and minimum inhibitory concentration (MIC)

Antimicrobial susceptibility of parent strains as well as transformants was determined by Kirby-Bauer disc diffusion method against β-lactam and non-β-lactam antibiotics (Hi-Media, India). MIC was also determined by agar dilution method for the isolates and the transformants carrying $P^{\text{VIM}-2}$ and $P^{\text{NDM}-1}$ towards imipenem (Merck, France), meropenem (AstraZeneca, UK), cefepime, aztreonam (Aristo, India), amikacin (Zuche pharmaceuticals, India), gentamicin (Pharmakem, India), ciprofloxacin(Ranbaxy, India), piperacillin-tazobactam (Alkem, India) and polymixin-B (Samarth, India) and interpreted as per CLSI guidelines [13].

Stability of $bla_{\text{VIM-2}}$ and $bla_{\text{NDM-1}}$

Stability of $bla_{\text{VIM-2}}$ and $bla_{\text{NDM-1}}$ gene was determined by serial passage of the isolates as well as of the transformants in 1:1000 ratios without antibiotic pressure [14]. After each passage the test isolates were subjected to phenotypic detection of MBL and further confirmed the presence of bla_{VIM} and bla_{NDM} by PCR assay.

Pulsed field gel electrophoresis

bla_{VIM} and bla_{NDM} positive isolates were typed by pulsed field gel electrophoresis where chromosomal DNA was prepared in agarose blocks and digested with restriction enzyme *Xba*1 (Promega, USA). DNA fragments were separated with CHEF-DR III apparatus (Bio-Rad, USA) and the electrophoresis conditions used were for 24 h at 6 V/cm with pulse rate of 10–40 s as described previously [15]. Clonal relatedness within the isolates was determined by comparing the band patterns.

Ethical approval

The work was approved by Institutional Ethical committee of Assam University, Silchar vide Reference Number: IEC/AUS/C/2014-001. The authors confirm that participants provided their written informed consent to participate in this study.

Results

Two clinical isolates of *P. aeruginosa* (PA-37 and PA-131) harboring bla_{VIM} were recovered from Silchar Medical College and Hospital, India. The gene was further sequenced and confirmed as $bla_{\text{VIM-2}}$ variant. The first isolate (PA-37) was recovered from pus samples of a 55 year old female patient suffering from wound infection admitted in surgery ward in December 2012 while the second one (PA-131) was isolated from urine of a 40 years old female patient with UTI, who attended gynecology outpatient department (OPD) in the month of February 2013. $bla_{\text{VIM-2}}$ was found to be horizontally transferable as the gene could be successfully conjugatively transferred from transformed *E. coli* JM107 to recipient *E. coli* strain B through an Inc F type plasmid having approximate size of 30 kb. These findings were further confirmed by Southern hybridization results. However, conjugative transfer of plasmids from *P. aeruginosa* to *E. coli* was not successful with our experiment. In both the isolates $bla_{\text{VIM-2}}$ was located within integron gene cassette and was flanked by other antimicrobial resistant determinant like gene for aminoglycoside resistance (Fig. 1). The two different types of cassette arrays observed were $bla_{\text{VIM-2}}$-*aad*B-*dhfr*A-orfC-*qac*E-*sul*1 (PA-37) and *aad*B-*aac*A7-$bla_{\text{VIM-2}}$-*dhfr*A1-orfC-*qac*E-sul1 (PA-131). Both the isolates were co-harboring $bla_{\text{NDM-1}}$ and further ESBL screening revealed the presence of $bla_{\text{VEB-1}}$ gene in these isolates. However, $bla_{\text{NDM-1}}$ gene could not be hybridized with 30 kb plasmid that was harboring $bla_{\text{VIM-2}}$, but with a 24 kb plasmid which was successfully hybridized with $bla_{\text{NDM-1}}$ specific probe (Fig. 2). Linkage of IS*Aba125* was observed in the upstream region of $bla_{\text{NDM-1}}$ whereas no association with integron gene cassette could be established. Interestingly on analyzing the stability of MBL genes i.e. $bla_{\text{VIM-2}}$ and $bla_{\text{NDM-1}}$, in case of wild type isolates these resistant genes were stable even after hundred consecutive passages but among their transformants, complete plasmid was lost after fifty-six passages in case of $bla_{\text{VIM-2}}$ while $bla_{\text{NDM-1}}$was retained till ninety passages without any antibiotic pressure. These $bla_{\text{VIM-2}}$ positive

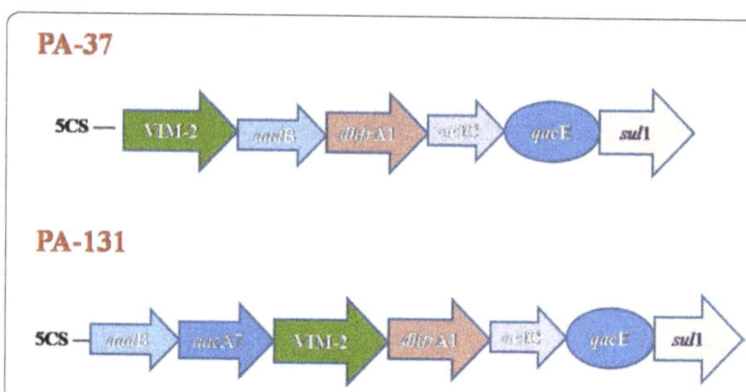

Fig. 1 Genetic Context of $bla_{\text{VIM-2}}$

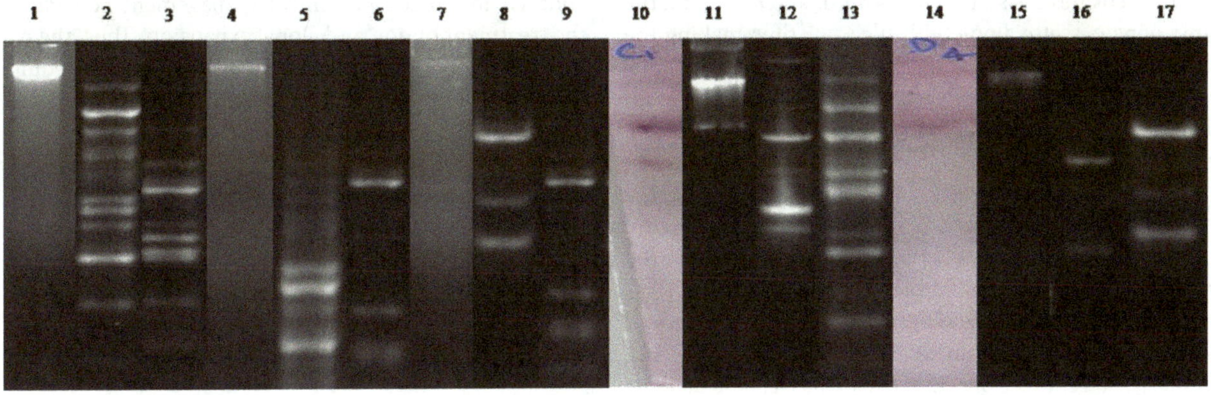

Fig. 2 PFGE and hybridization analysis of bla_{NDM-1}. *Lane 1* and *4* The undigested total DNA of PA 37 and PA 131 respectively; *Lane 2* and 3 The PA 37 total DNA is digested with S1 and *Xba* I respectively; *Lane 5* and *6* PA 131 total DNA digested with S1 and *Xba* I respectively; *Lane 7* The undigested plasmid of PA 37; *Lane 8* and *9 E. coli* transconjugant carrying plasmid of PA 37 digested with S1 and *Xba* I respectively; *Lane 10* Hybridized $P^{PA\ 37}$ with probe; *Lane 11* The undigested plasmid of PA 131; *Lane 12* and *13 E. coli* transconjugant carrying plasmid of PA 131 digested with S1 and *Xba* I respectively; *Lane 14* Hybridized $P^{PA\ 131}$ with probe; *Lane 15* The total DNA of recipient *E. coli* without plasmid; *Lane 16* and *17* The total DNA of recipient *E. coli* without plasmid digested with S1 and *Xba* I respectively

isolates showed resistance towards most of the antibiotics including piperacillin/tazobactam, co-trimoxazole, amikacin, gentamicin, netilmicin and quinolone group of drugs. MIC values obtained for both the isolates were above breakpoint towards ciprofloxacin, aminoglycosides, β-lactam-β-lactamase inhibitor as well as to polymixin B (Table 1). The two bla_{VIM-2} harboring isolates of *P. aeruginosa* were found to be clonally different from each other on the basis of their PFGE banding pattern (Fig. 2).

Discussion

It has been evidenced that the rapid emergence and dissemination of carbapenemase producing bacteria in this subcontinent is mainly due to the acquisition of bla_{NDM} [4]. But in the present study, we described an additional carbapenem resistance determinant i.e. bla_{VIM-2} which played a significant role in carbapenem resistance. Although bla_{VIM-2} with integron gene cassette is reported in previous studies [8], while in the present study, the genetic context of bla_{VIM-2} underscores their diverse origin and persistence along with other resistant genes. In the present study bla_{VIM-2} was found to be associated with the gene cassette along with other resistance determinants which is in agreement to the reports of Toleman et al. [16]. The association of other resistance determinants along with VIM type MBL confers the phenotype to become resistant to most of the available antimicrobial agents. The study reports the presence of

Table 1 MIC (μg/ml) of the bla_{VIM-2} and bla_{NDM-1} harboring isolates and their transformants

Organisms	Imipenem	Meropenem	Cefepime	Aztreonam	Amikacin	Gentamicin	Ciprofloxacin	Piperacillin-tazobactam	Polymixin B
PA-37[a]	>256	>256	>256	>256	>256	>256	256	>256	>256
E. coli JM107 (p^{VIM-2}/37)[b]	64	32	128	64	128	64	64	64	32
E. coli JM107 (p^{NDM-1}/37)[c]	64	64	128	64	128	128	64	64	32
PA-131[a]	>256	128	>256	>256	>256	>256	256	>256	256
E. coli JM107 (p^{VIM-2}/131)[b]	16	16	64	64	64	64	64	64	32
E. coli JM107 (p^{NDM-1}/131)[c]	32	16	128	64	64	64	64	64	16
E. coli JM107	0.06	0.012	0.06	0.12	0.06	0.125	0.06	0.12	0.006

[a] Donor strain

[b] Recipient *E. coli* carrying plasmid of bla_{VIM-2}

[c] Recipient *E. coli* carrying plasmid of bla_{NDM-1}

aminoglycosides resistance genes *aad*B and *aac*A7 on the same gene cassette along with bla_{VIM-2}, thus making the phenotype resistance to amikacin and gentamicin as well. In the year 2012, Toleman et al. [11] reported the association of insertion sequence IS*Aba125* in the upstream region of bla_{NDM-1} in *Acinetobacter baumanii*, we too observed the same insertion sequence present in the upstream region of bla_{NDM-1} in *P. aeruginosa*. Presence of NDM-1 in *P. aeruginosa* was for first time recorded in 2011 from patients in Serbia [17] and the same working group has reported that resistance determinant is chromosomally located in this particular organism [18]. Similarly, a report from India also has established its chromosomal location [19]. However, in our recent study we found presence of bla_{NDM-1} on plasmid DNA indicating a possible shift from one to another genetic location [20]. Future experiments will show which direction (chromosome to plasmid or vice versa) of the transfer took place in the organism. High MIC range as well as reduced susceptibility rate against majority of the tested antibiotics was observed in case of bla_{VIM-2} and bla_{NDM-1} harboring wild strains and transformants of bla_{VIM-2} and bla_{NDM-1}. Earlier studies reported [16] that carbapenemase producing isolates remain susceptible to polymixin B whereas both of our study isolates were found to be resistant to this antibiotic, which could be a challenging situation with no or too limited treatment option. The association of mobile genetic element with bla_{VIM-2} may facilitate their mobilization to other susceptible organisms. On performing the transmission dynamics of the strains and it was evident that bla_{VIM-2} and bla_{NDM-1} was horizontally transferable. It may be noted that in our study, the plasmid of *P. aeruginosa* encoding the NDM-1 was conjugally transferred from the *E. coli* transformants to recipient *E. coli* strain although conjugation of the same plasmid was not successful from original host *P. aeruginosa* to *E. coli*. The reason for absence of plasmid conjugation could be due to presence of some physiological barriers within these two strains or we did not find the appropriate laboratory conditions for initiation of conjugation or present plasmid do not carry functional Tra operon in *P. aeruginosa*. Serial passage of transformants harboring both bla_{VIM-2} and bla_{NDM-1} showed that bla_{NDM-1} gene is more stable compare to bla_{VIM-2}, may be because *E. coli* is an unnatural host for bla_{VIM-2}. The distinguishable pulsotypes of the two strains along with their different genetic arrangements indicates horizontal acquisition from diverse source and antibiotic pressure in this hospital setting.

Conclusions

Co-existence of multiple carbapenem resistance determinants in hospital isolate is worrisome and a matter of concern for infection control management considering the treatment option and clonal expansion. Thus, the current finding is of epidemiological interest, which requires immediate steps to initiate proper treatment option.

Abbreviations

VIM: Verona integron-encoded MBL; NDM: New Delhi metallo-β-lactamase; MBLs: metallo-β-lactamases; *Bla*: beta-lactamase; MHT: modified Hodge test; PCR: polymerase chain reaction; SIM: Seoul imipenemase; GIM: German imipenemase; SMB: Serratia metallo-β-lactamase; ESBL: extended spectrum beta-lactamase; 5CS & 3CS: 5′ & 3′-conserved segments; ISCR: insertion sequence common region; MIC: minimum inhibitory concentration; PFGE: pulse field gel electrophoresis; UTI: urinary tract infection; CLSI: Clinical and Laboratory Standards Institute.

Authors' contributions

DP: Design and performed the experimental work, literature search, data collection, analysis and prepared the manuscript. DD: Participated in experiment designing and manuscript correction. APM: Participated in sample collection and part of experiments. SM: Carried out the Southern hybridization experiment and result analysis. AC: Participated in experiment designing and manuscript correction. GDS: Participated in drafting the manuscript. AB: Supervised the research work and participated in designing the study and drafting the manuscript. All authors read and approved the final manuscript.

Author details

[1] Department of Microbiology, Assam University, Silchar, India. [2] Department of Microbiology, Silchar Medical College and Hospital, Silchar, India. [3] Department of Microbiology, Institute of Medical Sciences, Banaras Hindu University, Varanasi, India. [4] Department of Life Science and Bioinformatics, Assam University, Silchar, India.

Acknowledgements

The authors would like to acknowledge the support of HOD, Microbiology, Assam University for providing infrastructural facility. The authors sincerely acknowledge the financial support provided by Council of Scientific and Industrial Research and Department of Biotechnology (DBT-NER twinning Scheme) to carry out the work. Authors also acknowledge the help from Assam University Biotech Hub for providing laboratory facility to complete this work.

Competing interests

The authors declare that they have no competing interests.

Funding

Council of Scientific and Industrial Research (CSIR Grant Number: 37(1632)/14/EMR-II) and Department of Bio-technology (DBT-NER Twinning Scheme, BT/215/NE/TBP/2011 dtd.15/11/2011) Government of India.

References

1. Patel G, Bonomo RA. "Stormy waters ahead": global emergence of carbapenemases. Front Microbiol. 2013;48:1–17.
2. Cornaglia G, Giamarellou H, Rossolini GM. Metallo-β-lactamase: a last frontier for β lactams? Lancet Infect Dis. 2011;11:381–93.
3. Tato M, Coque TM, Baquero F, Canton R. Dispersal of carbapenemase bla_{VIM-1} gene associated with different Tn402 variants, mercury transposons and conjugative plasmids in enterobacteriaceae and *Pseudomonas aeruginosa*. Antimicrob Agents Chemother. 2010;54:320–7.
4. Yong D, Toleman MA, Giske CG, Cho HS, Sundman K, Lee K. Characterization of a New Metallo-β-Lactamase Gene, bla_{NDM-1}, and a Novel Erythromycin Esterase Gene Carried on a Unique Genetic Structure in

Klebsiella pneumoniae Sequence Type 14 from India. Antimicrob Agents Chemother. 2009;53:5046–54.

5. Castanheira M, Bell JM, Turnidge JD, Mathai D, Jones RN. Carbapenem resistance among *Pseudomonas aeruginosa* strains from India: evidence for nationwide endemicity of multiple metallo-beta-lactamase clones (VIM-2,-5,-6, and -11 and the newly characterized VIM-18). Antimicrob Agents Chemother. 2009;53:1225–7.
6. Kumarasamy KK, Toleman MA, Walsh TR, Bagaria J, Butt F, Balakrishnan R, Chaudhary U, Doumith M, Giske CG, Irfan S, Krishnan P, Kumar AV, Maharjan S, Mushtaq S, Noorie T, Paterson D, Pearson A, Perry C, Pike R, Rao B, Ray U, Sarma JB, Sharma M, Sheridan E, Thirunarayan MA, Turton J, Upadhyay S, Warner M, Welfare W, Livermore DM, Woodford N. Emergence of a new antibiotic resistance mechanism in India, Pakistan, and the UK: a molecular, biological, and epidemiological study. Lancet Infect Dis. 2010;10:597–602.
7. Colee JG, Diguid JP, Mackie Fraser AG, Microbiology McCartney Practical Medical. 14th edn. Edinburgh: Churchill, Livingstone; 1996.
8. Jh Y. Yi K, Lee H, Yong D, Lee K, Kim JM, Rossolini GM, Chong Y. Molecular characterization of metallo-β-lacatamase-producing *Acinetobacter baumannii* and *Acinetbacter genomospecies* 3 from Korea: identification of two new integrons carrying the bla_{VIM-2} gene cassettes. J Antimicrob Chemother. 2002;49:837–40.
9. Lee S, Park YJ, Kim M, Lee HK, Han K, Kang CS. Prevalence of Ambler class A and D β- lactamases among clinical isolates of *Pseudomonas aeruginosa* in Korea. J Antimicrob Chemother. 2005;56:122–7.
10. Koeleman JGM, Stoof J, Der Bijl MWV, Vandenbroucke-grauls CMJE, Savelkoul PHM. Identification of Epidemic Strains of *Acinetobacter baumannii* by Integrase Gene PCR. J Clin Microbiol. 2001;39:8–13.
11. Toleman MA, Spencer J, Jones L, Walsh TR. bla_{NDM-1} is a chimera likely constructed in *Acinetobacter baumannii*. Antimicrob Agents Chemother. 2012;56:2773.
12. Carattoli A, Bertini A, Villa L, Falbo V, Hopkins KL, Threlfall EJ. Identification of plasmids by PCR-based replicon typing. J Microbiol Methods. 2005;63:219–28.
13. Clinical Laboratory Standard Institute. Performance Standards for Antimicrobial Susceptibility Testing; Twenty-Third Informational Supplement. 2013; M100-S23. CLSI, Wayne.
14. Locke JB, Rahawi S, LaMarre J, Mankin LS, Shawa KJ. Genetic Environment and Stability of *cfr* in Methicillin-resistant *Staphylococcus aureus* CM05. Antimicrob Agents and Chemother. 2012;56:332–40.
15. Tato M, Coque TM, Ruiz-Garbajosa P, Pintado V, Cobo J, Sader HS, Jones RN, Baquero F. Complex clonal and plasmid epidemiology in the first outbreak of enterobacteriaceae infection involving VIM-1 metallo-β-lactamase in Spain: towards endemicity? Clin Infect Dis. 2007;45:1171–8.
16. Toleman MA, Vinodh H, Sekar U, Kamat V, Walsh TR. bla_{VIM-2}- harboring integrons isolated in India, Russia, and the United States arise from an ancestral class 1 integron predating the formation of the 3′conserved sequence. Antimicrob Agents and Chemother. 2007;51:2636–8.
17. Jovcic B, Lepsanovic Z, Suljagic V, Rackov G, Begovic J, Topisirovic L, Kojic M. Emergence of NDM-1 metallo-β-lactamase in *Pseudomonas aeruginosa* clinical isolates from Servia. Antimicrob Agents Chemother. 2011;55:3929–31.
18. Jovcic B, Lepsanovic Z, Begovic J, Rakonjac B, Perovanovic J, Topisirovic L, Kojic M. The clinical isolate *Pseudomonas aeruginosa* MMA83 carries two copies of the bla_{NDM-1} gene in a novel genetic context. Antimicrob Agents Chemother. 2013;57:3405–7.
19. Mishra S, Upadhyay S, Sen MR, Maurya AP, Choudhury D, Bhattacharjee A. Genetic Acquisition of NDM Gene Offers Sustainability among Clinical Isolates of *Pseudomonas aeruginosa* in Clinical Settings. PLoS ONE. 2015;10(1):e0116611. doi:10.1371/journal.pone.0116611.
20. Paul D, Dhar Chanda D, Maurya AP, Mishra S, Chakravarty A, Sharma GD, Bhattacharjee A. Co-Carriage of bla_{KPC-2} and bla_{NDM-1} in Clinical Isolates of *Pseudomonas aeruginosa* Associated with Hospital Infections from India. PLoS ONE. 2015;10(12):e0145823. doi:10.1371/journal.pone.0145823.

The potential of bacteriophage cocktail in eliminating Methicillin-resistant *Staphylococcus aureus* biofilms in terms of different extracellular matrices expressed by *PIA*, *ciaA-D* and *FnBPA* genes

Ahmed Sahib Abdulamir[1*], Sabah A. A. Jassim[2,3], Rand R. Hafidh[4] and Fatimah Abu Bakar[5*]

Abstract

Background: This study assessed novel approach of using highly lytic phages against methicillin-susceptible *Staphylococcus aureus* (MSSA) and methicillin-resistant *Staphylococcus aureus* (MRSA) biofilms with and without biofilm extracellular matrix- disrupting chemical.

Method: The resultant phage-based control was assessed in relation to the type of biofilm extracellular matrix namely, polysaccharide intercellular adhesion (PIA) or proteinacious fibronectin-binding protein A (FnBPA). The biofilms were formed in vitro by 24 h incubation of bacteria in 96 wells microtiter plates at room temperature. The formed biofilms were assessed by tissue culture plate (TCP). Moreover, the nature of the biofilm was assessed by scanning electron microscopy (SEM) and PCR assay for detecting PIA genes, *ciaA-D* and FnBPA genes.

Results: this study showed that applied phages with 0.08 % benezenthonium chloride, for PIA biofilms, and 0.06 % ethanol, for proteinacious FnBPA biofilms, exerted 100 % eradication for MSSA biofilms and about 78 % of MRSA biofilms. The phage-based control of biofilms with chemical adjuvant showed significantly higher efficiency than that without adjuvant ($P < 0.05$). Moreover, FnBPA biofilms were more common in MRSA than in MSSA while PIA biofilms were more common in MSSA than in MRSA. And the most resistant type of biofilms to phage-based control was FnBPA in MRSA where 50 % of biofilms were reduced but not eradicated completely.

Conclusions: It is concluded that PIA-disturbing agent and protein denaturing alcohol can increase the efficiency of attacking phages in accessing host cell walls and lysing them which in turn lead to much more efficient MRSA and MSSA biofilm treatment and prevention.

Keywords: Methicillin-resistant *Staphylococcus aureus*, MRSA, MSSA, Biofilm, Bacteriophages, PIA, FnBPA

Background

Staphylococcus aureus (*S. aureus*) is the prime cause of hospital-associated infections. According to antibiotic resistance profiling, *Staphylococcus aureus* is divided into Methicillin-susceptible *S. aureus* (MSSA) and Methicillin-resistant *S. aureus* (MRSA) which represents an especially big threat to the public-health system [1]. Traditionally, MRSA infections have been limited to hospitals and predisposed individuals, such as the elderly, immunocompromised and patients undergoing surgery [2, 3]. More recently, however, MRSA infections have occurred outside of the hospital setting [4]. Community-associated (CA)-MRSA were first reported in the Northern USA,

*Correspondence: ahmed.sahib@colmed-alnahrain.edu.iq; fatim@upm.edu.my
[1] Microbiology Department, College of Medicine, Alnahrain University, 14222 Baghdad, Iraq
[5] Faculty of Food Science, University Putra Malaysia, Serdang, 43400 Selangor, Malaysia
Full list of author information is available at the end of the article

where they caused fatal infections in otherwise healthy children [5]. Later, CA-MRSA has become a global problem, with the most serious epidemic seen in the USA [6]. According to recent estimates, MRSA infections cause more deaths annually in the USA than HIV/AIDS [7].

Staphylococci are usually related to infections of implanted medical devices. The predominant species isolated in these infections are *Staphylococcus epidermidis* and *Staphylococcus aureus.* Moreover, most of the attached *S. aureus* are in fact MRSA. The main virulent factor of these bacteria is the ability to form biofilm on polymeric surfaces to which it adheres and colonizes artificial materials [4, 8]. Biofilms are a population of multilayered cells growing on a surface and enclosed in exopolysaccharide matrix. Biofilm formations are considered to be a four step process: (a) attachment, (b) colonization and multiplication, (c) maturation and (d) dispersion.

Antibiotic resistance and biofilm-forming capacity contribute to the success of Staphylococcus aureus as a human pathogen in both healthcare and community settings [9]. The biofilm matrix is a complex mixture of macromolecules, including exopolysaccharides, proteins, and DNA. These virulence factors do not function independently of each other and the biofilm phenotype expressed by clinical isolates of *S. aureus* is influenced by acquisition of the methicillin resistance gene mecA. Methicillin-sensitive *S. aureus* strains commonly produce an icaADBC operon-encoded polysaccharide intercellular adhesin (PIA)-dependent biofilm. In contrast, the release of extracellular DNA (eDNA) and cell surface expression of a number of sortase-anchored proteins, and the major autolysin have been implicated in the biofilm phenotype of MRSA isolates [9]. The main exopolysaccharide of the SA biofilm matrix is a polymer of poly-*N*-acetylglucosamine, termed polysaccharide intercellular adhesin (PIA) or poly-*N*-acetylglucosamine (PNAG), whose synthesis depends on the enzymes encoded by the *icaADBC* operon in ica locus [10, 11]. Among ica genes, *icaA* and *icaD* have been reported to play a significant role in biofilm formation in MSSA and MRSA [12, 13].

However, the presence of PIA/PNAG exopolysaccharide is not found in all biofilms of MSSA or MRSA strains. Several studies have uncovered the existence of *S. aureus* isolates able to produce alternative biofilm matrixes [14–16]. When this occurs, it appears that proteins usually take the responsibility for mediating cell-to-cell interactions and multicellular behavior. More recently, two independent research groups have described a novel *S. aureus* biofilm phenotype mediated by the fibronectin-binding proteins, FnBPA and FnBPB, being FnBPA is more important and more constantly associated with proteinacious biofilm of MSSA or MRSA [17, 18]. Therefore, there are two types of biofilms for MSSA and MRSA bacteria, polysaccharide- or PIA- based biofilm and proteinacious, or FnBPA-based, biofilms. Nevertheless, the behaviour of these two types of biofilms was not studied well.

The rate at which *S. aureus* can develop or acquire resistance to new antibiotics seems to be higher than the rate at which new antibiotics are discovered and developed. Accordingly, new control measures, rather than antibiotics, are needed in action to contain the increasing hazard of MRSA [19]. Moreover, there is a need to a safe, widely accepted, and revolutionary measures for the control and therapy of MRSA. Worldwide, an estimated 2 billion people carry some form of *S. aureus*; of these, up to 53 million (2.7 % of carriers) are thought to carry MRSA [20]. One of the promising new measures of MRSA control is bacteriophages (phages). Phages are present abundantly in the environment and humans ingest billions of phages daily without harm; therefore, they are considered safe for humans and animals [21].

However, the most challenging problem for MRSA control, either using phages or other agents, is their ability to produce highly protective biofilms. Biofilms of MRSA are considered the main source for providing virulent bacterial cells ready to spread infection in hospitals and in community. Therefore, in our opinion, there is a need to formulate an effective non-antibiotic phage-based control for MRSA and MSSA biofilms. In the current study, anti-MSSA and anti-MRSA phages were optimized and designed and were used to assess phage control to MSSA and MRSA biofilms. Moreover, the nature of intercellular adhesion of MSSA and MRSA biofilms, PIA or FnBPA-based biofilms, were studied and their response to phage-based control was accordingly evaluated.

Methods

Sampling of bacteria

Seven isolates of MRSA and 10 isolates of MSSA were chosen to be used in the current study. These isolates were collected, as part of the routine hospital work, from clinical wound samples in three hospitals in Slenagor state in Malaysia, Hospital Serdang, Hospital Kajang and Hospital HUKL using Microbact GNB 12A system (Oxoid, UK) with 99 % confirmatory rate. The diagnosed *S. aureus* bacteria were then subjected to a series of selective and differential media to identify MRSA bacteria which are the most important target of this study. The current study has been approved by the ethical committee of University Putra Malaysia.

Isolation, identification, and propagation of MSSA and MRSA

Bacteria were swabbed from infected regions and were inoculated into nutrient broth (NB) (Merck, Germany) for 18 h at 37 °C. Next day, grown bacteria in NB were

ABC streaked onto nutrient agar (NA) (Merck, Germany) and incubated for 18 h at 37 °C. Next day, different colonies were grown, the suspected colonies of *S. aureus* were streaked onto a selective and differential medium namely, Mannitol salt agar (MSA) (Merck, Germany) for 18 h at 35 °C. Next day, the grown bacteria in yellow colonies were confirmed as *S. aureus*. In addition, light microscopy was used as a supportive tool for *S. aureus* diagnosis. In order to identify MRSA strains, MRSA chromogenic agar or MRSA agar (Merck, Germany) was used. MRSA agar is composed of 11 g peptone mixture, 1.9 g chromogenic substrate, 78 g growth factors and 12.5 biological agar. In addition, MRSA agar was used with added oxacillin (6 mg/L) (Sigma, USA) in the preparation of MRSA agar. MRSA agar was used as a screening medium for the determination of methicillin resistance and oxacillin resistance in *Staphylococcus aureus*. The presence of growth indicated oxacillin and methicillin resistance. Lack of growth indicated that the strain lacks the *mec*A resistance gene. Only the non-inhibited colonies in MRSA selective agar were considered MRSA.

Reference strains of MRSA and MSSA

Reference strains of MRSA and MSSA were involved in the current study along with the isolated and identified clinical samples. Two reference strains of MRSA were used namely, ATCC 700699 and ATCC 43300 and two MSSA reference strains were used, namely, ATCC 11987 and ATCC 27691.

The strategy of the current study

First, the biofilm formation is compared between MSSA and MRSA bacteria. Second, the type of biofilms produced are assessed and categorized into PIA-based biofilms or proteinacious FnBPA-based biofilms in both MSSA and MRSA using SEM and PCR detection for *icaA-D* genes, which are responsible for PIA synthesis, and *FnBPA* gene, which is responsible for fibronectin-binding protein synthesis. Third, the MSSA and MRSA biofilms are challenged with high titre of specific lytic phages for disintegrating the biofilm matrix and lysing the integrated bacteria. Fourth, the effectiveness of the phage-based control for MRSA and MSSA biofilms is assessed in comparison with MSSA versus MRSA and PIA-based versus FnBPA-based biofilms. In addition, the augmentation of the efficiency of phage-based control was assessed by coupling attacking phages with PIA-disturbing or protein-denaturing chemical adjuvants.

Isolation of wild phages to MSSA and MRSA

Phages to MSSA and MRSA were isolated from 3 different sources; Hospital environmental dirt, sewage disposal, and cattle waste. Crude specimens of approximately 50 g of environmental dirt, sewage disposal, or cattle waste were each collected in a sterile sample collection tube (100 ml). The procedure pursued was done according to [22] with some modification. One to three grams of each specimen were transferred into 90 ml of nutrient broth (NB) and vortexed for 30 s. Then 1 ml of 8 h NB cultures of the target MRSA clinical isolate or reference strains was added and incubated at 37 °C. After 18 h, 10 ml of the mixture were withdrawn into a sterile 15 ml test tube and centrifuged for 5 min at 5000×*g* at room temperature. Supernatant was aspirated into new sterile 15 ml test tubes. To the supernatant, 1 ml of chloroform (Sigma, USA) was added with gentle shaking of tubes for 5 min then all tubes were incubated on crushed ice for 5 min. A milky solution appears due to bacterial proteins digestion by chloroform. Centrifugation at 5000×*g* for 5 min at room temperature was carried-out. Top aqueous supernatant was collected into 15 ml sterile tube and stored at 4 °C as a possible phage solution.

Testing for the presence of wild phages (phage spot lysis assay)

Thin bacterial lawns of clinical isolates or reference strains were prepared by adding 500 μl of NB 18 h cultures on NA plates, allowing the liquid to soak into the plate. The plates were kept for 1 h at room temperature. Ten μl of the prepared phage suspension were spotted on bacterial lawns and incubated at 37 C. Plaques or lysis spot were observed after 6 h and 18 h. The detection of phage presence was based on visual appearance of lysis zone. Positive results were expressed by either clear or semi-clear (turbid) lysis zone while negative results were expressed by the absence of such lysis zones [23].

The approach of phage isolation and propagation

A series of optimization steps were used in order to augment the efficacy of phage hunting/isolation techniques. The optimization manoeuvres that were taken into account are:

The collection of crude phage samples was diversified in a way that 1 g of as minimal as 10 different samples from hospital dirt, sewage, and cattle waste was used to form the crude mixture. Samples of crude mixture (10 g) were placed in 100 ml Erlenmeyer flask with cotton-plugged filled with 80 ml of NB. Then, 10 MRSA isolates were used together to inoculate the phage mixture with 1 ml from each 18 h MRSA culture. After 18 h of incubation at 37 °C, 10 ml were dispensed into a sterile 15-mL plastic culture tubes. After centrifugation at 5000×*g* for 5 min at room temperature, the supernatant was transferred into 1.5 ml sterile microcentrifuge. Then 1:10 chloroform to lysate ratio was added with gentle shaking for 5 min at room temperature in order to lyse the bacterial cells followed by further 3 min incubation in crushed ice. The mixture was then centrifuged 5000×*g* for 15 min at room temperature and the supernatant was transferred into a 1.5 ml sterile microcentrifuge tubes. To this step, the isolated phages mixture was produced. The produced mixture of the isolated phages was propagated on the desired target bacteria lawn as it is earlier mentioned in the procedure of the phage spot lysis test [23].

Production of the transient phage stock

The produced mixture of the isolated phages was propagated on each target bacterial lawn as it is earlier mentioned in the procedure of the phage spot lysis assay. Lysis zones, if any, were cut by a sterile scalpel and plunged into 300 μl of Lambda buffer in 1.5 ml sterile microcentrifuge tubes for 20 min with intermittent gentle shaking. 1:10 chloroform to lysate ratio was added with gentle shaking for 5 min at room temperature in order to elute the phages from the agar and to lyse the bacterial cells. After further 3 min incubation in crushed ice the mixture centrifuged at 5000×*g* for 15 min at room temperature and the supernatant transferred in a 1.5 ml sterile microcentrifuge tubes [22].

Biofilm formation

The MRSA and MSSA biofilm formation assays were performed as described [24]. Sterile 96-well polystyrene microtiter plates were used throughout the study. Each assay was performed in triplicate and repeated at least three times. Briefly, bacterial isolates from fresh agar plates were inoculated in nutrient broth and incubated for 24 h at 37 °C in stationary condition and diluted (1 in 50) with fresh medium. Individual wells of sterile, polystyrene, flat-bottom tissue culture plates were filled with 200 μl aliquots of the diluted cultures (10^8 cfu/ml). The negative control was composed of broth only to check sterility and non-specific binding of media. The tissue culture plates were incubated for 24 h at 37 °C. After incubation, the content of each well was gently removed by tapping the plates. The wells were washed three times with 200 μl of phosphate buffer saline (PBS pH 7.2) to remove non-attached floating bacteria.

Detection of biofilm formation by tissue culture plate method (TCP)

The TCP assay is most widely used and was considered as standard test for the detection of biofilm formation. All isolates were screened for their ability to form biofilm by the TCP method as described by Christensen et al. [25] with a modification in duration of incubation which was extended to 24 h, according to O'Toole and Kolter [26]. After the formation of the biofilm in tissue culture wells, 25 μl of 1 % solution of crystal violet were added to each well (this dye stains the cells but not the polystyrene) plates. The plates were incubated at room temperature for 15 min, rinsed thoroughly and repeatedly with water. Adherent cells, which usually formed biofilm on all side wells, were uniformly stained with crystal violet. Crystal violet-stained biofilm was solubilized in 200 μl of ethanol-acetone (80:20, vol/vol) (Merck, Germany). Afterwards, 100 μl were transferred to a new polystyrene microtiter dish which was subjected to micro ELISA auto reader at 570 nm wavelength. Optical densities (OD) of stained adherent bacteria were determined and were considered as indices for bacterial potential to adhere to surfaces and form biofilms. Experiments for each strain were performed in triplicate and repeated three times. To compensate for background absorbance, OD readings of wells with ethanol were used as blank and subtracted from all tests' values. Biofilm production is considered high, moderate, weak, or zero according to the measurements of OD570 nm as shown in Table 1.

Phage application on MSSA and MRSA biofilms

Optimized and isolated phages to MSSA, 12 phages, and MRSA, 9 phages, in lambda buffer were applied on the formed biofilms of 10 clinical isolates and two reference strains of MSSA and 7 clinical isolates and 2 reference strains of MRSA. Ten (10) μl of anti-SA or anti-MRSA 10^{12} PFU/ml phages were applied on the formed biofilms in the tissue culture plates with and without adjuvant substances. Sublethal concentrations of chemical adjuvants together with applied phages were used in order to increase the permeability of the matrix of the biofilm as well as to increase the exposure of phage-binding receptors on the cell walls of MSSA and MRSA bacteria. For PIA type biofilms, after numerous trials and errors using a panel of PIA/PNAG-disturbing chemicals [data not shown], a sublethal dose, 0.08 %, of Benzethonium chloride was found to be the best in disintegrating PIA type biofilms when is mixed with applied phages; however, this dose was of no effect on either biofilms or phages when Benzethonium chloride was used alone. For FnBPA type biofilms, after numerous trial and error steps using a panel of protein-denaturing chemicals, sublethal dose, 0.06 %, of ethanol was found to be the best

Table 1 Classification of biofilms formation according to TCP method [8]

Biofilm formation	Mean OD values
Zero	<0.05
Weak	0.05–0.12
Moderate	0.12–0.24
High	>0.24

in disintegrating the proteinacious matrix of FnBPA type biofilms when is mixed with applied phages [data not shown]; however, this dose was of no effect on biofilms or phages when ethanol was used alone. Assessment of biofilm formation was conducted by using TCP method. The phage-based reduction of biofilm formation was scored from 0 to 3.

It is noteworthy to mention that plates were kept, without cover, stationary up to 24 h at room temperature. Microtiter plates were kept at room temperature without lid cover in order to mimic the sterilization conditions in hospitals where the sterilizing agents dry up after 30 min.

Scanning Electron Microscopy (SEM)

Formed biofilms of MSSA and MRSA were fixed in 2.5 % (vol/vol) glutaraldehyde (Sigma, USA) in Dulbecco PBS (PH 7.2) for 1.5 h, rinsed with PBS, and then dehydrated through an ethanol series. Samples were dried and gold–palladium coated. SEM examinations were made on a JSM-840 SEM (JEOL Ltd., Tokyo, Japan) [27]. SEM was used in the current study for visualizing the formed biofilms and most importantly for assessing visually the type of the formed biofilms whether polysaccharide- or protein- based biofilm. The IPA-based biofilm appears usually with rough crystallized surface while FnBPA-based biofilm appears as smooth non-crystallized surface.

PCR for the detection of *icaA, icaD,* and FnBPA genes

Bacterial DNA extraction

Chromosomal and plasmid DNA of the MSSA and MRSA bacteria were extracted using Wizard® Genomic DNA Purification Kit with accessory reagents (Promega, USA); the method of extraction was done according to the manufacturer's instructions. The obtained genomic DNA was rehydrated by adding 100 µl DNA Rehydration solution. Extracted DNA 260/280 nm ratio was >1.8 and quality was assessed by gel electrophoresis. Then, a 5 µl aliquot was used as a template for PCR amplification.

PCR protocols

The primers used were synthesized by the laboratories of Biotechnology institute of Malaysia. For *icaA-D* and FnBPA, PCR master mixture consisted of 2 µl of 10× PCR buffer, 0.8 µl of a 10 mM deoxynucleoside triphosphate mixture, 0.7 µl of forward and reverse primers at concentration of 10 pmol/µl, 1.5 µl of 25 mM MgCl2, and 0.2 µl of 0.5 U Taq DNA polymerase, and 50 ng of template DNA; the remaining volume consisted of distilled water. The PCR reaction was conducted in a thermocycler PCR system (PTC-110TM Model, MJ Research, Inc., USA). The PCR conditions, primres sequences are shown in Table 2.

Afterwards, 5 µl of PCR products, *icaA*, *icaD* and FnBPA, were electrophoresed on 2 % agarose gel using QIAGEN GelPilot DNA Molecular Weight Marker as a ladder. PCR products were separated by an electrophoresis system at a constant voltage of 80 V for 50 min and were stained with 0.25 µg/ml ethidium bromide (Sigma, USA). PCR products were photographed under UV transilluminator (Vilber Lourmat, Cedex, France) and the photos were taken using gel documentation system, Bio Rad Gel Doc 2000 Model Imaging System (Bio-Rad, USA). The resulted bands of the PCR product for FnBPA, *icaA*, and *icaD* were expressed as positive and negative expression.

Statistical analysis

Data of the current study was analyzed by SPSS version 12.0.1. For qualitative nominal data, Fisher exacts test was used. For quantitative nonparametric data, Mann–Whitney test was used. P values less than 0.05 was considered significant.

Results

Biofilm formation

All tested MRSA and MSSA isolates and reference strains developed various levels of biofilm expressed as weak, moderate, and high. The tested MSSA and MRSA isolates and reference strains showed variable tendencies for biofilm formation using TCP method (Table 3). In order to compare the level of biofilm formation between MSSA and MRSA, high/moderate versus weak groups of biofilm production was assessed in MSSA versus MRSA. Although tested MRSA showed higher tendency for

Table 2 PCR conditions, primer sequences, and PCR products of *icaA, icaD,* and *FnBPA* genes

The gene	Primers sequences	PCR product (bp)	Reference	Thermal cycles
icaA	F-5′-GAC CTC GAA GTC AAT AGA GGT A R-5′-CCC AGT ATA ACG TTG GAT ACC	814	[28]	95 °C for 5 min, 35 cycles 94 °C 30 s, 59.5 °C 30 s, 72 °C 50 s, and 72 °C 5 min after conclusion of the 35 cycles [29]
icaD	F-5′-AGG CAA TAT CCA ACG GTA A R-5′-GTC ACG ACC TTT CTT ATA TT	371		
FnBPA	F-5′-AGGGATCCGATGGTGGAGGTGGATA-3′ R-5′-AGCCCGGGTGGCGTTGGTGGCACGATTGGAG	1274	[30]	95 °C 5 min, 35 cycles 94 °C 30 s, 65.5 °C 30 s, 72 °C 1 min and 72 °C 5 min after conclusion of the 35 cycles [30]

Table 3 The frequency of MRSA and MSSA isolates/reference strains in forming different levels of biofilm

Bacteria	High, N (%)	Moderate, N (%)	Weak, N (%)
MRSA	4 (44.4)	3 (33.3)	2 (22.2)
MSSA	3 (25)	3 (25)	6 (50)

biofilm production, no significant difference was found in biofilm production level between SA and MRSA (P = 0.36).

Types of biofilms produced

The type of biofilms produced was assessed according to the PCR-based detection of PIA genes, *ica* A and D, or FnBPA gene (Fig. 1). In addition, SEM screening was used to visualize the morphology of the produced biofilm and to help assess the type whether PIA- or FnBPA-based biofilm (Fig. 2). The results of both SEM and PCR were in harmony. The PIA, rough crystalline morphology as shown in SEM, was congruous with the positive detection of both genes, *icaA* and *icaD* while the smooth proteinacious morphology of the produced biofilms was congruous with the positive detection of FnBPA gene. However, only one MRSA isolate showed simultaneous positivity for both *icaA-D* and FnBPA genes but it was seen in SEM as smooth-surfaced proteinacious biofilm; therefore, it was categorized as FnBPA-based biofilm producing bacteria (Table 4).

According to Table 3, MRSA showed higher tendency to produce FnBPA type biofilms; 6 isolates with FnBPA type biofilms and 3 isolates with PIA type biofilms at ratio 2: 1. On the contrary, SA showed higher tendency to produce PIA type biofilms, 8 isolates, FnBPA type biofilm, 4 isolates at ratio 2: 1. This important finding might provide evidence for the different responses of MRSA and MSSA biofilms to antibiotics, antiseptics, or biological antibacterial agents such as bacteriophages which were used in the current study. In addition, in MRSA, FnBPA biofilm type was found to be mainly of high/moderate score while PIA- biofilm type was mainly of weak score of biofilm formation; however, these differences did not reach statistical significance in the level of biofilm production (high/moderate versus weak) between PIA and FnBPA types of biofilms in both MSSA and MRSA bacteria (P = 0.65).

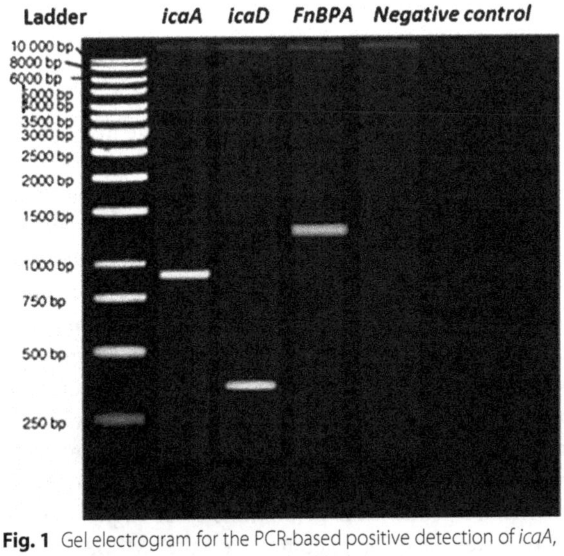

Fig. 1 Gel electrogram for the PCR-based positive detection of *icaA*, *icaD*, and *FnBPA* genes in MRSA and MSSA bacteria

Phage-based biocontrol for MRSA and SA biofilms

Two sets of phage application experiments were assessed, phage application with and without chemical adjuvant on both types of biofilms, namely PIA and FnBPA in MRSA and MSSA bacteria. The magnitude of phage-based reduction of biofilm was measured as reduction score which was from 0 to 3. For both types of biofilms in both MSSA and MRSA bacteria, it was found that phage application reduced effectively the formed biofilms (Table 5). By using phages alone without adjuvant chemical, 6/8 (75 %), 1/4 (25 %), 1/3 (33.3 %), and 1/6 (16.6 %) of biofilms were reduced one score in MSSA PIA, MSSA FnBPA, MRSA PIA, and MRSA FnBPA, respectively (Table 5). The current findings revealed that phage-based reduction is more remarkable in MSSA than in MRSA and in PIA than in FnBPA. Accordingly, MRSA FnBPA group was the least responsive to phage-based reduction of biofilms when phages without chemical adjuvant were used. On the other hand, by using phages with chemical adjuvant, 100 % of biofilms, whether MSSA or MRSA, were reduced at least one score. Moreover, 3/8 (37.5 %), 2/4 (50 %), 2/3 (66.6 %), and 3/6 (50 %) of biofilms were reduced two score and more in MSSA PIA, MSSA FnBPA, MRSA PIA, and MRSA FnBPA, respectively (Table 5). Hence, it appears clearly that MRSA biofilms responded to the addition of the chemical adjuvant to the applied phages more obviously than MSSA biofilms.

By using Mann–Whitney test for comparing the median scores of phage reduction of biofilms among different groups of the study, it was found that the median reduction score by phages with chemical adjuvant was higher than by counterpart phages without chemical adjuvant in biofilms of MSSA PIA (P = 0.034), MSSA FnBPA (P = 0.047), MRSA PIA (P = 0.11), and MRSA FnBPA (P = 0.0067). The current statistical design specified precisely the most responsive group to phages with chemical adjuvant, namely MRSA FnBPA. Since 6/9 (66.6 %) of MRSA samples studied in the current study

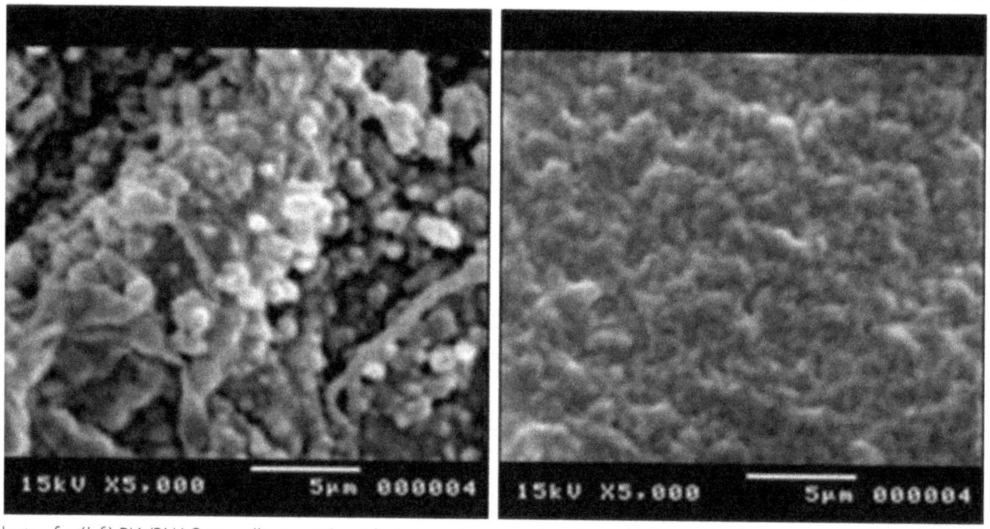

Fig. 2 SEM photos for (*left*) PIA/PNAG crystalline rough surface *cagA-D*-positive biofilm of MRSA and (*right*) smooth proteinacious FnBPA-positive biofilm of MRSA

Table 4 The type of produced biofilms in MRSA and MSSA bacteria assessed by SEM and PCR along with their corresponding level of biofilm production

Bacteria	PIA-based biofilm via PCR and rough crystalline biofilm via SEM			FnBPA-based biofilm via PCR and smooth proteinacious biofilm via SEM		
	High, N (%)	Moderate, N (%)	Weak, N (%)	High, N (%)	Moderate, N (%)	Weak, N (%)
MRSA	1 (11.1)	1 (11.1)	1 (11.1)	3 (33.3)	2 (22.2)	1 (11.1)
MSSA	2 (16.6)	2 (16.6)	4 (33.3)	1 (8.3)	1 (8.3)	2 (16.6)

produced FnBPA type biofilms, so using phage-based reduction of biofilms with chemical adjuvant seems interesting. Accordingly, the use of anti-MRSA and anti-MSSA phages in the reduction of MRSA and MSSA biofilms, respectively, was shown to be successful especially when coupled with chemical adjuvant helping denature and disintegrate the treated biofilm matrix.

The treated wells in which biofilms were not eliminated completely in the first treatment via phage application with chemical adjuvant were subjected to a second round of treatment. In this instance, the anti-MSSA and anti-MRSA phages, coupled with chemical adjuvant, were applied on the corresponding bacterial biofilms. It was found that all the SA biofilms which were remained after the first round, 3 weak MSSA PIA and 1 weak MSSA FnBPA, were eliminated completely via the second round of phages application with chemical adjuvant. Nevertheless, for MRSA biofilms which were remained after the first round, only 1 weak MRSA PIA and 1 weak MRSA FnBPA biofilm were completely eliminated by the second round of phages application with chemical adjuvant. This indicated the development of resistance by 2/9 (22.2 %) of MRSA biofilms and 2/6 (33.3 %) of FnBPA MRSA biofilms in particular to the attacking phages and this resistance impeded the complete eradication of biofilms in the first and second rounds of phages application.

Discussion

Microbial biofilms are considered one of the major health problem because they cause chronic infections which are difficult to treat, lead to longer hospitalization time, and can result in much higher treatment costs [29, 31]. Hence, a new approach, rather than the counterproductive antibiotics, must be used. In the current study, interestingly, all the 9 samples of MRSA and 12 samples of MSSA developed biofilms after 24 h. This indicated the highly potent ability of both MSSA and MRSA in developing rapidly biofilms. Moreover, weak production of biofilms in MSSA was half of the all biofilms produced while in MRSA were only 22.2 %. This provided evidence that MRSA production of biofilms is of higher efficacy and of faster pace. Ursic et al. stated that MRSA bacteria

Table 5 Phage-based reduction of biofilms, with or without using adjuvant chemical, in PIA and FnBPA types of both MRSA and SA

Bacteria	Type of biofilm	Phage application without chemical adjuvant Level of biofilm before: after (score of reduction)	Phage application with chemical adjuvant Level of biofilm before: after (score of reduction)
SA-1	PIA	High: high (0)	High: weak (2)
SA-2	PIA	Mod: weak (1)	Mod: zero (2)
SA-3	PIA	weak: zero (1)	weak: zero (1)
SA-10	PIA	weak: zero (1)	weak: zero (1)
SA-5	PIA	High: High (0)	High: weak (2)
SA-6	PIA	weak: zero (1)	weak: zero (1)
ATCC 11987	PIA	Mod: weak (1)	Mod: weak (1)
SA-8	PIA	weak: zero (1)	weak: zero (1)
Average score of reduction		0.75	1.38
SA-9	FnBPA	Mod: Mod (0)	Mod: zero (2)
SA-4	FnBPA	High: high (0)	High: weak (2)
SA-7	FnBPA	weak: weak (0)	weak: zero (1)
ATCC 27691	FnBPA	weak: zero (1)	weak: zero (1)
Average score of reduction		0.25	1.5
MR-4	PIA	Mod: Mod (0)	Mod: zero (2)
MR-5	PIA	High: High (0)	High: weak (2)
MR-7	PIA	weak: zero (1)	weak: zero (1)
Average score of reduction		0.33	1.67
MR-1	FnBPA	High: high (0)	High: zero (3)
MR-2	FnBPA	Mod: mod (0)	Mod: weak (1)
MR-3	FnBPA	High: high (0)	High: weak (2)
MR-6	FnBPA	weak: zero (1)	weak: zero (1)
ATCC 700699	FnBPA	Mod: Mod (0)	Mod: zero (2)
ATCC 43300	FnBPA	High: high (0)	High: mod (1)
Average score of reduction		0.17	1.67

Mod represents moderate production of biofilms, *Zero* describes mean OD values of TCP method less than 0.01

have an unrivalled potential of biofilm formation when compared with non-MRSA bacteria [30, 32]. Hence, special care for treating MRSA biofilms is highly needed.

In the current study, we analyzed the formed biofilms of MSSA and MRSA bacteria depending on the nature of the biofilm matrix whether it is PIA/PNAG or proteinacious FnBPA type. FnBPA biofilms in MRSA were found as double frequency as PIA biofilms while in MSSA biofilms the reverse was observed, the frequency of PIA biofilms was double that of FnBPA. These findings are congruous with findings of several previous studies which revealed that protein- mediated biofilm formation capacity seems to be particularly frequent among the highly virulent MRSA isolates, emphasizing the importance of this type of biofilm structure and its capacity for survival and antimicrobial resistance [16, 33]. Therefore, FnBPA type biofilm which is found mainly in highly virulent MRSA can be the key factor for the resilient biofilms produced by MRSA which lay heavy burden on the community medicine, hospital environment, and general health issues. From SEM photos, the proteinacious biofilms were shown with more rigid and compact matrix than PIA biofilms. Hence, the proteinacious FnBPA biofilms of MRSA appear to be difficult for anti-MRSA antibiotic because most of these antibiotics can not get through this compact matrix. In a study, it was found that even a highly effective drug like Vancomycin failed to produce a 2 log reduction in the biofilm embedded MRSA bacterial count and most antiseptics were found unable to completely eliminate MRSA biofilms on plastic or metal surfaces found in hospitals [34].

Accordingly, phage-based approach was taken into consideration for the treatment of MSSA and MRSA biofilms. A previous study revealed that a staphylococcal phage, GH15, was isolated and the endogenous lytic enzyme (LysGH15) was expressed and purified. The lysin LysGH15 displayed a broad lytic spectrum; in vitro treatment killed a number of Staphylococcus aureus strains rapidly and completely, including the methicillin-resistant Staphylococcus aureus (MRSA) [35]. In addition, phages can propagate in their bacterial host and phages produce depolymerases that hydrolyze biofilm extracellular polymers [36] therefore, phage mixtures or engineered phages could provide effective strategies to overcome bacterial biofilms. Lytic bacteriophages could become a new class of anti-biofilm agents. In the current study, when anti-MRSA and anti-MSSA phages without chemical adjuvant were used, findings revealed that phage-based reduction was more remarkable in MSSA than in MRSA and in PIA than in FnBPA; moreover, MRSA FnBPA group was the least responsive to phage-based reduction of biofilms. This showed the difficulty in addressing the problem of MRSA biofilms when phages are used alone. This might be attributed to the limited capacity of phages' depolymerases to hydrolyze extracellular matrix of MRSA biofilms especially the proteinacious FnBPA type.

As a result of the relatively poor eradication of MRSA and MSSA biofilms by applied phages, it was concluded that the main obstacle is the extracellular matrix of biofilms. Hence, a set of chemical reagents were tried to disrupt the PIA/PNAG or FnBPA protein matrices in parallel with attacking phages to pave the way for phages to access the cell wall of bacterial hosts. After a series of experiments, 0.08 % Benzenthonium chloride and 0.06 % ethanol were used along with applied phages against PIA and FnBPA biofilms, respectively. The resultant mixture of lytic phages and chemical adjuvant granted satisfactory outcomes. After 2 rounds of phages application, 100 % of MSSA PIA and MSSA FnBPA biofilms were removed completely and for MRSA, only 22.2 % of biofilms showed incomplete eradication via resistance against attacking phages with chemical adjuvant. The current findings gave clue to the best way for enabling lytic phages to eradicate efficiently bacterial hosts' biofilms. Unfortunately, no previous report was found conducting the same principle of phage-chemical biocontrol of MRSA and MSSA. The pioneering findings of the current study imply to new, practical, and cheap approaches to contain, reduce, or eliminate biofilms which are the main refractory source of MRSA and MSSA spread in both hospitals and environment. Moreover, the current phage: chemical mixture can be used in gel base for the prevention of biofilm production on inserted devices into human body such as urinary catheters leading to lowering the use of antimicrobial agents.

The successful control and treatment of MRSA and MSSA biofilms using phages: chemical mixtures have important health advantages. Doolittle et al. [37] demonstrated that the radial movement of T4 phage particles through a biofilm is similar to the process of plaque formation on a lawn of host bacteria, indicating that a single dose of phage could treat a biofilm-related infection. On the contrary, biofilm organisms are tolerant to antimicrobial drugs, disinfectants and biocides [38] and high concentrations of antimicrobials for prolonged treatment durations are normally required to achieve biofilm reduction or eradication [39]. Another drawback of antimicrobial agents is that higher antimicrobial concentrations are required to inactivate or eradicate the biofilm cells as the biofilm ages [40] while this is not found in the case of phages. Moreover, the biofilm extracellular matrix could also affect the efficacy of antimicrobial agents because of diffusion limitations [38] while phages diffuse more easily through alginate gels and extracellular matrix of biofilms. Collectively, all the mentioned advantages of phage-based control of bacterial biofilms when coupled with the currently discovered phage-sparing and biofilm matrix- disrupting chemical agent, the resultant weapon would be so deadly for biofilms of most notorious bugs such as MRSA.

Conclusions

Taken together, it was concluded that the application of highly lytic anti-MSSA and anti-MRSA phages along with biofilm matrix- disrupting chemicals led to highly successful eradication of host biofilms. The used mixtures of phages: chemical adjuvants are recommended to be used in a large scale evaluation study in order to prepare for the introduction of the current approach of MRSA biofilm control into the routine sanitary procedures done in hospitals. Moreover, the current approach can be used in the prevention of devices-related infections for the in vivo medical instruments, such as urinary catheters.

Authors' contributions

ASA designed and conducted the research, SAAJ, RRH and FAB designed the research. All authors read and approved the final manuscript.

Author details

[1] Microbiology Department, College of Medicine, Alnahrain University, 14222 Baghdad, Iraq. [2] Applied Bio Research Inc., Windsor, Canada. [3] Environmental Engineering, University of Windsor, Windsor, Canada. [4] Microbiology Department, College of Medicine, Baghdad University, Baghdad, Iraq. [5] Faculty of Food Science, University Putra Malaysia, Serdang, 43400 Selangor, Malaysia.

Acknowledgements

Appreciation for the University Putra Malaysia for incubating this research.

Competing interests

The authors declare that they have no competing interests.

References

1. Johnson AP, Pearson A, Duckworth G. Surveillance and epidemiology of MRSA bacteraemia in the UK. J Antimicrob Chemother. 2005;56(3):455–62.
2. Embleton ML, Nair SP, Heywood W, Menon DC, Cookson BD, Wilson M. Development of a novel targeting system for lethal photosensitization of

antibiotic-resistant strains of Staphylococcus aureus. Antimicrob Agents Chemother. 2005;49(9):3690–6.

3. Vergara-Irigaray M, Valle J, Merino N, Latasa C, Garcia B, Ruiz de Los Mozos I, Solano C, Toledo-Arana A, Penades JR, Lasa I. Relevant role of fibronectin-binding proteins in Staphylococcus aureus biofilm-associated foreign-body infections. Infect Immun. 2009;77(9):3978–91.
4. Chambers HF. The changing epidemiology of *Staphylococcus aureus*? Emerg Infect Dis. 2001;7(2):178–82.
5. CDC. From the Centers for Disease Control and Prevention. Four pediatric deaths from community-acquired methicillin-resistant *Staphylococcus aureus*—Minnesota and North Dakota 1997–1999. JAMA. 1999;282:1123–5.
6. Diep BA, Otto M. The role of virulence determinants in community-associated MRSA pathogenesis. Trends Microbiol. 2008;16(8):361–9.
7. Klevens RM, Morrison MA, Nadle J, Petit S, Gershman K, Ray S, Harrison LH, Lynfield R, Dumyati G, Townes JM, et al. Invasive methicillin-resistant *Staphylococcus aureus* infections in the United States. JAMA. 2007;298(15):1763–71.
8. Gad GFM, El-Feky MA, El-Rehewy MS, Hassan MA, Abolella H, El-Baky RMA. Detection of icaA, icaD genes and biofilm production by Staphylococcus aureus and Staphylococcus epidermidis isolated from urinary tract catheterized patients. J Infect Dev Ctries. 2009;3(5):342–51.
9. McCarthy H, Rudkin JK, Black NS, Gallagher L, O'Neill E, O'Gara JP. Methicillin resistance and the biofilm phenotype in *Staphylococcus aureus*. Front Cell Infect Microbiol. 2015;5:1.
10. McKenney D, Pouliot KL, Wang Y, Murthy V, Ulrich M, Doring G, Lee JC, Goldmann DA, Pier GB. Broadly protective vaccine for *Staphylococcus aureus* based on an in vivo-expressed antigen. Science. 1999;284(5419):1523–7.
11. O'Gara JP, Humphreys H. *Staphylococcus epidermidis* biofilms importance and implications. H Med Microbiol. 2001;50:582–7.
12. Yazdani R, Oshaghi M, Havayi A, Salehi R, Sadeghizadeh M, Foroohesh H. Detection of icaAD gene and biofilm formation in *Staphylococcus aureus* isolates from wound infections. Iranian J Publ Health. 2006;35:25–8.
13. Ammendolia MG, Rosa RD, Montanaro L, Arciola CR, Baldassarri L. Slime production and expression of slime–associated antigen by staphylococcal clinical isolates. J Clin Microbiol. 1999;37:3235–8.
14. Beenken KE, Dunman PM, McAleese F, Macapagal D, Murphy E, Projan SJ, Blevins JS, Smeltzer MS. Global gene expression in *Staphylococcus aureus* biofilms. J Bacteriol. 2004;186(14):4665–84.
15. Corrigan RM, Rigby D, Handley P, Foster TJ. The role of *Staphylococcus aureus* surface protein SasG in adherence and biofilm formation. Microbiology. 2007;153(Pt 8):2435–46.
16. Fitzpatrick F, Humphreys H, O'Gara JP. Evidence for icaADBC-independent biofilm development mechanism in methicillin-resistant *Staphylococcus aureus* clinical isolates. J Clin Microbiol. 2005;43(4):1973–6.
17. O'Neill E, Pozzi C, Houston P, Humphreys H, Robinson DA, Loughman A, Foster TJ, O'Gara JP. A novel *Staphylococcus aureus* biofilm phenotype mediated by the fibronectin-binding proteins, FnBPA and FnBPB. J Bacteriol. 2008;190:3835–50.
18. Shanks RMQ, Meehl MA, Brothers KM, Martinez RM, Donegan NP, Graber ML, Cheung AL, O'Toole GA. Genetic evidence for an alternative citrate-dependent biofilm formation pathway in *Staphylococcus aureus* that is dependent on fibronectin binding proteins and the GraRS two-component regulatory system. Infect Immun. 2008;76(6):2469–77.
19. Tacconelli E, De Angelis G, Cataldo MA, Pozzi E, Cauda R. Does antibiotic exposure increase the risk of methicillin-resistant *Staphylococcus aureus* (MRSA) isolation? A systematic review and meta-analysis. J Antimicrob Chemother. 2008;61(1):26–38.
20. Graham PL, Lin SX, Larson EL. A US population-based survey of *Staphylococcus aureus* colonization. Ann Intern Med. 2006;144(5):318–25.
21. Superbugs, MRSA, Phages and Bdellovibrio. Naked Scientists Podcast. http://www.thenakedscientists.com/HTML/podcasts/show/2004.12.12.
22. Jassim SA, Abdulamir AS, Abu Bakar F. Novel phage-based bio-processing of pathogenic Escherichia coli and its biofilms. World J Microbiol Biotechnol. 2012;28(1):47–60.
23. Abdulamir AS, Jassim SA, Abu Bakar F. Novel approach of using a cocktail of designed bacteriophages against gut pathogenic *E. coli* for bacterial load biocontrol. Ann Clin Microbiol Antimicrob. 2014;13:39.
24. Francois P, Tu Quoc PH, Bisognano C, Kelley WL, Lew DP, Schrenzel J, Cramton SE, Gotz F, Vaudaux P. Lack of biofilm contribution to bacterial colonisation in an experimental model of foreign body infection by *Staphylococcus aureus* and *Staphylococcus epidermidis*. FEMS Immunol Med Microbiol. 2003;35(2):135–40.
25. Christensen GD, Simpson WA, Younger JA, Baddour LM, Barrett FF, Melton DM, Beachey EH. Adherence of coagulase negative Staphylococci to plastic tissue cultures: a quantitative model for the adherence of staphylococci to medical devices. J Clin Microbiol. 1985;22:996–1006.
26. O'Toole GA, Kolter R. Initiation of biofilm formation in Pseudomonas fluorescens WCS365 proceeds via multiple, convergent signalling pathways: a genetic analysis. Mol Microbiol. 1998;28(3):449–61.
27. Soboh F, Khoury AE, Zamboni AC, Davidson D, Mittelman MW. Effects of ciprofloxacin and protamine sulfate combinations against catheter-associated Pseudomonas aeruginosa biofilms. Antimicrob Agents Chemother. 1995;39(6):1281–6.
28. Diemond-Hernandez B, Solorzano-Santos F, Leanos-Miranda B, Peregrino-Bejarano L, Miranda-Novales G. Production of icaADBC-encoded polysaccharide intercellular adhesin and therapeutic failure in pediatric patients with Staphylococcal device-related infections. BMC Infect Dis. 2010;10:68.
29. Arciola CR, Baldassarri L, Montanaro L. Presence of icaA and icaD genes and slime production in a collection of staphylococcal strains from catheter-associated infections. J Clin Microbiol. 2001;39(6):2151–6.
30. Piroth L, Que Y-A, Widmer E, Panchaud A, Piu S, Entenza JM, Moreillon P. The fibrinogen- and fibronectin-binding domains of *Staphylococcus aureus* fibronectin-binding protein A synergistically promote endothelial invasion and experimental endocarditis. Infect Immun. 2008;76(8):3824–31.
31. Desgrandchamps F, Moulinier F, Doudon M, Teillac P, Le Duc A. An in vitro comparison of urease induced encrustation of JJ stents in human urine. Br J Urol. 1997;79:24–7.
32. Ursic V, Tomic V, Kosnik M. Effect of different incubation atmospheres on the production of biofilm in methicillin-resistant Staphylococcus aureus (MRSA) grown in nutrient-limited medium. Curr Microbiol. 2008;57(4):386–90.
33. O'Neill E, Pozzi C, Houston P, Smyth D, Humphreys H, Robinson DA, O'Gara JP. Association between methicillin susceptibility and biofilm regulation in *Staphylococcus aureus* isolates from device-related infections. J Clin Microbiol. 2007;45:1379–88.
34. Dancer SJ. The effect of antibiotics on methicillin-resistant *Staphylococcus aureus*. J Antimicrob Chemother. 2008;61(2):246–53.
35. Gu J, Xu W, Lei L, Huang J, Feng X, Sun C, Du C, Zuo J, Li Y, Du T, et al. LysGH15, a novel bacteriophage lysin, protects a murine bacteremia model efficiently against lethal methicillin-resistant *Staphylococcus aureus* infection. J Clin Microbiol. 2011;49(1):111–7.
36. Donlan RM. Preventing biofilms of clinically relevant organisms using bacteriophage. Trends Microbiol. 2009;17(2):66–72.
37. Doolittle MM, Cooney JJ, Caldwell DE. Tracing the interaction of bacteriophage with bacterial biofilms using fluorescent and chromogenic probes. J Ind Microbiol. 1996;16(6):331–41.
38. Stewart PS. Biofilm antimicrobial resistance. In: Ghannoum M, O'Toole GA, editors. Microbial Biofilms. ASM Press; 2004, p. 250–268.
39. Ceri H, Olson ME, Stremick C, Read RR, Morck D, Buret A. The Calgary Biofilm Device: new technology for rapid determination of antibiotic susceptibilities of bacterial biofilms. J Clin Microbiol. 1999;37(6):1771–6.
40. Amorena B, Gracia E, Monzon M, Leiva J, Oteiza C, Perez M, Alabart JL, Hernandez-Yago J. Antibiotic susceptibility assay for *Staphylococcus aureus* in biofilms developed in vitro. J Antimicrob Chemother. 1999;44(1):43–55.

15

The occurrence of ESBL-producing *Escherichia coli* carrying aminoglycoside resistance genes in urinary tract infections in Saudi Arabia

Essam J. Alyamani[1*], Anamil M. Khiyami[2], Rayan Y. Booq[1], Majed A. Majrashi[1], Fayez S. Bahwerth[3] and Elena Rechkina[4]

Abstract

Background: The infection and prevalence of extended-spectrum β-lactamases (ESBLs) is a worldwide problem, and the presence of ESBLs varies between countries. In this study, we investigated the occurrence of plasmid-mediated ESBL/AmpC/carbapenemase/aminoglycoside resistance gene expression in *Escherichia coli* using phenotypic and genotypic techniques.

Methods: A total of 58 *E. coli* isolates were collected from hospitals in the city of Makkah and screened for the production of ESBL/AmpC/carbapenemase/aminoglycoside resistance genes. All samples were subjected to phenotypic and genotypic analyses. The antibiotic susceptibility of the *E. coli* isolates was determined using the Vitek-2 system and the minimum inhibitory concentration (MIC) assay. Antimicrobial agents tested using the Vitek 2 system and MIC assay included the expanded-spectrum (or third-generation) cephalosporins (e.g., cefoxitin, cefepime, aztreonam, cefotaxime, ceftriaxone, and ceftazidime) and carbapenems (meropenem and imipenem). Reported positive isolates were investigated using genotyping technology (oligonucleotide microarray-based assay and PCR). The genotyping investigation was focused on ESBL variants and the AmpC, carbapenemase and aminoglycoside resistance genes. *E. coli* was phylogenetically grouped, and the clonality of the isolates was studied using multilocus sequence typing (MLST).

Results: Our *E. coli* isolates exhibited different levels of resistance to ESBL drugs, including ampicillin (96.61%), cefoxitin (15.25%), ciprofloxacin (79.66%), cefepime (75.58%), aztreonam (89.83%), cefotaxime (76.27%), ceftazidime (81.36%), meropenem (0%) and imipenem (0%). Furthermore, the distribution of ESBL-producing *E. coli* was consistent with the data obtained using an oligonucleotide microarray-based assay and PCR genotyping against genes associated with β-lactam resistance. ST131 was the dominant sequence type lineage of the isolates and was the most uropathogenic *E. coli* lineage. The *E. coli* isolates also carried aminoglycoside resistance genes.

Conclusions: The evolution and prevalence of ESBL-producing *E. coli* may be rapidly accelerating in Saudi Arabia due to the high visitation seasons (especially to the city of Makkah). The health authority in Saudi Arabia should monitor the level of drug resistance in all general hospitals to reduce the increasing trend of microbial drug resistance and the impact on patient therapy.

Keywords: ESBL, *E. coli*, *K. pneumonia*, Phenotyping, Genotyping, Saudi Arabia

*Correspondence: eyamani@kacst.edu.sa
[1] National Center for Biotechnology, King Abdulaziz City for Science and Technology, P.O. Box 6086, Riyadh 11442, Saudi Arabia
Full list of author information is available at the end of the article

Background

Gram-negative bacteria that produce β-lactamases are a major concern in healthcare due to their ability to spread globally [1]. β-lactamases are produced by bacteria to hydrolyze the β-lactam ring in antibiotics, which results in ineffective drug treatment. Extended-spectrum β lactamases (ESBLs) are a major group of enzymes that confer resistance to several generations of β-lactam antibiotics, including third-generation cephalosporins [2, 3]. ESBL-producing Gram-negative bacteria are thought to be an important reason for cephalosporin therapy failure [4, 5]. Therefore, these bacteria should be monitored and reported by clinical laboratories to minimize their impact on patient therapy. ESBL resistance genes are primarily carried by plasmids. Plasmids may also carry genes encoding resistance to other antibiotic classes, such as ampA, ampC, aminoglycosides, chloramphenicol, macrolides, or quinolone. Therefore, treatment options are limited for bacteria that produce ESBLs due to the multiple resistance genes encoded in the plasmids. ESBL genes that are primarily encoded in plasmids include TEM, SHV, and CTX-M. Multiple variants of each gene are produced by altering the configuration of amino acids within the β-lactamase active site. Enterobacteriaceae, such as *Klebsiella pneumoniae* and *Escherichia coli*, are the major ESBL producers frequently isolated in clinical laboratories [6]. *Acinetobacter baumannii* is also an important ESBL-producing bacteria that has been reported globally [7]. Newer antibiotic classes, such as carbapenems, have been introduced by the pharmaceutical industry as treatment options for infections caused by ESBL-producing bacteria. Nevertheless, carbapenemase-producing bacteria have also been documented [8, 9]. Due to the increasing threat of multidrug-resistant bacteria, laboratory personnel, physicians, and clinical practitioners should implement a program to detect and report ESBLs as part of their infection control to limit the therapeutic failures caused by ESBL-producing bacteria. Molecular genotyping has been used concurrently with phenotyping techniques to detect and confirm antimicrobial drug resistance data and to detect Gram-negative ESBL producing bacteria [10]. PCR, multiplex PCR and oligonucleotide microarray-based assays have been developed and used to monitor the emergence of ESBLs and many other drug-resistant genes from *E. coli, K. pneumonia* and *A. baumannii* [11–15]. Strain characterization by multilocus sequence typing (MLST) is the method of choice in many clinical and research laboratories due to its high discriminatory power [16, 17]. The increased prevalence of ESBLs is being monitored and reported globally. Due to a lack of a solid data regarding the emergence of ESBLs from major Saudi general hospitals in the region of Makkah, this study reports the characterization of drug resistance genes for 58 *E. coli* isolates from an in-patient ward using phenotypic and genotypic approaches. Understanding the phenotypic and molecular nature of Enterobacteriaceae during the busy visitation Hajj season (pilgrimage season) in the city of Makkah, Saudi Arabia, is essential to reducing ESBL-strains prevalence.

Methods

Bacteriological culture

A total of 58 bacterial isolates were collected from two different general hospitals in the city of Makkah during the 2014–2015 Hajj (pilgrimage) season from patients with urinary tract infections. The bacterial isolates were phenotypically and genotypically investigated in microbiology laboratories at the King Abdulaziz City for Science and Technology (KACST). Single pure *E. coli* colonies were obtained from the all isolates. The bacteria were isolated from urine specimens using the clean-catch midstream urine sampling technique. Urine samples were inoculated using a calibrated 0.01 mL urine plastic loop on 5% sheep blood agar and MacConkey agar plates. The plates were incubated at 37 °C for 24 h. Urine samples were considered positive for UTIs if the number of colonies equaled or exceeded 10^5 CFU/mL. Gram staining was performed to identify urine specimens that contained more than 10^5 colony forming units (CFU)/mL of bacteria. A drop of well-mixed urine was fixed on a glass slide, stained, and examined under oil immersion (1000×) for the presence of at least one organism per oil immersion field.

Bacterial identification and antibiotic susceptibility testing

Bacterial identities were confirmed with a Vitek 2 GN ID card using the Vitek 2 system (bioMérieux, Marcy l'Etoile, France). Antibiotic susceptibility testing (AST) was completed using Vitek 2 cards (AST-N292) according to the manufacturer's recommendations (bioMérieux, Marcy l'Etoile, France). The Vitek ESBL susceptibility tests were interpreted according to the Clinical and Laboratory Standards Institute (CLSI) criteria using the Vitek system. *E. coli* ATCC 25922 was included in each Vitek testing step for quality control. The minimum inhibitory concentrations (MICs) were determined in Mueller–Hinton broth using microdilution plates [18]. The MICs of cefoxitin, ciprofloxacin, aztreonam, ceftazidime, meropenem, cefepime, cefotaxime, imipenem and ampicillin for all *E. coli* isolates were interpreted according to previous protocols (CLSI, 2014) [18]. Serial dilutions of the nine drugs were prepared (0.5, 1, 2, 4, 8, 16, 32, 64, 128, 256, 512 and 1024 μg/mL) in Mueller–Hinton broth and added to 96-well plates. Then, the bacterial suspensions were added to each well to achieve a final inoculum of

5×10^5 CFU/mL. The endpoint MIC was read visually and by spectrophotometer at 600 nm. The lowest concentration of antibiotic that inhibited visible bacterial growth after 24 h at 37 °C was defined as the MIC.

Amplification and sequencing of the 16S rRNA gene

The *E. coli* identity was confirmed using PCR and sequencing of the 16S rDNA gene [19–21]. Illustra PuReTaq Ready-To-Go PCR beads were used in the PCR reaction (GE Health Biosciences, USA). The 25-μL reaction was set up as follows: 2 μL of 10 pmol of each forward and reverse primer (IDT, Integrated DNA Technologies) were used with the 8-forward primer (AGA GTT TGA TCC TGG CTC AG) and 805-reverse primer (GAC TAC CAG GGT ATC TAA TC) [22]. Exactly 1 μL of DNA template was added to the beads, and the reaction was completed using 22 μL of nuclease-free ddH_2O (Promega). The amplification cycling conditions were 3 min for the initial incubation at 95 °C, followed by 35 cycles of 1 min at 95 °C, 1 min at 55 °C, and 2 min at 72 °C and a final extension at 72 °C for 7 min. All PCR amplicons were fractionated using 1% agarose gel electrophoresis prior to staining with ethidium bromide. Images were obtained with a gel documentation system under a UV transilluminator. The PCR amplicons were purified and sequenced in an ABI 3130 Genetic Analyzer (Life Technologies, Carlsbad, CA, USA) using the 16S rDNA forward primer with the ABI BigDye terminator cycle sequencing ready reaction kit according to the manufacturer's recommendations (Applied Biosystem, Foster City, CA, USA). The sequencing data were analyzed using the basic local alignment search tool BLAST-n (http://www.ncbi.nlm.nih.gov/BLAST) or the RDP database [23]. Unequivocal identification was obtained using 16S ribosomal DNA sequences.

Genetic background grouping of *E. coli* strains

The genetic background grouping of the *E. coli* isolates was explored. The grouping was performed based on Clermont phylo-typing method [24]. The majority of the pathogenic extra-intestinal *E. coli* strains belonged to groups B2. In contrast, the commensal *E. coli* strains belonged to groups A, B1, C, and F. The strains were subsequently phylogenetically inferred based on the presence or absence of the gene markers as follows: For group A, arpA+, chuA−, yjaA−, and TspE4.C2−, for group B1, arpA+, chuA−, yjaA−, and TspE4.C2+, for group F, arpA−, chuA+, yjaA−, and TspE4.C2−, for group B2, arpA−, chuA+, yjaA+, and TspE4.C2−, for group A or C, arpA+, chuA−, yjaA+, and TspE4.C2−, for group D or E, arpA+, chuA+, yjaA−, and TspE4.C2−. A standard 25-μL PCR reaction was used to investigate the genetic background of the *E. coli* strains used in our study. Illustra PuReTaq Ready-To-Go PCR beads were used in the PCR reaction (GE Health Biosciences, USA) as described by Clermont to amplify the arpA (400 bp) ChuA (288 bp), YjaA (211 bp), TspE4C2 (152 bp), and an internal control trpA (489 bp). Primers and PCR cycling conditions were described in (Table 1).

Detection of ESBL, ampC and carbapenemase genes

Global genotyping utilizing an oligonucleotide microarray-based assay and PCR genotyping were applied to identify and confirm the presence of drug resistance genes. For the microarray DNA analysis (Alere Technologies, Jena, Germany) [15], the ESBL/AmpC/carbapenemase genes were evaluated based on the manufacturer's protocols (bla_{ACC}, bla_{ACT}, bla_{CMY}, bla_{KHM}, $bla_{MOX\text{-}CMY9}$, $bla_{CTX\text{-}M\text{-}1}$, $bla_{CTX\text{-}M\text{-}15}$, $bla_{CTX\text{-}M\ 2}$, $bla_{CTX\text{-}M\text{-}8}$, $bla_{CTX\text{-}M\text{-}9}$, $bla_{CTX\text{-}M\text{-}26}$, $bla_{DHA\text{-}1}$, bla_{FOX}, $bla_{GES\text{-}1}$, $bla_{G1M\text{-}1}$, $bla_{MI\text{-}3}$, bla_{IMP}, bla_{KPC}, $bla_{LAP\text{-}1}$, $bla_{LEN\text{-}1}$, bla_{MOX}, $bla_{OXA\text{-}1}$, $bla_{OXA\text{-}2}$, $bla_{OXA\text{-}7}$, $bla_{OXA\text{-}9}$, $bla_{OXA\text{-}23}$, $bla_{OXA\text{-}23}$, $bla_{OXA\text{-}40}$, $bla_{OXA\text{-}48}$, $bla_{OXA\text{-}51}$, $bla_{OXA\text{-}54}$, $bla_{OXA\text{-}55}$, $bla_{OXA\text{-}58}$, $bla_{OXA\text{-}60}$, bla_{PER1}, bla_{PER2}, $bla_{PSE\text{-}1}$, $bla_{SHF\text{-}1}$, bla_{SHV}, $bla_{SEM\text{-}1}$, $bla_{SPM\text{-}1}$, bla_{TEM}, $bla_{VEB\text{-}1}$, and bla_{VIM}). For the PCR analysis, DNA templates were obtained by boiling 500 μL of bacterial cells ($OD_{600} = 1.0$) in a sterile single 1.5 mL Eppendorf tube in a water bath at 100 °C. The DNA lysate was diluted 1:10 with ddH_2O and frozen at −20 °C before use for bacterial genotyping confirmation with gene-specific primers (Table 2) [10]. The primers detected the β-lactamase genes and their variants (TEM, SHV, and CTX-M groups 1, 15, 2, 8, 9, and 26). The PCRs were performed using a 9800 Thermal Cycler (Applied Biosystem, USA) in a total volume of 25 μL containing 10 pmol of primers, 25 μmol of dNTPs, 10 μL of gDNA/plasmid lysate, 2.5 μL of 10X *Taq* buffer, 2.5 mM $MgCl_2$ and 2.5 U of *Taq* polymerase. The cycling conditions used for the PCR were an initial denaturation at 94 °C for 10 min, 35 cycles of 94 °C for 40 s, 60 °C for 40 s and 72 °C for 1 min and a final extension step at 72 °C for 7 min [10]. All PCR amplicons were fractionated by 1% agarose gel electrophoresis prior to staining with ethidium bromide. Images were obtained with a gel documentation system under a UV transilluminator.

Bacterial genotyping by multilocus sequence typing

Fifty-eight *E. coli* isolates were subjected to multilocus sequence typing (MLST) as previously described [25]. The MLST schemes used to type *E. coli* were conducted using internal fragments of the following seven housekeeping genes: *Adk* (adenylate kinase), *fumC* (fumarate hydratase), *gyrB* (DNA gyrase), *mdh* (malate dehydrogenase), *purA* (adenylosuccinate dehydrogenase), *icd* (isocitrate/isopropylmalate dehydrogenase), *recA* (ATP/GTP binding motif) (ID Genomics Inc, Seattle, WA, USA). The primers

Table 1 Primer sequences and PCR conditions for quadruplex phylo-grouping of *E. coli*

Target gene	Primer sequence	Size (bp)	PCR conditions	Reference
arpA (phylogenetic grouping)	F (5-AACGCTATTCGCCAGCTTGC-3) R (5-TCTCCCCATACCGTACGCTA-3)	400	PCR reactions were performed in a total volume of 25 μL by ready-to go PCR beads using 20 pmol of each primers for all targets except arpA (40 pmol) and trpA (12 pmol). The cycling conditions were as follow: denaturation 4 min at 94 °C, 30 cycles of 5 s at 94 °C and 20 s at 59 °C, 20 s at 72 °C and a final extension step of 5 min at 72 °C	[24]
chuA (phylogenetic grouping)	F (5-GACGAACCAACGGTCAGGAT-3) R (5-TGCCGCCAGTACCAAAGACA-3)	288		
yjaA (phylogenetic grouping)	F (5-TGAAGTGTCAGGAGACGCTG-3) R (5-ATGGAGAATGCGTTCCTCAAC-3)	211		
TspE4C2 (phylogenetic grouping)	F (5-GAGTAATGTCGGGGCATTCA-3) R (5-GCGCCAACAAAGTATTACG-3)	152		
Internal control trpA	F (5-CGGCGATAAAGACATCTTCAC-3) R (5-GCAACGCGGCCTGGCGGAAG-3)	489		

Table 2 Multiplex PCR-specific primers for ESBL gene detection in *Enterobacteriacaea*

Primer name	β-Lactamase target	Sequence (5′–3′)	Length (bases)	Amplicon size (bp)	Reference
Multiplex I TEM, SHV	TEM variants including TEM-1 and TEM-2	Multi- F CATTTCCGTGTCGCCCTTATTC Multi- R CGTTCATCCATAGTTGCCTGAC	22	800	[10]
	SHV variants including SHV-1	Multi-F AGCCGCTTGAGCAAATTAAAC Multi-R ATCCCGCAGATAAATCACCAC	21	713	
Multiplex II CTX-M group 1	Variants of CTX-M group 1 including CTX-M-1, CTX-M-3 and CTX-M-15	MultiCTX-M Gp1-F TTAGGAARTGTGCCGCTGYA MultiCTX-MGP1-R CGATATCGTTGGTGGTRCCAT	20 21	688	
Multiplex II CTX-M group 2	Variants of CTX-M group 2 including CTX-M-2	MultiCTX-MGp2-F CGTTAACGGCACGATGAC MultiCTXMGp2-R CGATATCGTTGGTGGTRCCA	18 21	404	
Multiplex II CTX-M group 9	Variants of CTX-M group 9 including CTX-M-9 and CTX-M-14	MultiCTX-MGp9-F TCAAGCCTGCCGATCTGGT MultiCTX-MGp9-R TGATTCTCGCCGCTGAAG	19 18	561	
Multiplex III CTX-M group 8/25	CTX-M-8, CTX-M-25, CTX-M-26 and CTX-M-39 to CTX-M-41	MultiCTX-MGg8/25-F AACRCRCAGACGCTCTAC MultiCTX-MGg8/25-R TCGAGCCGGAASGTGTYAT	18 19	326	

used for amplification and sequencing are illustrated in (Table 3) [25]. The PCR amplifications were performed using a 9800 Thermal Cycler (Applied Biosystem, USA) with the following conditions: initial denaturation at 94 °C for 7 min, followed by 35 cycles of denaturation at 94 °C for 30 s and an annealing temperature of 56 °C for 30 s, extension at 72 °C for 2 min and a final 7-min extension at 72 °C. The PCR amplicons were checked with 1% agarose gel electrophoresis prior to purification for sequencing. Forward and reverse sequencing reactions were performed for every isolate. Different allele sequences were assigned for each locus with an arbitrary allele number for identification. Each bacterial isolate was characterized by a pattern of numbers defining its sequence type (ST). The sequencing data of the MLST genes were analyzed using the *E. coli* MLST Database (Warwick Medical School, Coventry, UK database; http://mlst.warwick.ac.uk/mlst/dbs/Ecoli) [25]. The similarities of the allelic profiles were assessed using the Molecular Evolutionary Genetics Analysis (MEGA 6) software.

Phylogenetic analysis

Phylogenetic trees based on the concatenated alleles of seven MLST genes were constructed using the Molecular Evolutionary Genetics Analysis (Mega6) software for the *E. coli* dataset. The maximum likelihood trees were based on neighbor-joining (NJ) starting trees with Nearest-Neighbor Interchange branch swapping. The tree stability was assessed using the bootstrap method [26].

Results

Bacterial identification and antibiotic susceptibility testing

All obtained clinical *E. coli* isolates (n = 58) were phenotypically studied using the Vitek system and the microbroth dilution method to determine the MIC values against various antimicrobial drugs (cefoxitin, ciprofloxacin, aztreonam, ceftazidime, meropenem, cefepime, cefotaxime, imipenem and ampicillin), (Table 4). The greatest number of *E. coli* isolates was resistant to ampicillin (96.61%), followed by cefotaxime (76.27%), cefepime (74.58%), ceftazidime (81.36%), aztreonam (89.83%), and

Table 3 Primers used to amplify and sequence the seven housekeeping genes in the *E. coli* isolates for the MLST analysis

Gene	Primer sequences	Usage
adk	F 5′-ATTCTGCTTGGCGCTCCGGG -3′ R 5′-CCGTCAACTTTCGCGTATTT-3′	Amp/seq
fumC	F 5′-TCACAGGTCGCCAGCGCTTC-3′ R 5′-GTACGCAGCGAAAAAGATTC-3′	Amp/seq
gyrB	F 5′-TCGGCGACACGGATGACGG-3′ R 5′-ATCAGGCCTTCACGCGCATC-3′	Amp/seq
icd	F 5′-ATGGAAAGTAAAGTAGTTGTTCCGGCACA-3′ R 5′-GGACGCAGCAGGATCTGTT-3′	Amp/seq
mdh	F 5′-ATGAAAGTCGCAGTCCTCGGCGCTGCTGGCGG-3′ R 5′-TTAACGAACTCCTGCCCCAGAGCGA-TATCTTTCTT-3′	Amp/seq
purA	F 5′-CGCGCTGATGAAAGAGATGA-3′ R 5′-CATACGGTAAGCCACGCAGA-3′	Amp/seq
recA	F 5′-CGCATTCGCTTTACCCTGACC-3′ R 5′-TCTCGATCAGCTTCTCTTTT-3′	Amp/seq

cefoxitin (15.25%). Meropenem and imipenem had rates of 0%, and the non-β-lactam ciprofloxacin had a rate of 79.66%. All *E. coli* isolates were sensitive to meropenem and imipenem (Fig. 1).

ESBL-producing *E. coli* genotyping

The genotyping of ESBL-producing *E. coli* isolates by the global analysis of an oligonucleotide microarray-based assay and PCR identified a high proportion of β-lactamase genes among the *E. coli* isolates. The *bla*CTX-M1, *bla*CTX-M15, blaOXA1 and *bla*TEM genotypes were more frequently identified and were more predominant among the *E. coli* isolates than the *bla*CTX-M, *bla*OXA and *bla*SHV variants. The prevalence was 46.7% for *bla*CTX-M1 and *bla*CTX-M15, 48.3% for *bla*OXA1, and 38.7% for *bla*TEM. The genotypic prevalence of *bla*SHV was 3.2% among all isolates, which was considerably lower than the prevalence for *bla*CTX-M1, *bla*CTX-M15, *bla*OXA1 and *bla*TEM. No carbapenem-resistant *E. coli* isolate was detected (Fig. 2).

Distribution of ESBL genes in *E. coli*

The β-lactam genes were studied to evaluate the distribution of the genes among our isolates. We found that 13.7% (8/58) of the *E. coli* isolates harbored four major ESBL genes (bla_{CTX-M1}, $bla_{CTX-M15}$, bla_{OXA1}, and bla_{TEM}) and 17.2% (10/58) contained three ESBL genes (bla_{CTX-M1}, $bla_{CTX-M15}$, and bla_{OXA1}). Additionally, two positive ESBL genotypes (3.4%; 2/58) contained bla_{OXA1} and bla_{TEM} and two isolates contained only bla_{SHV} (3.4%; 2/58). No carbapenemase genes were detected among the isolates according to the phenotypic and genotypic testing.

The phylogenetic grouping of *E. coli* strains

The genetic background grouping of the *E. coli* isolates was assigned based on the Clermont method which is very specific for *E. coli* phylo-typing groups [24]. It has shown that 46.55% (27) of the ESBL-producing *E. coli* isolate collection belonged to group B2, and 6.9% (4) belonged to group D or E, while 12% (7) belonged to group B1, 3.4% (2) belonged to group A, 24% (14) belonged to group A or C and 6.9% (4) belonged to group F. The majority of the pathogenic extra-intestinal *E. coli* strains belonged to groups B2 (Fig. 3).

Prevalence of genes associated with aminoglycoside resistance in the *E. coli* isolates

The prevalence of genes associated with aminoglycoside resistance among the 58 *E. coli* isolates was investigated. A total of 44.8% of the *E. coli* isolates carried the *aac6* gene, 43% harbored *aac6Ib*, 42% contained *aadA4*, and 36% contained *strB*; these prevalences represented high proportions and were more common than the other aminoglycoside genes (15% for *aadA1*, 12% for *aadA2*, 4% for *aadB*, 4% for *ant2*, 12% for *aphA* and 1% for *strA*) (Fig. 4).

Bacterial genotyping by MLST

In this study, 58 *E. coli* isolates were assigned sequence types (ST) and ST complexes (STc) using a standard multi-locus sequence typing method (Fig. 5) [25]. Of the 58 *E. coli* isolates, 7 isolates (12%) belonged to STc 10, 20 isolates (34.5%) to STc 131, and 4 isolates (7%) to STc 648 and STc 38. Other ST complexes (46, 448, 156, 155, 23, 12 and 73) were represented by 1–3 isolates (2–5%). The ST complex could not be determined for 14 isolates (24%). A new allele of the *rec*A gene was identified in isolate ID 4. This allele had one nucleotide substitution compared to allele 2 at position 40 from the beginning of the allele (C substituted by T). The allelic profile of one isolate (isolate ID 12) was not previously reported (Fig. 5).

Phylogenetic analysis

We conducted a phylogenetic analysis to examine the clonal diversity and phylogenetic relationships among the *E. coli* isolates. The *E. coli* isolates clustered in several monophyletic clades that corresponded to known phylogenetic groups. The majority of the *E. coli* isolates fell into the phylogenetic groups B2: ST131 (20 isolates), ST1193 (3 isolates) [27], ST73 (1 isolate), ST12 (1 isolate) and ST127 (1 isolate). In this study, four *E. coli* isolates appeared to belong to group E: ST38 (3 isolates) [27] ST315 (1 isolate), of which all isolates were from STc 38. Of the rest, one isolate belonged to phylogroup A, thirteen to phylogroup C, eight to phylogroup B1, two to phylogroup C, and four to phylogroup F. Most of the known virulent extraintestinal strains primarily belong to group

Table 4 Minimum inhibitory concentration (MIC) values of antimicrobial agents against ESBL-producing *E. coli*

Strains	Cefoxitin (μg/mL) R ≥ 32 MIC	Cefepime (μg/mL) R ≥ 16 MIC	Aztreonam (μg/mL) R ≥ 4 MIC	Ceftazidime (μg/mL) R ≥ 16 MIC	Cefotaxime (μg/mL) R ≥ 64 MIC	Ciprofloxacin (μg/mL) R ≥ 4 MIC	Meropenem (μg/mL) R ≥ 4 MIC	Imipenem (μg/mL) R ≥ 4 MIC	Ampecillin (μg/mL) R ≥ 32 MIC
1059	8	32	256	128	1024	1024	<0.5	<0.5	>1024
1129	8	<0.5	<0.5	<0.5	<0.5	16	<0.5	<0.5	1024
1060	4	64	64	64	>1024	>1024	<0.5	<0.5	>1024
1097	4	64	128	32	>1024	<0.5	<0.5	<0.5	>1024
4110	8	8	128	16	64	32	<0.5	<0.5	1024
7055	1	16	<0.5	32	1024	1	<0.5	<0.5	>1024
1015	16	16	32	8	64	1024	<0.5	<0.5	512
2001	4	<0.5	128	64	1024	64	<0.5	<0.5	>1024
1114	8	256	512	128	>1024	128	<0.5	<0.5	>1024
1007	8	16	128	32	128	128	<0.5	<0.5	>1024
1111	256	128	128	128	>1024	64	<0.5	<0.5	>1024
1128	16	16	64	16	256	1024	<0.5	<0.5	1024
1005	4	4	64	16	1024	16	<0.5	<0.5	>1024
1116	8	16	32	8	>1024	64	<0.5	<0.5	>1024
1010	2	<0.5	<0.5	<0.5	2	32	<0.5	<0.5	>1024
1041	512	1024	>1024	1024	>1024	1024	<0.5	1	>1024
1089	8	128	128	32	1024	64	<0.5	<0.5	>1024
1031	16	32	128	32	256	32	<0.5	<0.5	>1024
1055	16	256	256	256	>1024	1024	<0.5	<0.5	>1024
1057	16	64	512	128	1024	1024	<0.5	<0.5	>1024
1075	8	8	512	64	32	64	<0.5	<0.5	1024
1065	8	128	512	256	1024	<0.5	<0.5	<0.5	>1024
1085	32	64	64	16	512	64	<0.5	<0.5	>1024
1053	16	256	512	128	>1024	1024	<0.5	<0.5	>1024
1054	32	256	256	128	>1024	1024	<0.5	<0.5	>1024
1013	16	16	64	32	512	16	<0.5	<0.5	>1024
1011	16	64	256	64	1024	1024	<0.5	<0.5	>1024
1034	16	64	256	128	256	128	<0.5	<0.5	>1024
1028	8	32	256	64	512	<0.5	<0.5	<0.5	>1024
1045	16	4	128	8	32	1024	<0.5	<0.5	1024
1118	32	32	128	32	256	1024	<0.5	<0.5	1024
1096	1	<0.5	>1024	<0.5	<0.5	<0.5	<0.5	<0.5	<0.5
1110	8	128	256	64	512	1024	<0.5	<0.5	>1024
1025	8	16	>1024	32	256	32	<0.5	<0.5	>1024
1016	16	16	128	64	256	16	<0.5	<0.5	>1024
4003	8	16	256	64	512	1024	<0.5	<0.5	>1024
90003	32	128	>1024	512	>1024	64	<0.5	<0.5	>1024
1020	128	<0.5	4	32	8	<0.5	<0.5	<0.5	>1024
1094	16	32	256	64	512	64	<0.5	<0.5	>1024
1019	8	128	>1024	512	>1024	64	<0.5	<0.5	>1024
1012	16	<0.5	<0.5	4	<0.5	32	<0.5	<0.5	8
2002	8	16	1024	32	256	32	<0.5	<0.5	>1024
4045	8	8	128	32	256	64	<0.5	<0.5	>1024
1081	8	32	256	32	512	1024	<0.5	<0.5	>1024
1018	4	32	128	64	1024	<0.5	<0.5	<0.5	>1024
3043	4	<0.5	<0.5	<0.5	<0.5	16	<0.5	<0.5	1024
1091	16	128	512	256	>1024	1024	<0.5	<0.5	>1024

Table 4 continued

Strains	Cefoxitin (μg/mL) R ≥ 32	Cefepime (μg/mL) R ≥ 16	Aztreonam (μg/mL) R ≥ 4	Ceftazidime (μg/mL) R ≥ 16	Cefotaxime (μg/mL) R ≥ 64	Ciprofloxacin (μg/mL) R ≥ 4	Meropenem (μg/mL) R ≥ 4	Imipenem (μg/mL) R ≥ 4	Ampecillin (μg/mL) R ≥ 32
	MIC	MIC	MIC	MIC	MIC	MIC	MIC	MIC	MIC
3067	32	<0.5	16	64	64	<0.5	<0.5	<0.5	>1024
2003	16	64	256	64	512	4	<0.5	<0.5	>1024
1103	32	32	16	2	64	1024	<0.5	<0.5	>1024
1120	16	32	64	32	256	32	<0.5	<0.5	>1024
1119	8	64	256	64	1024	1024	<0.5	<0.5	>1024
1098	8	8	128	32	128	64	<0.5	<0.5	1024
1124	8	64	512	256	1024	32	<0.5	<0.5	>1024
1104	16	16	16	1	64	<0.5	<0.5	<0.5	>1024
1125	8	32	128	64	512	<0.5	<0.5	<0.5	>1024
1102	8	64	256	64	512	128	<0.5	<0.5	>1024
1117	16	128	256	128	1024	<0.5	<0.5	<0.5	>1024
1105	8	<0.5	<0.5	<0.5	<0.5	<0.5	<0.5	<0.5	>1024

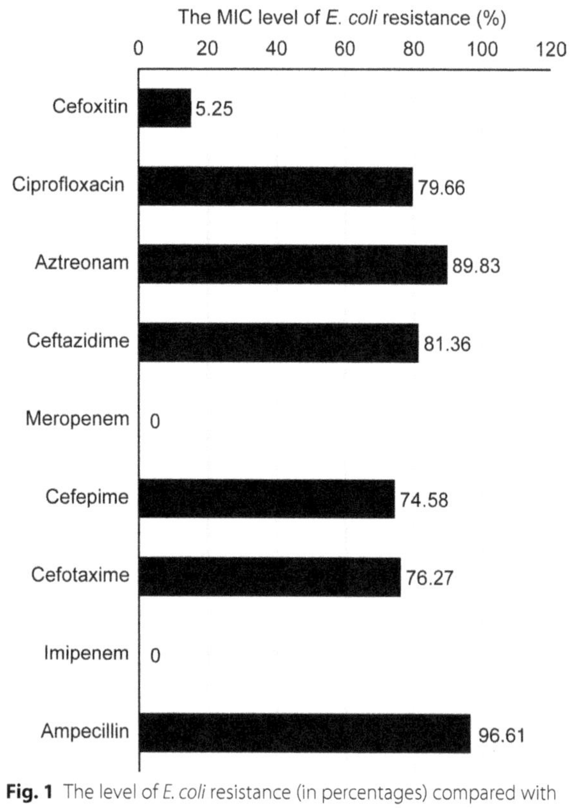

Fig. 1 The level of *E. coli* resistance (in percentages) compared with the major ESBL drugs based on the MIC tests. No carbapenase phenotype was detected but Ciprofloxacin-resistance (fluoroquinolone resistance) was identified among the *E. coli* isolates

B2 and to a lesser extent to group D or E (4). Group A together with group B1, F, and C are considered predominant among commensal *E. coli* strains (5).

Discussion

During congested visitation seasons, especially during the religious pilgrimage (Hajj), the risk of spreading multidrug-resistant microbes increases substantially [28]. Therefore, this study investigated the prevalence of ESBL-producing *E. coli* in local general hospitals in Makkah during Hajj and the correlation between the ESBL phenotype and antimicrobial drug resistance using genotyping approaches. This study also explored multilocus sequence typing (MLST) to characterize these isolates and to enhance our understanding of the epidemiology of ESBL-producing *E. coli* in our region. Our data had demonstrated that our *E. coli* isolates exhibited varying levels of resistance to ESBL drugs and carried genes associated with aminoglycoside resistance. No carbapenem resistance genes were identified in any of the collected and investigated *E. coli* isolates (n = 58). All uropathogenic *E. coli* isolates in this study are classified as multidrug-resistant (MDR) according to the criteria by Magiorakos [29].

The distribution of ESBL-producing *E. coli* was consistent with the data obtained from an oligonucleotide microarray-based assay and PCR genotyping against genes associated with β-lactam resistance. The dominant sequence type lineage of the isolates was ST131, which is

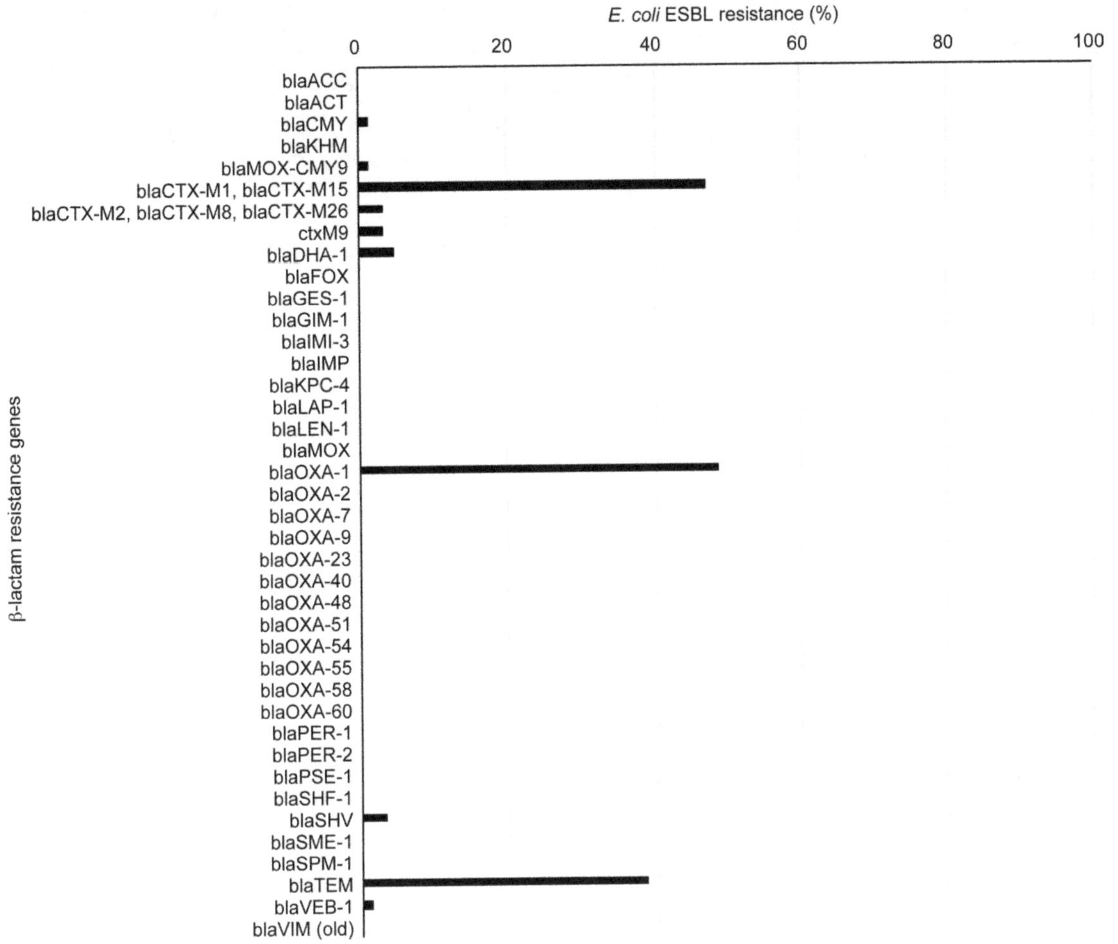

Fig. 2 The distribution of the 58 ESBL-producing *E. coli* isolates investigated via oligonucleotide microarray-based assay and PCR genotyping against genes associated with β-lactam resistance

the most uropathogenic *E. coli* lineage. The most commonly isolated bacterium from patients with urinary tract infections is *E. coli*. These isolates usually harbor different plasmids. Therefore, they have a tendency to acquire multidrug-resistant phenotypes and are difficult to treat.

Consistent with our study, studies have associated ST131/CTX-M15 human uropathogenic *E. coli* with ST410/CTX-M15, and ST648/CTX-M15. However, it was shown that ST410/CTX-M15, and ST648/CTX-M15 were also isolated from uropathogenic *E. coli* of cats and dogs (feline and canine) in Switzerland [30, 31]. These circulating STs may suggest that disease transmission between companion animals and humans may occur by direct contact. Furthermore, three isolates of *E. coli* ST1193 were evident in this study. *E. coli* ST1193 is associated with urinary tract infection and fluoroquinolone-resistance, namely ciprofloxacin-resistance (Figs. 1, 5) [32, 33]. *E. coli* ST1193 may also be transmitted through household contact as suggested by a study from Japan [34].

It was demonstrated that multidrug-resistance (MDR) *E. coli* clone ST131 was globally disseminated in six different geographical countries. The rapid spread and emergence among countries may be due to high virulence factor gene-content, the presence of ESBL CTX-M-15, and fluoroquinolones resistance. Notably, the *E. coli* clone ST131 fluoroquinolone resistance phenotype was

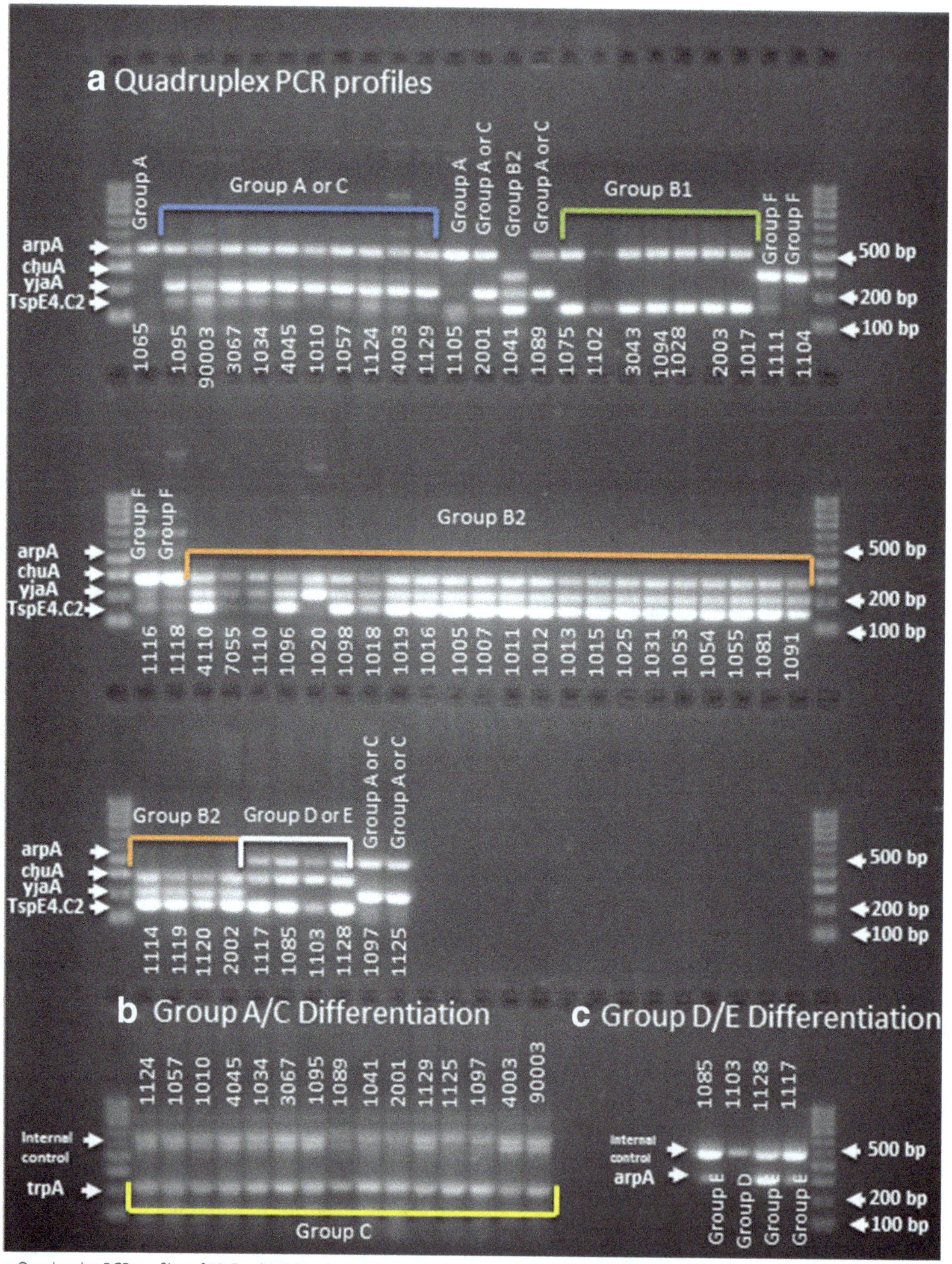

Fig. 3 **a** Quadruples PCR profiles of 58 *E. coli* MDR isolates. Isolate IDs shown under *each lane*. Data assignment were performed according to the presence or absence of signals of the following gene order arpA, chuA, yjaA, TspE4.C2. *Row 1*, *lanes 1*, *12*—group A (+−−−); *lanes 2–11*, *13*, *15*—groups A or C (+−+−), *lanes 16–22*—group B1 (+−+), *lane 14*—group B2 (−+++), *lanes 23–24*—group F (−+−); *Row 2*, *lanes 1–2*—group F (−+−), *lanes 3–24*—group B2 (−+++) or (−++−) in *lane 7*; *Row 3*, *lanes 1–4*—group B2 (−+++), *lanes 5–8*—groups E or D (++−+), *lanes 9–10*—groups A or C (+−+−). **b** Groups A/C differentiation. In all *lanes*, both bands for internal control and Group C specific trpA fragment (219 bp) are present. **c** Groups D/E differentiation. *Lanes 1*, *3* and *4*—both bands for internal control and Group E specific arpA fragment (301 bp) are present. *Lane 2*—only internal control present

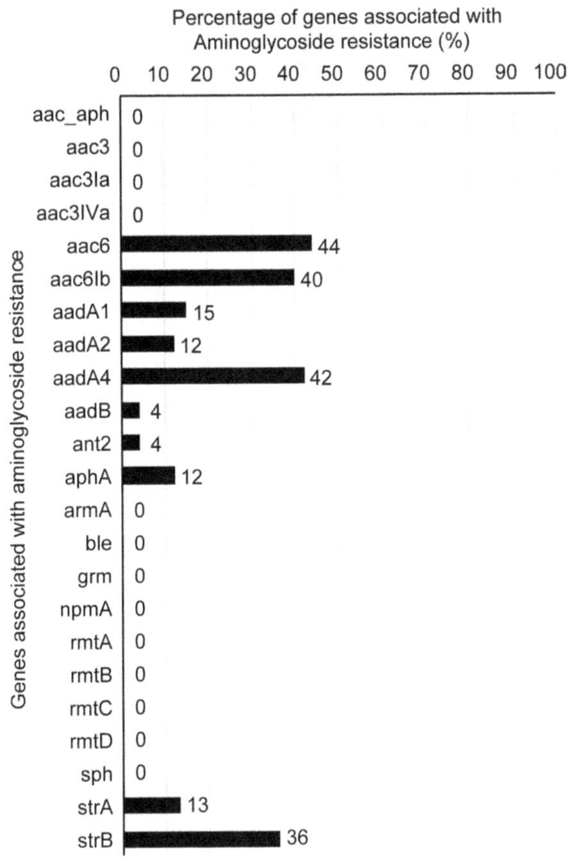

Fig. 4 Prevalence of genes associated with aminoglycoside resistance

the most prevalent geographically and was detected in this current study in Saudi Arabia (Figs. 1, 5) [35].

Studies have shown that pathogenicity island acquisition by uropathogenic *E. coli* may worsen urinary tract infections and aid in evasion of the host immune response, resulting in spreading in the bloodstream. Gene acquisition by intestinal pathogenic bacteria promotes their colonization in different intestinal regions; these genes may also alter the mechanism of bacterial-host interactions, causing distinct gastrointestinal pathology [27]. It was shown that a urinary sepsis niche for *E. coli* ST131 compared to bacteremia in non-ST131 *E. coli* clones [32, 36]. However, this niche could not be linked to the clinical manifestation of renal tract infections in humans. No clinical focus to other sites of infection, such as intra-abdominal abscess, ascitic fluid, bones/joints, respiratory tract or bacteremia, has been established for the ST131 clone [37, 38]. There is evidence for a direct human-to-human route of transmission for ST131. For instance, an elderly father with pyelonephritis transmitted ST131 *E. coli* to his daughter, which initiated a similar illness in her. Similarly, an identical clone was identified from a young child with osteoarticular infection and a fecal sample from his mother [39, 40]. ST131 may contain genes for multiple antimicrobial resistance mechanisms, which may make therapy difficult. Carbapenems alone or in combination with amikacin were successfully used to treat infections caused by clones harboring CTX-M genes [32, 39]. A study demonstrated ESBL-producing *E. coli* acquisition among Makkah visitors after the Hajj (pilgrimage) season, especially CTX-M genes [28].

Molecular epidemiological studies have focused on the characterization and spread of the ST131 clone; however, global studies on the distribution and spread between humans and animals are limited, particularly in the developing world. There is a high frequency of infection by the drug-resistant ST131 clone in developing countries and a lack of timely countermeasures resulting in high morbidity and mortality rates [41–43].

Conclusion

In this study, 58 *E. coli* isolates were collected from patients with urinary tract infections from two local hospitals in the city of Makkah during the 2014–2015 Hajj (pilgrimage) season and screened for the production of ESBL/AmpC/carbapenemase/aminoglycoside resistance genes using phenotypic and genotypic analyses. Our data had demonstrated that our isolates primarily carried various ESBL and aminoglycoside resistance genes. The dominant sequence type lineage of the isolates was ST131, which was the most uropathogenic *E. coli* lineage. A genetic analysis of multiple isolates from the Middle Eastern regions may contribute to the development of rapid molecular detection methods and may lead to new therapies. Furthermore, controlling the endemicity of emerging MDR and decreasing the occurrence and prevalence of drug-resistant uropathogenic *E. coli* during heavy visitation seasons in the city of Makkah may involve the implementation of a stringent antidrug treatment policy.

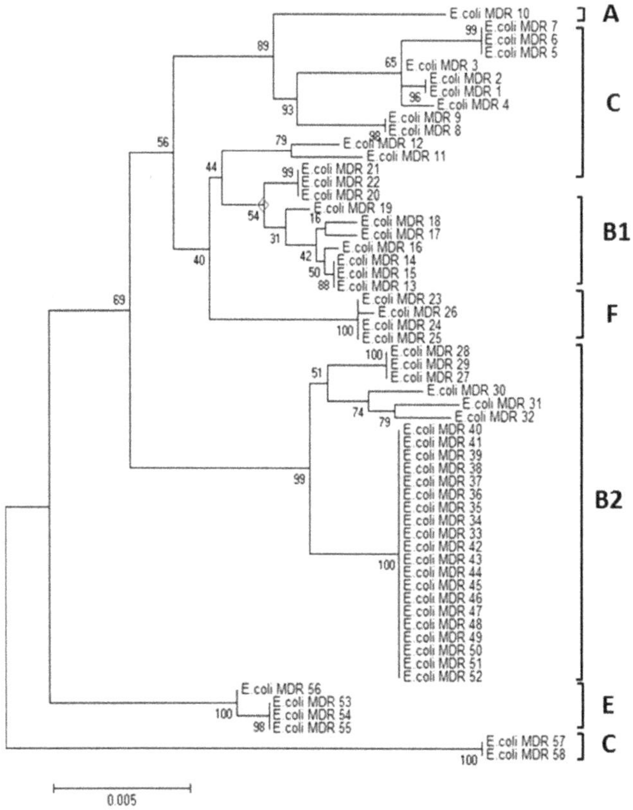

Isolate ID	Phylogroup	Isolate name	fumC	adk	icd	mdh	gyrB	purA	recA	ST	STc
10	A	1065	7	8	8	8	1	8	6	46	46
7	C	4003	11	10	8	8	4	13	73	617	10
6	C	1124	11	10	8	8	4	13	73	617	10
5	C	1057	11	10	8	8	4	13	73	617	10
3	C	1010	11	10	8	8	4	8	2	10	10
2	C	4045	11	10	8	8	4	8	7	44	10
1	C	1034	11	10	8	8	4	8	7	44	10
4	C	3067	11	10	1	8	4	8	2*NEW	NEW	10
9	C	90003	4	10	8	8	4	13	73	1284	none
8	C	1095	4	10	8	8	4	13	73	1284	none
12	C	1129	19	6	18	8	4	8	2	NEW	none
11	A	1105	29	6	18	11	178	8	41	1324	none
21	C	1089	4	6	1	20	12	18	7	410	23
22	C	2001	4	6	1	20	12	18	7	410	23
20	B2	1041	4	6	1	20	12	18	7	410	23
19	B1	1075	4	6	16	24	4	8	14	58	155
18	B1	1102	29	6	16	11	32	8	44	156	156
17	B1	3043	4	6	16	11	33	8	6	224	none
16	B1	1094	6	6	16	11	5	8	7	448	448
14	B1	1028	6	6	16	11	22	1	7	940	none
15	B1	2003	6	6	16	11	22	1	7	940	none
13	B1	1017	6	6	16	11	22	1	7	940	none
23	F	1111	4	92	96	70	87	58	2	648	648
26	F	1104	4	92	96	70	87	58	91	624	648
24	F	1116	4	92	96	70	87	58	2	648	648
25	F	1118	4	92	96	70	87	58	2	648	648
28	B2	4110	14	14	200	17	10	7	10	1193	none
29	B2	7055	14	14	200	17	10	7	10	1193	none
27	B2	1110	14	14	200	17	10	7	10	1193	none
30	B2	1096	14	13	36	23	19	11	10	127	none
31	B2	1020	13	13	13	16	9	10	9	12	12
32	B2	1098	24	36	13	17	9	11	25	73	73
40	B2	1018	40	53	13	36	47	28	29	131	131
41	B2	1019	40	53	13	36	47	28	29	131	131
39	B2	1016	40	53	13	36	47	28	29	131	131
38	B2	1005	40	53	13	36	47	28	29	131	131
37	B2	1007	40	53	13	36	47	28	29	131	131
36	B2	1011	40	53	13	36	47	28	29	131	131
35	B2	1012	40	53	13	36	47	28	29	131	131
34	B2	1013	40	53	13	36	47	28	29	131	131
33	B2	1015	40	53	13	36	47	28	29	131	131
42	B2	1025	40	53	13	36	47	28	29	131	131
43	B2	1031	40	53	13	36	47	28	29	131	131
44	B2	1053	40	53	13	36	47	28	29	131	131
45	B2	1054	40	53	13	36	47	28	29	131	131
46	B2	1055	40	53	13	36	47	28	29	131	131
47	B2	1081	40	53	13	36	47	28	29	131	131
48	B2	1091	40	53	13	36	47	28	29	131	131
49	B2	1114	40	53	13	36	47	28	29	131	131
50	B2	1119	40	53	13	36	47	28	29	131	131
51	B2	1120	40	53	13	36	47	28	29	131	131
52	B2	2002	40	53	13	36	47	28	29	131	131
56	E	1117	26	4	25	5	2	8	19	315	38
53	E	1085	26	4	25	5	2	5	19	38	38
54	D	1103	26	4	25	5	2	5	19	38	38
55	E	1128	26	4	25	5	2	5	19	38	38
57	C	1097	54	52	48	438	46	40	38	5584	none
58	C	1125	54	52	48	438	46	40	38	5584	none

Fig. 5 Phylogenetic tree of 58 MDR *E. coli* strains constructed using the maximum likelihood algorithm in the MEGA6 software [27] and based on the concatenated alleles of 7 housekeeping genes according to Achtman's scheme (*columns 4–10*). The *numerals* on the branches represent bootstrap values. The phylogenetic analysis identified 24 ST (*column 11*) that corresponded to 11 ST complexes (STc, *column 12*). Phylogenetic groups in *column 2* were identified using phylo-typing method [24] by quadruplex PCR using four target genes (*arpA*±, *chuA*±, *yjaA*±, *TspE4.C2*±). Strains incorrectly assigned using the extended quadruplex method are indicated in *red*. The phylo-group memberships of two isolates (1097, 1125) were ambiguous. Notably, *E. coli* Clone ST131, ST410, and ST1193, which are disseminated globally, were among the identified STs in this study

Abbreviations

MDR: multi drug resistance; ESBL: extended-spectrum-β-lactamase; AmpC: AmpC beta-lactamases; MIC: minimum inhibitory concentration; MLST: multilocus sequence typing; ST: sequence typing; STc: sequence typing complex.

Authors' contributions

EA and AK contributed to the study design. RB, FB, MM, and ER collected the samples, and all authors contributed equally to the laboratory experiments. All authors contributed to the data interpretation. EA and AK drafted and revised the manuscript. All authors read and approved the final manuscript.

Author details

[1] National Center for Biotechnology, King Abdulaziz City for Science and Technology, P.O. Box 6086, Riyadh 11442, Saudi Arabia. [2] College of Medicine, Princess Nora Bint Abdul Rahman University, Riyadh 12484, Saudi Arabia. [3] Hera Hospital, Makkah, Saudi Arabia. [4] ID Genomics, Seattle, WA, USA.

Acknowledgements

All authors wish to acknowledge the Life Science & *Environment Research Institute and* the National Center for Biotechnology at KACST for supporting and facilitating this work.

Competing interests

All authors declare that they have no competing interests.

Consent for publication

All authors approve the publication of this work.

Funding

This work was funded by an internal grant from the Life Science & *Environment Research Institute and from* the National Center for Biotechnology at KACST.

References

1. Pitout JD, Laupland KB. Extended-spectrum beta-lactamase-producing Enterobacteriaceae: an emerging public-health concern. Lancet Infect Dis. 2008;8(3):159–66.
2. Knothe H, Shah P, Krcmery V, Antal M, Mitsuhashi S. Transferable resistance to cefotaxime, cefoxitin, cefamandole and cefuroxime in clinical isolates of *Klebsiella pneumoniae* and *Serratia marcescens*. Infection. 1983;11(6):315–7.
3. Philippon A, Labia R, Jacoby G. Extended-spectrum beta-lactamases. Antimicrob Agents Chemother. 1989;33(8):1131.

4. Drawz SM, Papp-Wallace KM, Bonomo RA. New beta-lactamase inhibitors: a therapeutic renaissance in an MDR world. Antimicrob Agents Chemother. 2014;58(4):1835–46.
5. Rawat D, Nair D. Extended-spectrum beta-lactamases in Gram Negative Bacteria. J Glob Infect Dis. 2010;2(3):263–74.
6. Livermore DM. Bacterial resistance: origins, epidemiology, and impact. Clin Infect Dis. 2003;36(Suppl 1):S11–23.
7. Antunes LC, Visca P, Towner KJ. *Acinetobacter baumannii*: evolution of a global pathogen. Pathog Dis. 2014;71(3):292–301.
8. Gupta N, Limbago BM, Patel JB, Kallen AJ. Carbapenem-resistant Enterobacteriaceae: epidemiology and prevention. Clin Infect Dis. 2011;53(1):60–7.
9. Kanj SS, Kanafani ZA. Current concepts in antimicrobial therapy against resistant gram-negative organisms: extended-spectrum β-lactamase—producing Enterobacteriaceae, carbapenem-resistant Enterobacteriaceae, and multidrug-resistant *Pseudomonas aeruginosa*. Mayo Clin Proc. 2011;86(3):250–9.
10. Dallenne C, Da Costa A, Decre D, Favier C, Arlet G. Development of a set of multiplex PCR assays for the detection of genes encoding important beta-lactamases in Enterobacteriaceae. J Antimicrob Chemother. 2010;65(3):490–5.
11. Trung NT, Hien TT, Huyen TT, Quyen DT, Binh MT, Hoan PQ, Meyer CG, Velavan TP, le Song H. Simple multiplex PCR assays to detect common pathogens and associated genes encoding for acquired extended spectrum betalactamases (ESBL) or carbapenemases from surgical site specimens in Vietnam. Ann Clin Microbiol Antimicrob. 2015;14(1):23.
12. Valverde A, Turrientes MC, Norman F, San Martín E, Moreno L, Pérez-Molina JA, López-Vélez R, Cantón R. CTX-M-15-non-ST131 *Escherichia coli* isolates are mainly responsible of faecal carriage with ESBL-producing Enterobacteriaceae in travellers, immigrants and those visiting friends and relatives. Clin Microbiol Infect. 2015;21(3):252.e251–4.
13. Tawfik AF, Alswailem AM, Shibl AM, Al-Agamy MH. Prevalence and genetic characteristics of TEM, SHV, and CTX-M in clinical *Klebsiella pneumoniae* isolates from Saudi Arabia. Microb Drug Resist. 2011;17(3):383–8.
14. Alyamani EJ, Khiyami MA, Booq RY, Alnafjan BM, Altammami MA, Bahwerth FS. Molecular characterization of extended-spectrum beta-lactamases (ESBLs) produced by clinical isolates of *Acinetobacter baumannii* in Saudi Arabia. Ann Clin Microbiol Antimicrob. 2015;14(1):38.
15. Braun SD, Monecke S, Thurmer A, Ruppelt A, Makarewicz O, Pletz M, Reibetaig A, Slickers P, Ehricht R. Rapid identification of carbapenemase genes in gram-negative bacteria with an oligonucleotide microarray-based assay. PLoS ONE. 2014;9(7):e102232.
16. Kitchel B, Rasheed JK, Patel JB, Srinivasan A, Navon-Venezia S, Carmeli Y, Brolund A, Giske CG. Molecular epidemiology of KPC-producing *Klebsiella pneumoniae* isolates in the United States: clonal expansion of multilocus sequence type 258. Antimicrob Agents Chemother. 2009;53(8):3365–70.
17. Salerno A, Deletoile A, Lefevre M, Ciznar I, Krovacek K, Grimont P, Brisse S. Recombining population structure of *Plesiomonas shigelloides* (Enterobacteriaceae) revealed by multilocus sequence typing. J Bacteriol. 2007;189(21):7808–18.
18. CLSI. Performance standards for antimicrobial susceptibility testing; twenty-fourth informational supplement (M100-S24). Wayne, PA: Clinical and Laboratory Standard Institute; 2014.
19. Weisburg WG, Barns SM, Pelletier DA, Lane DJ. 16S ribosomal DNA amplification for phylogenetic study. J Bacteriol. 1991;173(2):697–703.
20. Wilson KH, Blitchington RB, Greene RC. Amplification of bacterial 16S ribosomal DNA with polymerase chain reaction. J Clin Microbiol. 1990;28(9):1942–6.
21. James G. Universal bacterial identification by PCR and DNA sequencing of 16S rRNA gene. In: Schuller M, Sloots TP, James GS, Halliday CL, Carter IWJ, editors. PCR for clinical microbiology: an Australian and international perspective. New York: Springer; 2010. p. 209–14.
22. Srinivasan R, Karaoz U, Volegova M, MacKichan J, Kato-Maeda M, Miller S, Nadarajan R, Brodie EL, Lynch SV. Use of 16S rRNA gene for identification of a broad range of clinically relevant bacterial pathogens. PLoS ONE. 2015;10(2):e0117617.
23. Maidak BL, Olsen GJ, Larsen N, Overbeek R, McCaughey MJ, Woese CR. The ribosomal database project (RDP). Nucl Acids Res. 1996;24(1):82–5.
24. Clermont O, Christenson JK, Denamur E, Gordon DM. The Clermont *Escherichia coli* phylo-typing method revisited: improvement of specificity and detection of new phylo-groups. Environ Microbiol Rep. 2013;5(1):58–65.
25. Wirth T, Falush D, Lan R, Colles F, Mensa P, Wieler LH, Karch H, Reeves PR, Maiden MC, Ochman H. Sex and virulence in *Escherichia coli*: an evolutionary perspective. Mol Microbiol. 2006;60(5):1136–51.
26. Tamura K, Stecher G, Peterson D, Filipski A, Kumar S: MEGA6: molecular evolutionary genetics analysis version 6.0. Mol Biol Evol. 2013;30(12):2725–9.
27. Welch RA, Burland V, Plunkett G 3rd, Redford P, Roesch P, Rasko D, Buckles EL, Liou SR, Boutin A, Hackett J, et al. Extensive mosaic structure revealed by the complete genome sequence of uropathogenic *Escherichia coli*. Proc Natl Acad Sci USA. 2002;99(26):17020–4.
28. Leangapichart T, Dia NM, Olaitan AO, Gautret P, Brouqui P, Rolain JM. Acquisition of extended-spectrum beta-lactamases by *Escherichia coli* and *Klebsiella pneumoniae* in gut microbiota of pilgrims during the Hajj Pilgrimage of 2013. Antimicrob Agents Chemother. 2016;60(5):3222–6.
29. Magiorakos AP, Srinivasan A, Carey R, Carmeli Y, Falagas M, Giske C, Harbarth S, Hindler J, Kahlmeter G, Olsson-Liljequist B. Multidrug-resistant, extensively drug-resistant and pandrug-resistant bacteria: an international expert proposal for interim standard definitions for acquired resistance. Clin Microbiol Infect. 2012;18(3):268–81.
30. Huber H, Zweifel C, Wittenbrink MM, Stephan R. ESBL-producing uropathogenic *Escherichia coli* isolated from dogs and cats in Switzerland. Vet Microbiol. 2013;162(2–4):992–6.
31. Giufrè M, Graziani C, Accogli M, Luzzi I, Busani L, Cerquetti M: Escherichia coli of human and avian origin: detection of clonal groups associated with fluoroquinolone and multidrug resistance in Italy. J Antimicrob Chemother. 2012;67(4):860–7.
32. Johnson JR, Johnston B, Clabots C, Kuskowski MA, Pendyala S, DebRoy C, Nowicki B, Rice J. *Escherichia coli* sequence type ST131 as an emerging fluoroquinolone-resistant uropathogen among renal transplant recipients. Antimicrob Agents Chemother. 2010;54(1):546–50.
33. Rubin JE, Pitout JD. Extended-spectrum β-lactamase, carbapenemase and AmpC producing Enterobacteriaceae in companion animals. Vet Microbiol. 2014;170(1):10–8.
34. Kojima Y, Harada S, Aoki K, Ishii Y, Sawa T, Hasegawa K, Saji T, Yamaguchi K, Tateda K. Spread of CTX-M-15 extended-spectrum β-lactamase-producing *Escherichia coli* isolates through household contact and plasmid transfer. J Clin Microbiol. 2014;52(5):1783–5.
35. Petty NK, Zakour NLB, Stanton-Cook M, Skippington E, Totsika M, Forde BM, Phan M-D, Moriel DG, Peters KM, Davies M. Global dissemination of a multidrug resistant *Escherichia coli* clone. Proc Natl Acad Sci. 2014;111(15):5694–9.
36. Pitout JDD, Gregson DB, Campbell L, Laupland KB. Molecular characteristics of extended-spectrum-β-lactamase-producing *Escherichia coli* isolates causing bacteremia in the Calgary Health Region from 2000 to 2007: emergence of clone ST131 as a cause of community-acquired infections. Antimicrob Agents Chemother. 2009;53(7):2846–51.
37. Suzuki S, Shibata N, Yamane K, Wachino J, Ito K, Arakawa Y. Change in the prevalence of extended-spectrum-beta-lactamase-producing *Escherichia coli* in Japan by clonal spread. J Antimicrob Chemother. 2009;63(1):72–9.
38. Bert F, Johnson JR, Ouattara B, Leflon-Guibout V, Johnston B, Marcon E, Valla D, Moreau R, Nicolas-Chanoine MH. Genetic diversity and virulence profiles of *Escherichia coli* isolates causing spontaneous bacterial peritonitis and bacteremia in patients with cirrhosis. J Clin Microbiol. 2010;48(8):2709–14.
39. Lee MY, Choi HJ, Choi JY, Song M, Song Y, Kim SW, Chang HH, Jung SI, Kim YS, Ki HK, et al. Dissemination of ST131 and ST393 community-onset, ciprofloxacin-resistant *Escherichia coli* clones causing urinary tract infections in Korea. J Infect. 2010;60(2):146–53.
40. Ender PT, Gajanana D, Johnston B, Clabots C, Tamarkin FJ, Johnson JR. Transmission of an extended-spectrum-beta-lactamase-producing *Escherichia coli* (sequence type ST131) strain between a father and daughter resulting in septic shock and emphysematous pyelonephritis. J Clin Microbiol. 2009;47(11):3780–2.
41. Manges AR, Johnson JR, Foxman B, O'Bryan TT, Fullerton KE, Riley LW. Widespread distribution of urinary tract infections caused by a multidrug-resistant *Escherichia coli* clonal group. N Engl J Med. 2001;345(14):1007–13.
42. Schaeffer AJ. Global molecular epidemiology of the O15:K52:H1 extraintestinal pathogenic *Escherichia coli* clonal group: evidence of distribution beyond Europe. J Urol. 2003;169(4):1612.

16

The evaluation and application of multilocus variable number tandem repeat analysis (MLVA) for the molecular epidemiological study of *Salmonella enterica* subsp. *enterica* serovar Enteritidis infection

Yao Liu[1†], Xiaolu Shi[2†], Yinghui Li[2], Qiongcheng Chen[2], Min Jiang[2], Wanli Li[1], Yaqun Qiu[2], Yiman Lin[2], Yixiang Jiang[2], Biao Kan[4], Qun Sun[1*] and Qinghua Hu[2,3*]

Abstract

Background: *Salmonella enterica* subsp. *enterica* serovar Enteritidis (*S.* Enteritidis) is one of the most prevalent *Salmonella* serotypes that cause gastroenteritis worldwide and the most prevalent serotype causing *Salmonella* infections in China. A rapid molecular typing method with high throughput and good epidemiological discrimination is urgently needed for detecting the outbreaks and finding the source for effective control of *S.* Enteritidis infections.

Methods: In this study, 194 strains which included 47 from six outbreaks that were well-characterized epidemiologically were analyzed with pulse field gel electrophoresis (PFGE) and multilocus variable number tandem repeat analysis (MLVA). Seven VNTR loci published by the US Center for Disease Control and Prevention (CDC) were used to evaluate and develop MLVA scheme for *S.* Enteritidis molecular subtyping by comparing with PFGE, and then MLVA was applied to the suspected outbreaks detection. All *S.* Enteritidis isolates were analyzed with MLVA to establish a MLVA database in Shenzhen, Guangdong province, China to facilitate the detection of *S.* Enteritidis infection clusters.

Results: There were 33 MLVA types and 29 PFGE patterns among 147 sporadic isolates. These two measures had Simpson indices of 0.7701 and 0.8043, respectively, which did not differ significantly. Epidemiological concordance was evaluated by typing 47 isolates from six epidemiologically well-characterized outbreaks and it did not differ for PFGE and MLVA. We applied the well established MLVA method to detect two *S.* Enteritidis foodborne outbreaks and find their sources successfully in 2014. A MLVA database of 491 *S.* Enteritidis strains isolated from 2004 to 2014 was established for the surveillance of clusters in the future.

Conclusions: MLVA typing of *S.* Enteritidis would be an effective tool for early warning and epidemiological surveillance of *S.* Enteritidis infections.

Keywords: *S.* Enteritidis, MLVA, PFGE, Epidemiological study

*Correspondence: qunsun@scu.edu.cn; huqinghua03@163.com
†Yao Liu and Xiaolu Shi contributed equally to this work
[1] Key Laboratory of Bio-resources and Eco-environment of the Ministry of Education, College of Life Sciences, Sichuan University, 29# Wangjiang Road, Chengdu 610064, Sichuan, People's Republic of China
[2] Shenzhen Major Infectious Disease Control Key Laboratory, Shenzhen Center for Disease Control and Prevention, Shenzhen 518055, Guangdong, People's Republic of China
Full list of author information is available at the end of the article

Background

The bacterium *Salmonella* causes acute gastroenteritis and it is one of the most common and widely distributed foodborne pathogens. There are two species of *Salmonella*: *Salmonella bongori* and *Salmonella enterica*. Over 2500 different serotypes of *Salmonella enterica* species have been identified to date [1]. The global burden of non-typhoidal *Salmonella* gastroenteritis is heavy—there are 93.8 million cases annually leading to 155,000 deaths, of which 80.3 million cases are foodborne [2]. Despite the great number of serotypes, the most common foodborne pathogens in human *Salmonella* infections are *S.* Enteritidis and *S.* Typhimurium, which account for 57 % of all isolates from human cases, while *S.* Enteritidis is the most prevalent serotype in China [3].

Molecular typing methods for discriminating different bacterial isolates of the same species are essential epidemiological tools for detecting the outbreak of foodborne diseases [4]. An approprite molecular typing method must provide both strong discriminatory power and high epidemiological concordance. Discriminatory power is the probability that two unrelated isolates can be distinguished from one another, while epidemiological concordance is the probability to determine whether two outbreaks are due to a common source and whether two isolates are part of the same outbreak. When a typing method can offer these two critical abilities, additional characteristics including rapidity, high throughput, and good reproducibility are expected. The molecular typing methods that are used commonly to detect bacterial disease outbreaks include PFGE, MLVA, and clustered regularly interspaced short palindromic repeat and multiple-virulence-locus sequence typing (CRISPR-MVLST). Recently, powered by whole-genome-sequencing (WGS) technologies, whole-genome single-nucleotide polymorphism (SNP) typing (WGST) has been applied to resolve outbreak clusters of *S.* Enteritidis [5].

PulseNet [6], a national molecular subtyping network for the surveillance of foodborne disease, was established by the US CDC in 1996. It uses PFGE to identify clusters of patients infected with enteric bacteria that have indistinguishable PFGE patterns and hence possibly represent a common source of outbreaks. The initial PFGE method was used to type a single pathogen (*Escherichia coli* O157:H7) [7], and then further developed to enable typing of various clinically important bacteria, including *Listeria monocytogenes, Vibrio parahaemolyticus* and *Salmonella*. Combined with epidemiological investigations, PFGE has been used as an elementary typing tool for the analysis of transmission events of foodborne pathogens and used successfully in detection of outbreaks and effective control of the infections [8–11]. Although PFGE is currently considered as the gold standard for subtyping *Salmonella*, it is labor-intensive, time-consuming, and offers low throughput. Furthermore the standardized PFGE protocols require a trained and skilled technician and its implementation takes approximately three days.

MLVA is a molecular subtyping method based on amplification and fragment size analysis of tandem sequence repeats that are found in microbial genome of most bacterial species. It utilizes the naturally occurring variation in the number of tandem repeat DNA sequences. MLVA is rapid and highly reproducible, and the results can be easy to be interpreted and standardized among laboratories. Bacteria that have been typed by MLVA include *S.* Typhimurium [12, 13], *S.* Enteritidis [14, 15], *E. coli* O157:H7 [16, 17], and *Vibrio parahaemolyticus* [18]. In recent years, MLVA has been proposed as a supplement to PFGE for subtyping *S.* Enteritidis in many countries. It can connect suspected, fast-evolving bacterial strains to an outbreak even when they might look the same when analyzed by PFGE. In Europe, a standardized protocol is being used for *S.* Enteritidis based on a scheme with five VNTR loci [14, 19, 20]. In contrast, the standardized protocol for *S.* Enteritidis in the US uses seven VNTR loci [21]. The two standardized protocols share five VNTR loci.

A latest study compared four subtyping methods including WGST, CRISPR-MVLST, MLVA and PFGE to analyze outbreak clusters of *S.* Enteritidis [5]. MLVA outperformed CRISPR-MVLST and PFGE in delineating outbreak clusters. WGST provides superior discriminatory power and accurate phylogenetic inferences with high epidemiological correlation; however this technology relies on detailed bioinformatics analysis. Among the four subtyping methods, WGST was the most expensive and not feasible to be a routine subtyping method.

In Guangdong province in China, the *S.* Enteritidis serotype is the second most common cause of human salmonellosis [22]. Data from the laboratory-based diarrheal disease sentinel surveillance network collected in Shenzhen, Guangdong province, China since 2007 show that the peak positive rate of *Salmonella* infection increased from 3.82 % in 2007 to 14.36 % in 2014, and that *S.* Enteritidis was the second most prevalent serotype causing *Salmonella* infection in Shenzhen (Shenzhen CDC, unpublished data). Considering the rapidity, high throughput, moderate discriminatory ability and simple operation, MLVA holds the potential to be suitable for detecting the clusters of foodborne pathogens in provincial and local labs. The feasibility of using MLVA typing method for the epidemiological study and the detecting of local outbreaks has not yet been evaluated systematically in China so far.

In our study, we described the development, evaluation, and application of MLVA. Furthermore, we applied

MLVA successfully to issue reports on *S.* Enteritidis infection outbreaks in 2014 and find their sources, and also established a MLVA database in Shenzhen for the surveillance of *S.* Enteritidis clusters. The results demonstrated that MLVA could be used to improve the efficiency of subtyping and the effectiveness of epidemiologically investigating *S.* Enteritidis infections.

Methods

Bacterial strains and DNA extraction

Bacterial strains used in this study were obtained from Shenzhen CDC in China between 2004 and 2014. The laboratory-based diarrheal disease sentinel surveillance network that established by the Shenzhen CDC collected patients information, including demographic characteristics (name, sex, age, nation and so on), recent travel, food consumption prior to becoming sick and clinical characteristics (date of accident, sampling date, isolation date and so on). Considering *S.* Enteritidis isolates' epidemiological information, a total of 147 sporadic isolates (Additional file 1: Table S1) were selected for evaluating seven VNTR loci, developing MLVA and comparing discriminatory power between PFGE and MLVA. The 47 strains (Additional file 2: Table S2) from six epidemiologically well-characterized outbreaks (outbreaks 1, 2, 3, 4, 5 and 6; involving 6, 20, 4, 4, 8, and 5 isolates, respectively) were used to evaluate epidemiological concordance. All isolates were stored at −80 °C in 25 % glycerol, until they were allowed to grow overnight in 2 mL Luria–Bertani (LB) broth in a shaking incubator at 37 °C. Suspensions of bacterial cells were boiled for 5 min and used directly in the PCR reactions after a brief centrifugation at 12,000 rpm for 5 min.

Measurement of systematic error in the genetic analysis

We used the CEQ 8800 Genetic Analysis System (Beckman Coulter Inc., Fullerton, CA, USA) to analyze the product size resulting from the amplification of VNTR loci. Sequences of all seven VNTR loci primers and characteristics are shown in Additional file 3: Table S3. To measure systematic error for the seven loci that we used, 31 *S.* Enteritidis strains were selected for PCR amplification and DNA sequencing. The following formula was used in MLVA to calculate the actual size of the repeat:

$$\text{Size of the repeat} = [(A \pm B) - C]/D$$

where A is observed PCR product size, B is the systematic error, C is the flank that does not contain repeats, and D is the length of one repeat unit.

Modification of the MLVA method

The amplification of SE6 described by the US CDC [21] was weak in our laboratory, so we modified the multiplex amplifications. Briefly, one multiplex amplification including SE1, SE2, SE6, and SE8 was carried out in a 20 μL volume containing 1 μL of template DNA, 2 μL of 10× PCR buffer, 1.6 μL of 2.5 mM dNTPs, 1.6 μL of 25 mM $MgCl_2$, and 10 mM primer pairs: 0.08 μL SE1, 0.2 μL SE2, 0.6 μL SE6, and 0.25 μL SE8. Another multiplex amplification including SE3, SE5 and SE9 was carried out in a 20 μL volume containing 1 μL of template DNA, 2 μL of 10× PCR buffer, 1.6 μL of 2.5 mM dNTPs, 1.2 μL of 25 mM $MgCl_2$, and 10 mM primer pairs: 0.3 μL SE3, 0.15 μL SE5, and 0.05 μL SE9. "S13130" was a clinical strain that presented in 31 sequenced isolates and used as a positive control in MLVA. Reaction mixtures without the DNA template were used as negative controls. After multiplex PCR, each multiplex reaction product was diluted 1:50 with PCR grade water. The next steps were performed according to the standardized protocols used by the US CDC on a Beckman Coulter CEQ 8800 GeXP for PCR fragment length analysis. The resulting data were imported into BioNumerics v5.1 software (Applied Maths) for clustering analysis, using categorical coefficients of zero tolerance and the unweighted pair-group method with arithmetic mean (UPGMA).

PFGE

Sample preparation, restriction digestion, electrophoresis, and gel staining for PFGE followed the standardized protocols [23]. To provide a universal size standard, DNA from *Salmonella* Braenderup H9812 was restricted with XbaI [24]. All *S.* Enteritidis isolates were digested with the restriction endonuclease XbaI and the results were analyzed by BioNumerics v5.1 software (Applied Maths) then submitted to PulseNet China. PFGE patterns were compared on dendrograms generated in BioNumerics using the Dice coefficient and a 1.5 % band position tolerance. Patterns with no noticeable differences were considered indistinguishable and were assigned the same PFGE pattern.

Statistical analysis

Diversity of each VNTR locus was assessed using Nei's measure of allelic diversity [25]. Simpson's diversity and Shannon-Weiner (Shannon) diversity indices were calculated to compare the discriminatory power of PFGE and MLVA. Variances and confidence intervals (CIs) of Simpson indices were calculated as described previously [26], and a *t* test was used to compare indices for MLVA versus PFGE.

Results

VNTR analysis

Diversity indices were calculated for individual locus based on 147 sporadic *S.* Enteritidis isolates, and the values ranged from 0.027 for SE8–0.722 for SE5 (Table 1). Among the seven VNTR loci, four of them (SE1, SE2, SE5 and SE9) showed appropriate discriminating abilities that were similar to previous reports [27–29]. In contrast, SE3, SE6 and SE8, were less polymorphic, with indices less than 0.1.

Diversity of MLVA and PFGE among the sporadic isolates

There were 33 MLVA types and 29 PFGE patterns among the sporadic isolates (Table 2), with a Simpson index of 0.7701 and 0.8043, respectively. Both the Simpson's and Shannon's indices were higher for PFGE than for MLVA, but there was no statistical difference between the two methods in terms of either index (*t* tests, $P > 0.05$). In contrast, most previous reports except one [30] found that the MLVA typing method showed much higher discriminatory power. There were common types for each method. JEGX01.CN0001 and JEGX01.CN0003 were common PFGE patterns in Shenzhen city and were also common in PulseNet China [31], while JEGMT0002 and JEGMT0003 were common MLVA types in Shenzhen.

Epidemiological concordance of MLVA among isolates from well-characterized outbreaks

The 47 strains from six epidemiologically well-characterized outbreaks were divided into four MLVA types and four PFGE patterns. All isolates within a single outbreak were indistinguishable by both methods (Fig. 1). JEGX01.CN0001 and JEGX01.CN0003 were common PFGE patterns in outbreak isolates and were also common among the sporadic isolates. JEGMT0002 and JEGMT0004 were common MLVA types in the isolates from outbreaks, and strains linked to outbreak four, five and six had the common MLVA types among the sporadic isolates.

Table 1 Genetic diversity of seven VNTR loci in sporadic *S.* Enteritidis isolates

Locus	Repeat size (bp)	No. of variants[a]	Nei's diversity index[b]
SE1	7	10	0.294
SE2	7	11	0.274
SE3	12	3	0.040
SE5	6	10	0.722
SE6	33	4	0.053
SE8	87	2	0.027
SE9	9	2	0.245

[a] number of different fragment size polymorphisms detected among 147 sporadic *S.* Enteritidis isolates

[b] Nei's diversity index as $1 - \Sigma$ (allele frequency)^2

Applying MLVA to detect *S.* Enteritidis infection outbreaks

We applied MLVA to detect two *S.* Enteritidis infection outbreaks in 2014 and find their sources successfully (Fig. 2).

In June 2014, a cluster of seven *S.* Enteritidis isolates with the common MLVA type JEGMT0003 was detected (Fig. 2). Epidemiological investigations showed that it was an outbreak of *S.* Enteritidis infection with the six strains being epidemiologically related and we confirmed that a bread countertop prepared with contaminated cakes was the food vehicle. As a result, the infectious source was decontaminated.

In September 2014, the Xixiang People's Hospital reported two food-related outbreaks: two different groups of people (3 and 5 individuals, respectively) became sick after eating lunch in the same restaurant within one week. From patients' stool samples, we isolated and identified the pathogen as *S.* Enteritidis, and used MLVA to type the isolates. A cluster of eight *S.* Enteritidis isolates with the same uncommon MLVA type, JEGMT0001, was detected (Fig. 2). The epidemiologists from Shenzhen CDC did the field investigation to confirm whether two outbreaks were epidemiologically related and where the sources were from. Based on the epidemiological investigation, 49 samples including 14 from foods, 10 environment swabs from kitchen and 25 anal swabs from 25 staffs who worked in the restaurant were collected and were sent to our laboratory for isolation and MLVA typing. As a result, three strains from anal swabs of three chefs shared the same JEGMT0001 MLVA type. Results of the epidemiological investigation and MLVA showed that two outbreaks were epidemiologically related and shared the same source.

Table 2 Comparison of MLVA and PFGE in sporadic *S.* Enteritidis isolates ($n = 147$)

Method	No. of types	Common types (n)	Diversity index[a]	
			Simpson's (CI)	Shannon's[b]
PFGE	29	JEGX01.CN0001 (33) JEGX01.CN0003 (55)	0.8043 (0.7536–0.8550)	2.2647
MLVA	33	JEGMT0002 (61) JEGMT0003 (33)	0.7701 (0.7146–0.8257)	2.1313

[a] *P* values were > 0.05 for PFGE vs MLVA comparison of both diversity indices

[b] Shannon's index is an indicator of species richness

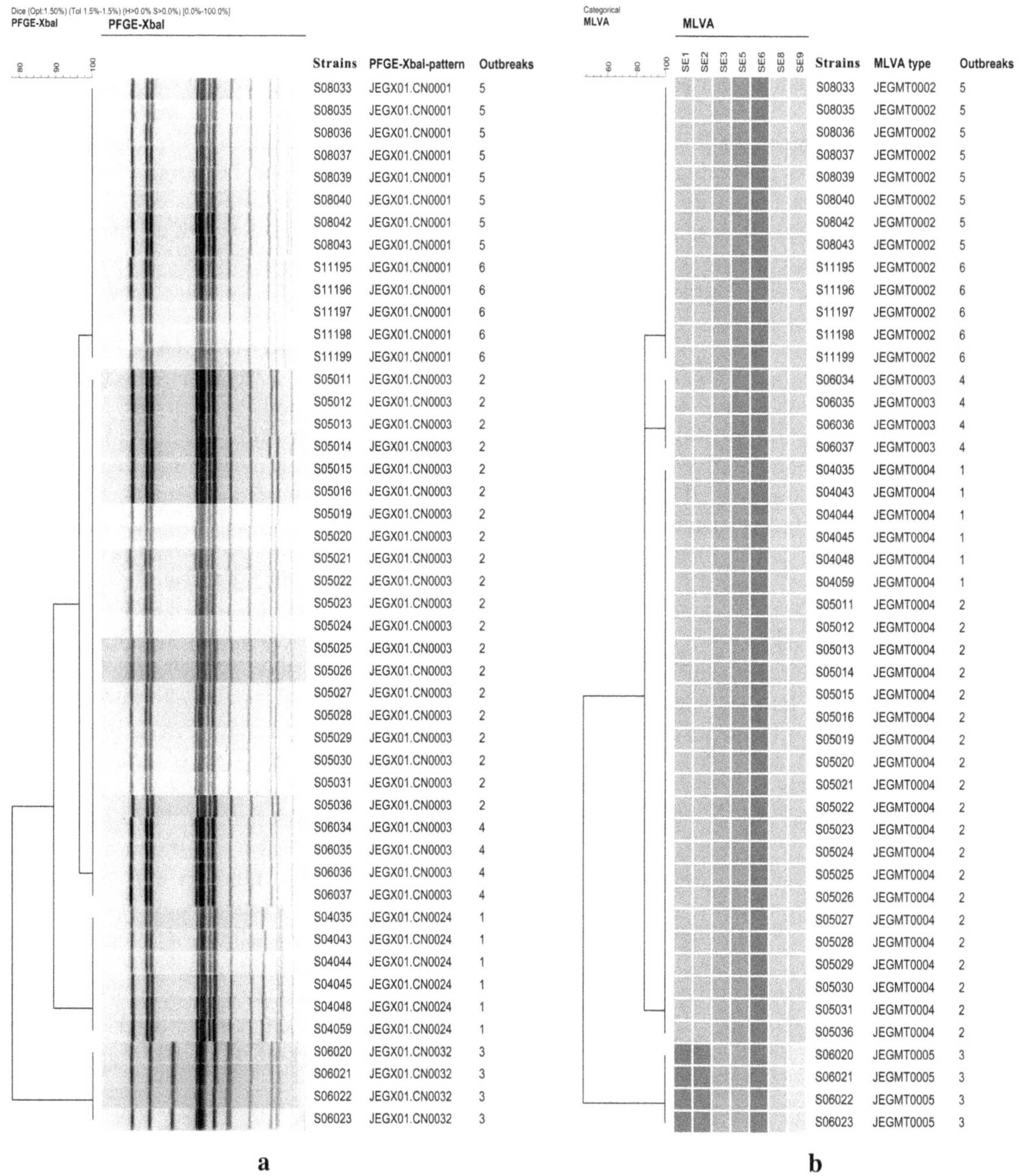

Fig. 1 Dendrograms for PFGE **a** using restriction enzyme XbaI and MLVA **b** performed on six *S.* Enteritidis outbreaks. The PFGE dendrogram was generated using the Dice coefficient (optimization 1.5 % and position tolerance 1.5 %) and unweighted-pair group method with arithmetic averages algorithm (UPGMA) algorithm. The MLVA dendrogram was generated using the categorical coefficient and UPGMA algorithm

Establishment of a MLVA database

We established a MLVA database of 491 strains that were isolated from 2004 to 2014 for the surveillance of *S.* Enteritidis clusters (Fig. 3). There were 70 MLVA types among all *S.* Enteritidis isolates, with JEGMT0002, JEGMT0003 and JEGMT0004 being the top three most common (Fig. 3). Although JEGMT0004 was a common type in the database, it was most common in 2004 and 2005 and the proportion of this type decreased in 2006.

Discussion

Shenzhen is a coastal region of China that has expanded meteorically, from a village of 30,000 people in 1978 to a large city of more than 10 million people in 2010 [32].

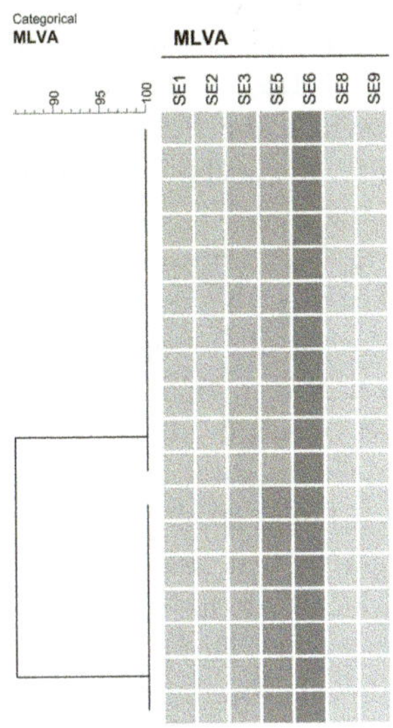

Strains	Epidemiologic information	Outbreaks	MLVA type	SE1	SE2	SE3	SE5	SE6	SE8	SE9	Allele string of VNTR loci
				The fragment length							
S14417	Patient, Baoan District, Sep., 2014	B	JEGMT0001	190	310	201	203	478	347	195	5-6-3-8-10-1-3
S14418	Patient, Baoan District, Sep., 2014	B	JEGMT0001	190	310	201	203	478	347	195	5-6-3-8-10-1-3
S14419	Patient, Baoan District, Sep., 2014	B	JEGMT0001	190	310	201	203	478	347	195	5-6-3-8-10-1-3
S14420	Patient, Baoan District, Sep., 2014	B	JEGMT0001	190	310	201	203	478	347	195	5-6-3-8-10-1-3
S14421	Chef A, Baoan District, Sep., 2014	B	JEGMT0001	190	310	201	203	478	347	195	5-6-3-8-10-1-3
S14422	Chef B, Baoan District, Sep., 2014	B	JEGMT0001	190	310	201	203	478	347	195	5-6-3-8-10-1-3
S14423	Chef C, Baoan District, Sep., 2014	B	JEGMT0001	190	310	201	203	478	347	195	5-6-3-8-10-1-3
S14424	Patient, Baoan District, Sep., 2014	B	JEGMT0001	190	310	201	203	478	347	195	5-6-3-8-10-1-3
S14425	Patient, Baoan District, Sep., 2014	B	JEGMT0001	190	310	201	203	478	347	195	5-6-3-8-10-1-3
S14518	Patient, Baoan District, Sep., 2014	B	JEGMT0001	190	310	201	203	478	347	195	5-6-3-8-10-1-3
S14519	Patient, Baoan District, Sep., 2014	B	JEGMT0001	190	310	201	203	478	347	195	5-6-3-8-10-1-3
S14072	Patient, Guangming District, Jun., 2014	A	JEGMT0003	190	310	201	221	478	347	195	5-6-3-11-10-1-3
S14073	Patient, Guangming District, Jun., 2014	A	JEGMT0003	190	310	201	221	478	347	195	5-6-3-11-10-1-3
S14074	Patient, Guangming District, Jun., 2014	A	JEGMT0003	190	310	201	221	478	347	195	5-6-3-11-10-1-3
S14075	Patient, Guangming District, Jun., 2014	A	JEGMT0003	190	310	201	221	478	347	195	5-6-3-11-10-1-3
S14076	Patient, Guangming District, Jun., 2014	A	JEGMT0003	190	310	201	221	478	347	195	5-6-3-11-10-1-3
S14077	Patient, Guangming District, Jun., 2014	A	JEGMT0003	190	310	201	221	478	347	195	5-6-3-11-10-1-3
S14078	Bakery, Guangming District, Jun., 2014	A	JEGMT0003	190	310	201	221	478	347	195	5-6-3-11-10-1-3

Fig. 2 Dendrogram of 18 isolates evaluated by MLVA on two *S.* Enteritidis outbreaks in 2014. The MLVA dendrogram was generated using the categorical coefficient and unweighted pair group method with arithmetic means. "Allele string of VNTR loci" in the figure means a string of the actual number of repeats at each locus (in order of SE1–SE2–SE3–SE5–SE6–SE8–SE9)

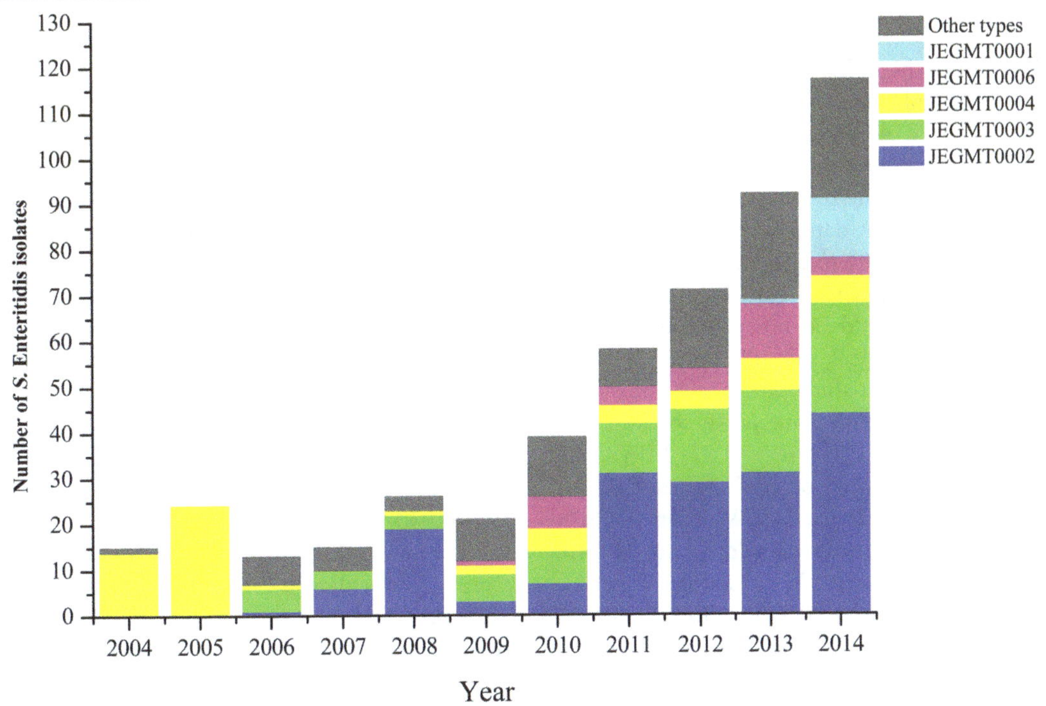

Fig. 3 Annual distribution of Shenzhen *S.* Enteritidis isolates over an 11-year period (2004–2014) according to the MLVA database. Other types: all MLVA types with less than 2.8 % occurrence in the database. The number of JEGMT0001 type was 14 in the MLVA database and the proportion of the type was 2.8 %, so we defined other types as all MLVA types with less than 2.8 % occurrence in the MLVA database

The floating population is larger than the registered permanent population of this city. Data from the laboratory-based diarrheal disease sentinel surveillance network in Shenzhen showed that the rate of *S.* Enteritidis infection increased annually (the peak positive rate of *Salmonella* infection increased from 3.82 % in 2007 to 14.36 % in 2014; Shenzhen CDC, unpublished data) and that *S.* Enteritidis infection was the second most prevalent serotype causing *Salmonella* infections. It is essential to type pathogens as soon as possible, in order to detect suspected infection outbreaks and to find the source in this kind of situation. The standardized PFGE protocol for subtyping *Salmonella* takes approximately three days; in contrast, the MLVA typing can be finished within 6 h. Although PFGE is widely considered to be the gold standard for subtyping *Salmonella*, implementation of this typing method for massive strains is not feasible. Hence, evaluating and developing MLVA for *S.* Enteritidis is very important for detecting outbreaks and tracing their sources.

The Simpson's and Shannon's diversity indices were higher for PFGE than for MLVA. However, the MLVA typing method showed much higher discriminatory power than PFGE in studies from other countries [5, 15, 27, 28]. Although the two indices were higher for PFGE than for MLVA, the values were not significantly different. To raise discriminatory power of MLVA, four more loci (SENTR2, SENTR3, SE-7, SE-10) described by previous studies [27, 29] were added into MLVA, but it did not result in a further discrimination (data not shown). Compared with discriminatory power, clustering concordance with epidemiological data is an equally important measure for evaluation of the utility of the molecular subtyping method. Epidemiological concordance did not differ for PFGE and MLVA in our assessment.

We succeeded in applying the MLVA typing to detect two *S.* Enteritidis foodborne outbreaks in 2014 and find their sources, and a MLVA database of all *S.* Enteritidis isolated from the years 2004 to 2014 was established for the surveillance of *S.* Enteritidis clusters. These results indicated that MLVA would be a useful tool for early warning and epidemiological surveillance of *S.* Enteritidis infection. In the latest study, whole-genome WGST showed the highest discriminatory power of four subtyping methods (WGST, CRISPR-MVLST, MLVA and PFGE), and the discriminatory power between CRISPR-MVLST and MLVA was similar [5]. We used CRISPR-MVLST to analyze three outbreaks (data not shown), and the typing result of CRISPR-MVLST was the same as MLVA. Two outbreaks shared the same CRISPR-MVLST type, while they shared the same MLVA type. Although epidemiological concordance between CRISPR-MVLST and MLVA was same, the expense of CRISPR-MVLST was tripled compared with MLVA. MLVA may be the most time-saving and the least expensive method for subtyping *S.* Enteritidis.

Whether PFGE or MLVA typing was used, there were common types for each method. It seems that regardless of the primary molecular subtyping method, a secondary subtyping method would be needed to differentiate the common *S.* Enteritidis subtypes. Hence, MLVA has been proposed as a supplementary method to PFGE for subtyping *S.* Enteritidis in previous studies. In July 2010, the US CDC calculated the average of JEGX01.0004 that was the most common PFGE pattern in the PulseNet USA database and identified a nationwide sustained increase in the number of the type, and the epidemiological investigation then showed that it was a nationwide *S.* Enteritidis infection outbreak associated with shell eggs [33]. In this study, we propose MLVA as an alternative to PFGE for subtyping *S.* Enteritidis. Typically, an epidemiological investigation would be initiated when the MLVA type of three or more strains within 30 days is shown to be identical. However, JEGMT0002 and JEGMT0003 were common MLVA types in Shenzhen, so that practice might increase the investigation workload of the epidemiologists. The average of JEGMT0002 and JEGMT0003 based on our MLVA database can be calculated, and average of the two types is 5 and 4 respectively. When cases of common MLVA types are larger than the average within 30 days, an epidemiological investigation would then be initiated to confirm whether or not it is an outbreak. An epidemiological investigation is needed when three or more clinical strains with same uncommon MLVA types or new types that do not appear previously are detected within 30 days. JEGMT0001 was an uncommon MLVA type that appeared in 2013 along with one clinical isolate and the type of 13 strains were detected in 2014, and then the epidemiological investigation confirmed that it was the outbreak.

Although all of the *S.* Enteritidis isolates evaluated in this study were from Shenzhen city, the common PFGE patterns of isolates were representative of the most common PFGE patterns in PulseNet China [31]. Nevertheless, in this study there was a limitation in the number of illness cases. Still, further investigation is necessary to estimate the average of two common MLVA types for detecting the clusters.

Conclusion

In conclusion, MLVA for *S.* Enteritidis showed a satisfactory performance, in terms of simplicity, speed, and reproducibility. The method can be applied as a routine subtyping method for early warning of outbreaks and initiating epidemiological investigations.

Additional files

Additional file 1: Table S1. Clinical isolates from sporadic cases used in this study.

Additional file 2: Table S2. Forty-seven isolates from six epidemiologically well-characterized outbreaks in this study.

Additional file 3: Table S3. Primer sequences and PCR product size used for *S.* Enteritidis MLVA typing.

Abbreviations

S. Enteritidis: *Salmonella enterica* subsp. *enterica* serovar Enteritidis; *S.* Typhimurium: *Salmonella enterica* subsp. *enterica* serovar Typhimurium; VNTR: variable number tandem repeat; MLVA: multilocus variable number tandem repeat analysis; PFGE: pulse field gel electrophoresis; PCR: polymerase chain reaction; CDC: Center for Disease Control and Prevention; CRISPR-MVLST: clustered regularly interspaced short palindromic repeat and multiple-virulence-locus sequence typing; WGS: whole-genome-sequencing; SNP: single-nucleotide polymorphism; WGST: whole-genome single-nucleotide polymorphism typing; LB: Luria–Bertani.

Authors' contributions

All authors contributed to this work. All authors read and approved the final manuscript.

Author details

[1] Key Laboratory of Bio-resources and Eco-environment of the Ministry of Education, College of Life Sciences, Sichuan University, 29# Wangjiang Road, Chengdu 610064, Sichuan, People's Republic of China. [2] Shenzhen Major Infectious Disease Control Key Laboratory, Shenzhen Center for Disease Control and Prevention, Shenzhen 518055, Guangdong, People's Republic of China. [3] School of Life Sciences, Shenzhen University, Shenzhen 518000, Guangdong, People's Republic of China. [4] Key Laboratory of Surveillance and Early-warning on Infectious Disease, Division of Infectious Disease, Chinese Center for Disease Control and Prevention, Beijing, People's Republic of China.

Acknowledgements

We thank staff of sentinel hospitals for collecting *Salmonella* isolates. This research was supported by the China National Science and Technology Major Projects Foundation (2012ZX10004215-003-005), the Department of Science and Technology of Sichuan Province of China (2014NZ0106), the Shenzhen Municipal Science and Technology Program (CXZZ20140411105636301), and the Natural Science Foundation of China (81071433; J1103518).

Competing interests

The authors declare that they have no competing interests.

References

1. Hong Y, Liu T, Lee MD, Hofacre CL, Maier M, White DG, Ayers S, Wang L, Berghaus R, Maurer J. A rapid screen of broth enrichments for *Salmonella enterica serovars enteritidis*, Hadar, Heidelberg, and Typhimurium by Using an allelotyping multiplex PCR that targets O- and H-antigen alleles. J Food Prot. 2009;72(10):2198–201.
2. Majowicz SE, Musto J, Scallan E, Angulo FJ, Kirk M, O'Brien SJ, Jones TF, Fazil A, Hoekstra RM. The global burden of nontyphoidal *Salmonella gastroenteritis*. Clin Infect Dis. 2010;50(6):882–9.
3. Ran L, Wu S, Gao Y, Zhang X, Feng Z, Wang Z, Kan B, Klena JD, Lo Fo Wong DM, Angulo FJ, et al. Laboratory-based surveillance of nontyphoidal Salmonella infections in China. Foodborne Pathog Dis. 2011;8(8):921–7.
4. Sabat AJ, Budimir A, Nashev D, Sa-Leao R, van Dijl J, Laurent F, Grundmann H, Friedrich AW. Overview of molecular typing methods for outbreak detection and epidemiological surveillance. Euro Surveill. 2013;18(4):20380.
5. Deng X, Shariat N, Driebe EM, Roe CC, Tolar B, Trees E, Keim P, Zhang W, Dudley EG, Fields PI, et al. Comparative analysis of subtyping methods against a whole-genome-sequencing standard for *Salmonella enterica* serotype Enteritidis. J Clin Microbiol. 2015;53(1):212–8.
6. Swaminathan B, Barrett TJ, Hunter SB, Tauxe RV. PulseNet: the molecular subtyping network for foodborne bacterial disease surveillance, United States. Emerging Infect Dis. 2001;7(3):382–9.
7. Barrett TJ, Lior H, Green JH, Khakhria R, Wells JG, Bell BP, Greene KD, Lewis J, Griffin PM. Laboratory investigation of a multistate food-borne outbreak of *Escherichia coli* O157:H7 by using pulsed-field gel electrophoresis and phage typing. J Clin Microbiol. 1994;32(12):3013–7.
8. Cavallaro E, Date K, Medus C, Meyer S, Miller B, Kim C, Nowicki S, Cosgrove S, Sweat D, Phan Q, et al. Salmonella typhimurium infections associated with peanut products. N Engl J Med. 2011;365(7):601–10.
9. Gaffga NH, Behravesh CB, Ettestad PJ, Smelser CB, Rhorer AR, Cronquist AB, Comstock NA, Bidol SA, Patel NJ, Gerner-Smidt P, et al. Outbreak of salmonellosis linked to live poultry from a mail-order hatchery. N Engl J Med. 2012;366(22):2065–73.
10. Behravesh CB, Mody RK, Jungk J, Gaul L, Redd JT, Chen S, Cosgrove S, Hedican E, Sweat D, Chavez-Hauser L, et al. 2008 outbreak of Salmonella Saintpaul infections associated with raw produce. N Engl J Med. 2011;364(10):918–27.
11. Sandt CH, Krouse DA, Cook CR, Hackman AL, Chmielecki WA, Warren NG. The key role of pulsed-field gel electrophoresis in investigation of a large multiserotype and multistate food-borne outbreak of Salmonella infections centered in Pennsylvania. J Clin Microbiol. 2006;44(9):3208–12.
12. Sintchenko V, Wang Q, Howard P, Ha CW, Kardamanidis K, Musto J, Gilbert GL. Improving resolution of public health surveillance for human *Salmonella enterica* serovar Typhimurium infection: 3 years of prospective multiple-locus variable-number tandem-repeat analysis (MLVA). BMC Infect Dis. 2012;12(1):78.
13. Wuyts V, Mattheus W, de Bex GL, Wildemauwe C, Roosens NH, Marchal K, De Keersmaecker SC, Bertrand S. MLVA as a tool for public health surveillance of human Salmonella Typhimurium: prospective study in Belgium and evaluation of MLVA loci stability. PLoS ONE. 2013;8(12):e84055.
14. Bertrand S, de Bex GL, Wildemauwe C, Lunguya O, Phoba MF, Ley B, Jacobs J, Vanhoof R, Mattheus W. Multi locus variable-number tandem repeat (MLVA) typing tools improved the surveillance of *Salmonella* Enteritidis: A 6 Years retrospective study. PLoS ONE. 2015;10(2):e0117950.
15. Kim J, Hyeon JY, Lee E, Lee D, Kim YJ, Kim S. Molecular epidemiological analysis of five outbreaks associated with *Salmonella enterica* serovar Enteritidis between 2008 and 2010 on Jeju Island, Republic of Korea. Foodborne Pathog Dis. 2014;11(1):38–42.
16. Jay MT, Cooley M, Carychao D, Wiscomb GW, Sweitzer RA, Crawford-Miksza L, Farrar JA, Lau DK, O'Connell J, Millington A, et al. *Escherichia coli* O157:H7 in feral swine near spinach fields and cattle, central California coast. Emerg Infect Dis. 2007;13(12):1908–11.
17. Perry N, Cheasty T, Dallman T, Launders N, Willshaw G. Application of multilocus variable number tandem repeat analysis to monitor Verocytotoxin-producing *Escherichia coli* O157 phage type 8 in England and Wales: emergence of a profile associated with a national outbreak. J Appl Microbiol. 2013;115(4):1052–8.
18. Kimura B, Sekine Y, Takahashi H, Tanaka Y, Obata H, Kai A, Morozumi S, Fujii T. Multiple-locus variable-number of tandem-repeats analysis distinguishes Vibrio parahaemolyticus pandemic O3: K6 strains. J Microbiol Methods. 2008;72(3):313–20.
19. Hopkins KL, Peters TM, de Pinna E, Wain J. Standardisation of multilocus variable-number tandem-repeat analysis (MLVA) for subtyping of *Salmonella enterica* serovar Enteritidis. Euro Surveill. 2011;16(32):19942.
20. Lindstedt BA, Torpdahl M, Vergnaud G, Le Hello S, Weill FX, Tietze E, Malorny B, Prendergast DM, Ghallchoir EN, Lista RF, et al. Use of multilocus variable-number tandem repeat analysis (MLVA) in eight European countries, 2012. Euro Surveill. 2013;18(4):20385.
21. PulseNet Standard Operating Procedure for Analysis of. MLVA Data of Salmonella enterica serotype Enteritidis in. BioNumerics– Beckman Coulter CEQ 8000/8800/GeXP Data (http://www.cdc.gov/pulsenet/PDF/salmonella-mlva-e-beckman-508c.pdf).
22. Ke B, Sun J, He D, Li X, Liang Z, Ke CW. Serovar distribution, antimicrobial resistance profiles, and PFGE typing of *Salmonella enterica* strains isolated from 2007–2012 in Guangdong, China. BMC Infect Dis. 2014;14:338.
23. Ribot EM, Fair MA, Gautom R, Cameron DN, Hunter SB, Swaminathan B, Barrett TJ. Standardization of pulsed-field gel electrophoresis protocols for the subtyping of *Escherichia coli* O157:H7, Salmonella, and Shigella for PulseNet. Foodborne Pathog Dis. 2006;3(1):59–67.
24. Hunter SB, Vauterin P, Lambert-Fair MA, Van Duyne MS, Kubota K, Graves L, Wrigley D, Barrett T, Ribot E. Establishment of a universal size standard strain for use with the PulseNet standardized pulsed-field gel electrophoresis protocols: converting the national databases to the new size standard. J Clin Microbiol. 2005;43(3):1045–50.
25. Hudson RR. Genetic Data Analysis. Methods for Discrete Population Genetic Data. Bruce S. Weir. Sinauer, Sunderland, MA, 1990. xiv, 377 pp. illus. $48; paper, $27. Science. 1990;250(4980):575.
26. Grundmann H, Hori S, Tanner G. Determining confidence intervals when measuring genetic diversity and the discriminatory abilities of typing methods for microorganisms. J Clin Microbiol. 2001;39(11):4190–2.

27. Boxrud D, Pederson-Gulrud K, Wotton J, Medus C, Lyszkowicz E, Besser J, Bartkus J. Comparison of multiple-locus variable-number tandem repeat analysis, pulsed-field gel electrophoresis, and phage typing for subtype analysis of *Salmonella enterica* serotype Enteritidis. J Clin Microbiol. 2007;45(2):536–43.
28. Cho S, Boxrud DJ, Bartkus JM, Whittam TS, Saeed M. Multiple-locus variable-number tandem repeat analysis of Salmonella Enteritidis isolates from human and non-human sources using a single multiplex PCR. FEMS Microbiol Lett. 2007;275(1):16–23.
29. Malorny B, Junker E, Helmuth R. Multi-locus variable-number tandem repeat analysis for outbreak studies of *Salmonella enterica* serotype Enteritidis. BMC Microbiol. 2008;8:84.
30. Campioni F, Davis M, Medeiros MIC, Falcao JP, Shah DH. MLVA typing reveals higher genetic homogeneity among < i > S </i > Enteritidis strains isolated from food, humans and chickens in Brazil in comparison to the North American strains. Int J Food Microbiol. 2013;162(2):174–81.
31. Jing L, Bao-wei D, Jie L, Biao K, Mei-ying Y. Characterization of *Salmonella* enteritidis with pulsed-field gel electrophoresis in China. Dis Surveill. 2013;8(6):434–8 **(in Chinese)**.
32. Song P, Zhu Y, Mao X, Li Q, An L. Assessing spatial accessibility to maternity units in Shenzhen, China. PLoS ONE. 2013;8(7):e70227.
33. Multistate Outbreak of Human *Salmonella* Enteritidis Infections Associated with shell eggs (Final Update) (http://www.cdc.gov/salmonella/2010/shell-eggs-12-2-10.html).

17

Profiling of antibiotic resistance of bacterial species recovered from routine clinical isolates in Ethiopia

Robert-Jan ten Hove[1*], Melaku Tesfaye[1], Witold Frederik ten Hove[2] and Mesfin Nigussie[1]

Abstract

Background: With the alarming rise in antibiotic resistance in African countries, the need for a surveillance system in the region has become pressing. The rapid expansion of data networks makes it possible to set up healthcare applications that can be both cost-efficient and effective. Large data sets are available for assessment of current antibiotic resistance among Ethiopian patients. Based on the data-presentation, a practical approach is proposed on how diagnostic laboratories can participate remedial action against antibiotic resistance in Ethiopia.

Methods: In Addis Ababa (Ethiopia), raw data comprising bacterial species name, specimen type and antibiograms covering the period January 2014 to May 2015 was accessed from the laboratory information management system. Using R code, the data was read and fitted into data-frames and analyzed to assess antibiotic resistance in the Ethiopian patient population.

Results: Susceptibility to an antibiotic was tested with 14.983 cultures of 54 different bacterial species or subgroups, isolated from 16 types of specimen. Half of the cultures (n = 6444) showed resistance to an antibiotic. Resistance against penicillin was highest with, on average, 91.1% of 79 bacterial cultures showing resistance. Very high resistance rates were also observed for ampicillin, whereas resistance was lowest with cefoxitin.

Conclusions: Extraction and analysis of raw-data from the laboratory database is relatively simple and can provide valuable insight into the relationships between type of sample and drug-resistance in countries where such data is still scarce. With the largest number of antibiotic resistance tests described for Ethiopia, a tool is proposed for consistent data collection with specified core variables. Trends in antibiotic resistance can be revealed and treatment failures avoided when used as an easy accessible reference application for healthcare providers.

Keywords: Antibiogram, Antibiotic, Ethiopia, R, Resistance, Surveillance

Background

Irrational use of antibiotics has been perceived to be a major problem worldwide and in particular in the African continent [1–3]. To improve rational drug use in Ethiopia, national standard treatment guidelines were issued to assist health care workers in their treatment of infectious diseases [4]. Treatment guidelines must be continuously revised as susceptibility to antibiotic drugs is constantly threatened due to an empirical approach to treatment and high self-medication of humans and animals without a medical prescription [5, 6]. Enforcing a strict adherence policy in the healthcare sector to reduce the development and spread of drug-resistant bacterial strains goes hand in hand with nationwide antimicrobial surveillance. Routine clinical diagnostic laboratories can contribute to the national surveillance network by sharing routine antibiograms from clinical samples [7, 8]. At the International Clinical Laboratories, routine diagnostic analyses are performed on clinical samples collected at patient service centers across the country and the results are reported back automatically via a virtual private network. The laboratory seeks to extend its services

*Correspondence: robert@theparasitologist.com
[1] International Clinical Laboratories, Addis Ababa, Ethiopia
Full list of author information is available at the end of the article

by promoting a healthy life-style to the general public and setting up network applications allowing clinicians to prescribe using mobile networks. Extracting raw data from the laboratory information system and then entering it into a customized data-frame requires some knowledge of programming. In this study, the open source R computing language was used to visualize the prevalence of antibiotic resistance in routine clinical samples in Ethiopia on the basis of raw data extracted from the laboratory information management system, which is the first step towards automated real-time presentation of antibiograms.

Methods

Data and sites

Retrospective data from January 2014 to May 2015 was exported from the Polytech laboratory information management system (LIMS) (Comp Pro Med Inc., Santa Rosa, USA) at International Clinical Laboratories, Addis Ababa, Ethiopia. Parameters in the raw data included bacterial species name, type of specimen and antibiotic sensitivity of the bacterial cultures. The data was obtained from routine analysis of clinical specimens collected from individual patients visiting the patient service site, and from clinics and hospitals. All specimens were received and analyzed at the central laboratory in Addis Ababa, Ethiopia.

Type of specimens

All types of specimen were included in the data query. From patient service sites outside Addis Ababa, only urine specimens were considered feasible for transportation and bacterial analysis at the central laboratory. Specimens that did not match the set categories in the LIMS were renamed as routine samples.

Bacterial species identification

Preliminary identification was based on number of colonies, types of colonies, morphological appearance and gram staining after growth on both selective and non-selective media. Further bacterial characterization involved biochemical testing and specific growth characteristics under different conditions. All identification tests were carried out according to validated standard operation procedures [9, 10]. After appropriate incubation and based on the site from which the specimen was obtained, the bacterial species were classified as pathogenic or contaminant bacteria. The group of bacteria classified as *Streptococcus* spp. includes all streptococcal species with the exception of the beta-hemolytic streptococcal species, which are categorized as a separate group.

Antimicrobial susceptibility testing

Antimicrobial susceptibility testing was performed using the Kirby Bauer disk diffusion technique. Standard discs were used to detect and measure induced inhibition for specified antibiotic concentrations, placed on Mueller–Hinton agar supplemented with 5% sheep blood seeded with 0.5 McFarland of bacteria. The plates were incubated overnight under specified conditions (e.g. temperature and atmosphere depending on bacteria species and type of specimen). After incubation was complete, the zone inhibition diameter, in mm, was measured. The zones were interpreted as susceptible, intermediate or resistant [11].

Quality control

Commercial pre-plated and quality control-passed media were used with 15 different ATCC strains and blank incubation controls to check the transportation and storage conditions of the pre-plated media. The quality control was based on retesting of retained strains and correlation between results of different characteristics of a strain. New batches of ATCC strains for media were checked and compared with previously used ATCC strains and gram stained control slides were used to check the quality of the staining reagents.

Data analysis

Scripts were written in R (version 3.2.2) to read and fit the raw data into data frames. Test results from *Mycobacterium* cultures were deleted from the data set. The remaining data was summarized and plotted. Anaerobic and aerobic blood cultures were merged in one group. Drug resistance was calculated by dividing the number of resistant cultures by the sum of resistant and sensitive cultures, disregarding the intermediate sensitivity results. The R scripts and raw data are accessible in the Github repository [12].

Results

Drug susceptibility was tested on 14.983 cultures excluding *Mycobacterium* spp. over the period from January 2014 until May 2015. The total numbers of resistant, intermediate and sensitive cultures were 7440, 1099 and 6444, respectively. Specimens were obtained from urine (n = 11.034), wounds (n = 1346), blood (n = 672), body fluid (n = 466), pediatric blood (n = 411), ear (n = 322), pus (n = 154), stool (n = 136), sputum (n = 134), cerebral spinal fluid (CSF) (n = 94), routine samples (n = 78), eye (n = 45), throat (n = 62), nasal swab (n = 11), nasal discharge (n = 10) and urethral discharge (n = 8) (Table 1).

In total, 54 different bacterial species or subgroups were identified (Appendix 1). To visualize resistance

Table 1 Eighteen months of retrospective bacterial analyses showing the most prevalent bacterial species for each sample

Source	Bacterial species most frequently isolated	Frequency of bacterial species	Percentage of bacterial species (%)
Blood	Coagulase-negative *Staphylococcus* species	214	31.8
Blood-pediatric	Coagulase-negative *Staphylococcus* species	157	38.2
Body fluid	*Escherichia coli*	183	39.3
Cerebral spinal fluid	*Staphylococcus aureus*	23	24.5
Ear culture	*Staphylococcus aureus*	79	24.5
Eye culture	*Streptococcus pneumoniae*	26	57.8
Nasal discharge	Group G *Streptococcus*	10	100.0
Nasal swab	Coagulase-negative *Staphylococcus* species	11	100.0
Pus	*Escherichia coli*	73	47.4
Routine	*Escherichia coli*	36	46.2
Sputum	*Klebsiella oxytoca*	49	36.6
Stool	*Salmonella* group non *paratyphi* A/B	43	31.6
Throat	*Streptococcus pyogenes* (Group A)	22	35.5
Urethral discharge	*Escherichia coli*	8	100.0
Urine	*Escherichia coli*	7140	64.7
Wound	*Staphylococcus aureus*	565	36.0

patterns, data was further tailored by merging bacterial species into genus groups. Antibiogram groups containing few cultures and bacterial cultures with intermediate resistance levels were considered not representative of the general antibiotic drug resistance (ADR) profiles and therefore omitted from further analyses. As a result, 1836 cultures were filtered out when the sum of resistant plus sensitive cultures was less than 7 within a group of bacterial species and for a given antibiotic. The remaining 13.147 antibiograms contained 927 intermediate cultures, which were subsequently excluded from the calculation of antibiotic resistance rates. The bacterial antibiotic resistance rate was calculated for each group of bacteria for the 21 different antibiotics (Fig. 1).

The highest resistance rates were observed for penicillin (P10) with on average 91.1% of 79 bacterial cultures showing resistance, with coagulase negative *Staphylococcus* (CNS) (92.9%; n = 42), *Staphylococcus aureus* (90.0%; n = 20) and *Enterococcus* spp. (88.2%; n = 17). High percentages of resistant cultures were also observed for ampicillin (AMP10) with the highest four *Klebsiella* spp. (100%; n = 30), CNS (90.2%; n = 51), *Pseudomonas* spp. (93.3%; n = 60) and *Escherichia coli* (91.5%; n = 331). The lowest resistance rates were observed with cefoxitin in *S. aureus* cultures (FOX30) (0%; n = 10). For imipenem (IMP), no or low resistance rates were observed in cultures with CNS (0%; n = 34), *Klebsiella* spp. (0%; n = 10), *S. aureus* (0%; n = 10), *E. coli* (1.3%, n = 224) and *Pseudomonas* spp. (13.3%; n = 15). Resistance to vancomycin (VA30) was observed with *Enterococcus* spp. (3.3%; n = 30), CNS (13.4%; n = 119), *S. aureus* (14.0%; n = 57) and *Streptococcus* spp. (16.7%; n = 12). A table showing percentages of resistance rates and numbers of cultures from this study is presented in Appendix 2.

Discussion

This study describes the results from almost fifteen thousand antibiograms analyzed with open-source software; it is the largest number of ADR test results to have been described in Ethiopia. As is the case throughout the rest of Africa, data on antibiotic resistance levels in Ethiopia is minimal and mostly derived from literature. Estimates of ADR percentages are rendered ambiguous as a result of quality assurance issues, small sample sizes and biases related to hospital-based studies with isolates from specific patient groups [6, 13, 14]. Although the interpretation of the data presented in this study must be taken with caution, it does provide a general overview of the current situation, showing similarities with ADR described in other recent studies.

One of the study limitations is the fact that the query in the laboratory database converged one time-period and was restricted to sample source, bacteria species and antibiotic susceptibility result. With the available LIMS query method, it was impossible to distinguish whether multiple specimens originated from one patient. Samples obtained from hospitals might have included patients hospitalized >48 h, which makes it impossible

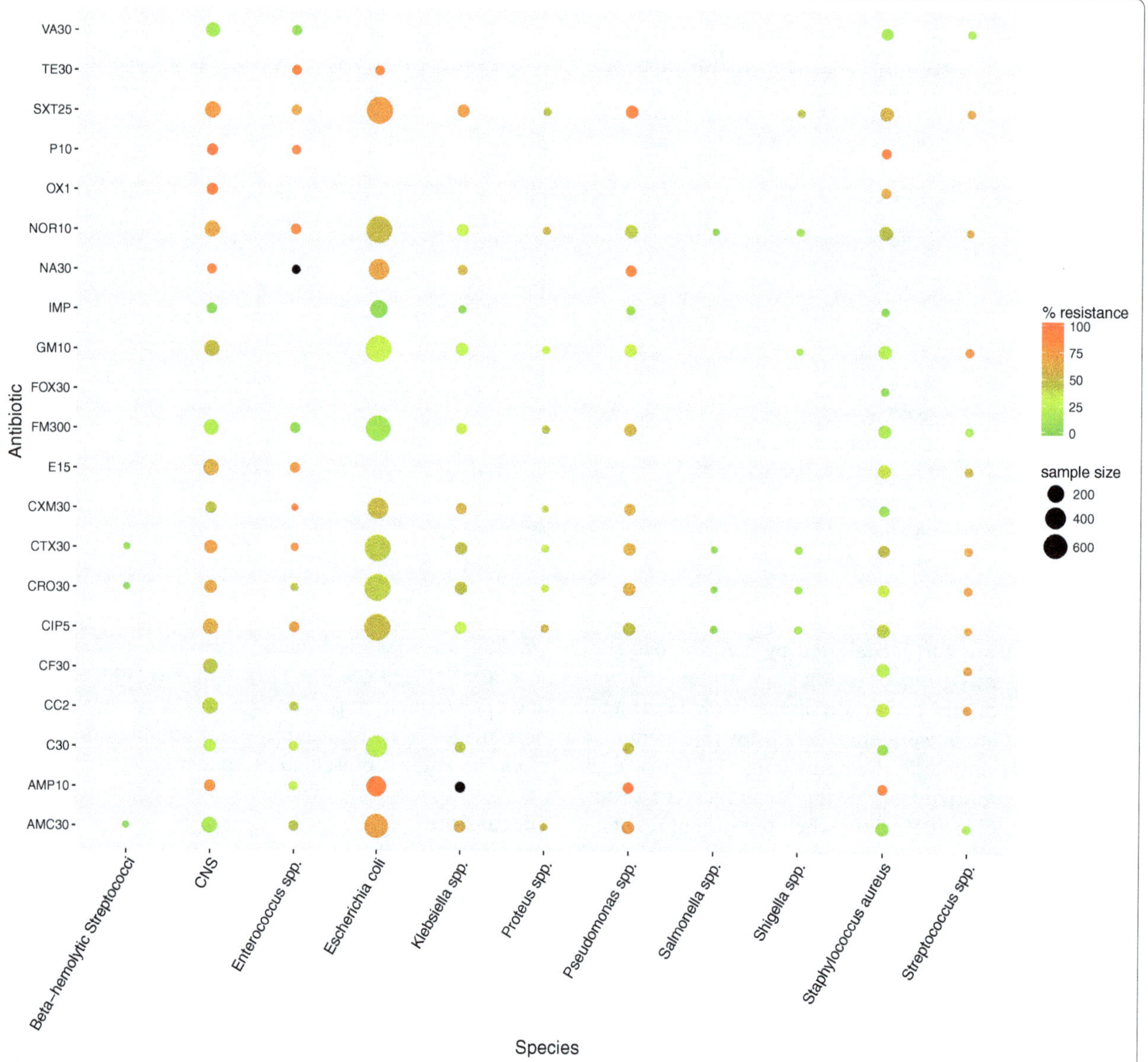

Fig. 1 Percentages of resistance of bacterial species (n = 12.220) against antibiotics represented by *color* and number of tested samples represented by *dot-size* (January 2014–May 2015). *CNS* coagulase negative staphylococci, *SAMC30* amoxicillin/clavulanic acid, *AMP10* ampicillin, *C30* chloramphenicol, *CC2* clindamycin, *CF30* cephalophin, *CIP5* ciprofloxacin, *CRO30* ceftriaxone, *CTX30* cefotaxime, *CXM30* cefuroxime, *E15* erythromycin, *FM300* nitrofurantoin, *FOX30* cefoxitin, *GM10* gentamicin, *IMP* imipenem, *NA30* nalidixic acid, *NOR10* norfloxacin, *OX1* oxacillin, *P10* penicillin, *SXT25* sulfamethoxazole, *TE30* tetracycline, *VA30* vancomycin

in this study to distinguish between hospital acquired infections and resistance patterns at community level. In addition, because information on antibiotic use prior to the bacterial culture was not available it is not possible to distinguish between patients who had been treated with antibiotics and those who were not. The tradition of empirical antibiotic treatment of presumed infectious illnesses in Ethiopia is such that it can be expected that patients will seek medical advice after treatment failure, which explains the high ADR levels described in this study.

The majority of antibiograms in this study were derived from urine samples in which *E. coli* was most often determined. More than 80% of the cultures showed resistance to ampicillin and tetracycline, while resistance rates to chloramphenicol, nitrofurantoin and imipenem were less than 27%. Overall, the resistance patterns were similar to the results described by Abejew et al. for the Dessie regional health research laboratory [15] in which also high rates was described for ampicillin and tetracycline while susceptible to nitrofurantoin. High rates of multi-drug resistant extended-spectrum beta-lactamase (ESBL) producing enterobacteriaceae uropathogens were described in Gondor hospital [16]. The results of the ESBL tests could not be entered in the LIMS during the study timeframe and were directly reported to physicians. Examination of these reports from the study time also suggests high prevalence of ESBL. After the recent installation of the BD Phoenix 100 instrument at International Clinical Laboratories (ICL) and with the data now being stored in the LIMS, suspected and confirmed ESBL-producing microorganisms are now encountered almost daily (private communication with ICL microbiologist).

The second most numerous specimens received at the laboratory were obtained from wounds, with most infections due to *S. aureus*. These bacteria demonstrated less than 21% resistance to most antibiotics, with the exception of penicillin (n = 20; resistance rate = 90.0%), ampicillin (n = 24; resistance rate = 87.5%) and oxacillin (n = 25; resistance rate = 64.0%). Presence of methicillin-resistant *S. aureus* (MRSA) could not be proven in this study. Other studies indicate high rates of MRSA in the community and amongst health-care workers, however, reliance on phenotypic tests usually provides an overestimation [17–19]. There are no recent estimates of the prevalence of MRSA in the Ethiopian community, therefore, making molecular confirmation methods more accessible in Ethiopia to be crucial for future national surveillance programs.

A comparison of the data obtained with the recommendations in the Ethiopian standard treatment guidelines [4] clearly shows that a high treatment failure rate can be expected when drugs are administered according to national protocols. There are extensive differences in the rates of resistance observed for different bacterial species within one type of specimen. It is therefore important to back up treatment consultations with bacterial species identification accompanied by antibiograms.

Resistance to antibiotics poses serious threats not only in the developing world, but internationally [20]. National and international surveillance initiatives are ongoing to identify and publicize trends in resistance rates and, in some instances, have resulted in rapid changes to national treatment guidelines [21, 22]. The crucial ingredient lacking in Ethiopian health policy is the availability of reliable data. The Ethiopia Food, Medicine, Healthcare Administration and Control Authority (EFMHACA) is currently establishing a five strategic plan to decrease antibiotic resistance. This strategy is based on awareness, evidence-based information, infection prevention, optimized use of antimicrobials in human and animal health and strengthening national partnerships. Microbiology laboratories are the first line of identification of antibiotic resistance among the general public. Besides delivering awareness to its clients, the laboratories play a key role in providing evidence-based data for antimicrobial surveillance. Reliable trends are directly correlated with reliable data input. The World Health Organisation published a manual on how to aggregate and validate national ADR files [23]. Additional guidance on how to structure raw data into correct data frames and how to visualize the data into clarifying figures could facilitate and encourage microbiology laboratories to assist in data collection. With currently available information technology, it takes relatively little effort to set up the application with real-time data feed as an additional service from diagnostic laboratories towards all levels: diagnostic laboratories providing the additional service of a real-time data feed that reaches all levels ranging from the clinicians prescribing antibiotics to national surveillance programs.

Conclusions

The extraction and analysis of raw-data from the laboratory database provides valuable insights into the relationships between type of sample and drug-resistance in countries where such data is still scarce. When used as an easy accessible reference application for healthcare providers, computer-based surveillance can reveal trends in antibiotic resistance levels and thus prevent treatment failures.

Abbreviations

ADR: antibiotic drug resistance; ATCC: American Type Culture Collection; CNS: coagulase negative *Staphylococcus*; CSF: cerebral spinal fluid; ESBL: extended-spectrum beta-lactamase; EFMHACA: Ethiopia Food, Medicine, Healthcare Administration and Control Authority; ICL: International Clinical Laboratories; LIMS: laboratory information management system; MRSA: methicillin-resistant *S. aureus*.

Authors' contributions

RTH: writing script, data analysis and drafting the manuscript; MT: laboratory work and drafting manuscript and Methods; WTH: writing script and data analysis. MN: supervision and drafting the manuscript. All authors read and approved the final manuscript.

Author details
[1] International Clinical Laboratories, Addis Ababa, Ethiopia. [2] HAN University of Applied Sciences, Nijmegen, The Netherlands.

Acknowledgements
We thank Mr. Kebede Fufa and the staff of the microbiology section for their input on microbiology diagnostics, and the International Clinical Laboratories for making the data accessible. Thanks also to Miss. Asnakech Alemu who was so kind as to elucidate us on the EFMHACA strategy plan. We extend our sincere appreciation to Sara Chauvin for reviewing the manuscript.

Competing interests
The authors declare that they have no competing interests.

Appendix 1
See Table 2.

Table 2 Identified bacteria with frequency in and percentage of the total number of isolates

Bacteria isolated	Frequency	Percentage (%)
Acinetobacter species	12	0.08
Actinomyces viscosus	9	0.06
Bacteroides fragilis	2	0.01
Beta hemolytic non-group A	7	0.05
Citrobacter braakii	1844	12.31
Citrobacter farmeri	16	0.11
Citrobacter freundii	8	0.05
Citrobacter koseri	8	0.05
Coagulase-negative *Staphylococcus* species	16	0.11
Enterobacter cloacae	59	0.39
Enterobacter species	15	0.10
Enterococcus faecalis	362	2.42
Enterococcus species	12	0.08
Escherichia coli	8057	53.77
Group A *Streptococcus*	33	0.22
Group B *Streptococcus*	85	0.57
Group C *Streptococcus*	26	0.17
Group F *Streptococcus*	9	0.06
Group G *Streptococcus*	10	0.07

Table 2 continued

Bacteria isolated	Frequency	Percentage (%)
Haemophilus influenzae biotype I	11	0.07
Haemophilus influenzae	5	0.03
Klebsiella ornithinolytica	36	0.24
Klebsiella oxytoca	446	2.98
Klebsiella pneumoniae	279	1.86
Klebsiella species	54	0.36
Klebsiella terrigena	24	0.16
Moraxella lacunata	8	0.05
Morganella morganii	8	0.05
Pantoea species 4 (*Erwina* species)	8	0.05
Proteus mirabilis	20	0.13
Proteus penneri	8	0.05
Proteus species	50	0.33
Proteus vulgaris	32	0.21
Pseudomonas aeruginosa	154	1.03
Pseudomonas species	771	5.15
Salmonella group	18	0.12
Salmonella paratyphi A	8	0.05
Salmonella paratyphi B	11	0.07
Salmonella species	41	0.27
Serratia species	13	0.09
Shigella boydii	19	0.13
Shigella dysenteriae	8	0.05
Shigella group A1	9	0.06
Shigella sonnei	16	0.11
Shigella species	22	0.15
Staphylococcus aureus	1554	10.37
Staphylococcus lugdunensis	294	1.96
Staphylococcus saprophyticus	80	0.53
Streptococcus agalactiae (group B)	11	0.07
Streptococcus anginosus/milleri	21	0.14
Streptococcus pneumoniae	63	0.42
Streptococcus pyogenes (group A)	76	0.51
Streptococcus species	210	1.40
Viridans streptococci	5	0.03
Total	14.983	100.00

Appendix 2
See Table 3.

Table 3 Percentage resistance and number of bacterial cultures (in brackets) per antibiotic after merging bacterial species and filtering out antibiogram groups containing less than 7 observations

	β-Hemolytic Streptococci	CNS	*Enterococcus* spp.	*Escherichia coli*	*Klebsiella* spp.	*Proteus* spp.	*Pseudomonas* spp.	*Salmonella* spp.	*Shigella* spp.	*Staphylococcus aureus*	*Streptococcus* spp.
VA30		3.4 (119)	3.3 (30)							3.5 (57)	8.3 (12)
TE30			4.8 (21)	5.3 (19)							
SXT25		2.6 (156)	3.7 (27)	0.7 (740)	4.6 (65)	11.1 (9)	4.6 (65)		11.1 (9)	3.4 (87)	8.3 (12)
P10		4.8 (42)	5.9 (17)							5.0 (20)	
OX1		6.7 (30)								4.0 (25)	
NOR10		2.6 (151)	3.6 (28)	0.7 (726)	3.5 (57)	11.1 (9)	5.4 (74)	14.3 (7)	11.1 (9)	3.4 (89)	12.5 (8)
NA30		5.0 (40)	7.7 (13)	0.6 (363)	4.0 (25)		5.6 (36)				
IMP		6.7 (30)		1.3 (224)	10.0 (10)		6.7 (15)			10.0 (10)	
GM10		2.7 (150)		0.7 (726)	4.5 (66)	11.1 (9)	4.6 (65)		14.3 (7)	3.5 (86)	7.7 (13)
FOX30										10.0 (10)	
FM300		2.8 (143)	3.1 (32)	0.6 (643)	5.1 (39)	11.1 (9)	3.4 (59)			2.7 (73)	8.3 (12)
E15		2.7 (149)	3.4 (29)							3.7 (81)	7.7 (13)
CXM30		5.0 (40)	14.3 (7)	1.0 (388)	5.6 (36)	14.3 (7)	4.7 (43)			3.8 (26)	
CTX30	14.3 (7)	2.4 (82)	11.1 (9)	0.7 (735)	4.6 (65)	12.5 (8)	5.9 (68)	14.3 (7)	11.1 (9)	6.4 (47)	8.3 (12)
CRO30	14.3 (7)	1.4 (71)	11.1 (9)	0.7 (746)	4.5 (67)	12.5 (8)	5.9 (68)	14.3 (7)	11.1 (9)	6.1 (49)	7.7 (13)
CIP5		2.8 (143)	3.4 (29)	0.7 (739)	3.6 (55)	11.1 (9)	4.5 (66)	12.5 (8)	11.1 (9)	3.5 (86)	11.1 (9)
CF30		3.1 (129)								3.6 (83)	7.7 (13)
CC2		2.6 (152)	5.9 (17)							3.6 (84)	7.7 (13)
C30		4.8 (62)	5.3 (19)	1.0 (400)	5.9 (34)		5.0 (40)			6.3 (32)	
AMP10		6.8 (44)	6.7 (15)	0.9 (331)	6.7 (30)		5.6 (36)			4.2 (24)	
AMC30	14.3 (7)	2.6 (152)	4.0 (25)	0.9 (559)	5.9 (51)	12.5 (8)	5.0 (60)			3.7 (3.7)	7.7 (13)

CNS coagulase negative staphylococci, *SAMC30* amoxicilline/clavulate acid, *AMP10* ampicillin, *C30* chloroamphenicol, *CC2* clindamycin, *CF30* cephalophin, *CIP5* ciprofloxacin, *CRO30* ceftriaxone, *CTX30* cefotaxime, *CXM30* cefuroxime, *E15* erythromycin, *FM300* nitrofurantoin, *FOX30* cefoxitin, *GM10* gentamicin, *IMP* imipenem, *NA30* nalidixic acid, *NOR10* norfloxacin, *OX1* oxacillin, *P10* penicillin, *SXT25* sulfamethoxazole, *TE30* tetracycline, *VA30* vancomycin

References

1. Essack SY, Desta AT, Abotsi RE, Agoba EE. Antimicrobial resistance in the WHO African region: current status and roadmap for action. J. Public Health. 2016. doi:10.1093/pubmed/fdw015.
2. Global action plan on antimicrobial resistance. WHA68.7. Sect. Agenda item 15.1 May 26. 2015. p 1–4. http://apps.who.int/gb/ebwha/pdf_files/WHA68/A68_R7-en.pdf.
3. Draft political declaration of the high-level meeting of the General Assembly on antimicrobial resistance. 16-16108 Sep 21. 2016. p 1–5. http://www.un.org/pga/71/wp-content/uploads/sites/40/2016/09/DGACM_GAEAD_ESCAB-AMR-Draft-Political-Declaration-1616108E.pdf.
4. Drug Administration and Control Authority of Ethiopia. Standard Treatment guidelines for health centers; 2010.
5. Groot MJ, van't Hooft KE. The hidden effects of dairy farming on public and environmental health in the Netherlands, India, Ethiopia, and Uganda, considering the use of antibiotics and other agro-chemicals. Front Public Health. 2016;4:1–9.
6. Zenebe T, Kannan S, Yilma D, Beyene G. Invasive bacterial pathogens and their antibiotic susceptibility patterns in Jimma Specialized Hospital, Jimma, Southwest Ethiopia. Ethiop J Health Sci. 2011;21:1–8.
7. Huang SS, Yokoe DS, Stelling J, Placzek H, Kulldorff M, Kleinman K, et al. Automated detection of infectious disease outbreaks in hospitals: a retrospective cohort study. PLoS Med. 2010;7:e1000238.
8. O'Brien TF, Stelling J. Integrated multilevel surveillance of the world's infecting microbes and their resistance to antimicrobial agents. Clin Microbiol Rev. 2011;24:281–95.
9. Isenberg H. Clinical microbiology procedures handbook. American Society for Microbiology; 2004.
10. Murray PA. Manual of clinical microbiology. 7th ed; 1999.
11. Clinical and Laboratory Standards Institute. Performance standards for antimicrobial disk susceptibility tests; approved standard; 2012.
12. ten Hove R-J, ten Hove W, Tesfayem M. Github repository for the antibiogram data set and R scripts. 2016. https://github.com/grebbel/antibiogram.git.
13. Shiferaw B, Gelaw B, Assefa A, Assefa Y, Addis Z. Bacterial isolates and their antimicrobial susceptibility pattern among patients with external ocular infections at Borumeda hospital, Northeast Ethiopia. BMC Ophthalmol. 2015;15:103.
14. Wasihun AG, Wlekidan LN, Gebremariam SA, Dejene TA, Welderufael AL, Haile TD, et al. Bacteriological profile and antimicrobial susceptibility patterns of blood culture isolates among febrile patients in Mekelle Hospital, Northern Ethiopia. SpringerPlus. 2015;4:314.
15. Abejew AA, Denboba AA, Mekonnen AG. Prevalence and antibiotic resistance pattern of urinary tract bacterial infections in Dessie area, North-East Ethiopia. BMC Res Notes. 2014;7:687.
16. Eshetie S, Unakal C, Gelaw A, Ayelign B, Endris M, Moges F. Multidrug resistant and carbapenemase producing Enterobacteriaceae among patients with urinary tract infection at referral Hospital, Northwest Ethiopia. Antimicrob Resist Infect Control. 2015;4:12.
17. Falagas ME, Karageorgopoulos DE, Leptidis J, Korbila IP. MRSA in Africa : filling the global map of antimicrobial resistance. PloS ONE. 2013;8:e68024.
18. Shibabaw A, Abebe T, Mihret A. Nasal carriage rate of methicillin resistant *Staphylococcus aureus* among Dessie Referral Hospital Health care workers; Dessie, Northeast Ethiopia. Antimicrob Resist Infect Control. 2013;2:1.
19. Tibebu M, Embiyale W. Community acquired multi drug resistant *Staphylococcus aureus* in a rural setting of North Western Ethiopia: a tough challenge. Ethiop Med J. 2014;52:147–50.
20. World Health Organization. The evolving threat of antimicrobial resistance—options for action. 2012. http://www.who.int/patientsafety/implementation/amr/publication/en/.
21. Ison CA, Town K, Obi C, Chisholm S, Hughes G, Livermore DM, et al. Decreased susceptibility to cephalosporins among gonococci: data from the Gonococcal Resistance to Antimicrobials Surveillance Programme (GRASP) in England and Wales, 2007–2011. Lancet Infect Dis. 2013;13:762–8.
22. Johnson AP. Surveillance of antibiotic resistance. Phil Trans R Soc B. 2015;370:20140080.
23. World Health Organization. Antimicrobial resistance. GLASS documents and tools. 2017. http://www.who.int/antimicrobial-resistance/global-action-plan/surveillance/glass-documents/en/.

18

The draft genomes and investigation of serotype distribution, antimicrobial resistance of group B *Streptococcus* strains isolated from urine in Suzhou, China

Yong Guo[1†], Xiao Deng[1†], Yuan Liang[2], Liang Zhang[3], Guo-Ping Zhao[2,3] and Yan Zhou[2,3*]

Abstract

Background: The group B *Streptococcus* (GBS) is a human commensal bacterium, which is capable of causing several infectious diseases in infants, and people with chronic diseases. GBS has been the most common cause of infections in urinary tract of the elders, but relatively few studies reported the urine-isolated GBS and their antimicrobial susceptibilities. Hence, we decided to investigate GBS specially isolated from urine in Suzhou, China.

Methods: 27 GBS samples were isolated from urine in Suzhou, China. The PCR and agarose gel electrophoresis were used to identify the serotype distribution. Susceptibility tests were based on MIC test and Kirby–Bauer test. Genome were sequenced via Illumina Hiseq platform and assembled by SPAdes. Genomes of five isolates were sequenced and submitted to NCBI genome database. The sequencing files in fastq format were submitted to NCBI SRA database.

Results: Five serotypes were identified. The resistant rates measured for tetracycline, erythromycin, clindamycin and fluoroquinolones were 74.1, 63.0, 44.4 and 48.1%, respectively. 18.5% of the isolates were nonsusceptible to nitrofurantoin. The resistance to tetracycline was mainly associated with the gene *tetM*. The erythromycin resistance was mainly associated with the genes *ermB* and *mefE*. The genes *ermB* and *lnuB* were the prevalent genes in cMLSB type. No known nitrofurantoin resistance gene was found in nitrofurantoin-nonsusceptible GBS.

Conclusions: Five serotypes were identified in our study. High rates of GBS isolates were resistant to tetracycline, erythromycin, clindamycin and fluoroquinolones. The genes *ermB* and *lnuB* occupied high rates in cMLS$_B$ phenotype.

Keywords: Group B *Streptococcus*, Serotype, Antimicrobial susceptibility, Drug resistance gene, Genome

Background

Group B Streptococcus (GBS, i.e. *Streptococcus agalactiae*) is a gram-positive microbe with bacterial morphology of sphere and oval observed via microscope [1]. Tilapia mossambica and cow are susceptible to GBS, leading to the reduced milk production [2, 3]. GBS can be divided into ten serotypes, Ia, Ib, and II–IX, based on variant capsular polysaccharide. The serotypes Ia, Ib, III and V are the predominant pathogens, primarily liable for human infection [4]. GBS has traditionally been considered as a perinatal pathogen, in relation to certain infectious diseases in pregnant or postpartum women encomapassing endometritis, septicemia, chorioamnionitis and urinary tract infection [5]. Furthermore, GBS has been proved causing severe diseases in infants, such as pneumonia and meningitis [6]. Infectious pattern in infants were separated into two ways: mother-to-child vertically transmitted infection and birth canal transmission [7]. Screening for GBS in pregnant women via swabs taken from the vagina, of which the colonized GBS were mostly harmless, following by antibiotic treatment to prevent the transmission to the babies.

*Correspondence: zhouy@fudan.edu.cn
†Yong Guo and Xiao Deng contributed equally to this work
[2] State Key Laboratory of Genetic Engineering, School of Life Sciences, Fudan University, Shanghai 200433, China
Full list of author information is available at the end of the article

GBS can also cause asymptomatic bacteriuria, cystitis, pyelonephritis, urethritis and urosepsis in urinary tract [8]. In a series of studies, bacteremia and urinary tract infections caused by GBS were the most common diagnoses among people over the age of 70, with 13 of 33 cases (39.4%) [9]. Previous studies indicated that all serotypes of GBS are susceptible to penicillin and have high rates of resistance to tetracycline, clindamycin and erythromycin [10], but little attention was paid to molecular mechanisms underlying those antimicrobial susceptibilities of GBS in urinary tract. A total of 27 GBS samples were isolated from urine in this study to investigate the serotype distribution and antibiotic susceptibilities in Suzhou, China.

Methods

Samples collecting and typing

All the GBS samples were isolated from urine between November 2015 and March 2017 in Suzhou Hospital of Traditional Chinese Medicine, Suzhou, China. The isolates were cultured on Blood agar medium at 37 °C with 5% CO_2 for 24 h. The DNA was extracted via the Ezup Column Bacteria Genomic DNA Purification Kit. The polymerase chain reaction (PCR) and agarose gel electrophoresis were applied (the primer sequences are in Additional file 1: Table S1, the PCR amplification system is in Additional file 1: Table S2 and the procedure of PCR is in Additional file 1: Table S3) to determine the serotype according to the expectation of electrophoresis result (Additional file 1: Table S4).

Antimicrobial susceptibility test and drug resistance gene PCR

Susceptibility tests to tetracycline, erythromycin, clindamycin, fluoroquinolones, nitrofurantoin, vancomycin, linezolid, quinupristin–dalfopristin and tigecycline were based on the MIC test. Susceptibility to ceftriaxone and penicillin was based on the Kirby–Bauer test recommended by the clinical and laboratory standards institute (CLSI) guidelines [11]. The clindamycin-induced resistance was detected based on D test [12]. The PCR of drug resistance genes was applied to find 12 resistance genes for tetracycline, erythromycin and clindamycin (Additional file 1: Table S5).

Genome sequencing and bioinformatics analysis

Genomes of four isolates (No.8, No.11, No.17 and No.24) showing multiple resistances and one isolate (No.20) indicating susceptive to all antibiotic were sequenced. The DNA was extracted by QIAGEN DNeasy® Blood & Tissue and sequenced via Illumina Hiseq platform. The genomes were assembled by SPAdes [13] and the k-mer value was set to 127. The scaffolds < 1 kb in length were dropped. The genome sequences were submitted to Antibiotic Resistance Genes Database (ARDB, http://ardb.cbcb.umd.edu/) [14] to query drug resistance genes. The genes were predicted by Prokka (version 1.12).

Two protein sequences of nitrofurantoin-resistant genes, *nsfA* and *nsfB*, were received from The Comprehensive Antibiotic Resistance Database (CARD, https://card.mcmaster.ca/) [15] and then aligned to No.8 genome and No.11 genome sequences via TBLASTN (0.05 e-value) in order to find matching sequences.

The assembled draft genomes of the five isolates were submitted to NCBI genome and SRA database (SAMN08287475, SAMN08287476, SAMN08287477, SAMN08287478 and SAMN0828747). The sequencing files were submitted to NCBI SRA database (SRP128497).

Six complete serotype III genomes were download from NCBI (NZ_CP022537.1/CP022537.1, NZ_CP010874.1/CP010874.1, NZ_CP010875.1/CP010875.1, NZ_CP011327.1/CP011327.1, NZ_CP011329.1/CP011329.1 and NC_004368.1/AL732656.1), respectively. The orthologous list of isolates No.8, No.11 and genomes downloaded from NCBI was built via orthoMCL (v1.4). The orthologous families which contain genes in isolates No.8, No.11 genome and in at most one complete genome downloaded from NCBI, genes in isolates No.8 genome and in at most one complete genome downloaded from NCBI, genes in isolates No.11 and in at most one complete genome downloaded from NCBI, genes in isolates No.8 and No.11 that did not be recorded to orthologous list were extracted by our own PERL script. We also built another orthologous list between isolates No.8 and No.11.

The orthologous list of isolates No.8, No.11, No.17, No.20 and No.24 was built via orthoMCL (v1.4). The orthologous families which contain genes both in isolates No.8 and No.11 genome were also extracted by our own PERL script.

Results

Group B *Streptococcus* can cause urinary tract infections (UTI). From November 2015 to March 2017 in Suzhou Hospital of Traditional Chinese Medicine, there were 147 individuals had positive urine culture of gram-positive bacteria and 30 (20.4%) of them were positive for GBS. However, few studies reported the GBS in urinary tract. Hence, we presented 27 GBS samples isolated from urine to investigate potential clinical treatment of GBS infections in Suzhou, China.

Serotypes

Five serotypes were found in 27 samples, which were Ia, Ib, III, V and VI. The proportion and number were 18.5%

(5/27), 22.2% (6/27), 29.6% (8/27), 22.2% (6/27) and 7.4% (2/27) respectively (Table 1).

Resistance of tetracycline, erythromycin and clindamycin

All the 27 samples were susceptible to ceftriaxone, penicillin, vancomycin, linezolid, quinupristin–dalfopristin and tigecycline, while the highest percentage of 74.1% (20/27, Table 1 and Additional file 1: Table S6) samples were resistant to tetracycline. In previous studies, only the PCR primers of genes involved in resistance to tetracycline, erythromycin and clindamycin has been reported. In our PCR test of antibiotic resistance genes, *tetM* was the dominating resistance gene to tetracycline with 90.0% (18/20) occurrence. Other genes resistant to tetracycline were *tetO, tetK* and *tetL*, and the rates were 15.0% (3/20), 5.0% (1/20) and 5.0% (1/20) respectively.

The resistant rate measured for erythromycin was 63.0% (17/27). *ErmB, mefE* and *ermTR* were found and the rates are 47.1% (8/17), 41.2% (7/17) and 17.6% (3/17) respectively. About 44.4% (12/27) isolates were resistant to clindamycin. *ErmB* 75.0% (9/12), *lnuB* 58.3% (7/12) *and ermTR* 8.3% (1/12) were found in these isolates. Seven isolates were resistant to erythromycin but susceptible to clindamycin. Three of them were 'inducible resistance to macrolides, lincosamides and streptograminB, (iMLS$_B$) phenotype since they were positive in D test (Additional file 2: Figure S1). Four isolates were 'resistance to macrolides and susceptibility to lincosamides (MS)' phenotype. The *erm* (erythromycin ribosome

Table 1 PCR result of antibiotic resistance genes

Serotype	Sample	*tetM*	*tetO*	*tetK*	*tetL*	*ermA*	*ermB*	*ermC*	*ermM*	*ermTR*	*mefA*	*mefE*	*lnuB*	Resistance summary	D test
III	13	+	–	–	–	–	+	–	–	–	–	–	+	TET, FQNS, cMLS$_B$	/
III	18	+	–	–	–	–	–	–	–	–	–	–	+	TET, FQNS, cMLS$_B$	/
III	27	+	–	–	–	–	+	–	–	–	–	–	+	TET, FQNS, cMLS$_B$	/
III	1	+	–	–	–	–	–	–	–	–	–	+	+	TET, FQNS, cMLS$_B$	/
V	26	+	–	–	–	–	+	–	–	+	–	+	+	TET, FQNS, cMLS$_B$	/
Ib	8	–	+	–	–	–	+	–	–	–	–	+	+	TET, cMLS$_B$	/
Ib	24	+	–	+	+	–	+	–	–	–	–	–	+	TET, cMLS$_B$	/
Ia	3	–	+	–	–	–	+	–	–	–	–	–	–	TET, cMLS$_B$	/
III	14	+	–	–	–	–	–	–	–	–	–	–	–	TET, FQNS, MS	Negative
V	17	+	–	–	–	–	–	–	–	+	–	+	–	TET, FQNS, iMLS$_B$	Positive
V	10	+	–	–	–	–	–	–	–	+	–	+	–	TET, FQNS, iMLS$_B$	Positive
Ib	4	–	–	–	–	–	–	–	–	–	–	–	–	FQNS, cMLS$_B$	/
Ib	22	–	–	–	–	–	–	–	–	–	–	–	–	FQNS, cMLS$_B$	/
Ib	15	–	–	–	–	–	–	–	–	–	–	–	–	CLI, FQNS	/
III	11	+	–	–	–	–	–	–	–	–	–	–	–	TET, iMLS$_B$	Positive
Ia	16	+	–	–	–	–	–	–	–	–	–	–	–	TET, MS	Negative
Ia	2	+	–	–	–	–	–	–	–	–	–	–	–	TET, MS	Negative
III	6	+	–	–	–	–	–	–	–	–	–	–	–	TET, MS	Negative
Ia	5	+	–	–	–	–	–	–	–	–	–	–	–	TET, CLI	/
Ib	7	–	–	–	–	–	–	–	–	–	–	–	–	FQNS	/
III	9	+	–	–	–	–	–	–	–	–	–	+	+	FQNS	/
Ia	23	+	–	–	–	–	–	–	–	–	–	–	–	TET	/
V	25	–	+	–	–	–	–	–	–	–	–	+	–	TET	/
V	19	+	–	–	–	–	+	–	–	–	–	–	–	TET	/
V	21	+	–	–	–	–	–	–	–	–	–	–	–	TET	/
VI	12	–	–	–	–	–	–	–	–	–	–	–	–	–	/
VI	20	–	–	–	–	–	–	–	–	–	–	–	–	–	/
Total number		18	3	1	1	0	10	0	0	3	0	9	8		

The order was sorted based on Additional file 1: Table S6. *Tet* genes are resistant to tetracycline; *erm* genes are resistant to clindamycin, erythromycin and streptogramin_b; *mef* genes are resistant to erythromycin; *lnuB* gene is resistant to clindamycin. Erythromycin is a kind of macrolides; clindamycin a kind of lincosamides

TET tetracycline, *CLI* clindamycin, *E* erythromycin, *FQNS* fluoroquinolones. *cMLS$_B$* constitutive resistance to macrolides, lincosamides, and streptograminB, *iMLS$_B$* inducible resistance to macrolides, lincosamides, and streptograminB, *MS* resistance to macrolides and susceptibility to lincosamides

methylase) gene has been considered as the reason of resistance to erythromycin, clindamycin and streptograminB, or the $cMLS_B$. There were ten isolates resistant to erythromycin and clindamycin ($cMLS_B$) with a high rate of *ermB* (80.0%) and *lnuB* (70.0%) detection. Five $cMLS_B$ isolates have both *ermB* and *lnuB* genes. Three $cMLS_B$ isolates have *ermB* gene without *lnuB* gene, two isolates have *lnuB* gene without *ermB* gene.

The PCR tests of common drug resistance genes (resistance genes for tetracycline, erythromycin and clindamycin) could explain 74.1% phenotype of drug resistances, except for the seven isolates (No.2, No.5, No.9, No.11, No.14, No.19 and No.25, Table 1 and Additional file 1: Table S6). We sequenced the genome of No.11 isolate and found another known erythromycin resistance gene, *ermT* (Table 3), suggesting that potentially there were other known resistance genes in the remaining six isolates.

Multiple resistance and detection for novel antibiotic resistance genes

Isolates of No.8, No.11, No.17 and No.24 were non-susceptible to at least three antibiotics. As the control, No.20 isolate was susceptible to all antibiotics. These five isolates were sequenced. The draft genome sizes were from 2.06 to 2.20 MB, and the scaffold N50 s were from 107,763 to 468,051 bp (Table 2). As expected, none known resistance genes were found in PCR test and draft genome of No.20 isolate.

The No.8 isolate was resistant to tetracycline, erythromycin, clindamycin, and intermediate to nitrofurantoin. Genes *tetO* (tetracycline resistant), *ermB* (erythromycin and clindamycin resistant), *mefE* (erythromycin resistant) and *lnuB* (clindamycin resistant) were found in the PCR test. Genes *tetO* (tetracycline resistant), *mefA* (erythromycin resistant) and *lnuB* (clindamycin resistant) were found in the draft genome. No nitrofurantoin resistance gene was found (Tables 1, 3). No.11 isolate was resistant to tetracycline, erythromycin, and intermediate to nitrofurantoin. Tetracycline resistance gene *tetM* was found in PCR test and in the draft genome, but no erythromycin resistance gene was found in PCR test. An erythromycin and clindamycin resistance gene *ermB* was found in the draft genome. However, no nitrofurantoin resistance gene was found. About 48.1% (13/27, Additional file 1: Table S6) of the isolates were resistant to fluoroquinolones. One of them, No.17 isolate, was resistant to tetracycline, erythromycin and fluoroquinolones.

Table 2 Genome information

Strain	Serotype	Total scaffolds number	Total length (bp)	Gap length (N) (bp)	Average length (bp)	Minimum length (bp)	Maximum length (bp)	GC content (%)	N50 (bp)
8	Ib	32	2,200,680	190	68,771	1085	394,159	35.64	183,219
11	III	41	2,107,554	92	51,403	1045	247,508	35.53	107,763
17	V	34	2,106,885	0	61,967	1213	265,957	35.47	117,386
20	VI	11	2,061,455	104	187,405	1064	1,656,169	35.39	1,656,169
24	Ia	20	2,113,859	97	105,692	1036	712,759	35.38	468,051

Table 3 Known antibiotic resistance genes in draft genomes

Sample no.	Resistance of phenotype	Gene name	Resistance of genotype
8	Tetracycline, erythromycin, clindamycin	*lnuB*	Clindamycin
		mefA	Erythromycin
		tetO	Tetracycline
11	Tetracycline, erythromycin	*ermT*	Clindamycin, erythromycin
		tetM	Tetracycline
17	Tetracycline, erythromycin, fluoroquinolones	*tetM*	Tetracycline
		mefA	Erythromycin
		pmrA	Fluoroquinolone
20	None	none	None
24	Tetracycline, erythromycin, clindamycin	*tetL*	Tetracycline
		tetM	Tetracycline
		macB	Erythromycin

These genomes were submitted to ARDB database to query known resistance genes

Fluoroquinolones resistance gene was not included in the targets of PCR test, but the *pmrA* was found in the draft genome. The *tetM* (tetracycline resistant) was found in PCR test and in the draft genome. The *ermTR* (erythromycin and clindamycin resistant) and *mefE* (erythromycin resistant) were found in PCR test. The *mefA* (erythromycin resistant) was found in the draft genome. No.24 isolate was resistant to tetracycline, erythromycin and clindamycin. Tetracycline resistance genes *tetM*, *tetK* and *tetL*, erythromycin and clindamycin resistance gene *ermB* and clindamycin resistance gene *lnuB* were found in PCR test. Tetracycline resistance genes *tetM* and *tetL* and erythromycin resistance gene *macB* were found in the draft genome.

About 18.5% (5/27, Additional file 1: Table S6) of the isolates were intermediate to nitrofurantoin, among which four nitrofurantoin-intermediate isolates were serotype III and the other one was serotype Ib. So far, two nitrofurantoin-resistant genes, *nsfA* and *nsfB*, have been reported [16]. About two-thirds of the length of *nsfB* protein were aligned to all of the five draft genomes by TBLASTN search (E-value threshold 0.05, Additional file 1: Table S7), in which the genome area contained a 'Ribosomal large subunit pseudouridine synthase B' f in No.8 isolate, a 'glyoxal reductase' in No.11, a "putative NAD(P)H nitroreductase YfkO" in No.17, No.20 and No.24 isolates. So that the phenotype of nitrofurantoin intermediation was not caused by *nsfB* in our cases.

Based on the assumption that the mechanism of the nitrofurantoin intermediation in two isolates was similar, six complete serotype III genomes download from NCBI were included and built orthologous list with genomes of the nitrofurantoin-intermediate samples to search for candidate genes, given that the nitrofurantoin intermediation could not be explained by reported nitrofurantoin-resistant genes. Considering that a detailed information for nitrofurantoin resistance of these complete serotype III genomes is limited, we supposed that at most one of these genomes has a nitrofurantoin-resistant phenotype according to the reference resistance occurrence. Seventeen orthologous contain genes in genomes of No.8, No.11 isolates only or mixed with at most one complete genome downloaded from NCBI. There were 18 genes of isolate No.8 and 17 genes of isolate No.11 in these seventeen orthologous (Additional file 1: Table S8). Most of those genes (16 of 35) were annotated as "hypothetical proteins" since their biological function has still not been clarified. We also identified several genes associated with transposition (6 of 35) and bacteriolysis (2 of 35), which appear to be unessential for the nitrofurantoin intermediation. Therefore, the nitrofurantoin-resistant related genes probably exist in those "hypothetical proteins". There were 27 genes distributed in the orthologous which contain genes only in isolate No.8 or mixed with at most one NCBI genome. 60 genes were distributed in the orthologous which contain genes only in isolate No.11 or mixed with at most one NCBI genome. Totally 148 genes of No.8 and 53 genes of No.11 were not recorded in this orthologous list. These genes cannot be found in another orthologous list which built between No.8 genome and No.11 genome either, suggesting that these 148 genes in No.8 and 53 genes in No.11 are unique genes of their own.

To further investigate the nitrofurantoin intermediation related genes in isolates No.8 and No.11 genome, the orthologous list of isolates No.8, No.11, No.17, No.20 and No.24 was built, with the other three genomes as the nitrofurantoin-susceptible control. A high proportion of genes were annotated as "hypothetical proteins" (10 of 28, Additional file 1: Table S9), which was consistent with the above-mentioned observation. On the basis of our findings, it can be predicted that there is a higher possibility for the intersection of genes identified in both two orthologous lists to be the candidate genes, which were classified as hypothetical protein, helix-turn-helix domain protein and recombinase. With the range of candidates narrowed down, the four genes annotated as hypothetical proteins (Additional file 1: Table S9) were more likely to be the nitrofurantoin-resistant related genes, providing valuable reference for future experimental study.

Discussion

Five serotypes were detected in our research, encompassing Ia, Ib, III, V and VI. The serotype III, V and Ib were of the highest proportion. The serotype III GBS was the most common type detected in our isolates, which was in line with studies from other countries [17, 18].

All of the GBS isolates studied in this work were susceptible to penicillin, indicating that penicillin is still a considerable choice for treatment of GBS infection. There was high rate of resistance to tetracycline (74.1%) in the test. However, this rate was lower than that reported in Beijing city (83.9%, isolated from vagina or rectum) [19], Taiwan (97.2%, isolated from urine, genital tract, genital tract, wound or pus, blood and respiratory tract) [20] and North American (89.2%, isolated from vagina or rectum) [17]. Compared to Shanghai, a city close to Suzhou, the rate of resistance to erythromycin in Suzhou (63.0%) is higher than reported in Shanghai (51.9%), however the rate of resistance to clindamycin in Suzhou (44.4%) is lower than that of Shanghai (61.5%) [21]. Note that, 80% of the nitrofurantoin-nonsusceptible GBSs in Suzhou were serotype III isolates, much higher than the 29.6% proportion of serotype III occurrence in the studied samples.

The *tetM* gene was the prevalent resistance gene (18/20) in tetracycline resistance isolates. The other detected tetracycline-nonsusceptible related genes were *tetO, tetK* and *tetL*. Besides, *ermB* (8/17) was the prevalent gene related to erythromycin resistance, which had been reported in Korea (isolated from vagina) [22]. It has been reported that the predominant genes in $cMLS_B$ were *ermB* in Spain [23, 24] and *ermB* and *ermB-mef(A/F)* in Shanghai city [21]. Interestingly, except *ermB*, we found *lnuB* also showed a high proportion (7/10) in $cMLS_B$ in Suzhou (70.0%), five isolates have both *ermB* and *lnuB* genes, three isolates have *ermB* gene only and two isolates have *lnuB* gene only. Although this high rate of *lnuB* had not been reported in previous studies.

We suspected that new resistance genes probably exist in the genomes of isolates No.8 and No.11 since the phenotype of nitrofurantoin intermediation in our cases was not caused by *nsfA* and *nsfB*, nitrofurantoin-resistant genes that were recorded in CARD database. If the nitrofurantoin resistance mechanism is similar in the two samples, the 35 genes in the orthologous which contain genes both in the genomes of isolates No.8 and No.11 only or mixed with at most one NCBI genome would be potential candidates for the nitrofurantoin resistance. We also built another orthologous list with the other three genomes of the five isolates as the nitrofurantoin-susceptible control to integrate our finding. There is a greater likelihood for the four genes annotated as hypothetical proteins in the intersection of the two orthologous lists to be the nitrofurantoin-resistant related genes.

Conclusions

We isolated 27 GBS samples from urine in Suzhou, China. Five serotypes were identified (Ia, Ib, III, V and VI). The serotype III was the primary type. All of the samples were susceptible to ceftriaxone, penicillin, vancomycin, linezolid, quinupristin–dalfopristin and tigecycline. The resistance rates to tetracycline, erythromycin, clindamycin and fluoroquinolones were 74.1, 63.0, 44.4 and 48.1% respectively. The resistance to tetracycline was mainly associated with the gene *tetM* (18/20). The erythromycin resistance was mainly associated with the genes *ermB* (8/17) and *mefE* (7/17). The genes *ermB* (8/10) and *lnuB* (7/10) occupied high rates in $cMLS_B$ phenotype. We found five samples were nonsusceptible to nitrofurantoin, and four of them were serotype III, among which two genomes of isolates do not contain any reported nitrofurantoin resistance genes. Five isolates genomes were sequenced and submitted to NCBI genomes database (SAMN08287475, SAMN08287476, SAMN08287477, SAMN08287478 and SAMN0828747) and SRA database (SRP128497).

Additional files

Additional file 1: Table S1. The primers of serotype testing PCR. **Table S2.** The PCR amplification system of cps gene. **Table S3.** The procedure of PCR amplification system for cps gene. **Table S4.** The PCR amplification products of serotype Ia to IX. **Table S5.** The primers of drug resistance genes. **Table S6.** Antimicrobial susceptibility test result. **Table S7.** TBLAST result of nsfB against five draft genomes. **Table S8.** The function and numbers of genes in orthologous which contain genes in genomes of isolates both No.8 and No.11 only or mixed with at most one NCBI genome. **Table S9.** The function and numbers of genes in orthologous which contain genes in genomes of isolates No.8, No.11, No.17, No.20 and No.24.

Additional file 2: Figure S1. Positive results (iMLSB) in D-test. From left to right are No.10, No.11 and No.17, respectively.

Abbreviations

GBS: group B *Streptococcus*; UTI: urinary tract infections; cMLSB: constitutive resistance to macrolides, lincosamides, and streptograminB; iMLSB: inducible resistance to macrolides, lincosamides, and streptograminB; MS: resistance to macrolides and susceptibility to lincosamides; CLSI: clinical and laboratory standards institute guidelines; NCBI: National Center for Biotechnology Information; ARDB: Antibiotic Resistance Genes Database; CARD: Comprehensive Antibiotic Resistance Database; PCR: the polymerase chain reaction; MIC: minimal inhibit concentration.

Authors' contributions

GY collected the GBS samples, carried out the serotyping and drug testing experiment and sequenced genomes. DX carried out the bioinformatics analysis and drafted the manuscript. LY and ZL helped to draft the manuscript. ZGP raised useful suggestions. ZY conceived of the study, participated in its design and coordination, helped to draft the manuscript. All authors read and approved the final manuscript.

Author details

[1] Institutes of Biology and Medical Sciences, Medical College of Soochow University, Suzhou 215123, China. [2] State Key Laboratory of Genetic Engineering, School of Life Sciences, Fudan University, Shanghai 200433, China. [3] Shanghai-MOST Key Laboratory of Health and Disease Genomics, Chinese National Human Genome Center at Shanghai, Shanghai 201203, China.

Acknowledgements

We thank the Suzhou Hospital of Traditional Chinese Medicine kindly provided the GBS samples for this study.

Competing interests

The authors declare that they have no competing interests.

Consent for publication

Not applicable.

Funding

This work was funded in part by the National Key Research Program of China (2017YFC0907503), Shanghai Municipal Science and Technology Commission (16ZR1423900 and 17DZ2270800).

References

1. Delannoy CM, Crumlish M, Fontaine MC, Pollock J, Foster G, Dagleish MP, Turnbull JF, Zadoks RN. Human *Streptococcus agalactiae* strains in aquatic mammals and fish. BMC Microbiol. 2013;13:41. https://doi.org/10.1186/1471-2180-13-41.

2. Liu G, Zhang W, Lu C. Comparative genomics analysis of *Streptococcus agalactiae* reveals that isolates from cultured tilapia in China are closely related to the human strain A909. BMC Genomics. 2013;14:775. https://doi.org/10.1186/1471-2164-14-775.
3. Zuba S, de Villiers EP, Fuxelius HH, Andersson G, Johansson KE, Bishop RP, Bongcam-Rudloff E. Genome sequence of *Streptococcus agalactiae* strain 09mas018883, isolated from a Swedish cow. Genome Announc. 2013;1(4):e00456-13. https://doi.org/10.1128/genomeA.00456-13.
4. Poyart C, Tazi A, Réglier-Poupet H, Billoët A, Tavares N, Raymond J, Trieu-Cuot P. Multiplex PCR assay for rapid and accurate capsular typing of group B *Streptococci*. J Clin Microbiol. 2007;45(6):1985–8. https://doi.org/10.1128/JCM.00159-07.
5. Stoner TD, Weston TA, Trejo J, Doran KS. Group B streptococcal infection and activation of human astrocytes. PLoS ONE. 2015;10(6):e0128431. https://doi.org/10.1371/journal.pone.0128431.
6. Mhalu FS. Infection with *Streptococcus agalactiae* in a London hospital. J Clin Pathol. 1976;29(4):309–12. https://doi.org/10.1136/jcp.29.4.309.
7. Porta K, Rizzolo D. Preventing group B streptococcal infections in newborns. J Am Acad Phys. 2015;28(3):24–9. https://doi.org/10.1097/01.JAA.0000460915.52391.70.
8. Ulett KB, Benjamin WH, Zhuo FL, Xiao M, Kong FR, Gilbert GL, Schembri MA, Ulett GC. Diversity of group B *Streptococcus* serotypes causing urinary tract infection in adults. J Clin Microbiol. 2009;51(8):2806. https://doi.org/10.1128/JCM.01067-13.
9. Trivalle C, Martin E, Martel P, Jacque B, Menard JF, Lemeland JF. Group B streptococcal bacteraemia in the elderly. J Med Microbiol. 1998;47(7):649–52. https://doi.org/10.1099/00222615-47-7-649.
10. Church D, Carson J, Gregson D. Point prevalence study of antibiotic susceptibility of genital group B *Streptococcus* isolated from near-term pregnant women in Calgary, Alberta. Can J Infect Dis Med Microbiol. 2012;23(3):121–4. https://doi.org/10.1155/2012/876103.
11. Clinical and Laboratory Standards Institute. Performance standards for antimicrobial susceptibility testing. Clinical and Laboratory Standards Institute: Wayne; 2017 **(M100-S27)**.
12. Seppälä H, Nissinen A, Yu Q, Huovinen P. Three different phenotypes of erythromycin-resistant *Streptococcus pyogenes* in Finland. J Antimicrob Chemother. 1993;32(6):885–91. https://doi.org/10.1093/jac/32.6.885.
13. Bankevich A, Nurk S, Antipov D, Gurevich AA, Dvorkin M, Kulikov AS, Lesin VM, Nikolenko SI, Pham S, Prjibelski AD, Pyshkin AV, Sirotkin AV, Vyahhi N, Tesler G, Alekseyev MA, Pevzner PA. SPAdes: a new genome assembly algorithm and its applications to single-cell sequencing. J Comput Biol. 2012;19(5):455–77. https://doi.org/10.1089/cmb.2012.0021.
14. Liu B, Pop M. ARDB—antibiotic resistance genes database. Nucleic Acids Res. 2009;37:D443–7. https://doi.org/10.1093/nar/gkn656.
15. Jia BF, Raphenya AR, Alcock B, Waglechner N, Guo PY, Tsang KK, Lago BA, Dave BM, Pereira S, Sharma AN. CARD 2017: expansion and model-centric curation of the comprehensive antibiotic resistance database. Nucleic Acids Res. 2017;45(D1):D566–73. https://doi.org/10.1093/nar/gkw1004.
16. Shanmugam D, Esak SB, Narayanaswamy A. Molecular characterisation of nfsA gene in nitrofurantoin resistant uropathogens. J Clin Diagn Res. 2016;10(6):DC05–9. https://doi.org/10.7860/JCDR/2016/17280.7957.
17. Teatero S, Ferrieri P, Martin I, Demczuk W, McGeer A, Fittipaldi N. Serotype distribution, population structure, and antimicrobial resistance of group B *Streptococcus* strains recovered from colonized pregnant women. J Clin Microbiol. 2017;55(2):412–22. https://doi.org/10.1128/JCM.01615-16.
18. Mengist A, Kannan H, Abdissa A. Prevalence and antimicrobial susceptibility pattern of anorectal and vaginal group B *Streptococci* isolates among pregnant women in Jimma, Ethiopia. BMC Res Notes. 2016;91:351. https://doi.org/10.1186/s13104-016-2158-4.
19. Wang P, Tong JJ, Ma XH, Song FL, Fan L, Guo CM, Shi W, Yu SJ, Yao KH, Yang YH. Serotypes, antibiotic susceptibilities, and multi-locus sequence type profiles of *Streptococcus agalactiae* isolates circulating in Beijing, China. PloS ONE. 2015;10(3):e0120035. https://doi.org/10.1371/journal.pone.0120035.
20. Ko WC, Lee HC, Wang LR, Lee CT, Liu AJ, Wu JJ. Serotyping and antimicrobial susceptibility of group B Streptococcus over an eight-year period in southern Taiwan. Eur J Clin Microbiol Infect Dis. 2001;20(5):334–9. https://doi.org/10.1007/s10096-001-8115-7.
21. Yan YZ, Hu H, Lu TY, Fan HQ, Hu Y, Li G, Zhang XH, Shi Y, Xia R. Investigation of serotype distribution and resistance genes profile in group B *Streptococcus* isolated from pregnant women: a Chinese multicenter cohort study. APMIS. 2016;124(9):794–9. https://doi.org/10.1111/apm.12570.
22. Seo YS, Srinivasan U, Oh KY, Shin JH, Chae JD, Kim MY, Yang JH, Yoon HR, Miller B, DeBusscher J. Changing molecular epidemiology of group B *Streptococcus* in Korea. J Korean Med Sci. 2010;25(6):817–23. https://doi.org/10.3346/jkms.2010.25.6.817.
23. Gonzalez JJ, Andreu A. Multicenter study of the mechanisms of resistance and clonal relationships of *Streptococcus agalactiae* isolates resistant to macrolides, lincosamides, and ketolides in Spain. Antimicrob Agents Chemother. 2005;49(6):2525–7.
24. Betriu C, Culebras E, Gómez M, Rodríguez-Avial I, Sánchez BA, Agreda MC, Picazo JJ. Erythromycin and clindamycin resistance and telithromycin susceptibility in *Streptococcus agalactiae*. Antimicrob Agents Chemother. 2003;47(3):1112–4. https://doi.org/10.1128/AAC.47.3.1112-1114.2003.

19

Extended spectrum beta-lactamase and metallo beta-lactamase production among *Escherichia coli* and *Klebsiella pneumoniae* isolated from different clinical samples in a tertiary care hospital in Kathmandu, Nepal

Krishus Nepal[1], Narayan Dutt Pant[2*], Bibhusan Neupane[1], Ankit Belbase[1], Rikesh Baidhya[1], Ram Krishna Shrestha[3], Binod Lekhak[4], Dwij Raj Bhatta[4] and Bharat Jha[3]

Abstract

Background: Extended spectrum beta-lactamase (ESBL) and metallo beta-lactamase (MBL) production in *Klebsiella pneumoniae* and *Escherichia coli* are the commonest modes of drug resistance among these commonly isolated bacteria from clinical specimens. So the main purpose of our study was to determine the burden of ESBL and MBL production in *E. coli* and *K. pneumoniae* isolated from clinical samples. Further, the antimicrobial susceptibility patterns of *E. coli* and *K. pneumoniae* were also determined.

Methods: A cross-sectional study was conducted at Om Hospital and Research Centre, Kathmandu, Nepal by using the *E. coli* and *K. pneumoniae* isolated from different clinical samples (urine, pus, body fluids, sputum, blood) from May 2015 to December 2015. Antimicrobial susceptibility testing was performed by Kirby-Bauer disc diffusion technique. Extended spectrum beta-lactamase production was detected by combined disc method using ceftazidime and ceftazidime/clavulanic acid discs and cefotaxime and cefotaxime/clavulanic acid discs. Similarly, metallo beta-lactamase production was detected by combined disc assay using imipenem and imipenem/ethylenediaminetetracetate discs. Bacteria showing resistance to at least three different classes of antibiotics were considered multidrug resistant (MDR).

Results: Of total 1568 different clinical samples processed, 268 (17.1%) samples were culture positive. Among which, *E. coli* and *K. pneumoniae* were isolated from 138 (51.5%) and 39 (14.6%) samples respectively. Of the total isolates 61 (34.5%) were ESBL producers and 7 (4%) isolates were found to be MBL producers. High rates of ESBL production (35.9%) was noted among the clinical isolates from outpatients, however no MBL producing strains were isolated from outpatients. Among 138 *E. coli* and 39 *K. pneumoniae*, 73 (52.9%) *E. coli* and 23 (59%) *K. pneumoniae* were multidrug resistant. The lowest rates of resistance was seen toward imipenem followed by piperacillin/tazobactam, amikacin and cefoperazone/sulbactam.

Conclusions: High rate of ESBL production was found in the *E. coli* and *K. pneumoniae* isolated from outpatients suggesting the dissemination of ESBL producing isolates in community. This is very serious issue and can't be neglected.

*Correspondence: ndpant1987@gmail.com
[2] Department of Microbiology, Grande International Hospital, Dhapasi, Kathmandu, Nepal
Full list of author information is available at the end of the article

Regular monitoring of rates of ESBL and MBL production along with multidrug resistance among clinical isolates is very necessary.

Keywords: *E. coli, K. pneumoniae*, ESBL, MBL

Background

The drug resistance among the gram negative bacteria is present as a serious global problem [1]. ESBLs are the important members of beta-lactamases produced mainly by gram negative bacteria [2] and are responsible for mediating resistance to extended-spectrum cephalosporins and monobactam aztreonam [3]. These enzymes are commonly detected in the members of the enterobacteriaceae like *Klebsiella pneumoniae* and *Escherichia coli* [3]. ESBL producing bacteria do not show resistance only to penicillins, most cephalosporins and aztreonam but also to other classes of antibiotics such as aminoglycosides, cotrimoxazole, tetracycline and fluoroquinolones [4, 5]. Further, the easy transmission of the ESBLs coding plasmids between the species has become a major threat mainly in hospitalized patients, often the infections caused by organisms producing ESBL being involved in outbreaks [6, 7]. Carbapenems are the drugs of choice for the treatment of the infections caused by ESBL producing bacteria [8]. However over the past few years, carbapenem resistance due to metallo-beta-lactamases (MBLs) production has been increasingly reported among clinical isolates from all around the world [9]. Metallo-beta-lactamase needs bivalent metal ions mainly zinc for its activation and resistance to carbapenems is mainly mediated by this enzyme [10].

The rapid increasing rate of MBL production among the members of enterobacteriaceae, mainly *E. coli* and *K. pneumoniae*, which are the most common causes of infections among human is present as a serious global public health problem [9]. There are limited treatment options for the infections caused by ESBL and MBL producing bacteria [11] due to which the treatments of such infections are very difficult often resulting into treatment failure. The regular surveillance of the drug resistance among the clinical isolates will be helpful to know the actual gravity of the situation, hence to formulate the necessary policy to reduce the incidence of drug resistance among the bacteria. Further, the knowledge about the local antimicrobial susceptibility patterns will be helpful to start timely proper preliminary treatment. So, in this study we determined the burden of ESBL and MBL production in *E. coli* and *K. pneumoniae* isolated from clinical samples. In addition, we also determined their antimicrobial susceptibility patterns.

Methods

A cross-sectional study was conducted at Om Hospital and Research Centre, Kathmandu, Nepal, a 150 bedded hospital by using the *E. coli* and *K. pneumoniae* isolated from total of 1568 different clinical samples (urine, pus, body fluids, sputum, blood) from May 2015 to December 2015. The colonies grown after culturing of samples using standard microbiological techniques were identified with the help of biochemical tests [12, 13]. Antimicrobial susceptibility testing was performed by Kirby-Bauer disc diffusion technique following clinical and laboratory standards institute guidelines [14]. For performing antimicrobial susceptibility testing 90 mm diameter petriplates were used and in one plate 6 antibiotic discs were tested. The diameter of the susceptibility zone was measured with the help of Vernier caliper.

Screening and confirmation of ESBL producers

The isolates were screened for possible ESBL production using ceftazidime (30 μg) and cefotaxime (30 μg). According to the CLSI guidelines, the isolates showing reduced susceptibility to at least one of these drugs with zone of inhibition for ceftazidime $\leq$ 22 mm and cefotaxime $\leq$ 27 mm were considered as the possible ESBL producing strains. The suspected ESBL producing strains were confirmed for ESBL production by combined disc assay using ceftazidime (30 μg) and ceftazidime/clavulanic acid (30/10 μg) discs and cefotaxime (30 μg) and cefotaxime/clavulanic acid discs (30/10 μg). The zones of inhibition for the ceftazidime and cefotaxime discs were compared to those of the ceftazidime/clavulanic acid and cefotaxime/clavulanic acid discs. An increase in zone diameter of $\geq$ 5 mm in the presence of clavulanic acid was confirmed as positive for ESBL production [14]. Bacteria showing resistance to at least three different classes of antibiotics were considered multidrug resistant [15].

Detection of MBL producers

The isolates showing resistance to imipenem were subjected to confirmation for MBL production by combined disc assay using imipenem and imipenem/ethylenediaminetetracetate discs [16].

Results

Of total 1568 different clinical samples processed, 268 (17.1%) samples showed bacterial growth. Among which, *E. coli* and *K. pneumoniae* were isolated from 138 (51.5%)

and 39 (14.6%) samples respectively. Out of 138 *E. coli*, 84% isolates were from urine followed by pus (7.9%). Likewise, out of 39 *K. pneumoniae*, 51.3% isolates were from urine followed by sputum (17.9%) (Table 1).

Distribution of the isolates on the basis of type and department of the patients

A total of 128 (72.3%) isolates were from outpatients and 49 (27.7%) from inpatients. Among the isolates, 78.3% and 21.7% of *E. coli* were obtained from outpatients and inpatients respectively. Similarly, 51.3 and 48.7% of *K. pneumoniae* were obtained from outpatients and inpatients respectively. Highest percentage of the isolates were obtained from general medicine department (35.5%) followed by obstetrics and gynecology (31.1%). Maximum percentage (35.5%) of *E. coli* were isolated from general medicine followed by obstetrics and gynecology (33.3%). Most of the *K. pneumoniae* were isolated from intensive care unit (25.6%) (Table 2).

Table 1 Overall growth and distribution of *E. coli* and *K. pneumoniae* within different clinical samples

Samples	Total (%)	Bacterial isolates	
		E. coli (%)	*K. pneumoniae* (%)
Urine	184 (68.6)	116 (84.0)	20 (51.3)
Pus	22 (8.2)	11 (8)	2 (5.1)
Sputum	12 (4.5)	2 (1.4)	7 (17.9)
Catheter tips	7 (2.6)	2 (1.4)	5 (12.8)
Blood	20 (7.5)	3 (2.2)	3 (7.7)
Wound swab	14 (5.2)	4 (2.9)	0 (0)
ET suction tips	9 (3.4)	0 (0)	2 (5.1)
Total	268	138	39

Antibiotic resistance patterns of the isolates

The lowest rate of resistance was seen toward imipenem followed by piperacilli/tazobactam, amikacin and cefoperazone/sulbactam. All isolates were found to be resistant to amoxicillin (Table 3). Out of total 177 isolates, 96 (54.2%) were multidrug resistant. Among 138 *E. coli* and 39 *K. pneumoniae*, 73 (52.9%) *E. coli* and 23 (59%) *K. pneumoniae* were multidrug resistant.

ESBL and MBL production among the isolates

Out of 177 isolates, 121 isolates of *E. coli* and 33 isolates of *K. pneumoniae* were suspected as ESBL producers on primary screening test. Among them, 46 isolates of *E. coli* and 15 isolates of *K. pneumoniae* were confirmed as ESBL producers. Of the total isolates 61 (34.5%) were ESBL producers. Of total 61 ESBL positive strains detected, 51 were detected by both ceftazidime and ceftazidime/clavulanic acid discs and cefotaxime and cefotaxime/clavulanic acid discs, while 4 were detected by ceftazidime and ceftazidime/clavulanic acid discs only and 6 by cefotaxime and cefotaxime/clavulanic acid discs only.

Similarly, 9 isolates (3 *E. coli* and 6 *K. pneumoniae*) were suspected as MBL producers on the basis of resistance to imipenem. 7 (2 *E. coli* and 5 *K. pneumoniae*) (4%) isolates were found to be MBL producers.

Distribution of ESBL and MBL producing isolates on the basis of samples

The distribution of ESBL producing strains according to different samples is presented in Table 4. Similarly, 1 of MBL producing bacterium was isolated from each urine, catheter tip and pus samples, while 2 MBL producing bacteria were isolated from each sputum and suction tip.

Table 2 Distribution of the isolates on the basis of type and department of the patients

Patient types	Departments	Bacterial isolates (N = 177)		Total (%)
		E. coli (%)	*K. pneumoniae* (%)	
Outpatient	Emergency	7 (5.1)	1 (2.6)	8 (4.5)
	Obstetrics and gynecology	46 (33.3)	9 (23.1)	55 (31.1)
	Pediatrics	6 (4.3)	2 (5.1)	8 (4.5)
	General medicine	49 (35.5)	8 (20.5)	57 (32.2)
	Sub-total	108 (78.3)	20 (51.3)	128 (72.3)
Inpatient	Ward	16 (11.6)	9 (23.1)	25 (14.1)
	ICU	14 (10.1)	10 (25.6)	24 (13.6)
	Sub-total	30 (21.7)	19 (48.7)	49 (27.7)
	Total	138	39	177

ICU Intensive care unit

Table 3 Antibiotic resistance patterns of *E. coli* and *K. pneumoniae* isolated

Antibiotics used	Resistance patterns of the isolates		Total (%)
	E. coli (N = 138) (%)	*K. pneumoniae* (N = 39) (%)	
Amikacin	10 (7.2)	9 (23.1)	19 (10.7)
Amoxicillin	138 (100)	39 (100)	177 (100)
Cefalexin	124 (89.8)	37 (94.9)	161 (91)
Ceftriaxone	117 (84.8)	33 (84.6)	150 (84.7)
Cefotaxime	120 (87)	33 (84.6)	153 (86.4)
Ceftazidime	114 (82.6)	33 (84.6)	147 (83)
Cefoperazone/sulbactam	12 (8.7)	8 (20.5)	20 (11.3)
Imipenem	3 (2.2)	6 (15.4)	9 (5.1)
Ciprofloxacin	68 (49.3)	18 (46.2)	86 (48.6)
Ofloxacin	68 (49.3)	18 (46.2)	86 (48.6)
Piperacillin/tazobactam	9 (6.5)	10 (25.6)	19 (10.7)
Co-trimoxazole	75 (54.3)	20 (51.3)	95 (53.7)

Table 4 Distribution of ESBL producing isolates on the basis of samples

Samples	Overall ESBL (%)	ESBL (%)	
		E. coli (n = 46)	*K. pneumoniae* (n = 15)
Urine	43 (70.5)	38 (82.6)	5 (33.3)
Catheter tips	3 (4.9)	0 (0)	3 (20.0)
Sputum	4 (6.6)	0 (0)	4 (26.7)
ET suction tips	0 (0)	0 (0)	0 (0)
Pus	7 (11.5)	6 (13.0)	1 (6.7)
Blood	3 (4.9)	1 (2.2)	2 (13.3)
Wound swab	1 (1.6)	1 (2.2)	0 (0)
Total	61 (100)	46 (100)	15 (100)

Distribution of ESBL and MBL producing bacteria on the basis of type and department of patients

Most of the ESBL producing isolates were from outpatients. Among the outpatients, most of the isolates were from general medicine (43.3%) followed by obstetrics and gynecology department (27.9%). Similarly, among the inpatients, ESBL producing bacteria were more frequent in intensive care unit (16.4%) than wards (8.2%) (Table 5). MBL producing strains were not isolated from outpatients. 3 MBL producing bacteria were isolated from intensive care unit and 4 from wards.

Resistance patterns of ESBL and MBL producing isolates

No ESBL producing strains were found to be resistant to imipenem. Similarly, among other antibiotics tested lowest rate of resistance was seen toward cefoperazone/sulbactam, piperacillin/tazobactam and amikacin (Table 6). MBL producing strains showed high rates of resistance to the antibiotics tested.

Discussion

Similar rate of growth positivity as in our study was also reported by Poudyal et al. (16.9%) [17]. In our study, *E. coli* (51.5%) and *K. pneumoniae* (14.7%) were most frequently isolated gram negative bacteria. Similar isolation rates for *E. coli* and *K. pneumoniae* were also reported by Poudyal et al. [17]. *E. coli* and *K pneumoniae* are among the commonest bacteria isolated from clinical specimens. Majority of the isolates in our study were from urine samples. This may be due to the larger number of urine samples included in our study. Further, *E. coli* and *K. pneumoniae* are common cause of urinary tract infection [18].

Higher numbers of isolates were from outpatient department in comparison to inpatient department. This may be attributed to the larger number of samples being included from outpatients.

Misuse of antibiotic is responsible for higher incidence of antibiotic resistance among bacteria [19]. We found the incidence of multidrug resistant bacteria to be 54.2%, with 52.9% of *E. coli* and 59% of *K. pneumoniae* being multidrug resistant. Different studies in Nepal have found the rates of multidrug resistance among *E. coli* to be ranging from 38.2 to 95.52% and those for *K. pneumoniae* to be 25–100% [17, 20, 21]. Common risk factors associated with infection by multidrug resistant bacteria are hospitalization and previous use of antibiotics [22].

In our study the rate of ESBL production was 34.5 with 33.3% of the *E. coli* and 38.5% of the *K. pneumoniae* being ESBL positive. The prevalence of ESBL producing *E. coli* and *K. pneumoniae* was found as low as 18.2 and 4.1%

Table 5 Distribution of ESBL producing bacteria on the basis of type and department of patients

Patient types	Departments of patient	*E. coli* (%)	*K. pneumoniae* (%)	Total (%)
Outpatient	Emergency	2 (4.3)	0 (0)	2 (3.3)
	Obstetrics and gynecology	15 (32.6)	2 (13.3)	17 (27.9)
	Pediatric	2 (4.3)	1 (6.7)	3 (4.9)
	General medicine	20 (43.5)	4 (26.7)	24 (39.3)
	Sub-total	39 (84.8)	7 (46.7)	46 (75.4)
Inpatient	ICU	5 (10.9)	5 (33.3)	10 (16.4)
	Ward	2 (4.3)	3 (20.0)	5 (8.2)
	Sub-total	7 (15.2)	8 (53.3)	15 (24.6)
	Total	46 (100)	15 (100)	61 (100)

Table 6 Resistance patterns of ESBL producing isolates

Antibiotics	*E. coli* (%)	*K. pneumoniae* (%)	Total (%)
Co-trimoxazole	28 (60.9)	8 (53.3)	36 (59)
Cephalexin	46 (100)	15 (100)	61 (100)
Amoxicillin	46 (100)	15 (100)	61 (100)
Amikacin	3 (6.5)	2 (13.3)	5 (8.2)
Ciprofloxacin	28 (60.9)	8 (53.3)	36 (59)
Ofloxacin	28 (60.9)	8 (53.3)	36 (59)
Ceftriaxone	40 (87)	13 (86.7)	53 (86.9)
Ceftazidime	43 (93.5)	15 (100)	58 (95.1)
Cefotaxime	45 (97.8)	15 (100)	60 (98.4)
Cefoperazone/sulbactam	1 (2.2)	2 (13.3)	3 (4.9)
Pipercillin/tazobactam	2 (4.3)	2 (13.3)	4 (6.6)
Imipenem	0 (0)	0 (0)	0 (0)

respectively in a study conducted by Raut et al. [23] and as high as 80% for *E. coli* [17] and 90.9% for *K. pneumoniae* [24]. The worldwide prevalence of ESBL production among the clinical isolates is found to be ranging from < 1 to 74% [25].

In our study, cefotaxime-clavulante combination disc identified numerically more confirmed ESBL producers in comparison to ceftazidime-clavulanate, which was analogous to the findings by Poudyal et al. [17] and Ranjini et al. [26].

Lower rate of MBL production in comparison to the study by Bora et al. (*E. coli* = 18.98%, *K. pneumoniae* = 21.08%) was reported in our study [9]. However, in other studies conducted in different countries showed the rates of MBL production to be ranging from 13.4 to 61.5% for *E. coli* and 33–36% for *K. pneumoniae* [27–29].

In our study high rate of ESBL production was observed among the bacteria isolated from out patients, which is very serious and shows the dissemination of ESBL producing bacteria to the community. However, no MBL producing organism was isolated from outpatients.

The prevalence of drug resistant bacteria may not only vary from countries to countries but also from institutions to institutions and this can be partially explained by the difference in local antibiotic prescribing habits and difference in effectiveness of infection control program in different health institutes.

In our study, the highest rate of susceptibility of the bacteria was found toward imipenem followed by pipercillin/tazobactum, amikacin and cefoperazone/sulbactum. These findings were in harmony with the findings of other studies conducted by Ansari et al. [30], Kader and Kumar [31] and Shashwati et al. [32].

Conclusions

ESBL and MBL production along with multidrug resistance among *E. coli* and *K. pneumoniae* are presenting as the serious problem in Nepal. The high rate of ESBL production among the isolates from outpatients is very serious issue, which suggests the dissemination of ESBL producing isolates in community. Regular monitoring of rate of ESBL and MBL production along with multidrug resistance among these clinical isolates is very necessary. Further, to control the emergence of drug resistance strict policy to rationalize the use of antibiotics is necessary. On the basis of the drug resistance patterns we found in our study imipenem followed by piperacilli/tazobactam, amikacin and cefoperazone/sulbactam may be used for the preliminary treatment of the infections caused by *E. coli* and *K. pneumoniae* in our setting.

Abbreviations

ESBL: extended spectrum beta-lactamase; MBL: metallo beta-lactamase; MDR: multidrug resistant; ICU: intensive care unit.

Authors' contributions

NDP and KN designed and conceived the study, carried out the research works, analyzed data, and prepared the final manuscript. AB, BN and RB carried out the research works and analyzed the data. RKS, BL, DRB and BJ monitored the study. All authors read and approved the final manuscript.

Author details
[1] Department of Microbiology, GoldenGate International College, Battisputali, Kathmandu, Nepal. [2] Department of Microbiology, Grande International Hospital, Dhapasi, Kathmandu, Nepal. [3] Department of Laboratory Medicine, OM Hospital and Research Center, Chabahil, Kathmandu, Nepal. [4] Central Department of Microbiology, Tribhuvan University, Kirtipur, Kathmandu, Nepal.

Acknowledgements
The authors would like to thank, Golden Gate International College, Kathmandu, Nepal and OM Hospital and Research Center, Kathmandu, Nepal for providing the opportunity to conduct this research. The authors would also like to thank all the patients and the technical staffs for their help during the study.

Competing interests
The authors declare that they have no competing interests.

Consent for publication
Not applicable.

Funding
To conduct this study no fund was obtained from any sources.

References

1. Gniadkowski M. Evolution and epidemiology of extended-spectrum beta-lactamases (ESBLs) and ESBL-producing microorganisms. Clin Microbiol Infect. 2001;7(11):597–608.
2. Haque R, Salam MA. Detection of ESBL producing nosocomial gram negative bacteria from a tertiary care hospital in Bangladesh. Pak J Med Sci. 2010;26(4):887–91.
3. El-Baky RMA, El-Azeim NHA, Gad GFM. Prevalence of extended-spectrum beta-lactamase, AmpC Beta-lactamase, and metallo-beta-lactamase among clinical isolates of *Pseudomonas aeruginosa*. J Adv Biotechnol Bioeng. 2013;1:22–9.
4. Colodner R. Extended-spectrum beta-lactamases: a challenge for clinical microbiologists and infection control specialists. Am J Infect Control. 2005;33(2):104–7.
5. Rawat D, Nair D. Extended-spectrum ß-lactamases in gram negative bacteria. J Global Infect Dis. 2010;2:263–74.
6. Rangachari RK, Mathavi SK, Priyadharsini I. Detection of extended spectrum beta-lactamase producing gram negative bacilli in urinary isolates. Int J Biol Med Res. 2010;1(4):130–2.
7. Tonkic M, Goic-Barisic I, Punda-Polic V. Prevalence and antimicrobial resistance of extended-spectrum beta-lactamases-producing *Escherichia coli* and *Klebsiella pneumoniae* strains isolated in a university hospital in Split, Croatia. Int Microbiol. 2005;8(2):119–24.
8. Kanj SS, Kanafani ZA. Current concepts in antimicrobial therapy against resistant gram-negative organisms: extended-spectrum beta-lactamase-producing Enterobacteriaceae, carbapenem-resistant Enterobacteriaceae, and multidrug-resistant *Pseudomonas aeruginosa*. Mayo Clin Proc. 2011;86(3):250–9.
9. Bora A, Sanjana R, Jha BK, Mahaseth SN, Pokharel K. Incidence of metallo-beta-lactamase producing clinical isolates of *Escherichia coli* and *Klebsiella pneumoniae* in central Nepal. BMC Res Notes. 2014;7:557.
10. Manoharan A, Chatterjee S, Mathai D, SARI Study Group. Detection and characterization of metallo beta lactamases producing *Pseudomonas aeruginosa*. Indian J Med Microbiol. 2010;28(3):241–4.
11. Mishra SK, Acharya J, Kattel H, Pokhrel BM, Rijal BP. Extended-spectrum beta-lactamase and metallo-beta-lactamase-producing bacterial strains among the patients attending a tertiary care center in Nepal. Int J Infect Dis. 2012;16:e425.
12. Cheesbrough M. District laboratory practice in tropical countries, part II. 2nd ed. New York: Cambridge University Press; 2006.
13. Holt JG, Krieg NR, Sneath PHA, Staley JT, Williams ST. Bergey's manual of determinative bacteriology. Baltimore: Williamsons and Wilkins; 1994.
14. Clinical and Laboratory Standards Institute. CLSI document M100-S25. Performance standards for antimicrobial susceptibility testing: Twenty fifth informational supplement ed. Wayne: CLSI; 2015.
15. Magiorakos AP, Srinivasan A, Carey RB, Carmeli Y, Falagas ME, Giske CG, et al. Multidrug-resistant, extensively drug-resistant and pandrug-resistant bacteria: an international expert proposal for interim standard definitions for acquired resistance. Clin Microbiol Infect. 2012;18:268–81.
16. Yong D, Lee K, Yum JH, Shin HB, Rossolini GM, Chong Y. Imipenem-EDTA disk method for differentiation of metallo-beta-lactamase-producing clinical isolates of *Pseudomonas* spp. and *Acinetobacter* spp. J Clin Microbiol. 2002;40(10):3798–801.
17. Poudyal S, Bhatta DR, Shakya G, Upadhyaya B, Dumre SP, Buda G, et al. Extended Spectrum beta-lactamase producing multidrug resistant clinical bacterial isolates at National Public Health Laboratory, Nepal. Nepal Med Coll J. 2011;13(1):34–8.
18. Behzadi P, Behzadi E, Yazdanbod H, Aghapour R, Akbari Cheshmeh M, Salehian Omran D. A survey on urinary tract infections associated with the three most common uropathogenic bacteria. Maedica (Buchar). 2010;5(2):111–5.
19. Neupane S, Pant ND, Khatiwada S, Chaudhary R, Banjara MR. Correlation between biofilm formation and resistance toward different commonly used antibiotics along with extended spectrum beta lactamase production in uropathogenic *Escherichia coli* isolated from the patients suspected of urinary tract infections visiting Shree Birendra Hospital, Chhauni, Kathmandu, Nepal. Antimicrob Resist Infect Control. 2016;5:5.
20. Baral P, Neupane S, Marasini BP, Ghimire KR, Lekhak B, Shrestha B. High prevalence of multidrug resistance in bacterial uropathogens from Kathmandu, Nepal. BMC Res Notes. 2012;5:38.
21. Yadav KK, Adhikari N, Khadka R, Pant AD, Shah B. Multidrug resistant Enterobacteriaceae and extended spectrum β-lactamase producing Escherichia coli: a cross-sectional study in National Kidney Center, Nepal. Antimicrob Resist Infect Control. 2015;4:42.
22. Chaudhary NK, Murthy MS. Prevalence of multidrug resistance in uropathogenic *Klebsiella* species with reference to extended spectrum β-lactamases production. Res J Pharm Biol Chem Sci. 2013;4(3):728–35.
23. Raut S, Gokhale S, Adhikari B. Prevalence of extended spectrum beta-lactamases among *Escherichia coli* and *Klebsiella* spp. isolates in Manipal Teaching Hospital, Pokhara, Nepal. J Microbiol Infect Dis. 2015;5(2):69–75.
24. Pathak J, Pokharel N. Multidrug resistant and extended spectrum β-lactamase (ESBL) isolates from different clinical specimens. Int J Sci and Res Pub. 2015;5:1–5.
25. Thokar MA, Fomda BA, Maroof P, Ahmed K, Bashir D, Bashir G. Proliferation of extended spectrum ß–lactamase (ESBL) producing Gram negative bacteria, diagnostic inputs and impact on selection of Antimicrobial therapy. Phys Acad. 2010;4(3):25–31.
26. Ranjini CY, Kasukurthi LR, Madhumati B, Rajendran R. Prevalence of multidrug resistance and extended spectrum beta-lactamases among uropathogenic *Escherichia coli* isolates in a tertiary care hospital in South India: an alarming trend. Community Acquir Infect. 2015;2:19–24.
27. Enwuru NV, Enwuru CA, Ogbonnia SO, Adepoju-Bello AA. Metallo-**B**-lactamase production by *Escherichia Coli* and *Klebsiella* species isolated from Hospital and Community subjects in lagos, Nigeria. Nat Sci. 2011;9(11):1–5.
28. Mate PH, Devi KS, Devi KM, Damrolien S, Devi NL, Devi PP. Prevalence of carbapenem resistance among Gram-Negative bacteria in a Tertiary Care Hospital in North-East India. IOSR J Dent Med Sci. 2014;13(12):56–60.
29. Wadekar MD, Anuradha K, Venkatesh D. Phenotypic detection of ESBL and MBL in clinical isolates of *Enterobacteriaceae*. Int J curr Res Aca Rev. 2013;1(3):89–95.
30. Ansari S, Nepal HP, Gautam R, Shrestha S, Neopane P, Gurung G, et al. Community acquired multi-drug resistant clinical isolates of Escherichia coli in a tertiary care center of Nepal. Antimicrob Resist Infect Control. 2015;4:15.
31. Kader AA, Kumar AK. Prevalence of extended spectrum beta-lactamase among multidrug resistant gram-negative isolates from a general hospital in Saudi Arabia. Saudi Med J. 2004;25:570–4.

The frequency of *Klebsiella pneumonia* encoding genes for CTX-M, TEM-1 and SHV-1 extended-spectrum beta lactamases enzymes isolated from urinary tract infection

Masomeh Dehshiri[1], Seyed Sajjad Khoramrooz[1], Mohammad Zoladl[1], Seyed Abdolmajid Khosravani[1], Najmeh Parhizgari[1], Mohammad Hossein Motazedian[2], Soheyla Jahedi[3] and Asghar Sharifi[1*]

Abstract

Background: The extended- spectrum β-lactamase producing bacteria are widely spread worldwide. The productions of these enzymes cause bacterial resistance to a wide range of antibiotics. The aim of this study was to investigated the frequency of *K. pneumonia* encoding genes for CTX-M, TEM-1 and SHV-1 extended-spectrum beta lactamases enzymes isolated from urinary tract infection.

Methods: This study is cross-sectional study. All *K. pneumonia* isolates from urine samples, which had grown on media culture more than 105 were delivered to the medical microbiology laboratory. *K. pneumonia* susceptibility of 198 samples were confirmed by disk diffusion. The gene frequency of genes was determined using PCR, and analyzed using SPSS version 21 software.

Finding: Most of the *K. pneumonia* isolated from urine producing β-lactamase were resistant to cotrimoxazole (53.2%) followed by cefotaxime (50%), ceftazidime, ceftriaxone (40.3%), nalidixic acid (17.8%), amikacin and imipenem (1.6%) and meropenem (0%) respectively. Out of the 198 confirmed isolates of *K. pneumonia*, 62 cases (31.3%) have the gene phenotype of broad spectrum β-lactamase enzymes and highest frequency of gene phenotype was related to the SHV-1 gene (85.5%). Then in the terms of abundance from highest to lowest CTXM-3 (56.5%), CTXM-1 (27.4%), TEM-1 (16.1%) and CTXM-2 (8.1%), were respectively.

Conclusion: This study showed that *K. pneumonia* isolated from urine producing β-lactamase were resistance to a wide range of antibiotics. Due to the increasing resistance of most antibiotics, control and supervision in the use of antibiotics and identification of broad spectrum β-lactamase enzymes by phenotypic methods appears to be essential.

Keywords: Antibiotic resistance, Extended-spectrum β-lactamase, *K. pneumonia*, Urinary tract infection, Genes SHV, TEM, CTXM

Background

Klebsiella is a Gram negative, non-motile, facultative anaerobic, catalase positive, oxidase negative, and usually encapsulated bacteria. It ferments sugars such as lactose and sucrose. Most strains produce gas from fermentation and starch which is an important distinguishing feature of these bacteria. The bacteria are part of Enterobacteriaceae family and *K. pneumonia* strain is an indicator species of this genus of bacteria [1]. *K. pneumonia* is an opportunistic pathogen among enterobacteriacae family, Klebsiella The genus Klebsiella has two pathogenic species; *K. pneumonia* and *K. oxytoka* [2].

*Correspondence: asgharsharifi@yahoo.com
[1] Cellular and Molecular Research Centre, Yasuj University of Medical Sciences, Yasuj, Iran
Full list of author information is available at the end of the article

Klebsiella pneumonia is closely related to *K. oxytoka*, and recognized from the latter by being indole negative and its growth ability on 3-hydroxybutyrate [2, 3]. This bacterium is available in gasterointestinal, eye, respiratory, and urogenital tract in healthy human. It exists as saprophyte microorganisms in nasopharynx of 1–6% individuals. The prevalence increases up to 20% in patient who are admitted in hospitals. Infections are less common outside the hospitals, and routes of transmission are usually hospital staff hands, antiseptic solutions, working containers, and equipments [4]. Anesthesia and artificial respiration instruments are the best means of infection transport due to dampness. In general, patients over 40 years old those with immunodeficiency syndromes, and underlying medical conditions such as diabetes mellitus and chronic lung disease are the objective of this bacterium [4, 5].

β-Lactamases from TEM type are often found in *K. pneumonia*. These enzymes are derived from TEM-1 and TEM-2 enzymes. TEM-1 is the most important β-lactamase in Gram negative bacteria. Both TEM-1 and TEM-2 are capable of hydrolyzing penicillin and first generation cephalosporin but are not able to invade oxyimino–cephalosporin. Amino acid replacement can be created in many places of TEM-1. β-lactamase in vitro without losing the most activity. These changes are responsible for phenotypic extended spectrum β-lactamases (ESBL) change and enzyme activity site that gives access to oxy Mino β-lactamase. More than 130 common TEM enzymes have been identified, which provide a useful method for the distribution of resistant genes [6, 7].

β-Lactamase SHV type (class A)

These enzymes are derived from SHV-1. They are the first enzymes of SHV class which are found in *K. pneumonia* and are responsible for 20% of ampicillin resistance in the present samples [8, 9].

There exists a structural likeness between SHV-1 and TEM-1 in general, and a 68% amino acid similarity. More than 50 SHV varieties have come to be known based on the replacement of amino acid combinations.

β-Lactamases CTX-M type (class A)

CTX is representative of the high hydrolysis power of β-lactamase against cefotaxime. More than 40 CTX-M enzymes are known so far, which can be classified in five groups.

1. CTX-M group which contains 6 enzymes dependent on plasmid.

   A-CTX-M1, CTX-M3, CTX-M-10, CTX-M-12, CTX_M-15 and, FEC-4.
2. CTX-M-2 group which contains 8 CTX-M enzyme dependent on plasmid.
   CTX-M-2, CTX-M-4, CTX-M-4L, CTX-M-5, CTX-M-6, CTX-M-7, CTX-M-20 and Toto-1.
3. CTX-M-8 group which contains 1 member dependent on plasmid.
4. CTX-M-9 group which contains 9 enzymes dependent on plasmid.
   CTX-M-9, CTX-M-13, CTX-M-14, CTX-M-16, CTX-M-17, CTX-M-19, CTX-M-21, CTX-M-27 and Toho 2.
5. CTX-M-25 group containing CTX-M-25 and CTX-M-26, CTX-M-2, CTX-M-3 and CTX-M-14 which have the most dispersion (3, 32, 52, 53).

These enzymes are capable of cephalothin hydrolysis better than penicillin and cefaloxine, and more than Ceftazidime. CTXM type is predominantly found in three geographic areas; South America, The Far East, and Europe [10, 11].

The aim of present study was to indicate the frequency of Klebsiella isolates encoding SHV-1, TEM-1, CTXM genes and the broad spectrum β-lactamase enzymes in urinary tract infection (UTI) patients in Yasuj City, Kohgiluyeh and Boyer-Ahmad province, Iran, during 2014–2015.

Methods

This study sought to determine the prevalence of *K. pneumonia* isolates encoding SHV-1, TEM-1, CTXM genes and the broad spectrum β-lactamase enzymes in UTI patients in Yasuj City during 2014–2015. In this sense, statistical, cross sectional, and descriptive analysis methods were employed.

Ethics approval and consent to participate

Ethics approval (MEC: 93.05.06.07) was obtained prior to the start of this study.

Sampling and culture methods

This study was carried out during October 2014 to August 2015. Urinary samples of patients confirmed with UTI from three laboratories around the city were sent to microbiology laboratory of Yasuj University of Medical Science. Then, each sample was cultured on EMB media. Further diagnostic tests followed as described below:

Phenotyping test for ESBL production

Confirmatory tests for ESBL production based on CLSI standards were carried out on the bacteria. First, bacteria were inoculated on MHA media culture containing ceftazidime and cefotaxime disks. Both plates were inoculated alike and kept on incubator for 18–24 h. The zone of inhibition diameter (ZOID) was measured around each disk and ZOIDs more than 5 mm were considered positive [12].

Polymerase chain reaction (PCR)

Bacterial genome extraction by boiling method: One colony from fresh bacteria was solved in 300 ml distilled water and homogenized with vortex and kept on thermo block in 100° C for 10 min, and then centrifuged in 12,000 rpm for 10 min and the supernatant containing genome was used for PCR [13].

Mastermix preparation

Five micro litters of purified DNA, 1 μl FORWARD primer (20 pmol), 1 μl REVERSE primer (20 μmol), and 12.5 μl mastermixe were mixed and the volume was brought to 25 μl by adding distilled water.

Primary denaturation (92 °C for 2 min), 30 thermal cycles of denaturation (95 °C for 1 min), primer binding (57 °C for 30 s for β-lactamase SHV gene), 61 °C for 20 s for β-lactamase TEM gene, 55 °C for 30 s for β-lactamase CTXM-1, 55 °C for 30 s for β-lactamase CTX M2 gene, 59 °C for 20 s for bla CTXM2 gene, proliferation temperature 72 °C for 30 s, and final proliferation temperature (72 °C for 5 min) were performed [14].

Samples were put into gel wells which had already been prepared. Then the electrodes were connected (red wire was the sign of positive electric charge which was placed in the bottom and black wire was the sign of negative electric charge sign which was placed next to gel holes). After the connection of electrodes, the instrument was adjusted to 100 voltage for 1 h with 700 mA flow (current strength), and then turned on.

Photography from gel

The gel was placed inside the device and then the device was turned on with the correct setting (Table 1).

Data analysis method

For data analysis, SPSS software version 21 was applied. Both descriptive statistics such as frequency, mean, standard deviation, graph, and statistical inferential tests such as Chi square, fishers exact test, independent T test, and one-way variance analytic test were used. It is worth noting that in this study, before inferential statistical tests with Kolmogorov–Smirnov test, variable study from normal distribution was reviewed and approved.

Finding

Out of 986 samples suspicious to *K. pneumonia* UTI, 198 (20.1%) were confirmed based on Klebsiella diagnostic test. The results are summarized in Table 2.

Table 1 Primers used for ESBL genes presence in *Klebsiella*

Gene name	Primer sequence 5–3	Product size (bp)
SHV	F:5′ TCAGCGAAAAACACCTTG 3′ R:5′ TCCCGCAGATAAATCACC 3′	472
TEM	F: 5′ CTTCCTGTTTTTGCTCACC 3′ R: 5′ AGCAATAAACCAGCCAGC 3′	632
CTXM-1	F: 5′ GAC GAT GTC ACT GGC TGA GC 3′ R: 5′ AGC CG C CGA CGC TAA TAC A 3′	499
CTXM2	F: 5′ GCG ACC TGG TTA ACT ACA ATCC 3′ R: 5′ CGG TAG TAT TGC CCT TAA GCC 3′	351
CTXM3	F: 5′ CGC TTT GCC ATG TGC AGC ACC 3′ R: 5′ GCT CAG TAC GAT CGA GCC 3′	307

Based on Table 2 out of 198 samples, 138 were female patients and 60 were males. The minimum and maximum ages were 1 month to 68 years respectively with the standard deviation of 16.33 ± 17.92.

Susceptibility test of *K. pneumonia* to CLSI antibiotics

Klebsiella pneumonia in vitro susceptibility test against antibiotics such as Amikacin (AMK 30 mg), Ceftriaxone (CTK 30 mg), Meropenem (MRP 10 mg), Nalidixic acid (NAL 30 mg), Cefotaxim (CTX 30 mg), Ceftazidime (CAZ 30 mg), Cefotaxime (CTX + C 40 mg), and Ceftazidime (CAZ + C 40 mg) were examined Table 3.

Based on these findings, the maximum resistance of *K. pneumonia* isolates was against Co-trimoxazole (27.5%). The remaining resistance intensities from highest to lowest were as follows: Cefotaxime (15.5%), Ceftazidin, Ceftriaxone (12.5%), Nalidixic acid (9%), Amikacin, Imipenem (1%) and Meropenem (0%).

Frequency distribution of *K. pneumonia* isolates according to broad spectrum β-lactamase phenotype and sex are revealed in Table 4.

Frequency of β-lactamase genes TEM-1, SHV-1, CTXM-2, and CTXM-3 in 62 samples producing ESBL was estimated by PCR and shown in Figs. 1, 2, 3 and Table 5. As noticed, the most synchronizing pattern belonged to B lactamase genes SHV-1 and CTXM-3 (30.7%).

All *K. pneumonia* isolates were susceptible to meropenem and most antibiotic resistance in both genders were observed with Co-trimoxazole. No statistically significant difference was seen between antibiotic resistance of isolates by gender or age. Also, presence of β-lactamase genes such as TEM-1, SHV-1,CYXM-2, and CTXM-3 confirmed with PCR. No statistically significantly differ was observed among individuals of various ages. As Table 6 showed the most commonly ESBL producing gene was belonged to SHV-1(85.5%), followed by highest

Table 2 Frequency distribution *Klebsiella pneumoniae* isolated from UTI patients referred to clinical laboratories according to Gender in Yasuj city

Confirmed tests for K.p on samples urine sample according to gender	Sum		Non confirmed		Confirmed	
	Percent	Number	Percent	Number	Percent	Number
Male	48.4	477	42.3	417	6.1	60
Female	51.6	509	37.6	371	14	138
Sum	100	986	79.9	788	20.1	198

Table 3 Frequency distribution of *Klebsiella pneumoniae* isolation according to resistant to antibiotics

Antibiotic results	Sensitive		Semisensitive		Resistance		Total	
Antibiotic name	Percent	Number	Percent	Number	Percent	Number	Percent	Number
Amikacin	98	194	1	2	1	2	100	198
Ceftriaxon	86	170	1.5	3	12.5	25	100	198
Co-trimoxazol	71	141	1.5	3	27.5	54	100	198
Imipenem	99	196	0	0	1	2	100	198
Meropenem	100	198	0	0	0	0	100	198
Nalidixic acid	82.5	163	8.5	17	9	18	100	198
Cefotaxim	84	166	0.5	1	15.5	31	100	198
Cefazidim	84.5	167	3	6	12.5	25	100	198

Table 4 Frequency distribution of *Klebsiella pneumoniae* according to broad spectrum β-lactamase phenotype and sex

Broad spectrum β-lactamase phenotype from urine samples according to sex	ESBL+		ESBL−		Sum	
	Percent	Number	Percent	Number	Percent	Number
Male	13.6	27	16.7	33	30.3	60
Female	17.7	35	52	103	69.7	138
Sum	31.3	62	68.7	136	100	198

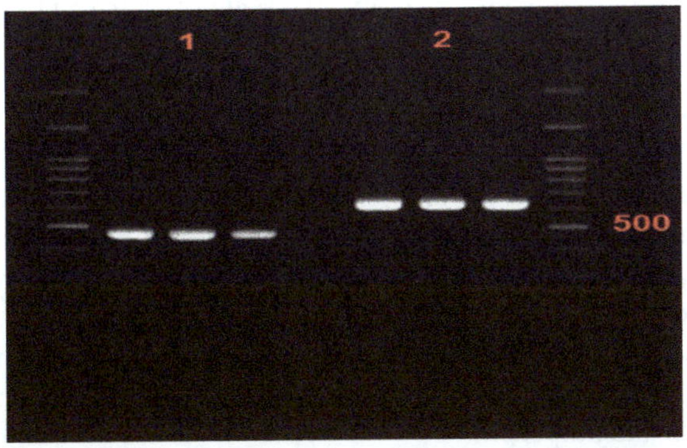

Fig. 1 Electrophoresis gel sample SHV-1 and TEM-1 in *Klebsiella pneumoniae* isolates producing broad spectrum β-lactamase (ESBL). Column No. 1 has SHV-1 with size band 472 and column No. 2 has TEM-1 gene with band size 632

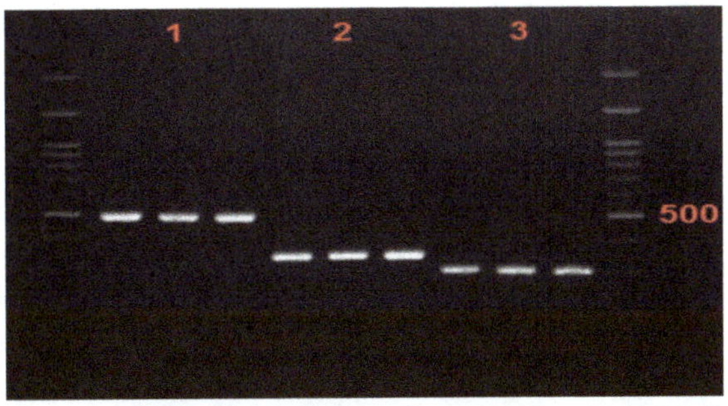

Fig. 2 Electrophoresis gel sample confirming CTXM-1, CTXM-2, and CTXM gene in *Klebsiella pneumoniae* isolation producing ESBL In this figure, column No. 1 belongs to CTXM-1 with 499 band size, column No II has CTXM-2 genes with 351 band size, and column No. III has CTXM-3 with 307 band size

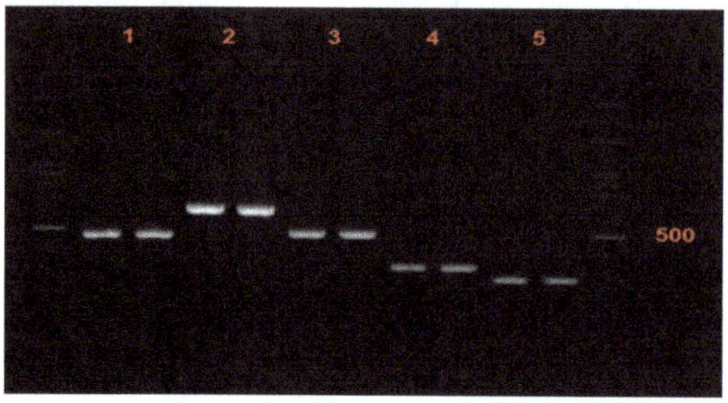

Fig. 3 Frequency distribution of *B. lactamase* genes TEM-1, SHV-1, CTXM-1, CTXM-2, and CTXM-3 in *Klebsiella pneumoniae* isolates producing ESBL Column No.1 has SHV-1 gene with 472 band size, column No. 2 has TEM-1 gene with 632 band size, column No. III has CTXM-1 with 499 band size, column No. III has CTXM-2 gene with 351 band size, and column No. 5 has CTXM-3 with 307 band size

Table 5 Frequency of β-lactamase genes synchronization in *Klebsiella pneumoniae* strains of producing ESBL

β-Lactamase pattern genes in K.p producing ESBL	Relative frequency %	Number absolute frequency
Wihtout β-lactamase	8.1	5
SHV-1 gene alone	24.3	15
CTXM-3 gene alone	4.8	3
β-Lactamase genes(SHV-1, CTXM-1 and CTXM-2) synchronization	6.4	4
β-Lactamase genes(SHV-1 and CTXM-3) synchronization	30.7	19
β-Lactamase genes(TEM-1, SHV-1, CTXM-1 and CTXM-3) synchronization	9.7	6
β-Lactamase genes(SHV-1, CTXM-1, CTXM-2 and CTXM-3) synchronization	1.6	1
β-Lactamase genes(CTXM-1 and CTXM-3) synchronization	1.6	1
β-Lactamase genes(SHV-1 and, CTXM-) synchronization	3.2	2
β-Lactamase genes(TEM-1, SHV-1, CTXM-1, CTXM-2 and CTXM-3) synchronization	1.6	1
β-Lactamase genes(SHV-1, CTXM-1 and CTXM-2) synchronization	1.6	1
β-Lactamase genes(TEM-1, SHV-1, CTXM-1 and CTXM-2) synchronization	1.6	1
β-Lactamase genes(TEM-1 and SHV-1) synchronization	3.2	2
β-Lactamase genes(SHV-1, CTXM-1 and CTXM-3) synchronization	1.6	1
Sum	100	62

to lowest CTXM-3(56.5%), CTXM-1(27.4%), TEM-1(16.1%) and CTXM-2(8.1%) respectively.

Discussion

Klebsiella pneumonia is a common cause of nosocomial infections such as UTI. The importance of UTI is that if not diagnosed or diagnosed too late it will lead to renal failure.

β-Lactam drugs are one of the most effective drugs in UTI treatment. The ESBL bacteria, with inactivation of a wide range of β-lactam drugs especially cephalosporin and monobactam, cause treatment failure and increase healthcare costs. Therefore, the study of gene resistance to β-lactamase is important. It seems that the emergence and spread of these bacteria are due to prolonged hospitalization, increased consumption of β-lactam antibiotics (especially ceftazidime), use of catheters, and experimental treatments against antibiotic-resistant [16].

The aim of this study was to determine the prevalence of *K. pneumonia* producing ESBL and molecular diagnosis of B lactamase genes such as β-lactamase CTX-M, β-lactamase TEM, and β-lactamase SHV).

In present study out of 198 samples, 62 (31.3%) were ESBL productive (27 separated from males and 35 from females). Published result from different scientific researches related to ESBL production in Iran is very diverse ranging from 9.8% to 75.7% depending on infection control system and therapeutic regimens. Another study from Bazaz et al. reported the prevalence of ESBLs in *K. pneumonia* and *E. coli* bacteria as high as 59.2%. In another research on 218 bacterial strains, 70 (32%) strains of Klebsiella and 49 (70%) strains of *K. pneumonia* contained ESBL [13]. Reports on ESBL production rate in *K. pneumonia* isolates from different countries also show significant variations. In a study in Japan and USA the prevalence rate was reported 40 and 44% respectively. However, in Southeast Asia, the prevalence rates of ESBL reported varied from 20% to more than 60%. ESBL production in India, Taiwan, Thailand, Pakistan, and Korea were reported 44, 8–29, 64, 36–56 and 22% respectively [14, 15].

The prevalence rate of ESBL production was reported by Ajas et al. in Lahore Pakistan 71% [16].

Due to emergence of bacterial resistance and ESBL production In a region compared to other regions is different. Also, the treatments of this infection with cephalosporins and other broad-spectrum antimicrobials have led to the emergence of multi-drug resistance. In this study, bacterial resistance was shown to be 30.4, 50, and 61.1% respectively in the case of cephalosporin-ceftriaxone and imipenem.

Mullana et al. demonstrated that the resistance of *K. pneumonia* strains in clinical samples of Babol city was against ceftriaxone (60%) cefotaxime (90%), and imipenem (60%) [17].

Table 6 Frequency distribution β-lactamase genes (TEM-1,SHV-1,CTXM-1, CTXM-2 and CTXM-3) *Klebsiella pneumoniae* strains producing broad spectrum ESBL genes

Presence of K.p genes strain situation producing ESBL	Having		Not having		Sum	
Gene name	Percent	Number	Percent	Number	Percent	Number
β-Lactamase gene TEM-1	16.1	10	83.9	52	100	62
β-Lactamase gene SHV-1	85.5	53	14.5	9	100	62
β-Lactamase gene CTXM-1	27.4	17	72.6	45	100	62
β-Lactamase gene CTXM-2	8.1	5	91.9	57	100	62
β-Lactamase gene CTXM-3	56.5	35	43.5	27	100	62
β-Lactamase gene TEM-1	16.1	10	83.9	52	100	62

In the present study resistance to amikacin was 61.1%, ceftazidime 32.40%, nalidixic acid 74.17% and sensitivity to imipenem was 38.98%.

Ishim in Japan determined that the imipenem as an effective antibiotic for *K. pneumonia* treatment [18].

PCR results in our research on β-lactamase Drug resistance to antibiotics in different regions of Iran and worldwide is differs due to genetic variations in causative strains and the use of antibiotics, access to broad spectrum and new antibiotics, and difference of climate conditions.

The genes presence in this study demonstrated as following prevalence rates as: lactamase TEM (16.1%), β-lactamase CTXM-3(56.5%), β-lactamase CTXM-2 (8.1%), β-lactamase CTXM-1 (27.4%), β-lactamase SHV (85.5%). Eftekhar et al. in 2012 reported the following prevalence rates: β-lactamase SHV 1.43%), β-lactamase TEM (2.35%), and β-lactamase CTXM (3.31%) in urinary *K. pneumonia* strains [19]. Nasehi et al. reported genes isolation rates of 18% and 26% for β-lactamase TEM and β-lactamase SHV which are lower compared to the present study [20]. In 2010 Faizabadi et al. reported abundance of genes of β-lactamase TEM and β-lactamase SHV as 67.4 and 46.5% respectively (11). The statistics show that Lactamase genes β-lactamase CTXM, β-lactamase SHV, and TEM are increasing and worrying. In most reports frequent Lactamases among *K. pneumonia* isolates was from SHV group derivatives which is consistent with the present study.

Conclusion

Due to insufficient information about ESBL gene plasmid abundance and genetic pattern in Iran, the diagnosis of *K. pneumonia* strains containing β-lactamase enzyme for better treatment and prevention of the spread of these genes to other bacteria is essential by genotyping and phenotyping methods. However, this study showed that this bacterium is one the most health problem in south west of Iran and more cure should be done for prevention of infection and resistance spread to other area.

Authors' contributions

AS designed the study. MD, carried out the experiments and collected the data. MZ and SJ performed the statistical analysis. SAK, SSK and NP interpreted the clinical data. MHM revised the result of PCR and approved the tests result. All authors read and approved the final manuscript.

Author details

[1] Cellular and Molecular Research Centre, Yasuj University of Medical Sciences, Yasuj, Iran. [2] Department of Parasitology and Mycology, Shiraz University of Medical Sciences, Shiraz, Iran. [3] Paradise shahid Bahonar, Farhangian University of Shiraz, Shiraz, Iran.

Acknowledgements

The authors would like to express their gratitude to (Dr. Azizi, Dr. Salehy, and Dr. Jannesar) that prepared and sent the samples from their laboratories. This project was financially supported by the Vice Chancellor for Research, Yasuj University of Medical Sciences, Iran.

Competing interests

The authors declare that they have no competing interests.

References

1. Brooks G, Carroll KC, Butel J, Morse S. Jawetz Melnick&Adelbergs Medical Microbiology 27th edition. McGraw Hill Professional; 2017. p. 231–244.
2. Wilson GS, Miles AA. Topley and Wilson's principles of bacteriology, virology and immunity. 1975.
3. Dutzler R, Rummel G, Albertí S, Hernández-Allés S, Phale P, Rosenbusch J, et al. Crystal structure and functional characterization of OmpK36, the osmoporin of *Klebsiella pneumoniae*. Structure. 1999;7(4):425–34.
4. Huang W, Petrosino J, Hirsch M, Shenkin PS, Palzkill T. Amino acid sequence determinants of β-lactamase structure and activity. J Mol Biol. 1996;258(4):688–703.
5. Nukaga M, Mayama K, Hujer AM, Bonomo RA, Knox JR. Ultrahigh resolution structure of a class A β-lactamase: on the mechanism and specificity of the extended-spectrum SHV-2 enzyme. J Mol Biol. 2003;328(1):289–301.
6. Bonomo RA, Szabo D. Mechanisms of multidrug resistance in Acinetobacter species and Pseudomonas aeruginosa. Clin Infect Dis. 2006;43(Supplement 2):S49–56.
7. Pitout JD, Nordmann P, Laupland KB, Poirel L. Emergence of Enterobacteriaceae producing extended-spectrum β-lactamases (ESBLs) in the community. J Antimicrob Chemother. 2005;56(1):52–9.
8. Tzouvelekis L, Tzelepi E, Tassios P, Legakis N. CTX-M-type β-lactamases: an emerging group of extended-spectrum enzymes. Int J Antimicrob Agents. 2000;14(2):137–42.
9. Radice M, Power P, Di Conza J, Gutkind G. Early dissemination of CTX-M-derived enzymes in South America. Antimicrob Agents Chemother. 2002;46(2):602–4.

10. Linscott AJ, Brown WJ. Evaluation of four commercially available extended-spectrum beta-lactamase phenotypic confirmation tests. J Clin Microbiol. 2005;43(3):1081–5.
11. Feizabadi MM, Delfani S, Raji N, Majnooni A, Aligholi M, Shahcheraghi F, et al. Distribution of bla TEM, bla SHV, bla CTX-M genes among clinical isolates of *Klebsiella pneumoniae* at Labbafinejad Hospital, Tehran, Iran. Microb Drug Resist. 2010;16(1):49–53.
12. Mirsalehian A, Akbari NF, Peymani A, Kazemi B, Jabal AF, Mirafshar S. Prevalence of extended spectrum β-lactamase-producing Enterobacteriaceae by phenotypic and genotypic methods in intensive care units in Tehran, Iran. Daru. 2008;16 (3):169–73.
13. Bazzaz B, Naderinasab M, Mohamadpoor A, Farshadzadeh Z, Ahmadi S, Yousefi F. The prevalence of extended-spectrum beta-lactamase-producing *Escherichia coli* and *Klebsiella pneumoniae* among clinical isolates from a general hospital in Iran. Acta Microbiol Immunol Hung. 2009;56(1):89–99.
14. Pitout JD. Multiresistant Enterobacteriaceae: new threat of an old problem. Expert Rev Anti Infect Ther. 2008;6(5):657–69.
15. Coque TM, Baquero F, Canton R. Increasing prevalence of ESBL-producing Enterobacteriaceae in Europe. Euro Surveill. 2008;13(47):144–53.
16. Ejaz H, Zafa A, Mahmood S, Javed MM. Urinary tract infections caused by extended spectrum β-lactamase (ESBL) producing *Escherichia coli* and *Klebsiella pneumoniae*. Afr J biotech Res. 2013;10(73):16661–6.
17. Molana Z, Ferdosi SE, Gharavi S, Shafii M, Norkhomami S, Ahangarkani F, et al. Molecular investigation of class I integron in *Klebsiella pneumoniae* isolated from intensive care unit. JBUMS. 2011;13(6):7–13.
18. Ishii Y, Alba J, Kimura S, Shiroto K, Yamaguchi K. Evaluation of antimicrobial activity of β-lactam antibiotics using E test against clinical isolates from 60 medical centers in Japan. Int J Antimicrob Agents. 2005;25(4):296–301.
19. Eftekhar F, Rastegar M, Golalipoor M, Mansoursamaei N. Detection of extended spectrum β-lactamases in urinary isolates of *Klebsiella pneumoniae* in relation to blaSHV, blaTEM and blaCTX-M gene carriage. Iran J Public Health. 2012;41(3):127.
20. Leila N, Fereshteh S, Nikbin VS, Shoeib N. PER, CTX-M, TEM and SHV Beta-lactamases in clinical isolates of *Klebsiella pneumoniae* isolated from Tehran, Iran. Iran J Basic Med Sci. 2010;13(3):111–8.

21

Association of virulence gene expression with colistin-resistance in *Acinetobacter baumannii*: analysis of genotype, antimicrobial susceptibility, and biofilm formation

Abbas Bahador[1,5,6], Zahra Farshadzadeh[1], Reza Raoofian[2,3], Masoumeh Mokhtaran[1], Babak Pourakbari[4], Maryam Pourhajibagher[1,5] and Farhad B. Hashemi[1*]

Abstract

Background: *Acinetobacter baumannii* causes difficult-to-treat nosocomial infections, which often lead to morbidity due to the development of antimicrobial drug resistance and expression of virulence genes. Data regarding the association of resistance to colistin, a last treatment option, and the virulence gene expression of *A. baumannii* is scarce.

Methods: We evaluated the MLVA genotype, antimicrobial resistance, and biofilm formation of 100 *A. baumannii* isolates from burn patients, and further compared the in vitro and in vivo expression of four virulence genes among five colistin-resistant *A. baumannii* (Cst-R-AB) isolates. Five Cst-R-AB isolates were tested; one from the present study, and four isolated previously.

Results: Our results showed that reduced expression of *recA*, along with increased in vivo expression of *lpsB*, *dnaK*, and *blsA*; are associated with colistin resistance among Cst-R-AB isolates. Differences in virulence gene expressions among Cst-R-AB isolates, may in part explain common discrepant in vitro vs. in vivo susceptibility data during treatment of infections caused by Cst-R-AB.

Conclusions: Our findings highlight the intricate relationship between colistin-resistance and virulence among *A. baumannii* isolates, and underscore the importance of examining the interactions between virulence and antimicrobial resistance toward efforts to control the spread of multidrug-resistant *A. baumannii* (MDR-AB) isolates, and also to reduce disease severity in burn patients with MDR-AB infection.

Keywords: *Acinetobacter baumannii*, Colistin resistance, Virulence gene expression, Murine burn model

Background

Acinetobacter baumannii is an opportunistic pathogen that can cause formidable infections among patients with burn wounds worldwide [1]. Also, the World Health Organization (WHO) has announced *A. baumannii* as "Critical" priority pathogenic bacteria that pose the greatest threat to human health. Treatment of *A. baumannii* wound infection is often difficult; primarily due to the pathogenic factors, which enable the establishment of persistent infections within burn patients leading to high morbidity and mortality [2–4]. These pathogenic factors mainly include the development of multi-drug resistance, and production of virulence determinants, such as biofilm formation [5–7]. Reports from various parts of the world have indicated a worrisome growing trend of isolating multi-, extensive- and pan-drug resistant (MDR, XDR, and PDR) strains of *A. baumannii*, some of which are even resistant to colistin, a last resort drug [8–13]. Whether the expression of virulence determinants, such as genes involved in biofilm formation, play an important

*Correspondence: farhadb.hashemi@gmail.com; bonakdar@tums.ac.ir
[1] Department of Microbiology, School of Medicine, Tehran University of Medical Sciences, 100 Poursina Ave., 100 Keshavarz Blvd, Tehran 14167-53955, Iran
Full list of author information is available at the end of the article

role in the high rate of treatment failure among wound infections caused by highly resistant *A. baumannii* isolates remains to be explored [14].

To date, the expression of several *A. baumannii* virulence genes has been linked to the persistence and enhanced survival of *A. baumannii* within the host, including quorum sensing genes [15], and genes that confer biofilm production, which ultimately lead to increased antimicrobial resistance [16, 17]. Furthermore, the activation of *A. baumannii* virulence determinant genes, such as *recA* and *dnaK*, can render robust strains, which are less vulnerable to host response stresses [18]. Moreover, the expression of *recA* by *A. baumannii* isolates increases resistance to stress [19], while *recA* inactivation increases susceptibility to a variety of antimicrobial agents [15, 20].

Then again, mounting evidence suggests that increased virulence gives rise to isolates that are less "fit" to survive in their host, and renders them more susceptible to antimicrobial agents [21]. For instance, the loss of glycosyl transferase gene (*lps*B)], essential for *A. baumannii* lipopolysaccharide (LPS) core biosynthesis, corresponds to the phenotypes of "reduced survival rate", attenuated biofilm formation, and increased antimicrobial susceptibility [22–24]. Similarly, the expression of blue light sensing (*blsA*) gene and production of BlsA protein has been demonstrated to inhibit biofilm formation, which also leads to increased susceptibility to antimicrobial agents [25, 26]. In addition, among *A. baumannii* clinical isolates, the development of colistin resistance (Cst^R) has been shown to enhance biofilm formation, but reduce their invasiveness [27, 28]. Although these reports present evidence of likely interactions between virulence and the antimicrobial susceptibility profile of *A. baumannii*, the association of the expression of specific virulence genes with antimicrobial susceptibility has not been thoroughly investigated. Likewise, data comparing the expression of virulence genes among colistin-resistant *A. baumannii* (Cst-R-AB) strains is scarce.

In the present study, we aim to examine whether resistance to colistin in *A. baumannii* isolates is associated with the expression of specific virulence genes. We also analyze the genotypes of the *A. baumannii* isolates, their biofilm formation ability, and antimicrobial susceptibility profiles. By revealing the interaction of virulence genes with Cst^R among *A. baumannii* isolates, we attempt to explain, at least in part, the apparent discrepancies between in vitro antimicrobial resistance data, and in vivo clinical outcomes in *A. baumannii* infected burn patients. Our findings may ultimately help devise strategies toward effective treatments of *A. baumannii* burn wound infections, as well as make prudent decisions regarding other infection control measures to thwart nosocomial outbreaks of MDR *A. baumannii*.

Methods

Specimens, bacterial isolates and cultures

One hundred non-repetitive clinical specimens were collected from the burn unit of the Burn Medical Center Complex in Tehran, Iran; during April–December 2014. After admission, written informed consent forms were obtained from either the patients, or their authorized representatives. This study was approved by Tehran University of Medical Sciences (TUMS) Research Ethics Committee (Application No. TREC-89. 01-30-10430). All 100 burn wound isolates were initially identified as *A. baumannii* using the API20NE system (bioMérieux, Marcy-l'Etoile, France), and later confirmed using the *gyrB* multiplex PCR, as described previously [29]. Mueller–Hinton Broth (MHB) and brain heart infusion (BHI) agar plates (both from Merck, Darmstadt, Germany) were used to culture the bacterial isolates under aerobic conditions for 24 h at 37 °C. In total, five Cst-R-AB isolates were analyzed including, a single Cst-R-AB isolates from this study, and four additional Cst-R-AB isolates from previous cohort studies.

Antimicrobial susceptibility testing

To assess antimicrobial susceptibility patterns of *A. baumannii* clinical isolates, we carried out the disk agar diffusion (DAD) method according to the Clinical and Laboratory Standards Institute (CLSI) procedures [30] and breakpoint interpretations, using antimicrobial disks containing the 17 antimicrobial agents: ampicillin–sulbactam, cefepime, ceftazidime, ciprofloxacin, colistin, gentamicin, imipenem, levofloxacin, meropenem, minocycline, piperacillin, piperacillin-tazobactam, rifampicin, tetracycline, tigecycline, tobramycin, and trimethoprim-sulfamethoxazole (Mast Diagnostics, Bootle, UK). The CLSI guideline for Broth microdilution test for minimum inhibitory concentration (MIC) was used to assess isolate susceptibility to colistin, rifampicin, and tigecycline. Colistin MICs were interpreted according to the CLSI breakpoints [30]. For tigecycline susceptibility tests, the criteria of the European Committee on Antimicrobial Susceptibility Testing (EUCAST) [31] for *Enterobacteriaceae* were used, in which an MIC of <1 µg/mL was defined as susceptible and >2 µg/mL was considered resistant [31]. Rifampicin susceptibility was interpreted according to CLSI criteria using breakpoint values suggested for *Staphylococcus aureus*, in which susceptible and resistant were defined as ≤ 1 and ≥ 4 µg/mL, respectively [30]. *A. baumannii* isolates were defined as multi-, extensive- and pan-drug resistant (MDR, XDR, and PDR) according to the definitions described previously [32]. Antimicrobial agents were categorized into three groups; namely, Group A that were agents deemed appropriate for primary testing panel; Group B agents, for which primary testing may be warranted, but they may be reported selectively (such as when the organism is resistant to agents of the same class, as in group A). Also, Group O (other) that comprised agents that had a clinical indication for *A. baumannii*, but were not candidates for primary testing panel in the USA [30]. Colistin resistance (Cst^R) among *A. baumannii* isolates was confirmed by the genetic analysis of the *pmr* operon showing mutations in *pmrA/pmrB* signal transduction system, which confers Cst^R by modifying lipid A phosphoethanolamine moiety of the lipopolysaccharide (LPS) layer in the outer membrane.

International clones, MLVA genotype analysis

International clone (IC) types of the isolates were determined based on the presence of *ompA*, *csu*E, and bla_{OXA-51}-like allele amplicons using two complementary multiplex PCR assays, as previously described [33]. Table 1 shows the primers used in the multiplex PCR assays, which selectively amplified the outer membrane protein A (ompA), chaperone-subunit usher E (csuE), and $bla_{OXA-51-like}$ intrinsic carbapenemase genes of the *A. baumannii* isolates. Isolates not assigned as either IC type I, II, or type III were reported as the variant clonal type (IC-V).

To examine the genotypic diversity of *A. baumannii* clinical isolates, multi-loci variable-number tandem repeat analysis (MLVA) was carried out, as previously described [34]. Briefly, DNA from the *A. baumannii* isolates was extracted using a GeneJET DNA purification kit and its concentration was assessed using a NanoDrop 1000 spectrophotometer (Thermo Scientific, USA). Genomic DNA (25 ng/µL) was assayed by PCR using a 30 µL final volume containing 5 ng of DNA, 10× reaction buffer (SinaClon BioScience, Iran), 1.5 mM MgCl [1, 2] U of Taq DNA polymerase, 200 µM each deoxynucleotides (dNTP), and 0.3 µM of each primer (all provided by SinaClon BioScience, Iran). Amplification cycles included an initial 94 °C denaturation for 5 min, followed by 35 cycles of 94 °C for 30, 30 s of annealing at 50 or 55 °C depend on melting temperature of the primers, elongation at 72 °C for 30 s, and a final elongation at 72 °C for 10 min. Then, 5 µL of each PCR amplicon solution were analyzed on a 25 cm 3% agarose gel (SinaClon BioScience, Iran) by electrophoresis (3 h at 6 V/cm) in 1× Tris–borate-EDTA (TBE) buffer. Size markers included a 100-bp (SinaClon Bioscience), and 50-bp DNA standards (Thermo Scientific) for L- and S-variable number tandem repeats (VNTRs), respectively. The amplicon bands were visualized with UV illumination after ethidium bromide (0.5 µg/mL) staining. Band sizes were determined using GeneTools v.3.08 automatic image analysis software (Syngene, Cambridge, United Kingdom). For cluster analysis, allele strings were analyzed by BioNumerics software v.7.0 as character values (Applied Maths, Sint-Martens-Latem, Belgium). Clusters were defined using cut-off values of 95% similarity, and MLVA type was determined using a 100% similarity cutoff, as previously described [35].

Table 1 Primer sequences used in this study

Primer name	Sequence (5′–3′)	Amplicon size (bp)
blsA-F	ACCTTTAACCCGCTTTTGCT	117
blsA-R	TCCCCTATTCACCATTCCAA	
lpsB-F	AGGCCATCAATCTTTGGTTG	137
lpsB-R	GCTGACGTAATGGACGGATT	
dnaK-F	GCGTTTAATTGGTCGTCGTT	105
dnaK-R	ACTTCAACCCAAGCATCACC	
recA-F	CACGCCCTAGACCCTCAATA	136
recA-R	CGATTAAATCAATTGCGCCT	
16srRNA-F	AAAGTTGGTATTCGCAACGG	117
16srRNA-R	ACCTTTAACCCGCTTTTGCT	

Semi-quantitative biofilm formation assay

The semi-quantitative assessment of biofilm formation was performed in triplicate using crystal violet staining, as previously described [36]. Briefly, *A. baumannii* isolates were cultured on BHI agar overnight, and an isolated colony was suspended in LB Broth (Himedia, India) for 4 h. Bacterial suspensions (200 µL) in logarithmic growth phase were adjusted to 0.5 McFarland's standard [1.5×10^8 colony forming units (CFU)/mL] and incubated at 35 °C in flat-bottomed 96-well plates. After 48 h, media was removed, and wells were washed three times with dH_2O. Then, 200 µL of 1% crystal violet dye was added and plates were incubated at room temperature (RT) for 20 min. The dye was then decanted, wells were washed twice with dH_2O and dried. Finally, 200 µL of 95% ethanol (200 µL/well) was added, and the optical absorbance (A) was measured at 570 nm (Thermo Scientific GmbH, Driesch, Germany). Reference strain (ATCC DH5α) was used as negative control (NC) to assign scores for biofilm formation, according to following formula: negative isolate (N) $= A_I \leq A_{NC}$; weakly positive isolate (W) $= A_{NC} < A_I \leq 2A_{NC}$; moderately positive isolate (M) $= 2A_{NC} < A_I \leq 4A_{NC}$; and strongly positive isolate (S) $= A_I > 4A_{NC}$.

Virulence genes detection

To detect virulence factor genes *dnaK*, *recA*, *lpsB* and *blsA*, a series of PCR assays were utilized using primers (Table 1; Primer 3 software v.4.0). Briefly, 1 µL of genomic DNA (25 ng) from Cst-R-AB strains was assessed by PCR using 12.5 µL of 2× PCR Master Mix, and 1 µL (2.5 pM) of each primer (both from SinaClon BioScience, Iran). Amplifications were performed using a Mastercycler

Personal (Eppendorf®, Germany), with initial denaturation for 5 min at 94 °C, and 35 cycles at 94 °C for 30 s, annealing for 30 s at 52 °C (Table 1), followed by elongation at 72 °C for 30 s, and a final step at 72 °C for 5 min. The presence of gene specific amplicons was verified visually by 2% agarose gel electrophoresis using ethidium bromide staining.

Animal study design

All animal experiments were carried out in accordance to the protocols approved by the Animal Ethics Committee of Tehran University of Medical Sciences (Application No. TUMS-AEC-89-0130-10430). Male C57BL/6 mice (6–8 week old; 18–23 g; Pasteur Institute, Tehran, Iran) were housed one mouse per cage, under sanitary conditions at 22–25 °C and at 12 h light/dark cycles, with access to sanitized pellet food and water. Mice were acclimated to room conditions for 1 week prior to each experiment. To increase the accuracy of microbiological assessments, the cages were disinfected with povidone iodine solution 10%, and the bedding materials were autoclaved, and replaced every day.

Based on mortality rates of burn wound infection from previous studies, the effect size (No. of mice in experimental groups) was estimated as five mice per each isolate, using power analysis with power arbitrarily set at 80%. Initially, two groups (five mice per group) were infected with the only Cst-R-AB (MT10) isolated in this study. One group was infected with colistin-treated Cst-R-AB isolate, and the other with Cst-R-AB isolate with no colistin treatment. Mock-infected burned mice (C-Burn) served as controls, and received physiological saline instead of *A. baumannii* infection (third group).

Similarly, groups of mice were later infected with additional four Cst-R-AB isolates (MIC 32–256 μg/mL), recovered from burn wounds in a previous study [37]. In order to expose the Cst-R-AB isolates to colistin, and evaluate the putative colistin-induced changes in virulence gene expression, the group of colistin-treated Cst-R-AB infected mice were administered with colistin (20 μg/g weight); which yielded sub-MIC serum levels of approximately 25 μg/μL [38]. For analysis of all five (i.e. 1 + 4) Cst-R-AB isolates, all in vivo data were combined and presented as Mean + SD.

Murine burn wound infection and bacterial quantification

Burn wounds were generated, as described previously [39]. Briefly, mice were anesthetized by an intraperitoneal (i.p.) injection of a ketamine–xylazine cocktail, after which the dorsal/posterior surface was shaved, and each mouse was then injected with 0.5 mL (i.p.) of sterile saline to prevent dehydration. A brass 10 mm × 10 mm block preheated to 95 °C was applied to the shaved area for a 10 s period. This procedure consistently generated a nonlethal, full-thickness, third-degree burn. Burn wound infections were established as previously described [40]. Briefly, 5 min after inducing the burn wound, using a sterile inoculating loop, a 50 μL suspension of each Cst-R-AB isolate containing $1.1–2.1 \times 10^5$ CFU/mL was smeared onto the burn wound site. After 72 h, bacterial concentrations in wound sites of mice infected with untreated Cst-R-AB were compared to mice infected with Cst-treated Cst-R-AB isolate (treated with sub-optimal i.e. <MIC). Viable bacteria quantitated by colony enumeration of bacteria harvests from the wound bed, and reported as CFU/mL by using biopsy punch method as previously described [41]. All mice were euthanized via an overdose of ketamine (250 mg/kg) and xylazine (25 mg/kg) prior to bacterial harvest from the wound site.

RNA extraction and cDNA synthesis and in vivo virulence gene expression

To measure in vivo virulence genes expression within the wound bed skin, tissue specimens were collected from the infected tissue from each sacrificed mouse were processed separately. Briefly, wound bed skin tissue specimens were aseptically excised (2 mm deep), placed in PBS, and frozen in liquid N_2 for immediate RNA extraction.

To compare the relative quantities of gene-specific mRNA of Cst-R-AB isolates under in vivo vs. in vitro conditions RNA extraction was carried out. For the "in vivo samples" mRNA was extracted from Cst-R-AB isolates in their respective burn wound sites, 72 h after inoculation. The in vitro mRNA samples were, however, prepared using Cst-R-AB isolates grown in culture media, as described above. In all comparative analyses, 16S rRNA gene mRNA served as control to normalize mRNA quantities among the samples. Total bacterial RNA of planktonic mid-log phase cultures of Cst-R-AB isolates were extracted using the Total RNA Extraction Kit (iNtRON Biotech Inc., Seoul, South Korea). To extract bacterial RNA from tissue, wound specimens were ground and homogenized in liquid nitrogen, and the cellular lysates were run through All Prep DNA/RNA columns. Total RNA extraction was performed using RNeasy Plus Mini Kit (QIAGEN, Hilden, Germany) following the manufacturer's recommendations. Bacterial mRNA enrichment was achieved by step-wise treatment of total RNA samples to eliminate mouse mRNA [NEBNext Poly(A) mRNA Magnetic Isolation Module, New England Biolabs, USA], followed by the removal of mouse and bacterial rRNA (Ribo-Zero Gold rRNA Removal Kit, Epicentre Biotechnologies, USA). RNA purity was determined by 260/280 and 260/230 nm absorbance ratio using a NanoDrop 1000 spectrophotometer (Thermo Scientific, USA), and size-verified by 2% agarose gel electrophoresis prior to RT-PCR and qRT-PCR assays. Before generating cDNA, bacterial mRNA samples were treated with DNase I (Thermo Scientific, USA) and RevertAid First Strand cDNA Synthesis Kit (Thermo Scientific, USA). Samples of 1 μg total RNA were used to generate cDNA libraries, for the reverse transcription (RT)-PCR, and quantitative real time RT-PCR (qRT-PCR) assays.

Reverse transcriptase (RT-PCR) and quantitative (qRT)-PCR assays

RT-PCR assay was used to assess the expression of *dnaK, blsA, recA,* and *lpsB* genes. Briefly, first-strand cDNA served as a template for the amplification of virulence genes, and qRT-PCR was used to measure the relative changes in mRNA levels as indicators of virulence gene expression. Samples of cDNA from Cst-R-AB isolates were analyzed by qRT-PCR assay using the primer sets shown in Table 1. The Line-Gene K Real Time PCR System (BIOER Technology Co., China) was used to perform the qRT-PCR according to the minimum information for publication of quantitative real-time PCR experiments (MIQE) guidelines [42] under the following conditions: 95 °C for 15 min, followed by 45 cycles of 95 °C for 15 s, annealing for 30 s at 60, and 72 °C for 30 s, using 10 μL of SYBR® Premix Ex Taq™ II (Tli RNaseH Plus) (TaKaRa Bio Inc., Japan), 2 μL of gene-specific forward and reverse primers (2.5 pmol), cDNA template (50 ng), and 7 μL of ddH_2O (total 20 μL). The quantity of gene-specific amplicons was determined by qPCR relative to an internal standard (16S rRNA) used as a calibrator. Target amplicons were checked for size and specificity by agarose gel electrophoresis and melting curve analysis, respectively. The changes in the expression level of each virulence gene was calculated by the $2^{-\Delta\Delta Ct}$ method using the Relative Expression Software Tool (REST) 2009 software (version 2.0.13; Qiagen, Valencia, CA, USA) [44]. Difference of >4-fold relative to basal gene expression levels was considered significant, and referred to as *n*-fold difference.

Statistical analysis

Data were analyzed using the Student's t-test, and the Chi square test using the SPSS software package (version 22). Results were considered significant if $P < 0.05$.

Results

Antimicrobial susceptibility profiles

As shown in Fig. 1, the majority (95%) of *A. baumannii* isolates had a MDR (31%) or XDR (64%) profile of antimicrobial resistance, while the frequency of non-MDR, or PDR isolates was 4%, and 1%, respectively. While most isolates (96%) were resistant to at least three classes of antimicrobial agents, nearly 90% were resistant to at least 10 tested antimicrobial agents including; cephalosporins, trimethoprim/sulfamethoxazole, tetracycline, piperacillin/tazobactam, and fluoroquinolones. Figure 1 also shows the susceptibility profile of *A. baumannii* isolates against seven antimicrobial agents representing the A, B, and O groups of antimicrobial agents [30]. The highest resistance rates were among group A (45–96%), followed by group B (19–97%), and group O antimicrobial agents (1%). The lowest rates of resistance were against colistin (1%), tigecycline (19%), and minocycline (42%). Moreover, resistance rates to ciprofloxacin, tobramycin, and imipenem were 89, 64 and, 60% respectively. Surprisingly, the rate of resistance to tobramycin was higher among MDR isolates (82%) than the XDR (87%) isolates ($P > 0.05$).

MLVA genotyping and international clone analysis

International clone (IC) type analysis showed that the majority of *A. baumannii* isolates were IC-V variants (43%), followed by IC-II (37%), IC-I (19%), and IC-III types (1%). Also, MLVA genotype analysis (95% allelic similarity) revealed eight different strain clusters, including strain clusters A, B, and C in one group, as well as clusters D through H in another group (Fig. 1).

Overall, we identified 32 MLVA types (MT), which consisted of 1–24 members each (at 100% similarity cutoff). While most MTs had a single member, the three main MTs were MT29 (n = 24), MT13 (n = 17), and MT14 (n = 10), which together comprised over 50% of all isolates (Fig. 1). The majority of MT29 (18/24) and MT14 (8/10) members were IC-V variants, which were predominantly XDR isolates. Specifically, 83% (15/18) of MT29 IC-V variants, and 50% (4/8) of MT14 variants showed XDR profiles. The small MT12 cluster (n = 4) was remarkable since all four were IC-V and XDR isolates. Approximately 75% of the MT29 isolates and 40% of the MT14 isolates were categorized as IC-V. Among the MT29, MT13, and MT14 isolates, XDR isolates predominated and showed similar frequencies. Most MT13 isolates (76%) were IC-II types with nearly 70% of these being XDR strains (Fig. 1).

Association of MDR profile with IC types and biofilm formation index

We further examined the association of the MDR profile of antimicrobial resistance of each isolate with the ability

(See figure on next page.)
Fig. 1 Comparison of MLVA genotype diversity of 100 *Acinetobacter baumannii* isolates (dendogram) with their biofilm formation phenotype, as well as resistance to CLSI antimicrobial groups, and international clonal lineage

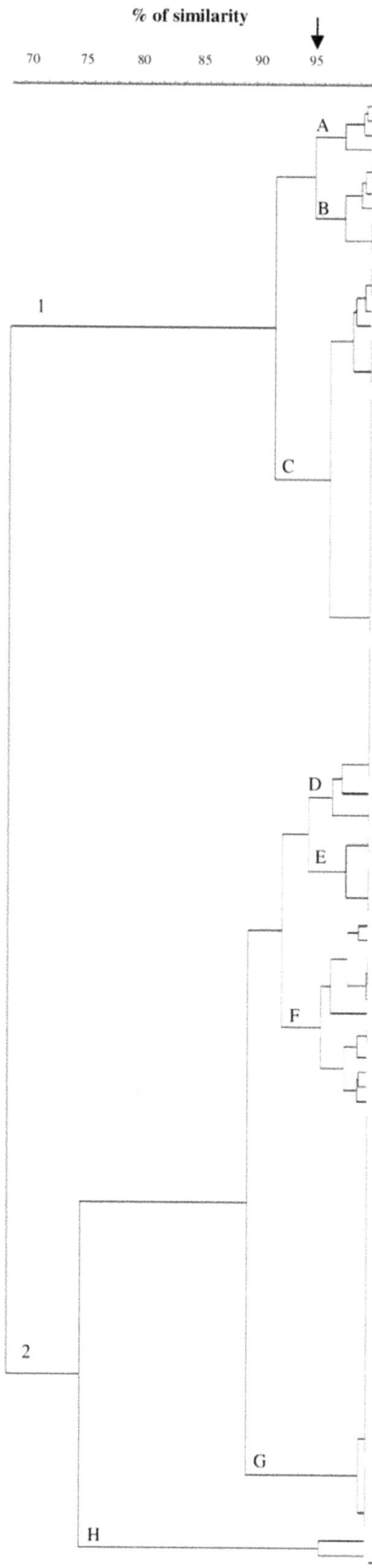

Strain ID	MLVA type	IC[a]	Biofilm[b]	Phenotype[c]	% Resistant to CLSI antimicrobial groups[d]						
					A				B		O
					CIP	TOB	IPM	SAM	MIN	TGC	CST
24	1	V	W	X	*	*	*	*			
76	2	1	W	N							
36	3	2	S	X	*						
80	4	V	M	X	*	*		*	*		
48	5	1	S	M	*						
1	5	1	S	M	*						
61	6	V	M	M	*						
12	7	V	S	X	*	*		*	*	*	
19	8	1	M	X	*	*	*	*			
62	8	1	W	M		*	*				
18	8	1	M	X	*		*	*	*		
9	9	2	S	M			*				
43	9	V	S	X	*		*	*			
47	9	2	S	M	*						
77	10	1	W	P	*	*	*	*	*	*	*
78	11	1	S	X	*						
64	12	V	S	X	*	*	*	*	*	*	
17	12	V	S	X	*	*	*	*	*	*	
35	12	V	S	X	*	*	*	*	*	*	
8	12	V	S	X	*	*	*	*	*	*	
46	13	2	W	M	*	*	*				
2	13	2	W	X	*						
38	13	V	S	M		*	*	*	*	*	
53	13	V	S	X	*		*				
52	13	2	M	M	*	*	*				
37	13	V	W	X	*	*					
55	13	2	M	X	*	*	*	*	*		
4	13	2	M	M	*	*	*	*			
6	13	2	S	X	*	*					
58	13	2	S	M	*	*	*	*	*		
25	13	2	S	X	*	*	*	*			
39	13	2	M	X	*	*	*	*	*		
54	13	2	M	X	*	*	*	*			
98	13	2	M	X	*	*	*	*			
86	13	2	M	X	*	*	*	*			
95	13	2	M	X	*	*	*	*			
11	13	V	M	X	*	*	*				
51	14	V	S	X	*	*	*	*	*	*	
49	14	2	W	M	*	*	*				
29	14	V	M	M	*	*					
42	14	V	S	X	*	*					
63	14	V	S	X	*	*	*	*	*	*	
23	14	2	W	M							
59	14	V	M	M	*	*	*				
33	14	V	M	M							
14	14	V	S	X	*	*	*		*	*	
31	14	V	M	M	*	*		*			
81	15	2	S	N							
56	16	1	M	X	*		*	*	*	*	
16	16	1	M	X	*		*	*	*	*	
28	17	2	S	M	*	*	*				
74	17	2	S	M		*	*				
70	18	V	M	X	*		*				
13	18	V	M	X	*		*				
21	18	2	M	X	*		*				
22	18	2	M	X	*				*		
67	19	1	M	X	*			*	*		
15	20	1	S	M	*						
68	21	2	M	M	*	*	*				
27	21	2	M	X	*	*	*	*	*	*	
45	21	2	M	M	*	*	*				
93	22	1	S	M	*						
60	23	2	M	X	*						
85	24	1	M	X	*			*	*		
90	24	1	M	X	*			*	*		
71	25	2	S	N							
34	26	2	M	X	*	*		*			
72	27	2	W	M	*						
73	28	2	M	X	*			*			
40	29	V	S	X	*	*	*	*	*	*	
32	29	2	M	M	*	*					
96	29	V	S	X	*	*	*	*	*	*	
91	29	V	S	X	*		*				
66	29	V	S	X	*	*	*	*	*		
92	29	V	W	X	*		*	*			
5	29	V	W	X	*	*	*	*	*	*	
100	29	V	W	N		*	*				
65	29	V	S	M	*	*	*				
99	29	V	S	X	*	*	*	*			
89	29	V	S	X	*	*	*	*	*	*	
84	29	2	M	X	*		*				
87	29	2	S	M	*		*				
79	29	V	S	X	*	*	*	*	*		
26	29	V	S	X	*	*	*	*	*		
83	29	V	S	X	*	*	*	*	*		
97	29	V	S	X	*		*				
94	29	2	W	X	*						
44	29	2	W	M	*	*					
20	29	V	S	X	*	*	*				
41	29	V	S	X	*	*	*	*	*		
57	29	2	M	M	*	*					
88	29	V	S	X	*						
82	29	V	S	X	*	*	*	*	*	*	
10	30	1	W	X	*						
50	30	1	W	M	*						
7	30	1	M	X	*						
69	30	1	M	X	*						
75	30	V	M	X	*			*	*		
3	31	V	M	M			*				
30	32	3	S	X	*	*	*		*	*	

to form biofilm as a virulence determinant, as well as the IC type of each isolate (Fig. 2a, b). Our analysis focused on comparing the biofilm formation index of each isolate with the isolate MDR and XDR profile, since 95% of all isolates had either an MDR or XDR profile. Figure 2a shows that the majority of XDR isolates were IC variants, whereas MDR isolates were predominantly IC-II type. The frequency of IC-II isolates with MDR profile (55%) was almost two folds higher than that of those with XDR profiles (28%; $P=0.031$). In contrast, the frequency of IC-V isolates with MDR profiles was nearly half the frequency of those with XDR profiles (23% vs. 53%; $P=0.021$). The frequencies of MDR vs. XDR profiles among IC-I and IC-III isolates was similar (Fig. 2a).

Comparison of the antimicrobial resistance profile of the isolates' with their biofilm strength index revealed that 77% of the W- and M-biofilm forming isolates had either an MDR, or XDR profile. While, the S-biofilm formers comprised only 23% of MDR isolates, the single PDR isolate was a W-biofilm former. All MT12 members (n = 4) were IC-V type and S-biofilm formers that showed an XDR antimicrobial susceptibility profile. Among XDR isolates, the frequency of S- and M-biofilm formers were 48 and 43%, respectively; while among the MDR isolates, W- and M-biofilm formers were isolated at an identical 39% rate (Fig. 2b). In contrast, the frequency of W-biofilm formers among MDR isolates was 39%, whereas only 12% of XDR isolates were W-biofilm formers ($P=0.009$). Similarly, the frequency of S-biofilm forming isolates with the XDR, or MDR antimicrobial susceptibility profile was 47 and 23%, respectively ($P=0.004$). Finally, all four non-MDR isolates were either W- or S-biofilm formers (50% frequency of isolation); i.e. they included no M-biofilm formers.

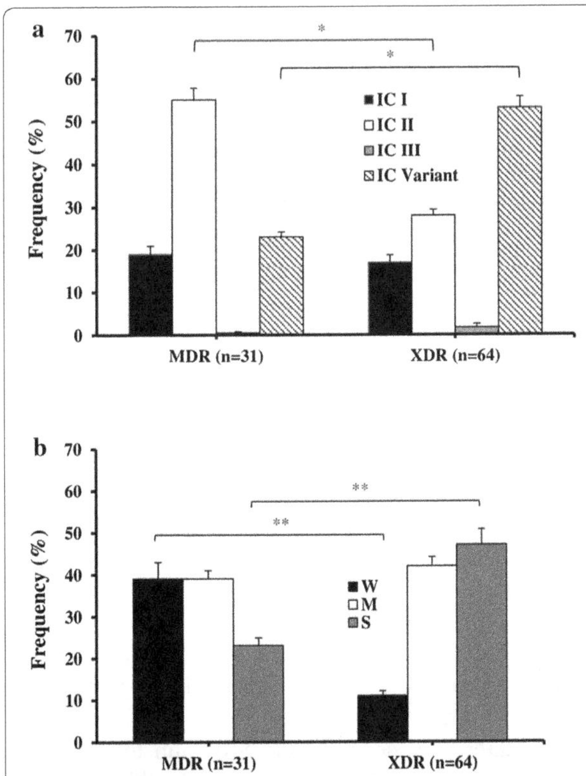

Fig. 2 Comparison of MDR and XDR isolates' frequency according to their IC type **a**; and, the frequency of MDR and XDR isolates with weak (W), moderate (M), and strong (S) biofilm formation **b**. Bars indicate Mean + SEM; *P < 0.05; **P < 0.01, between the indicated pairs

Association of IC type with biofilm formation

Additionally, we assessed whether the strength of biofilm formation was associated with the IC type of *A. baumannii* isolates. Figure 3 shows the frequency of W-, M- and S-biofilm formers among IC-I, IC-II, and IC-V isolates, which comprised 99% of all isolates. Among IC-V isolates, the frequency of S-biofilm formers (63%) was six folds higher than the W-biofilm formers (12%; $P=0.001$); while, among IC-I and IC-II isolates, the frequencies of W-, M-, and S-biofilm formers were comparable, showing only 4–7% variation: i.e. 26% vs. 19% for W-biofilm formers ($P=0.382$), and 26% vs. 30% for S-biofilm formers ($P=0.521$), and finally 47% vs. 51% for M-biofilm formers ($P=0.437$), in that order. As shown in Fig. 3, M-biofilm-forming isolates were almost twice as often seen among the IC-I and IC-II isolates compared to the IC-V isolates [47% vs. 26% for IC-I ($P=0.036$), and 51% vs. 26% for IC-II ($P=0.028$), respectively.

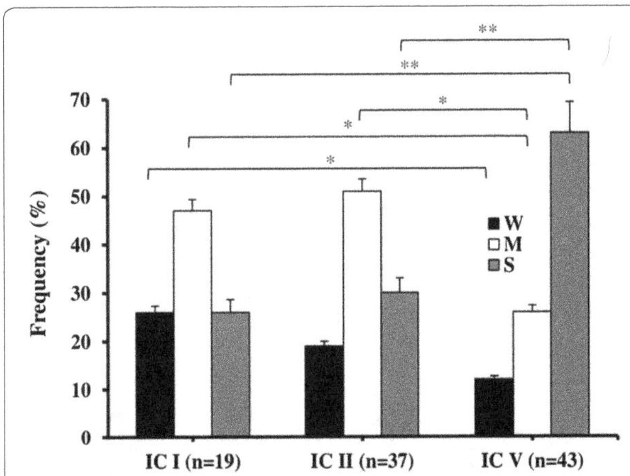

Fig. 3 Frequency comparison of weak (W), moderate (M), and strong (S) biofilm forming *A. baumannii* isolates according to their IC lineage. Analysis included semi-quantitative measurements of biofilm formation strength (see "Methods" section). Bars indicate Mean + SEM; *P < 0.05; **P < 0.01

Quantification of CFU concentration in wound bed tissues

There was no significant difference between the log CFU concentrations in the wound sites infected with untreated Cst-R-AB isolate (7.78 ± 6.0), versus the log CFU concentrations (6.99 ± 5.82; P > 0.05) in wound beds that were infected with Cst-R-AB, which was treated with sub-MIC colistin. Thus, Cst-R-AB isolate concentrations (i.e. growth) were unaffected by the Cst-treatment of wound bed infection site.

Virulence genes detection and expression in vitro and in vivo

Virulence factor genes *dnaK*, *recA*, *lpsB* and *blsA*, were detected in the Cst-R-AB strain by PCR. In order to examine whether the expression of virulence genes *dnaK*, *blsA*, *recA*, and *lpsB* is associated with Cst resistance among isolates, we compared the relative gene-specific mRNA quantities of Cst-R-AB isolates under in vivo, vs. in vitro conditions (Fig. 4). The final data analysis included five Cst-R-AB isolates; including a single Cst-R-AB isolate from the present study (Additional file 1: Figure S1), and four additional Cst-R-AB isolates from previous studies.

Overall, as shown in Fig. 4, the expression levels of *dnaK*, *recA*, and *lpsB* genes in Cst-R-AB isolates were markedly different between in vivo vs. in vitro conditions. The relative change over basal expression levels of the four virulence genes, in vivo vs. in vitro, among Cst-R-AB isolates was reported as the Mean ± SD (Fig. 4).

Among the Cst-R-AB isolates, the in vivo expression of *dnaK* and *lpsB* was 23 and 14 folds higher than basal; respectively (Fig. 4); while *recA* mRNA levels showed a slight 3-fold increase ($P < 0.05$). Conversely, Cst-R-AB in vitro cultures revealed no significant increase in the expression of *dnaK*, *blsA*, and *lpsB*, with only a modest 4-fold rise in *recA* expression. Interestingly, under either condition, *blsA* gene mRNA levels of the Cst-R-AB isolates was up-regulated by 3–4-fold.

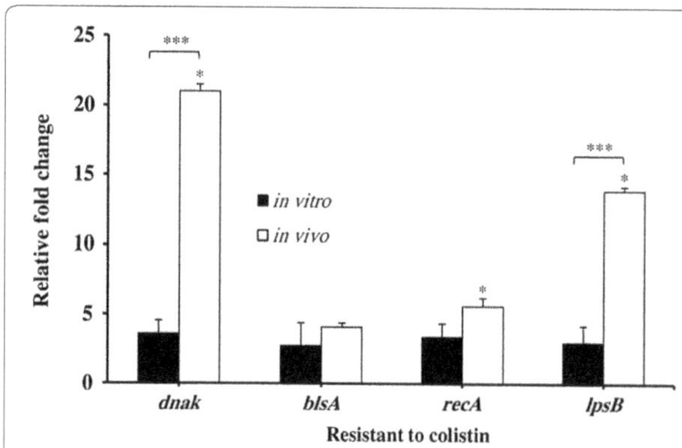

Fig. 4 Comparison of relative change in the mRNA levels of virulence determinant genes *dnaK*, *blsA*, *recA*, and *lpsB* in cultures of five Cst-R-AB isolates, under in vitro and in vivo conditions. Bar indicates mean ± SD; five mice in each group. #P < 0.01; *P < 0.05; ***P < 0.001

Discussion

The emergence of multidrug-resistant *A. baumannii* (MDR-AB), as a major nosocomial pathogen among patients with burn wound infections, has drawn clinical attention to an old antimicrobial agent that is active against MDR-AB, namely colistin (Cst) [43, 44]. Unfortunately, reports from several regions of the world, including Iran, indicate that the widespread use of Cst, as a last resort to control MDR-AB infections, has led to a worrisome growing trend of Cst-resistance (Cst^R) among MDR-AB strains [8, 45, 46]. Recurrently, the eradication of MDR-AB burn wound infections prove very challenging because, not only do clinical strains often develop antimicrobial resistance, but these strains also produce virulence factors (e.g. biofilm) that transform these MDR-AB into even more formidable wound pathogens [10, 12].

While, some studies have associated the presence of specific virulence genes with an increase in the pathogenic potential of clinical isolates [47, 48], the association between the virulence gene expression of *A. baumannii* and the susceptibility to specific antimicrobial agents has not been assessed. In fact, despite several reports regarding the increase in the prevalence of Cst-resistance among MDR-AB isolates worldwide [8–14, 45], few studies have focused on the possible link between Cst^R, and the expression of virulence genes that can potentially affect therapy outcome. We have used a murine burn infection model to demonstrate that mRNA levels of virulence genes *dnaK*, *blsA*, *recA*, and *lpsB* vary in Cst-R-AB isolates depending on whether they are cultured in vitro or in vivo. Moreover, to examine the genotypic diversity among *A. baumannii* isolates, we have characterized their MLVA genotypes, IC lineage. We further evaluated any associations between the isolates' IC lineage, susceptibility patterns, and their biofilm formation profiles.

Here, we also present evidence suggesting that the XDR or MDR profile of *A. baumannii* is associated with the biofilm strength. As shown in Fig. 2b, the frequency of W-biofilm formers among MDR isolates was about three times higher than among XDR isolates, which suggests that the strength of biofilm formation is related to the extended spectrum of antimicrobial resistance among isolates. Conversely, W- and M-biofilm formers were equally common (39%) among MDR isolates. That the XDR isolates had more M- and S-biofilm formers than MDR isolates suggests that the antimicrobial susceptibility profile is associated with biofilm strength among these isolates. However, since the rates of M-biofilm formation were similar among XDR and MDR isolates, the

M-biofilm formation phenotype does not seem to follow this association pattern.

Interestingly, the frequency of S- and M-biofilm formers among XDR isolates were similar (48% vs. 43%, respectively); whereas among the MDR isolates, the W- and M-biofilm formers were isolated at an identical 39% rate (Fig. 2b). Conversely, the frequency of W-biofilm formers among MDR isolates were about three times higher than XDR isolates ($P = 0.009$), which suggests that strength of biofilm formation is associated with the isolate antimicrobial profile. Likewise, isolates with XDR antimicrobial susceptibility profiles were more than twice as likely to be S-biofilm formers, as compared to the frequency of S-formers among MDR isolates ($P = 0.004$). This suggests that stronger biofilm formation may be associated with broader antimicrobial resistance. The remarkable finding that all MT12 members were S-biofilm formers, and shared the same IC-V type and antimicrobial susceptibility profile is suggestive of a common source of isolation.

Interestingly, while IC-V variants had the highest frequency of S-biofilm formers, they included lowest frequency of W-biofilm formers. In addition, our data revealed that most of S-biofilm forming IC-V isolates also had XDR profiles, which is contrary to the reports that indicate biofilm formation is a common attribute of clinical *A. baumannii* isolates, regardless of their IC minor or major clonal variation [49–52]. This apparent discrepancy might be due to the unique features of our local IC-V isolates that have neither been isolated, nor characterized elsewhere. Consequently, the conclusion of studies that have reported no correlation between *A. baumannii* biofilm formation and IC lineage may be limited to the IC-I, -II, and -III categories, which apparently do not encompass a global representation of all *A. baumannii* isolates.

Here, we present evidence suggesting that the development of Cst^R may also lead to changes in *A. baumannii* virulence determinant genes expression, which in turn might enhance the ability to establish, and persist in burn wound infections. In order to further strengthen the scope of our initial findings, which were based on a single Cst-R-AB isolate, we expanded our in vivo experimental data by using four additional Cst-R-AB isolates in a similar murine model (Fig. 4). Since Cst^R has been shown to cause increased outer membrane permeability, higher division rate, and structural changes in the cell wall of *A. baumannii* isolates, it could be proposed that during prolonged infections, persistent Cst^R can lead to reduced fitness, and lower *A. baumannii* virulence over time. However, our findings suggest that the opposite may occur, where enhanced *A. baumannii* virulence can be of greater benefit to some highly resistant local variants of MDR-AB. While the present study focused on the expression profile of four virulence genes among five Cst-R-AB isolates, the variation in the levels of virulence gene mRNA in vitro vs. in vivo conditions among Cst-R-AB isolates could be due to a myriad of additional factors, such as differences between the cellular environment of the wound site as compared to the cell-free culture conditions. Moreover, the role of tissue specific factors that dictate gene regulation, non-specific immune responses, remains to be investigated.

To our knowledge, this is the first report that attempts to establish an association between Cst^R among *A. baumannii* isolates and changes in the virulence genes expression. Our findings show the merits of a comprehensive investigation using a larger number of Cst-R-AB isolates from various regions of the world. Future detailed studies will shed light on the causal relationship between expression of a wider array of *A. baumannii* virulence genes, and genes that confer resistance to colistin, as well as other antimicrobial agents.

Finally, our findings highlight the intricate relationship between resistance to colistin, and the expression of *A. baumannii* virulence genes. It is commonly supposed that an increase in antimicrobial resistance leads, directly or indirectly, to reduced virulence of *A. baumannii* isolates. However, our data suggest that the opposite may occur, and it provides evidence that thorough investigations are warranted to directly measure the correlation between Cst^R, reduced virulence, and "fitness" of *A. baumannii* isolates. Virulence gene expression variations among Cst-R-AB isolates might gain further clinical importance in health care settings, where isolates often transfer from patient to patient. Moreover, that the virulence of Cst-R-AB isolates may depend on their in vitro or in vivo conditions can help explain, at least in part, commonly encountered discrepancies between in vivo and in vitro laboratory test results. For instance, the recurrent failure of therapeutic antimicrobial agents in eradicating *A. baumannii* in patients' burn wounds, despite the in vitro susceptibility of isolated pathogen to the same agents.

Conclusions

This study concludes that the development of resistance to colistin among *A. baumannii* may be associated with virulence gene expression, which fluctuates under in vivo and in vitro conditions. We also provide evidence to speculate that enhanced virulence may be of greater benefit to highly-resistant variants of MDR-AB, and may give rise to formidable pathogens that increase morbidity among burn patients, and threaten the public health systems worldwide. Our findings warrant detailed examination of the interactions between virulence and antimicrobial

resistance toward efforts to control the spread of multidrug-resistant *A. baumannii* (MDR-AB) isolates, and also to reduce disease severity in burn patients with MDR-AB infection.

Abbreviations

AB: *Acinetobacter baumannii* or *A. baumannii*; MDR-AB: multidrug-resistant *A. baumannii*; Cst-R-AB: colistin-resistant *A. baumannii*; *recA*: gene encoding the RecA protein; *lpsB*: gene encoding the lipopolysaccharide core biosynthesis mannosyltransferase protein LpsB; *dnaK*: gene encoding the chaperone protein DnaK; *blsA*: gene encoding the BlsA (blue-light-sensing) photoreceptor protein; MDR: multi-drug resistant; XDR: extensive-drug resistant; GmbH: Gesellschaft mit beschränkter Haftung, which means "company with limited liability"; Cst^R: colistin resistance; TUMS: Tehran University of Medical Sciences; *gyrB*: gene encoding the GyrB subunit of DNA gyrase protein; PCR: polymerase chain reaction; MHB: Mueller–Hinton Broth; DAD: disk agar diffusion; CLSI: Clinical and Laboratory Standards Institute; MIC: minimum inhibitory concentration; EUCAST: European Committee on Antimicrobial Susceptibility Testing; LPS: lipopolysaccharide; C-Burn: Mock-infected burned mice that serve as controls; *ompA*: gene encoding outer membrane protein A; bla_{OXA-51}: the gene encoding the carbapenemase OXA-51; ompA: outer membrane protein A; csuE: chaperone-subunit usher E; MLVA: multi-loci variable-number tandem repeat analysis; DNA: deoxyribonucleic acid; ng: nanogram; μL: microliter; mM: millimolar; $MgCl_2$: magnesium chloride; U: units; Taq: *Thermus aquaticus*; μM: micromolar; MIQE: minimum information for publication of quantitative real-time PCR experiments; dNTP: deoxyribonucleotide triphosphate; et al.: Et alii meaning "and other people"; s: second(s); cm: centimeter(s); %: percent; h: hour(s); V: volt(s); X: times; TBE: tris–borate-EDTA; bp: base pair(s); VNTRs: variable number tandem repeats; L-VNTRs: large variable number tandem repeats; S-VNTRs: small variable number tandem repeats; μg: microgram(s); v.: version; BHI: brain–heart-infusion; LB: Luria–Bertani; CFU: colony forming unit(s); dH_2O: distilled water; RT: room temperature; A: optical absorbance; Nm: nanometer(s); PDR: pan-drug resistant; ATCC: American Type Culture Collection; NC: negative control; N: negative isolate; M: moderately positive isolate; S: strongly positive isolate; A_i: initial absorbance; A_{NC}: absorbance of negative control; ®: registered trademark; wk: week; g: gram; No.: number; IC: international clone; i.p.: intraperitoneal; mm: millimeter; kg: kilogram; RNA: ribonucleic acid; cDNA: complementary DNA; PBS: phosphate-buffered saline; N_2: nitrogen; S: svedberg unit(s) (e.g. 16S); rRNA: ribosomal ribonucleic acid; mRNA: mitochondrial ribonucleic acid; USA: United States of America; RT-PCR: reverse transcription PCR; qRT-PCR: quantitative real-time RT-PCR; DNase I: deoxyribonuclease I; °C: degrees centigrade; pmol: picomolar; ng: nanogram(s); min: minute(s); ddH_2O: double distilled water; REST: Relative Expression Software Tool; >: greater than; *n*-fold difference: Relative fold difference as compared to the basal gene expression; MT: MLVA type(s); W-biofilm formers: weak biofilm formers; M-biofilm formers: moderate biofilm formers; S-biofilm formers: strong biofilm formers; Suppl.: supplement; SD: standard deviation.

Authors' contributions

FBH and AB analyzed and processed the data and drafted the manuscript. ZF and MM did the PCR and MLVA assays. MM did the specimen cultures, animal studies and biofilm assays. MP performed the antimicrobial assays. RR helped with the RNA extraction and virulence gene expression assays, BP helped with clinical coordination and obtaining the patient specimens from the hospitals. All authors read and approved of the final manuscript.

Author details

[1] Department of Microbiology, School of Medicine, Tehran University of Medical Sciences, 100 Poursina Ave., 100 Keshavarz Blvd, Tehran 14167-53955, Iran. [2] Legal Medicine Research Center, Legal Medicine Organization, Tehran, Iran. [3] Innovative Research Center, Islamic Azad University, Mashhad Branch, Mashhad, Iran. [4] Pediatrics Infectious Disease Research Center, Tehran University of Medical Sciences, Tehran, Iran. [5] Dental Research Center, Dentistry Research Institute, Tehran University of Medical Sciences, Tehran, Iran. [6] Laser Research Center, Dentistry Research Institute, Tehran University of Medical Sciences, Tehran, Iran.

Acknowledgements

We would like to thank all the medical staff, who assisted with collection of the specimens used in this study. We would also like to acknowledge Ms. Jocelyn C. Gile for her invaluable editorial assistance.

Competing interests

The authors declare that they have no competing interests.

Funding

This research was supported by Tehran University of Medical Sciences & Health Services Grant No. 89. 01-30-10430.

References

1. Girerd-Genessay I, Bénet T, Vanhems P. Multidrug-resistant bacterial outbreaks in burn units: a synthesis of the literature according to the ORION statement. J Burn Care Res. 2016;37(3):172–80.
2. Leseva M, Arguirova M, Nashev D, Zamfirova E, Hadzhyiski O. Nosocomial infections in burn patients: etiology, antimicrobial resistance, means to control. Ann Burns Fire Disasters. 2013;26(1):5–11.
3. Golberg A, Broelsch GF, Vecchio D, et al. Eradication of multidrug-resistant *A. baumannii* in burn wounds by antiseptic pulsed electric field. Technology (Singap World Sci). 2014;2(2):153–60.
4. Atilla A, Tomak L, Katrancı AO, Ceylan A, Kılıç SS. Mortality risk factors in burn care units considering the clinical significance of acinetobacter infections. Ulus Travma Acil Cerrahi Derg. 2015;21(1):34–8.
5. Mortensen BL, Skaar EP. Host-microbe interactions that shape the pathogenesis of *Acinetobacter baumannii* infection. Cell Microbiol. 2012;14(9):1336–44.
6. Longo F, Vuotto C, Donelli G. Biofilm formation in *Acinetobacter baumannii*. New Microbiol. 2014;37(2):119–27.
7. Weber BS, Harding CM, Feldman MF. Pathogenic acinetobacter: from the cell surface to infinity and beyond. J Bacteriol. 2015;198(6):880–7.
8. Bahador A, Taheri M, Pourakbari B, et al. Emergence of rifampicin, tigecycline, and colistin-resistant *Acinetobacter baumannii* in Iran; spreading of MDR strains of novel international clone variants. Microb Drug Resist. 2013;19(5):397–406.
9. Moradi J, Hashemi FB, Bahador A. Antibiotic resistance of *Acinetobacter baumannii* in Iran: a systemic review of the published literature. Osong Public Health Res Perspect. 2015;6(2):79–86.
10. Doi Y, Murray GL, Peleg AY. *Acinetobacter baumannii*: evolution of antimicrobial resistance-treatment options. Semin Respir Crit Care Med. 2015;36(1):85–98.
11. Inchai J, Liwsrisakun C, Theerakittikul T, Chaiwarith R, Khositsakulchai W, Pothirat C. Risk factors of multidrug-resistant, extensively drug-resistant and pandrug-resistant *Acinetobacter baumannii* ventilator-associated pneumonia in a Medical Intensive Care Unit of University Hospital in Thailand. J Infect Chemother. 2015;21(8):570–4.
12. Potron A, Poirel L, Nordmann P. Emerging broad-spectrum resistance in *Pseudomonas aeruginosa* and *Acinetobacter baumannii*: mechanisms and epidemiology. Int J Antimicrob Agents. 2015;45(6):568–85.
13. Gupta M, Lakhina K, Kamath A, et al. Colistin-resistant *Acinetobacter baumannii* ventilator-associated pneumonia in a tertiary care hospital: an evolving threat. J Hosp Infect. 2016;94(1):72–3.
14. Liu H, Wu YQ, Chen LP, et al. Biofilm-related genes: analyses in multi-antibiotic resistant *Acinetobacter Baumannii* isolates from Mainland China. Med Sci Monit. 2016;28(22):1801–7.
15. Zarrilli R. *Acinetobacter baumannii* virulence determinants involved in biofilm growth and adherence to host epithelial cells. Virulence. 2016;7(4):367–8.
16. Lee J, Page R, García-Contreras R, et al. Structure and function of the *Escherichia coli* protein YmgB: a protein critical for biofilm formation and acid-resistance. J Mol Biol. 2007;373(1):11–26.

17. Wroblewska MM, Sawicka-Grzelak A, Marchel H, Luczak M, Sivan A. Biofilm production by clinical strains of *Acinetobacter baumannii* isolated from patients hospitalized in two tertiary care hospitals. FEMS Immunol Med Microbiol. 2008;53(1):140–4.
18. Fiester SE, Actis LA. Stress responses in the opportunistic pathogen *Acinetobacter baumannii*. Future Microbiol. 2013;8(3):353–65.
19. Schröder W, Goerke C, Wolz C. Opposing effects of aminocoumarins and fluoroquinolones on the SOS response and adaptability in *Staphylococcus aureus*. J Antimicrob Chemother. 2013;68(3):529–38.
20. Aranda J, Bardina C, Beceiro A, et al. *Acinetobacter baumannii RecA* protein in repair of DNA damage, antimicrobial resistance, general stress response, and virulence. J Bacteriol. 2011;193(15):3740–7.
21. Beceiro A, Tomás M, Bou G. Antimicrobial resistance and virulence: a successful or deleterious association in the bacterial world? Clin Microbiol Rev. 2013;26(2):185–230.
22. Luke NR, Sauberan SL, Russo TA, et al. Identification and characterization of a glycosyltransferase involved in *Acinetobacter baumannii* lipopolysaccharide core biosynthesis. Infect Immun. 2010;78(5):2017–23.
23. McConnell MJ, Actis L, Pachón J. *Acinetobacter baumannii*: human infections, factors contributing to pathogenesis and animal models. FEMS Microbiol Rev. 2013;37(2):130–55.
24. Lean SS, Yeo CC, Suhaili Z, Thong KL. Comparative genomics of Two ST 195 carbapenem-resistant *Acinetobacter baumannii* with different susceptibility to polymyxin revealed underlying resistance mechanism. Front Microbiol. 2016;6:1445. https://doi.org/10.3389/fmicb.2015.01445.
25. Mussi MA, Gaddy JA, Cabruja M, et al. The opportunistic human pathogen *Acinetobacter baumannii* senses and responds to light. J Bacteriol. 2010;192(24):6336–45.
26. Golic A, Vaneechoutte M, Nemec A, Viale AM, Actis LA, Mussi MA. Staring at the cold sun: blue light regulation is distributed within the genus Acinetobacter. PLoS ONE. 2013;8(1):e55059. https://doi.org/10.1371/journal.pone.0055059.
27. Pournaras S, Poulou A, Dafopoulou K, et al. Growth retardation, reduced invasiveness, and impaired colistin-mediated cell death associated with colistin resistance development in *Acinetobacter baumannii*. Antimicrob Agents Chemother. 2014;58(2):828–32.
28. Dafopoulou K, Xavier BB, Hotterbeekx A, et al. Colistin-resistant *Acinetobacter baumannii* clinical strains with deficient biofilm formation. Antimicrob Agents Chemother. 2015;60(3):1892–5.
29. Higgins PG, Schneiders T, Hamprecht A, Seifert H. In vivo selection of a missense mutation in adeR and conversion of the novel blaOXA-164 gene into blaOXA-58 in carbapenem-resistant *Acinetobacter baumannii* isolates from a hospitalized patient. Antimicrob Agents Chemother. 2010;54(12):5021–7.
30. Clinical and Laboratory Standards Institute. Performance standards for antimicrobial susceptibility testing: twenty fourth informational supplement M100-S28. Wayne: CLSI; 2018.
31. The European Committee on Antimicrobial Susceptibility Testing. Breakpoint tables for interpretation of MICs and zone diameters Version 5.0. 2015. http://www.eucastorg/clinical_breakpoints. Accessed 01 Jan 2015.
32. Magiorakos AP, Srinivasan A, Carey RB, et al. Multidrug-resistant, extensively drug-resistant and pandrug-resistant bacteria: an international expert proposal for interim standard definitions for acquired resistance. Clin Microbiol Infect. 2012;18(3):268–81.
33. Turton JF, Gabriel SN, Valderrey C, Kaufmann ME, Pitt TL. Use of sequence-based typing and multiplex PCR to identify clonal lineages of outbreak strains of *Acinetobacter baumannii*. Clin Microbiol Infect. 2007;13(8):807–15.
34. Pourcel C, Minandri F, Hauck Y, et al. Identification of variable-number tandem-repeat (VNTR) sequences in *Acinetobacter baumannii* and interlaboratory validation of an optimized multiple-locus VNTR analysis typing scheme. J Clin Microbiol. 2011;49(2):539–48.
35. Nhu NT, Lan NP, Campbell JI, et al. Emergence of carbapenem-resistant *Acinetobacter baumannii* as the major cause of ventilator-associated pneumonia in intensive care unit patients at an infectious disease hospital in southern Vietnam. J Med Microbiol. 2014;63(Pt10):1386–94.
36. Zhang D, Xia J, Xu Y, et al. Biological features of biofilm-forming ability of *Acinetobacter baumannii* strains derived from 121 elderly patients with hospital-acquired pneumonia. Clin Exp Med. 2016;16(1):73–80.
37. Bahador A, Raoo An R, Farshadzadeh Z, et al. The prevalence of IS Aba 1 and IS Aba 4 in *Acinetobacter baumannii* species of different international clone lineages among patients with burning in Tehran, Iran. Jundishapur J Microbiol. 2015;8(7):e17167. https://doi.org/10.5812/jjm.17167v2.
38. Pachón-Ibáñez ME, Docobo-Pérez F, López-Rojas R, et al. Efficacy of rifampin and its combinations with imipenem, sulbactam, and colistin in experimental models of infection caused by imipenem-resistant *Acinetobacter baumannii*. Antimicrob Agents Chemother. 2010;54(3):1165–72.
39. Dai T, Tegos GP, Lu Z, et al. Photodynamic therapy for *Acinetobacter baumannii* burn infections in mice. Antimicrob Agents Chemother. 2009;53(9):3929–34.
40. Ha U, Jin S. Expression of the soxR gene of *Pseudomonas aeruginosa* is inducible during infection of burn wounds in mice and is required to cause efficient bacteremia. Infect Immun. 1999;67(10):5324–31.
41. Thompson MG, Black CC, Pavlicek RL, et al. Validation of a novel murine wound model of *Acinetobacter baumannii* infection. Antimicrob Agents Chemother. 2014;58(3):1332–42.
42. Bustin SA, Beaulieu JF, Huggett J, Jaggi R, Kibenge FSB, Olsvik PA, Penning LC, Toegel S. MIQE précis: practical implementation of minimum standard guidelines for fluorescence-based quantitative realtime PCR experiments. BMC Mol Biol. 2010;11:74.
43. Saun TJ, Rogers AD, Leis JA, Cartotto R. The use of intravenous and inhaled colistin therapy during a burn center outbreak of multidrug-resistant *Acinetobacter baumannii*. J Burn Care Res. 2017. https://doi.org/10.1097/BCR.
44. Fishbain J, Peleg AY. Treatment of acinetobacter infections. Clin Infect Dis. 2010;51(1):79–84.
45. Sepahvand S, Doudi M, Davarpanah MA, Bahador A, Ahmadi M. Analyzing pmrA and pmrB genes in *Acinetobacter baumannii* resistant to colistin in Shahid Rajai Shiraz, Iran Hospital by PCR: first report in Iran. Pak J Pharm Sci. 2016;29(4 Suppl):1401–6.
46. Garnacho-Montero J, Dimopoulos G, Poulakou G, et al. Task force on management and prevention of *Acinetobacter baumannii* infections in the ICU. Intensive Care Med. 2015;41(12):2057–75.
47. Eijkelkamp BA, Stroeher UH, Hassan KA, Paulsen IT, Brown MH. Comparative analysis of surface-exposed virulence factors of *Acinetobacter baumannii*. BMC Genomics. 2014;25(15):1020. https://doi.org/10.1186/1471-2164-15-1020.
48. Yoon EJ, Balloy V, Fiette L, Chignard M, Courvalin P, Grillot-Courvalin C. Contribution of the Ade resistance-nodulation-cell division-type efflux pumps to fitness and pathogenesis of *Acinetobacter baumannii*. MBio. 2016;7(3):pii: e00697–716. https://doi.org/10.1128/mbio.00697-16.
49. Lee NY, Chang TC, Wu CJ, et al. Clinical manifestations, antimicrobial therapy, and prognostic factors of monomicrobial *Acinetobacter baumannii* complex bacteremia. J Infect. 2010;61(3):219–27.
50. Azim A, Dwivedi M, Rao PB, et al. Epidemiology of bacterial colonization at intensive care unit admission with emphasis on extended-spectrum beta-lactamase- and metallo-beta-lactamase-producing Gram-negative bacteria–an Indian experience. J Med Microbiol. 2010;59(Pt 8):955–60.
51. Kang YS, Park W. Contribution of quorum-sensing system to hexadecane degradation and biofilm formation in *Acinetobacter* sp. strain DR1. J Appl Microbiol. 2010;109(5):1650–9.
52. Sanchez CJ, Kumar N, Lizcano A, et al. *Streptococcus pneumoniae* in biofilms are unable to cause invasive disease due to altered virulence determinant production. PLoS ONE. 2011;6(12):e28738. https://doi.org/10.1371/journal.pone.0028738.

22

Molecular determination of antimicrobial resistance in *Escherichia coli* isolated from raw meat in Addis Ababa and Bishoftu, Ethiopia

Yohannes Equar Messele[1*], Reta Duguma Abdi[2,3], Shimels Tikuye Yalew[1], Desiye Tesfaye Tegegne[1], Bezina Arega Emeru[1] and Gebremeskel Mamu Werid[1]

Abstract

Background: Consumption of meat contaminated by *E. coli* causes a serious illness and even death to affected individuals. Recently the emerging of antibiotic resistant foodborne *E. coli* poses serious public health risks worldwide. However, little is known about the antibiotic resistance profile of *E. coli* in Ethiopia. This study aimed to determine the prevalence and Antimicrobial resistance (AMR) status of *E. coli* isolated from different type of meat.

Methods: Overall 292 samples were collected from December 2015 to April 2016 from slaughterhouses to determine the prevalence and AMR of *E. coli* isolated from raw beef, mutton, chevon and chicken meat from Addis Ababa and Bishoftu, Ethiopia. The isolates were screened for AMR against commonly used antibiotics circulating in the Ethiopian market. Both phenotypic and genotypic approach were employed for AMR detection using disc diffusion test and PCR respectively.

Results: The prevalence of *E. coli* was 63 (21.6%), indicating one sample in every five samples harbors *E. coli*. Among these, the highest *E. coli* isolates was observed in chicken meat samples (37.0%; 27), followed by mutton (23.3%; 17), chevon (20.6%; 15) and beef (5.5%; 4). Results of disk diffusion test on the 63 isolates showed that only 4.8% of them were not resistance to all antimicrobials tested. Multiple drug resistance (resistance to ≥3 drugs) was 46.0%. Significantly high resistance to ampicillin (71.4%) and tetracycline (47.6%) was observed. Identification of genes associated with AMR was also done using PCR. The prevalence of *E. coli* isolates harboring resistance gene responsible for tetracycline *(tet(A))*, beta lactams *(blaCMY)* and sulphanamide (*sulI)* antibiotics were found 65.1, 65.1 and 54.0%, respectively. Twenty-five out of the 63 (39.7% %) *E. coli* isolates have got antimicrobial resistance gene to three or more classes of drugs. The associations of antimicrobial resistance phenotypes and resistance genes was also determined. The detection of resistance trait against tetracycline, sulphametazole and chloramphenicol measured either phenotypically or genotypically were high.

Conclusions: The rising levels of resistance *E. coli* to multiple antimicrobial dictate the urgent need to regulate and monitor antimicrobial use in both animals and humans.

Keywords: Antibiotic resistance, *Escherichia coli*, Meat, Ethiopia

*Correspondence: equarachin@gmail.com
[1] Ethiopian Institute of Agricultural Research, National Agricultural Biotechnology Research Center, P.O.Box 31, Holeta, Ethiopia
Full list of author information is available at the end of the article

Background

Meat and meat products serve as important source of proteins for humans. However, recently the emerging antibiotic resistant foodborne pathogens combined with the injudicious use of antibiotics in animals bears considerate public health threats worldwide. Usually, meat and meat products gets contaminated by pathogens during animal slaughter and food processing. *Escherichia coli (E. coli)* is the frequently isolated foodborne pathogens from meat and meat products. Meat can be contaminated by *E. coli* during animal slaughter due to unhygienic slaughter practices, through airborne, rodents, insects, and other animals [1]. Consumption of meat contaminated by *E. coli* causes a serious illness and even death to affected individuals [2].

Recently published reports indicated that the *E. coli* strains isolated from contaminated meat and meat products have become resistant to commonly used antibiotics. This is mainly due to injudicious usage of antibiotics in both humans and animals [3]. The wide spread and imprudent use of antibiotics in food animals is thought to be accountable for the emergence and wider spreading of antimicrobial resistant (AMR) bacteria in humans [3, 4]. In humans, positive selection for drug resistant bacteria have also been reported in the normal microflora of exposed individuals or populations. This indicates that antibiotic resistance can be developed in both commensal and pathogenic bacterial strains and can even be transferred to other bacterial strains, including other pathogenic and environmental bacteria [5].

Consumption of contaminated and/or uncooked meat poses the risks of acquiring foodborne *E. coli* strains [6] causing a serious public health concern. These bacterial strains easily harbors antibiotic resistant genes from one another. This is because genes encoding AMR determinants that are carried on mobile genetic elements such as plasmids and transposons of some bacterial strains could be transferred to other bacteria strains during contact [7], causing a threat to cure acute infections in man and animals. In Ethiopia, a review done by Alemu et al. [8] showed that several pathogen have established resistance against oxytetracycline drugs. Similarly, oxytetracycline and penstrep are the main prescribed antibiotics in Ethiopia [8, 9]. So far, no study has been carried out to identify the antibiotic resistance genes of *Escherichia coli* in Ethiopia.

In this paper, we explain the phenotypic and genotypic sources of MDR in *Escherichia coli* isolates recovered from different type of meat samples taken from Addis Ababa city abattoir and Alema farm poultry slaughter slab, Ethiopia. This enquiry pursues to deliver useful evidence on the prevalence and AMR profile of *E. coli* isolated from beef, mutton, chevon and chicken meat.

Methods

Sample collection and isolation of *E. coli*

The study was carried out from December 2015 to April 2016 to collect meat sample from Addis Ababa city abattoir enterprise and Alema farm slaughter slab found in Bishoftu town, Ethiopia. A total of 292 meat sample including beef meat (n = 73), sheep meat (n = 73), goat meat (n = 73) were collected from Addis Ababa municipal abattoir and chicken meat (n = 73) from Alema farm slaughter slab located in Bishoftu city. Sample were collected by swabbing from carcass gluteal muscle and inserted into 10 ml peptone water containing test tube. The samples were taken following the guidelines of the International Organization for Standardization [10]. The sample were transported to National Agricultural Biotechnology Research Center in an ice box for further processing. The *E. coli* isolates were identified by using standard bacteriological methods, comprising of colony structure determination, using different culture media and biochemical tests as previously indicated [11]. Isolates were preserved at −80 °C in a trypticase soy broth with 10% glycerol for further analysis.

Antimicrobial susceptibility testing

Antibiotic sensitivity was determined by disc diffusion method according to the guidelines of the Clinical and Laboratory Standards Institute [12]. Bacterial suspension was prepared by adding 2–4 colonies to a 5 ml tube containing 0.9% normal saline (NaCl), to achieve absorbance of 0.17–0.18 at wavelength of 600 nm (equivalent to 0.5 McFarland standards) [13]. The suspension was spread onto Mueller–Hinton agar media (HIMEDIA, India) using a sterile cotton swab, and the antibiotic disc (Oxoid, UK) were placed on the top of the agar plate. The inoculated plates were incubated aerobically at 37 °C for 18–24 h, after which all *E. coli* isolates were tested for susceptibility using the following antimicrobial discs and their corresponding concentrations: tetracycline (30 μg/disk); streptomycin (10 μg/disk); chloramphenicol (30 μg/disk), sulfamethoxazole–trimethoprim (25 μg/disk), gentamycin (10 μg/disk); ampicillin, (10 μg/disk); erythromycin (15 μg/disk); by the Kirby-Bauer disk diffusion method [14].

DNA extraction and PCR amplification of resistance genes

Bacterial strains were grown overnight in nutrient agar (HIMEDIA, India) at 37 °C. A loop full of the colonies was added to 100 μl of sterile water. Bacterial DNA was extracted by boiling a bacterial suspension in water. After boiling the suspension for 13 min, the suspension were frozen for 5 min in ice and centrifuged at 14,000 rpm for 15 min to pellet the cell debris [15]. The supernatant from the centrifuged tubes was transferred to new 1.5 ml clean plastic tube and used as a template for PCR amplification. The purified DNA were detected by electrophoresis in 1.5% agarose gel and then kept at −20 °C for further use. Primers for AMR genes such as streptomycin (*aadA1*), tetracycline [*tet*(A)], gentamicin [*aac(3)-IV*], sulfonamides (*sul1*), beta-lactams (*bla*SHV, *bla*CMY), erythromycin [*ere*(A)] and chloramphenicol (*catA1, cmlA*) were used from published article. The specific primer sequences (Bioneer, South Korea) and the estimated size of the amplified products for different resistance gene coding regions are found in Table 1. Amplification of antimicrobial resistance gene from *E. coli* isolates were performed as described by Fode et al. [16]. The amplification products were then separated by electrophoresis on a 1.5% agarose gel stained with gel red (Biotium Inc, USA) as described by Huang et al. [17] and visualized using UV illumination. A 100 bp DNA molecular marker (Bioneer, South Korea) were used to determine the size of the PCR product.

Statistical analysis

The prevalence of *E. coli* infection was quantified and compared among meat samples of different livestock species. Prevalence of AMR was quantified along with resistance patterns. The data were analyzed by using SPSS software version 20 and P value was calculated using Chi square and Fisher's exact tests to determine any significant correlation. P value less than 0.05 was considered statistically significant.

Results

Prevalence of *E. coli*

In this study, a total of 63 (21.6%) *E. coli* isolates were identified from the 292 raw meat samples examined (Table 2). Of these positive cases, chicken meat had the highest (37.0%) whilst beef meat had the lowest prevalence (5.5%) of *E. coli*. A significance difference in *E. coli* prevalence ($P < 0.05$) was observed among meat samples of different livestock species. In this regard, meat of chevon 2.8 times, mutton 3.2 times and chicken meat

Table 1 Primers used for detection of antimicrobial resistant genes in *Escherichia coli* isolates

Drug type	Antimicrobial resistance genes	Primers	Sequence 5′–3′	Amplicon size (Bp)	References
Streptomycin	Adenylyl transferases (*aadA1*)	*aadA1*F	TATCCAGCTAAGCGCGAACT	447	[18]
		*aadA1*R	ATTTGCCGACTACCTTGGTC		
Gentamicin	Aminoglycoside acetyltransferases (*aac(3)-IV*)	*aac(3)-IV*F	CTTCAGGATGGCAAGTTGGT	286	
		*aac(3)-IV*R	TCATCTCGTTCTCCGCTCAT		
Sulfonamide	Dihydropteroate synthase (*sul1*)	*sul1*F	TTCGGCATTCTGAATCTCAC	822	
		*sul1*R	ATGATCTAACCCTCGGTCTC		
Beta-lactams	β-lactamase encoding penicillin resistance (*bla*$_{SHV}$)	*bla*$_{SHV}$F	TCGCCTGTGTATTATCTCCC	768	
		bla$_{SHVR}$	CGCAGATAAATCACCACAATG		
	β-lactamase encoding cephalosporin resistance (*bla*$_{CMY}$)	*bla*$_{CMY}$F	TGGCCAGAACTGACAGGCAAA	462	
		bla$_{CMY}$R	TTTCTCCTGAACGTGGCTGGC		
Erythromycin	Erythromycin esterase (*ere*(A))	*ere*(A)F	GCCGGTGCTCATGAACTTGAG	419	
		ere(A)R	CGACTCTATTCGATCAGAGGC		
Chloramphenicol	Acetyltransferases (*catA1*)	*catA1*F	AGTTGCTCAATGTACCTATAACC	547	
		*catA1*R	TTGTAATTCATTAAGCATTCTGCC		
	Transporter resistance (*cmlA*)	*cmlA*F	CCGCCACGGTGTTGTTGTTATC	698	
		*cmlA*R	CACCTTGCCTGCCCATCATTAG		
Tetracycline	Efflux pump resistance (*tet*(A))	*tet*(A)F	GGTTCACTCGAACGACGTCA	577	[19]
		tet(A)R	CTGTCCGACAAGTTGCATGA		

Table 2 Prevalence of *E. coli* in meat samples of different livestock species

Meat sample	Total sample tested	No. of positives	Prevalence (%)	OR	P value
Chicken	73	27	37.0	Reference	<0.001
Mutton	73	17	23.3	0.51	
Chevon	73	15	20.6	0.44	
Beef	73	4	5.5	0.10	
Total	292	63	21.6		

5.7 times were more infected than beef meat by *E. coli* indicating a difference in *E. coli* infection risk to humans based on meat type.

Phenotypic antibiotic susceptibility test

The distribution of Antimicrobial resistance (AMR) among the *E. coli* isolates from meat samples of four livestock species was shown in Table 3. The lists of AMR was Ampicillin (71.4%), tetracycline (47.6%), erythromycin (42.8%), streptomycin (36.5%), sulfamethoxazole–trimethoprim (34.9%), chloramphenicol (23.8%) and gentamycin (4.8%). Among the *E. coli* isolates identified from meat of different food animals, resistance to ampicillin was highest in chevon (86.7%), followed by chicken (70.4%), mutton (64.7%) and beef meat (50%) as presented in Table 3.

Of 63 isolates, only 3 isolates (4.8%) were pan-sensitive and the rest were single drug resistance (12 isolates; 20.4%), double drug resistance (19; 30.2%) and multidrug (≥3 or more drugs) resistance (29; 46.0%). Two isolates demonstrated resistance to six different drugs. The AMR patterns and AMR frequencies were shown in Table 4. The most common AMR pattern found in the multiresistant isolates was ampicillin, tetracycline and erythromycin which jeopardizes the use of these drugs in the study area.

Molecular detection of antimicrobial resistance

All of the 63 *E. coli* isolates were confirmed by PCR to determine the existence of any AMR gene. The erythromycin esterase gene *ere*(*A*) and the aminoglycoside adenylyl transferases genes *aadA1* were not identified in any of the 63 *E. coli* isolates (Fig. 1). The *ere*(A) gene confers resistance to erythromycin whilst aadA1 gene confer resistance to streptomycin. The most commonly detected AMR genes were *blaCMY* (65.1%), *tetA* (65.1%) and *sul1* (54.0%). The distribution of resistance genes among *E. coli* isolates are summarized in Table 5. The bla_{SHV}, β-lactamase gene and bla_{CMY} genes were identified in 4.8 and 65.1% of the isolates, respectively. The *aac*(*3*)-*IV* gene which codes resistance against gentamycin was found also in 14.3% of isolates.

Overall, 39.7% (25/63) of isolates harbored resistance gene responsible to three or more drugs (Table 6). The most commonly detected genes were *tetA*, sul1, and bla_{CMY}. The most common pattern detected was *sulI* and *tet*(*A*) together (n = 23; 36.5%) followed by bla_{CMY} and *tetA* (n = 22; 35.0%) and bla_{CMY} and *sulI* (n = 20; 31.7%).

Relationship between drug resistance by disc diffusion and PCR methods

The most commonly drugs to which isolates demonstrated resistance by disk diffusion method were

Table 3 Antimicrobial sensitivity test of *E. coli* isolates (n = 63) sampled from meat of different livestock species

	E	AMP	GN	S	TE	Sxt	C
Beef (n = 4)							
R (%)	0	2 (50.0)	0	2 (50.0)	2 (50.0)	1 (25.0)	1 (25.0)
I (%)	2 (50.0)	1 (25.0)	0	1 (25.0)	0	0	1 (25.0)
S (%)	2 (50.0)	1 (25.0)	4 (100)	1 (25.0)	2 (50.0)	3 (75)	2 (50.0)
Mutton (n = 17)							
R (%)	9 (53.0)	11 (64.7)	2 (11.8)	7 (41.2)	4 (23.5)	3 (17.6)	2 (11.8)
I (%)	7 (41.2)	3 (17.6)	1 (5.9)	3 (17.6)	2 (11.8)	3 (17.6)	3 (17.6)
S (%)	1 (5.9)	3 (17.6)	14 (82.3)	7 (41.2)	11 (64.7)	11 (64.7)	12 (70.6)
Chevon (n = 15)							
R (%)	7 (46.7)	13 (86.7)	1 (6.7)	1 (6.7)	3 (20)	1 (6.7)	1 (6.7)
I (%)	8 (53.3)	0	1 (6.7)	5 (33.3)	2 (13.3)	2 (13.3)	0
S (%)	0	2 (13.3)	13 (86.7)	9 (60)	10 (66.7)	12 (80.0)	14 (93.3)
Chicken (n = 27)							
R (%)	11 (40.7)	19 (70.4)	0	13 (48.1)	21 (77.8)	17 (63.0)	11 (40.7)
I (%)	10 (37.0)	3 (11.1)	7 (26.0)	6 (22.2)	4 (14.8)	3 (11.0)	5 (18.5)
S (%)	6 (22.2)	5 (18.5)	20 (74.0)	8 (29.6)	2 (7.4)	7 (26.0)	11(40.7)
Overall							
R (%)	27 (42.9)	45 (71.4)	3 (4.8)	23 (36.5)	30 (47.6)	22 (34.9)	15 (23.8)
I (%)	27 (42.9)	7 (11.1)	9 (14.3)	15 (23.8)	8 (12.7)	8 (12.7)	9 (14.3)
S (%)	9 (14.3)	11 (17.5)	51 (81.0)	25 (39.7)	25 (39.7)	33 (52.4)	39 (61.9)

S sensitive, *I* intermediate, *R* resistant, *E* erythromycin, *AMP* ampicillin, *GN* gentamycin, *S* streptomycin, *TE* tetracycline, *Sxt* sulfamethoxazole–trimethoprim, *C* chloramphenicol

Table 4 Antimicrobial resistance pattern of *E. coli* isolates from meat samples of different livestock species

Number of antibiotic classes (number of isolates; %)	AMR pattern	Number of isolates (%)
No resistance		3 (4.7)
One (n = 13; 20.6%)	AMP	10 (15.9)
	E	1 (1.6)
	TE	1 (1.6)
	C	1 (1.6)
Two (n = 19; 30.2%)	AMP*C	1 (1.6)
	AMP*S	1 (1.6)
	AMP*Sxt	1 (1.6)
	AMP*TE	4 (6.3)
	E*AMP	6 (9.5)
	E*S	1 (1.6)
	E*TE	3 (4.8)
	TE*Sxt	1 (1.6)
Three (n = 11; 17.5%)	AMP*Sxt*C	1 (1.6)
	AMP*TE*C	1 (1.6)
	AMP*TE*Sxt	3 (4.8)
	E*AMP*S	1 (1.6)
	E*AMP*Sxt	1 (1.6)
	S*Sxt*C	1 (1.6)
	S*TE*Sxt	3 (4.8)
Four (n = 9; 14.3%)	AMP*S*TE*C	1 (1.6)
	AMP*S*TE*Sxt	1 (1.6)
	E*AMP*GN*S	3 (4.8)
	E*AMP*S*TE	2 (3.4)
	E*AMP*Sxt*C	1 (1.6)
	E*AMP*TE*C	1 (1.6)
Five (n = 7; 11.1%)	AMP*S*TE*Sxt*C	2 (3.4)
	E*AMP*S*TE*Sxt	2 (3.4)
	E*S*TE*Sxt*C	3 (4.8)
Six (n = 2; 3.2%)	E*AMP*S*TE*Sxt*C	2 (3.4)

E erythromycin, *AMP* ampicillin, *GN* gentamicin, *S* streptomycin, *TE* tetracycline, *Sxt* sulfamethoxazole–trimethoprim, *C* chloramphenicol

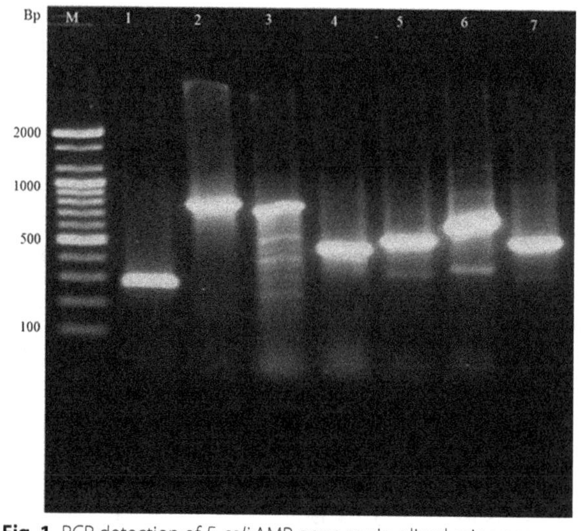

Fig. 1 PCR detection of *E. coli* AMR gene as visualized using agarose gel electrophoresis. *Bp* base pair, *M* molecular weight standard, *lane 1 aac(3)-IV* (286 Bp), *lane 2 sul1* (822 Bp), *lane 3* bla_{SHV} (768 Bp), *lane 4* bla_{CMY} (462 Bp), *lane 5 catA1* (547 Bp), *lane 6 cmlA* (698 Bp), *lane 7 tet(A)* (577 Bp)

consistent with the most common resistance genes detected (Table 7). Tetracycline, sulfamethoxazole and chloramphenicol were top three drugs recognized as being the most common for resistance measured either disk diffusion or molecular method. However, the phenotypic and genotypic resistance characterization of the isolates to erythromycin, streptomycin and gentamycin were not correlated.

Discussion

The magnitude of *E. coli* prevalence and its AMR patterns were investigated in raw meat samples of four livestock species at Addis Ababa and Bishoftu slaughter house. In our study, in raw meat, the prevalence of *E. coli* was 21.6%. The study indicated that *E. coli* was 2.8 times, 3.2 times, and 5.7 times more prevalent in chevon, mutton and chicken meat, respectively, than in beef meat. It implies that meat of livestock species types has a difference in magnitude of *E. coli* infection, therefore, has implications on the risk to public health. It has been reported that poor hygienic practices is responsible for contamination of meat by *E. coli* [20]. The magnitude of *E. coli* prevalence in this study was similar to the previous studies in different part of Ethiopia 22.2, 26.6 and 20.3% by Haileselassie et al. [21], Haimanot et al. [22] and Bitew et al. [23] respectively. However, Mekonen et al. [24] and Taye et al. [25] also reported higher prevalence of carcass contamination with an overall isolation rate of 40 and 30.97%, respectively. The current study deals with the magnitude of *E. coli* only at one point (i.e. slaughterhouse) of the food chain until it reaches the fork. It shouldn't be overlooked that there could be ample chances for *E. coli* to infect the meat released from the slaughterhouse during transport, handling and processing chains before it reaches the consumer (fork) as hygienic practices are substandard in Ethiopia. It has been reported that poor hygienic practices is responsible for contamination of meat by *E. coli* [20].

In the current study, the prevalence of *E. coli* was significantly higher in chicken meat than in chevon, mutton and beef meat. This might be attributed to husbandry and production systems where, small holder farmers prefer to rear their chickens in backyard to scavenge. Thus, *E. coli* could be transmitted from intestinal normal flora of

Table 5 Distribution of AMR genes in *E. coli* isolates (n = 63) using PCR test

Meat type	Number of isolates with AMR gene (%)								
	aadA1	*aac(3)-IV*	*sul1*	*bla*$_{SHV}$	*bla*$_{CMY}$	*ere*(A)	*catA1*	*cmlA*	*tet*(A)
Beef (n = 4)	0	0	1 (25.0)	0	0	0	1 (25.0)	0	0
Mutton (n = 17)	0	0	5 (29.4)	0	11 (64.7)	0	1 (5.9)	0	11 (64.7)
Chevon (n = 15)	0	1 (6.7)	9 (60.0)	0	14 (93.3)	0	0	0	5 (33.3)
Chicken (n = 27)	0	8 (29.6)	19 (70.4)	3 (11.1)	16 (59.2)	0	3 (11.1)	7 (26.0)	25 (92.6)
Total	0	9 (14.3)	34 (54.0)	3 (4.8)	41 (65.1)	0	5 (8.0)	7 (11.1)	41 (65.1)

aadA1 streptomycin, *aac(3)-IV* gentamicin, *sul1* sulfonamide, *bla*$_{SHV}$ and *bla*$_{CMY}$ beta lactams, *ere(A)* erythromycin, *catA1* and *cmlA* chloramphenicol, *tet(A)* tetracycline

livestock to the chicken via the food chain [26]. Over all, the variations observed among the reported prevalence could be emanated from difference in hygiene, breed, geographical origins of animals and history of treatment with antimicrobial.

Emergence and dissemination of antimicrobial resistance is on the increase trend among enteric bacteria [27]. In this research the overall result showed that significantly high resistance rate to ampicillin (71.4%) and tetracycline (47.6%). More importantly, in the current report, chicken meat harbored the highest number of drug resistant *E. coli* isolates compared to the other meat origins. As expected, the most common resistance were found to older drugs such as ampicillin (Introduced in 1961) followed by tetracycline (Introduced in 1948) [28]. Similarly, Momtaz et al. [29] observed that tetracycline, sulfamethoxazole, chloramphenicol and trimethoprim resistance was the most common finding with the prevalence rate of 91.2, 45.6 and 29.8% respectively. Likewise, studies conducted in Korem, Ethiopia on diarrheic patients showed that the highest *E. coli* resistance were found against ampicillin followed by chloramphenicol, and tetracycline [30]. Hiko et al. [31] also found that the isolated *E. coli* is highly resistant to streptomycin, cephlaothin, tetracycline, ampicillin and trimethoprim. Another study revealed that all *E. coli* isolates from beef were found 100% resistance to ampicillin and amoxicillin and 33.33% to tetracycline [25]. The observed higher level of antimicrobial resistance might be attributed to the widespread and indiscriminate use of antibiotics in animals for medication and other prophylaxis purposes. Although tetracycline has the second most resistance in this study, it is one of the most commonly used antibiotics for the treatment of different infections, including *E. coli* in Ethiopia.

Recently, among gram negative bacteria, multidrug resistant (MDR) phenotypes are spreading widely [32]. In the current study, the overall rate of multiple drug resistance was 46.0% and only 4.8% of the isolates were found sensitive to all antimicrobials tested (Table 4). This is in agreement with the findings of Schroeder et al. [33]

Table 6 Multiple antimicrobial resistance gene patterns of *E. coli* isolates

Number of AMR gene (%)	Resistance gene patterns	Number of isolates (%)
No resistance		7 (11.1)
One (n = 11; 17.5%)	*bla*$_{CMY}$	6 (9.5)
	tet(A)	3 (4.7)
	sul1	1 (1.6)
	catA1	1 (1.6)
Two (n = 20; 31.8%)	*aac(3)-IV* * *bla*$_{CMY}$	1 (1.6)
	aac(3)-IV * *tet*(A)	1 (1.6)
	cmlA * *tet*(A)	1 (1.6)
	bla$_{CMY}$ * *tet*(A)	7 (11.1)
	*sul1** *bla*$_{CMY}$	5 (7.9)
	*sul1** *catA1*	1 (1.6)
	*sul1** *tet*(A)	4 (6.3)
Three (n = 15; 23.8%)	*sul1** *bla*$_{CMY}$ * *tet*(A)	10 (15.9)
	*sul1** *cmlA* * *tet*(A)	2 (3.2)
	aac(3)-IV * *sul1** *tet*(A)	1 (1.6)
	bla$_{CMY}$ * *cmlA* * *tet*(A)	1 (1.6)
	bla$_{CMY}$ * *catA1** *tet*(A)	1 (1.6)
Four (n = 6; 9.5%)	*sul1** *bla*$_{CMY}$ * *catA1** *tet*(A)	2 (3.2)
	aac(3)-IV * *sul1** *bla*$_{CMY}$ * *tet*(A)	2 (3.2)
	*sul1** *bla*$_{CMY}$ * *cmlA* * *tet*(A)	1 (1.6)
	sul1 * *bla*$_{SHV}$ * *bla*$_{CMY}$ * *tet*(A)	1 (1.6)
Five (n = 4; 6.3%)	*aac(3)-IV* * *sul1** *bla*$_{CMY}$ * *cmlA* * *tet*(A)	2 (3.2)
	aac(3)-IV * *sul1** *bla*$_{SHV}$ **bla*$_{CMY}$* *tet*(A)	2 (3.2)

aadA1 streptomycin, *aac(3)-IV* gentamicin, *sul1* sulfonamide, *bla*$_{SHV}$ and *bla*$_{CMY}$ beta lactams, *ere(A)* erythromycin, *catA1* and *cmlA* chloramphenicol, *tet(A)* tetracycline

and Zhao et al. [34] from USA that reported that multiple resistance to tetracycline, kanamycin, streptomycin, ampicillin, and sulfamethoxazole. Similarly, among sulfonamide resistant *E. coli* isolates, Wu et al. [35] reported that ampicillin and streptomycin are the two

Table 7 Agreement between the two tests on resistance isolate detection from the 63 isolates tested

Antimicrobial resistance isolates (%)	Resistance gene detected (%)	Agreement (%)
Erythromycin (n = 27; 42.8)	*ere(A)* (n = 0)	0
Gentamicin (n = 3; 4.8)	*aac(3)-IV* (n = 9; 14.3)	0
Streptomycin (n = 23; 36.5)	*aadA1* (n = 0)	0
Tetracycline (n = 30; 47.6)	*tet(A)* (n = 41; 65.1)	23 (76.7)
Sulfamethoxazole–trimethoprim (n = 22; 34.9)	*sul1* (n = 34; 54.0)	14 (63.6)
Chloramphenicol (n = 15; 23.8)	*catA1* (n = 5; 8.0)	2 (13.3)
	cmlA (n = 7; 11.1)	4 (26.7)

most frequently co-transferred resistance phenotypes. However, Daniel et al. [28] reported a resistance profile of tetracycline (80%) and streptomycin (74%), among the sulfonamide-resistant *E. coli* isolates. The transfer of resistance among microorganisms has long been recognized as a serious threat, contributing to the evolution and emergence of antibiotic resistant bacteria, thereby reducing the therapeutic potential against pathogens [36].

After phenotypic screening, genes associated with antimicrobial resistance was analyzed using PCR. In this study, the most commonly detected resistance genes were *blaCMY* (65.1%), *tetA* (65.1%) and *sul1* (54.0%)) for cephalosporin, tetracycline and sulfonamide respectively. However, streptomycin and erythromycin resistance genes were not detected. In Iran, among the *E. coli* isolates, 52.6% of resistance to tetracycline as well as 47.4% for both sulfonamides and erythromycin was reported [31]. The prevalence of different resistance genes from pediatric patient *E. coli* isolate were also reported 85.06, 60.38, 57.79, 90.25, 40.25 and 54.54% positive for *tetA*, *cmlA*, *SHV β-lactamase*, *CITM*, *sul1* and *aac(3)-IV* resistance genes respectively [37].

The phenotypic and genotypic resistance patterns with in the same *E. coli* isolates might be strongly correlated [38]. In our research, detection of tetracycline resistance by disk diffusion test and identification of its resistance gene *tet(A)* by PCR test, sulfamethoxozole–trimethoprim and *sulI*, chloramphenicol and *cmlA* were strongly associated. But there was a lack of association between phenotypic erythromycin resistance and molecular detection of *ere(A)*, streptomycin and *aadA1*, chloramphenicol and *catA1* resistance gene. Similarly, reports from Thailand showed that, *E. coli* isolates from chickens were found to be resistant to tetracycline (90%) and erythromycin (73.3%) in Agar disk diffusion assays and these resistance properties were associated with *tet*(A) and *ere*(A) resistance genes respectively [4]. However, the presence of resistance phenotypes might not represent all the underlying resistance genes. Alternatively, the presence or absence of a resistance gene might not indicate the particular isolate is resistant or susceptible to an antimicrobial [39].

The observed discrepancy in the resistance level of genotypes and phenotypes might be attributed to either of or combination of the reasons including but not limited to the presence of unexpressed genes in the bacterial isolates, not containing the possible resistance genes in the test, use of incorrect cut points of test results used for resistance and susceptibility classification, or some of resistance phenotypes are caused by due to point mutations rather than gene transfer or acquisition [40].

Conclusions

This study revealed that raw meat available for consumers in Ethiopia was often contaminated with *E. coli*. We reported on a comprehensive study of the phenotypic and molecular basis for Multi Drug Resistance (MDR) in meat *E. coli* isolates recovered from Ethiopian Abattoir. Furthermore, a high rate of resistance to Ampicillin and resistance to more than one class of antibiotics among *E. coli* isolates was found. Additionally, several strains were found positive for the bla_{CMY}, *tet(A)*, and *sul1* antimicrobial resistance genes. All these findings suggest that the consumption of undercooked meat or food cross-contaminated with *E. coli* may pose a serious threat to consumer health.

Abbreviations

AMR: antimicrobial resistance; MDR: multidrug resistance; *aadA1*: streptomycin resistance gene; *tet(A)*: tetracycline resistance gene; *aac(3)-IV*: gentamycin resistance gene; *sulI*: sulphanamide resistance gene; *blaSHV*: betalactam resistance gene (pencillin); *blaCMY*: betalactam resistance gene (cephalosporin); *ere(A)*: erythromycin resistance gene; *catA1*: chloramphenicol resistance gene; *cmlA*: chloramphenicol resistance gene; PCR: polymerase chain reaction; $MgCl_2$: magnesium chloride; dNTP: deoxynucleotide tri phosphate; UV: ultra violet; Bp: base pair; OR: odds ratio; DNA: deoxynucleic acid; SPSS: statistical package for social science; χ2: Pearson chi square; P value: predictive value; R: resistance; I: intermediate; S: susceptible; E: erythromycin; Amp: ampicillin; GN: gentamycin; S: streptomycin; TE: tetracycline; Sxt: sulfamethoxazole–trimethoprim; C: chloramphenicol; ISO: International Organization for Standardization; CLIS: Clinical and Laboratory Standards Institute.

Authors' contributions

The research idea and study design was developed by YEM and GMW. Sample collection were done by YEM, STY, DTT and BAE. YEM supervised the study. YEM and RDA provided valuable information on data analysis and manuscript writing. All authors read and approved the final manuscript.

Author details

[1] Ethiopian Institute of Agricultural Research, National Agricultural Biotechnology Research Center, P.O.Box 31, Holeta, Ethiopia. [2] College of Veterinary Medicine and Agriculture, Addis Ababa University, P.O.Box 34, Bishoftu, Ethiopia. [3] University of Tennessee Institute of Agriculture Department of Animal Science, Rivers Drive, Knoxville, TN, USA.

Acknowledgements

I greatly appreciate the contribution made by the Ethiopian National Agricultural Biotechnology Research Center in funding this project and the staff of the Animal Biotechnology Laboratory, for assisting during the bench work which has led to the success of this work.

Competing interests

The authors declare that they have no competing interests.

Consent to publish

Not applicable.

References

1. Laury A, Echeverry A, Brashears M. Fate of *Escherichia coli* O157:H7 in meat Chapter 2. In: Toldra F, editor. Safety of meat and processed meat. New York: Springer; 2009. p. 31–53.
2. Pradel N, Livrelli V, De Champs C, Palcoux JB, Reynaud A, Scheutz F, et al. Prevalence and characterization of Shiga toxin producing *Escherichia coli* isolated from cattle, food, and children during a one-year prospective study in France. J Clin Microbiol. 2000;38:1023–31.
3. Molbak K. Spread of resistant bacteria and resistance genes from animals to humans, the public health consequences. J Vet Med. 2004;51:364–9.
4. Mooljuntee S, Chansiripornchai P, Chansiripornchai N. Prevalence of the cellular and molecular antimicrobial resistance against E. coli isolated from Thai broilers. Thai J Vet Med. 2010;40:311–5.
5. Lindsey RL, Frye SN, Thitaram RJ, Meinersmann PJ. Fedorka-Cray, Englen MD. Characterization of multidrug-resistant *Escherichia coli* by antimicrobial resistance profiles, plasmid replicon typing, and pulsed-field gel electrophoresis. Microb Drug Resist. 2011;17:157–63.
6. Frye JG, Jackson CR. Genetic mechanisms of antimicrobial resistance identified in *Salmonella enterica*, *Escherichia coli*, and *Enterococcus* spp. Isolated from U.S. food animals. Front Microbiol. 2013;4:135.
7. Van den Bogaard AE, Stobberingh EE. Epidemiology of resistance to antibiotics. Links between animals and humans. Int J Antimicrob Agents. 2000;14:327–35.
8. Alemu T, Eyasu M, Solomon G, Tenaw A, Yilkal A. Literature review on infectious diseases, antimicrobial use, resistance and containment. In: Antimicrobial use, resistance, and containment baseline survey syntheses of findings. Drug administration and control authority of ethiopia in collaboration with management sciences for health, strengthening pharmaceutical systems; 2009. p. 37–42.
9. Beyene T, Endalamaw D, Tolossa Y, Feyisa A. Evaluation of rational use of veterinary drugs especially antimicrobials and anthelmintics in Bishoiu, Central Ethiopia. BMC Res Notes. 2015;8:482.
10. International Organization for Standardization (ISO). Microbiology of food and animal feeding stuffs carcass sampling for microbiological analysis. Geneva: International Organization for Standardization; 2013.
11. Hitchins AD, Feng P, Watkins WD, Rippey SR, Chandler LA. *Escherichia coli* and the coliform bacteria. In: U.S. Food and Drug Administration, editor. Bacteriological analytical manual. Gaithersburg: AOAC International; 1998. p. 401–29.
12. Clinical and Laboratory Standards Institute (CLIS). Performance standards for antimicrobial susceptibility testing; twenty-second informational supplement. Wayne: M100-S21, CLS; 2012.
13. Walker RD. Antimicrobial susceptibility testing and interpretation of results. Antimicrobial therapy in veterinary medicine. Ames: RD Walker Iowa State Press, 2000. p. 12–26.
14. Bauer A, Kirby W, Sherris J, Turck M. Antibiotic susceptibility testing by a standardized single disk method. Am J Clin Pathol. 1966;45(4):493–6.
15. Reischl U, Youssef M, Kilwinski J, Lehn N, Zhang W, Karch H, et al. Real-time fluorescence PCR assays for detection and characterization of Shiga toxin, intimin, and enterohemolysin genes from Shiga toxin-producing *Escherichia coli*. J Clin Microbiol. 2002;40:2555–65.
16. Fode-Vaughan K, Maki J, Benson J, Collins M. Direct PCR detection of *Escherichia coli* O157:H7. Lett Appl Microbiol. 2003;37:239–43.
17. Huang Q, Baum L, Fu W. Simple and practical staining of DNA with gel red in agarose gel electrophoresis. Clin Lab. 2010;56(3–4):149–52.
18. Van TT, Chin J, Chapman T, Tran LT, Coloe PJ. Safety of raw meat and shellfish in Vietnam: an analysis of Escherichia coli isolations for antibiotic resistance and virulence genes. Int J Food Microbiol. 2008;124:217–23.
19. Randall LP, Cooles SW, Osborn MK, Piddock LJ, Woodward MJ. Antibiotic resistance genes, integrons and multiple antibiotic resistance in thirty-five serotypes of *Salmonella enterica* isolated from humans and animals in the UK. J Antimicrob Chemother. 2004;53:208–16.
20. Vahedi M, Nasrolahei M, Sharif M, Mirabi A. Bacteriological study of raw and unexpired pasteurized cow's milk collected at the dairy farms and super markets in Sari City in 2011. J Prev Med Hyg. 2013;54:120–3.
21. Haileselassie M, Taddele H, Adhana K. Source(s) of contamination of 'raw' and 'ready-to-eat' foods and their public health risks in Mekelle City, Ethiopia. J Food Agric Sci. 2012;2(2):20–9.
22. Haimanot T, Alemseged A, Getnet B, Solomon G. Microbial flora and food-borne pathogens on minced meat and their susceptibility to antimicrobial agents. Ethiop J Health Sci. 2010;20(3):137–43.
23. Bitew M, Tafere A, Tolosa T. Study on bovine mastitis in dairy farms of Bahir Dar town and its environment. J Anim Vet Adv. 2010;9:2912–7.
24. Mekonnen H, Habtamu T, Kelali A, Shewit K. Food safety knowledge and practices of abattoir and butchery shops and the microbial profile of meat in Mekelle city, Ethiopia. Asian Pac J Trop Biomed. 2013;3(5):407–12.
25. Taye M, Berhanu T, Berhanu Y, Tamiru F, Terefe D. Study on carcass contaminating *Escherichia coli* in apparently healthy slaughtered cattle in Haramaya University slaughter house with special emphasis on *Escherichia coli* O157:H7, Ethiopia. J Vet Sci Technol. 2013;4:132.
26. Ming-Cheng L, Fang W, Fan L. Identification and molecular characterization of antimicrobial-resistant shiga toxin-producing *Escherichia coli* isolated from retail meat products. Foodborne Pathog Dis. 2011;8(4):489–93.
27. Sawant AA, Hegde NV, Straley BA, Donaldson SC, Love BC, Knabel SJ, et al. Antimicrobial-resistant enteric bacteria from dairy cattle. Appl Environ Microbiol. 2007;73:156–63.
28. Daniel A, Shaohua Z, Emily T, Sherry A, Aparna S, Mary J, et al. Antimicrobial drug resistance in *Escherichia coli* from humans and food animals, united states, 1950–2002. Emer Infect Dis. 2012;18(5):741–9.
29. Momtaz H, Rahimi E, Moshkelani S. Molecular detection of antimicrobial resistance genes in *E. coli* isolated from slaughtered commercial chickens in Iran. Vet Med. 2012;57(4):193–7.
30. Meng J, Zhao S, Doyle M, Joseph S. Antibiotic resistance of *Escherichia coli* O157:H7 and O157: NM isolated from animals, food, and humans. J Food Prot. 1998;61:1511–4.
31. Hiko A, Daniel A, Girma Z. Occurrence of *Escherichia coli* O157:H7 in retail raw meat products in Ethiopia. Infect Dev Ctries. 2008;2(5):389–93.
32. Higgins CF. Multiple molecular mechanisms for multidrug resistance transporters. Nature. 2007;446:749–57.
33. Schroeder CM, Zhao C, DebRoy C, Torcolini J, Zhao S, White DG, et al. Antimicrobial resistance of *Escherichia coli* O157 isolated from humans, cattle, swine, and food antimicrobial resistance of *Escherichia coli* O157 isolated from humans, cattle, swine, and food. Appl Environ Microbiol. 2002;68:576–81.
34. Zhao S, White DG, Ge B, Ayers S, Friedman S, English L, et al. Identification and characterization of integron mediated antibiotic resistance among shiga toxin-producing *Escherichia coli* isolates. Appl Environ Microbiol. 2001;67:1558–64.
35. Wu S, Dalsgaard A, Hammerum A, Porsbo L, Jensen L. Prevalence and characterization of plasmids carrying sulfonamide resistance genes

among *Escherichia coli* from pigs, pig carcasses and human. Acta Vet Scand. 2010;52:47.

36. Hawkey P, Jones A. The changing epidemiology of resistance. J Antimicrobial Chemother Suppl. 2009;1:3–10.
37. Maryam H, Hassan M, Mahboobeh M. Characterization of diarrheagenic antimicrobial resistant *Escherichia coli* isolated from pediatric patients in Tehran, Iran. Red Crescent Med J. 2014;16(4):e12329.
38. Shaw K, Hare R, Sabatelli F, Rizzo M, Cramer C, Naples L, et al. Correlation between aminoglycoside resistance profiles and DNA hybridization of clinical isolates. Antimicrob Agents Chemother. 1991;35:2253–61.
39. Aarts, H, Guerra B, Malorny B. Molecular methods for detection of antimicrobial resistance in antimicrobial resistance in bacteria of animal origin F. Aarestrup M, editor. Washington DC: ASM press; 2006. p. 37–48.
40. Blake D, Humphry R, Scott K, Hillman K, Fenlon D, Low J. Influence of tetracycline exposure on tetracycline resistance and the carriage of tetracycline resistance genes within commensal *Escherichia coli* populations. J App Microbiol. 2003;94:1087–97.

Impact of the use of local fidaxomicin treatment algorithms for managing *Clostridium difficile* infection in hospitalized patients in southeastern United States

Jonathan C. Cho[1*], Sandy J. Estrada[2], Jamie J. Kisgen[3], Angelina Davis[4] and Laura Puzniak[5]

Abstract

Background: *Clostridium difficile*-associated diarrhea (CDAD) is a major public health threat that results in increased length of stay, hospital readmissions, deaths, and economic burden. CDAD treatment is often guided by severity of disease. Although various tools exist to determine CDAD severity, real-world data evaluating the use of such tools in treatment algorithms are sparse.

Methods: A local CDAD treatment pathway was developed independently to guide fidaxomicin prescribing at wellStar Health System (WellStar) and at Lee Health (LH) and Sarasota Memorial Hospital (SMH). Each algorithm was designed locally by the stewardship pharmacist and was utilized to identify patients at high risk for *C. difficile* recurrence. Patient and clinical data was retrospectively gathered to evaluate the utility and outcomes of the treatment pathway.

Results: There were 262 patients that received fidaxomicin at these three hospitals during the study time period. Only 30% at WellStar and 20% at LH or SMH met the study criteria and adhered to the pathway requirements. After completion of fidaxomicin, 30-day recurrence rates at WellStar was 0 and at LH and SMH 7%. Clinical cure rates were 83% in WellStar and 93% in LH and SMH.

Conclusions: The results from these two pathways show positive outcomes for the use of fidaxomicin in patients at high risk for CDAD recurrence. This data supports the potential utility of fidaxomicin against CDAD.

Background

Burden of *Clostridium difficile* infection

Diarrheal illness and complications caused by *Clostridium difficile* associated diarrhea (CDAD) constitute a substantial and increasing burden to patients and healthcare facilities in the United States (US) and throughout the world. In the US, it has been estimated that there may be over 450,000 incident infections annually, with 83,000 of these being first recurrences, and over 29,000 cases leading to mortality [1]. Of these cases, approximately 100,000 cases are acquired in hospitals [2]. *C. difficile* imposes numerous burdens on resources including the need for private rooms, isolation supplies, enhanced environmental cleaning, and vigilant hand hygiene, resulting in an estimated excess cost of as much as $4.8 billion to US acute care facilities, in addition to severe negative impact on patients' quality of life [3].

Current CDAD therapies

Historically, treatments for CDAD included vancomycin and metronidazole, with the choice of therapy usually dependent on disease severity; tigecycline can also be used in cases of CDAD colitis [4]. Updated guidelines for the treatment of CDAD from the Infectious Diseases Society of America and Society for Healthcare Epidemiology of America were recently published and highlight

*Correspondence: jcho@uttyler.edu
[1] College of Pharmacy, The University of Texas at Tyler, 3900 University Blvd., Tyler, TX 75799, USA
Full list of author information is available at the end of the article

the challenges in the prevention, diagnosis and treatment management of this condition. The guidelines recommend vancomycin and fidaxomicin over metronidazole for initial non-severe and severe episodes, initial recurrence and multiple recurrences and discusses the use of risk factors to identify patients that have increased likelihood for unfavorable outcomes [5].

Increasing incidence of treatment failure with traditional agents (i.e. metronidazole and vancomycin) prompted research into and development of new molecules. Fidaxomicin, an oral macrocyclic antimicrobial that inhibits *C. difficile* growth as well as sporulation through RNA transcription inhibition, and whose narrow spectrum minimizes alterations of the colonic microbiota compared to existing agents [6], was approved for treatment of non-severe CDAD in the US in 2011. Approval followed two large randomized controlled trials that showed fidaxomicin was non-inferior to vancomycin in terms of the rate of clinical cure, but it was associated with a lower recurrence rate at 6 weeks post-treatment [7, 8]. A recent Cochrane review of 22 studies encompassing 3215 patients found that 71% (407 of 572) of fidaxomicin patients achieved symptomatic cure, compared to 61% (361 of 592) of vancomycin patients (RR 1.17, 95% CI 1.04–1.31; moderate quality evidence) [9].

CDAD treatment pathways

Despite its demonstrated efficacy and effectiveness, however, it has been difficult to precisely define fidaxomicin's place in the CDAD armamentarium, due to unclear definitions of risk factors for recurrence or severe/complicated CDAD, lack of clinical data in multiple recurrences or complicated CDAD, and high economic cost [6]. For maximum benefit in terms of both patient outcomes and economic efficiency, it may be beneficial for institutions to develop and rigorously evaluate clinical pathways that can guide selection of fidaxomicin for those patients most likely to respond best to the drug, both in regard to acute symptom relief and prevention of recurrence. This is problematic, however, in that pathway centered efforts have met with only mixed success, due to problems such as prescriber noncompliance [10]. Achievement of adequate sample size so that reliable conclusions can be drawn can also present a difficulty in conducting such research. This paper presents an evaluation of the results of two fidaxomicin-directed treatment pathways implemented in two separate healthcare systems in the southeastern United States.

Various *C. difficile* disease scoring systems exist including a disease severity measure in the IDSA guidelines [11], the ATLAS system predicting cure [12], and the D'Agostino model for predicting recurrence [13]. The ATLAS scoring tool is a validated tool that takes into account the clinical factors of age, treatment with systemic antibiotics during CDAD therapy, leukocytosis, albumin, and serum creatinine at the time of diagnosis. This tool has been shown to be useful in predicting treatment response and mortality in CDAD and has potential to be a resource for evaluating severity and determining treatment selection [14]. The D'Agostino model is a simple scoring rule, developed to help predict the risk of developing CDAD recurrence based on the clinical features of age, number of unformed bowel movements, serum creatinine, episode of CDAD, and treatment choice [13]. Due to questionable reliability of documentation of unformed bowel movements, evaluation of the D'Agostino criteria, without assessing unformed bowel movements, as risk stratification measures is warranted. Each of these tools has the potential to help guide drug therapy for *C. difficile* infections; however, there is a lack of data evaluating the implementation of these tools in a real world setting. This study describes the local implementation and outcomes associated with two different fidaxomicin treatment pathways.

Methods

A local CDAD treatment pathway was developed independently to guide fidaxomicin prescribing at WellStar Health System (WellStar) in Georgia and at Lee Health (LH) and Sarasota Memorial Hospital (SMH) in Florida. Each algorithm was designed locally by the stewardship pharmacist and was utilized to identify patients at high risk for *C. difficile* recurrence. Patient and clinical data was retrospectively gathered to evaluate the utility of the treatment pathway.

WellStar is a not-for-profit system of eleven hospitals serving NW metropolitan Atlanta. Patients with a positive *C. difficile* PCR result from clinical microbiology testing with Xpert *C. difficile*/Epi (Cepheid, Sunnyvale, CA) and a clinical diagnosis consistent with CDAD between 12/1/12 and 3/31/14 from 5 of the hospitals in the WellStar system were included in this study. Patients over age 18 were included if it was their initial episode or first recurrence of CDAD with laboratory confirmed, non NAP1 strains with less than 24 h of enteral (PO) vancomycin or parenteral (IV) or PO metronidazole and at least one of the following conditions: age > 65 with severe disease, ulcerative colitis/Crohn's disease, creatinine clearance (CrCl) < 30 mL/min or end-stage renal disease (ESRD), active malignancy, concomitant systemic antibiotic therapy, or immunocompromised status (HIV/AIDS, active chemotherapy, organ or bone marrow transplant, moderate to high-dose steroids (≥ 0.3 mg/kg/day prednisone), or immunosuppressive agents (i.e. mycophenolate, methotrexate, adalimumab, etc.).

LH is an integrated delivery network consisting of four acute care hospitals and two specialty hospitals with a total of 1423 beds in Fort Myers and Cape Coral, FL. Patients with a positive *C. difficile* result based on Xpert *C. difficile*/Epi (Cepheid, Sunnyvale, CA) were included in the study.

SMH is an 806-bed regional medical center, including a network of outpatient, long-term care, and rehabilitation centers, serving approximately 800,000 patients each year. CDAD was assessed at SMH using Xpert *C. difficile*/Epi *C. diff* Quik Chek Complete® (TECHLAB, Blacksburg, VA) with reflex PCR using Xpert *C. difficile*/Epi (Cepheid, Sunnyvale, CA).

LH and SMH evaluated the impact of a treatment pathway targeting fidaxomicin for patients based on ATLAS Score and CDAD episode between 1/5/15 and 11/2/15 (Tables 1, 2). Patients were included if they were 18 years of age or older with laboratory confirmed CDAD admitted to the hospital, with a clinical diagnosis consistent with CDAD, seen by infectious diseases (ID) service and received at least 3 days of fidaxomicin. Patients with fulminant disease, ileus, toxic megacolon, receipt of alternative CDAD therapy such as tigecycline or IVIG, greater than 24 h of metronidazole or vancomycin or had missing ATLAS score criteria were excluded.

Patients in all centers were assessed to determine adherence to pathway protocol, recurrence at 30 and 60 days, readmission and clinical cure. Recurrence was defined as a new clinical diagnosis of CDAD or receipt of new CDAD therapy after completion of initial course after 14 days from start but within 30 and 60 days post treatment cessation. Clinical cure was based on assessment of one or more of the following criteria: resolution of diarrhea (less than or equal to three unformed stools for two consecutive days) maintained throughout the treatment course and 2 days afterward or until hospital discharge, documentation of clinical resolution in the medical record, no requirement for additional CDAD therapy (including the need for a switch in CDAD therapy) on or before Day 14.

Descriptive statistics were used to describe the patient population and the outcomes among patients adhering to the treatment pathway. Continuous variables were reported as means and standard deviations. Categorical variables were reported as frequency and percent.

The institutional review board at each participating institution approved the study.

Table 1 ATLAS scoring system (Florida)

Parameter	0 points	1 point	2 points
Age (years)	<60	60–79	≥80
Treatment with systemic antibiotics for ≥1 day upon CDAD diagnosis or 48 h prior	No	–	Yes
Leukocytosis	<16,000	16,000–25,000	>25,000
Albumin (g/dL)	>3.5	2.6–3.5	≤2.5
Serum creatinine (mg/dL)	≤1.3	1.4–2	>2

Results

WellStar

There were 120 patients who received fidaxomicin at a participating WellStar institution within the study timeframe, but only 36 (30%) met inclusion/exclusion criteria.

Table 2 *Clostridium-difficile* associated diarrhea treatment pathway using ATLAS scoring (Florida)

ATLAS score	ATLAS classification	First episode	First recurrence	≥2 recurrences
0	Mild CDAD	Metronidazole 500 mg PO/IV q8h	Vancomycin 125–250 mg PO q6h	Fidaxomicin 200 mg PO BID or Vancomycin taper[b]
1				
2				
3	Moderate CDAD	Vancomycin 125–250 mg PO q6h	Fidaxomicin 200 mg PO BID	Fidaxomicin 200 mg PO BID or Vancomycin taper[b]
4				
5	Severe CDAD	Fidaxomicin 200 mg PO BID	Fidaxomicin 200 mg PO BID	Fidaxomicin 200 mg PO BID or Vancomycin taper[b]
6				
7				
8				
9				
10				
Any	Fulminant CDAD[a]	Fidaxomicin 200 mg PO BID + Metronidazole 500 mg IV q8h	Fidaxomicin 200 mg PO BID + Metronidazole 500 mg IV q8h	(Fidaxomicin 200 mg PO BID or Vancomycin taper[b]) + Metronidazole 500 mg IV q8h

[a] CDAD in presence of hypotension/shock (SBP < 90 mmHg requiring vasopressor therapy), ileus, or toxic megacolon

[b] Vancomycin taper: vancomycin 125 mg PO q6h × 10 days, followed by vancomycin 125 mg PO q12h × 7 days, followed by vancomycin 125 mg PO q24h × 7 days, then vancomycin 125 mg PO every 3 days × 14 days

Exclusions were due to NAP1 strain (37, 31%), multiple recurrences (24, 20%), prior CDAD treatment (22, 18%), and absent/missing PCR (19, 16%) (Fig. 1). Mean age was 68.6 years (16.7 SD, range 24–91). Half of the patients were male and the majority (61%) was Caucasian. Most of the patients were admitted from the community (75%) and a small percentage had a previous hospitalization (14%) or ICU stay (8%) within the past 30 days. The patients included in the analysis had several comorbidities including moderate to severe renal disease (56%), diabetes (53%) and cardiovascular disease (47%) (Table 3).

This was the first CDAD episode for 32 (89%) of patients and the CDAD was present within 24 h of admission for 15 (42%) of the patients. Patients received an average of 8.4 ± 3.6 days of fidaxomicin. Most patients (83%) were considered clinical cure based on resolution of diarrhea (37%), clinical documentation (23%) and/or no additional CDAD treatment (50%). There were no recurrences at 30 or 60 days and there were five readmissions, but none were related to CDAD.

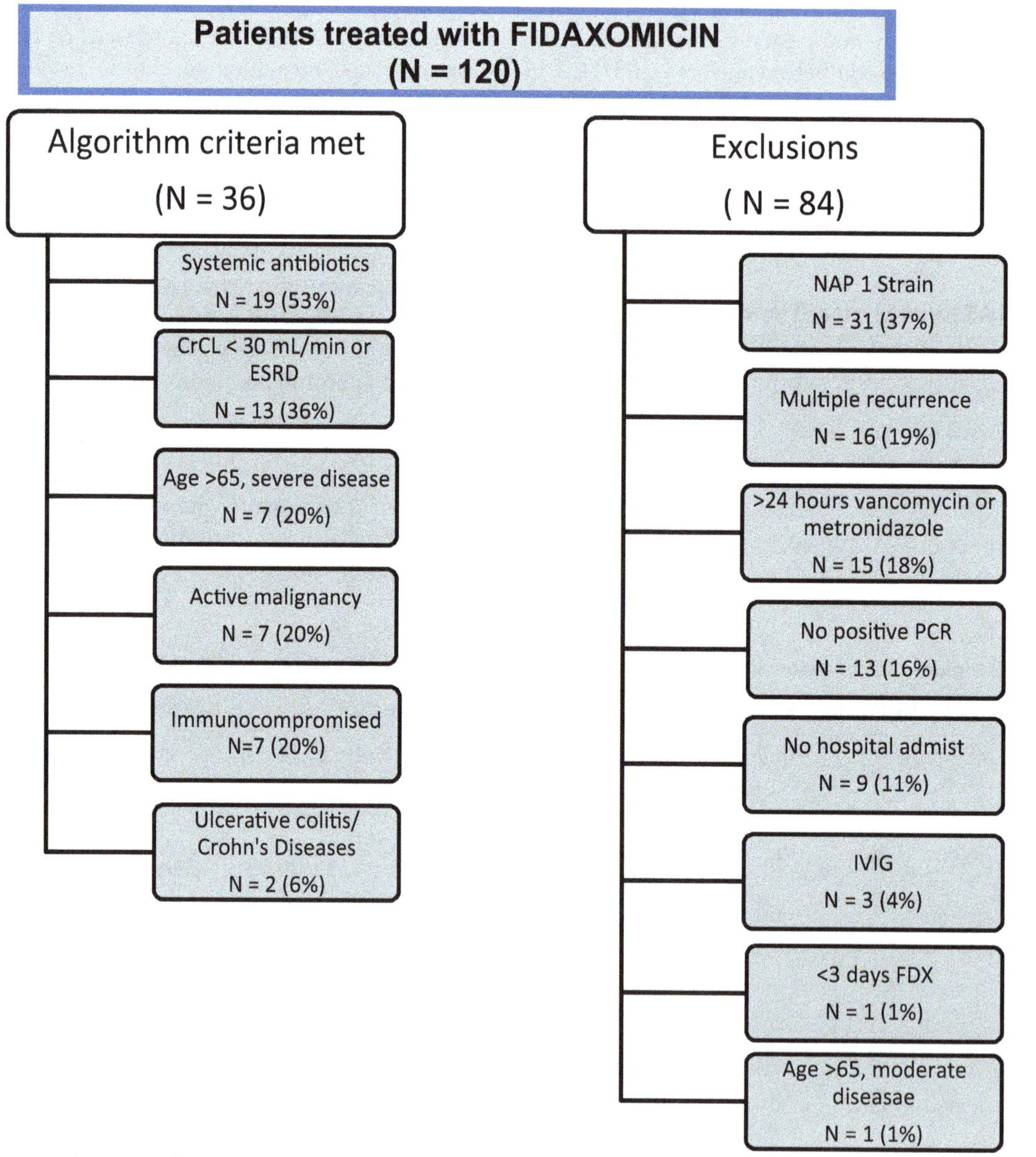

Fig. 1 Inclusion and exclusions for WellStar fidaxomicin pathway

Table 3 Patient demographics and *Clostridium difficile*-infection related outcomes

	WellStar	Florida
Patient characteristics	N=36	N=28
Age	68.6±16.7	82±10.2
Gender: Male	18 (50%)	14 (50%)
Race		
Caucasian	22 (61%)	23 (82%)
African American	5 (14%)	1 (3.0%)
Other	9 (25%)	4 (14%)
Admission source		
Community	27 (75%)	15 (57%)
Other healthcare facility	9 (25%)	12 (43%)
Previous hospitalization	5 (14%)	17 (61%)
Episode		
Initial episode	32 (89%)	20 (71%)
First recurrence	4 (11%)	6 (21%)
>2 recurrences	NA	2 (7%)
CDAD present within 24 h	15 (42%)	17 (61%)
Top comorbidities		
Moderate to severe renal disease	20 (56%)	6 (18%)
Diabetes	19 (53%)	9 (27%)
Cardiovascular disease	17 (47%)	15 (54%)
Fidaxomicin treatment (days)	8.4±3.6	7.9±5.2
Outcomes		
Pathway adherence	36/120 (30%)	28/142 (20%)
Recurrence 30 day	0	2 (7%)
Recurrence 60 day	0	3 (9.7%)
Readmission	5 (14%)	6 (21%)
Readmission related to CDAD	0	3 (50%)
Clinical cure	30 (83%)	26 (93%)

Florida

There were 142 patients who received fidaxomicin during the study period, but only 28 (20%) met study criteria. Patients were excluded due to receiving greater than 24 h of vancomycin or metronidazole (57, 40%), not meeting ATLAS pathway criteria (31, 22%), receiving less than 3 days of fidaxomicin (11, 8%), no ID consult (6, 4%), or having fulminant disease (6, 4%). Of the eligible patient population, the average age was 82 years (10.2 SD, range 57–100). Half were male and the majority was Caucasian (23, 82%). Many were admitted from another care facility (12, 43%) and the majority had a previous hospitalization (17, 61%). The patients included had several comorbidities including cardiovascular disease (54%), diabetes (27%) and moderate to severe renal disease (18%). The majority (26, 93%) of patients had an ATLAS score ≥ 5.

This was the first episode for 20 (71%) and the majority (17, 61%) had CDAD within 24 h of admission. Patients received an average of 7.9±5.2 days of fidaxomicin. Most patients (26, 93%) were considered to have a clinical cure, and two (6%) had recurrence at 30 days. Six (19%) patients were readmitted within 30 days, of whom three (50%) were related to CDAD. All three of these patients had at least one previous CDAD episode prior to the index event.

Discussion

The results from these two pathways show positive outcomes for the use of fidaxomicin in patients at high risk for CDAD recurrence. This data supports the benefits of fidaxomicin against CDAD. Although these two pathways used different criteria to identify patients at high risk, most of the patients included were older and had multiple comorbidities. Most patients presented with an initial CDAD episode (89% in WellStar, 71% in Florida) and first CDAD recurrent episodes (11%, 21%) and resulted in similar known recurrence rates [7, 15]. After completion of treatment, 30-day recurrence rates in the Florida pathway (7%) were similar to recurrence rates of studies that compared fidaxomicin to vancomycin [8] whereas the WellStar pathway resulted in no recurrent episodes. Clinical cure rates remained high in both pathways, 83% in WellStar and 93% in Florida.

These results are consistent with that of other CDAD studies [7, 15]. *C. difficile*-infection has become more prevalent and is a leading cause of morbidity and mortality in hospitalized patients [1, 15–18]. Due to its increased prevalence, there are significant financial burdens associated with the management of CDAD. These financial burdens are attributed to increases in treatment failures, recurrent disease and emergence of a hypervirulent strain [17, 19, 20]. Recurrent CDAD causes significantly increased mortality when compared to primary CDAD and can range from 20% from an initial episode to 60% after multiple recurrences [15, 16]. In order to decrease the burden of CDAD, alterations in current standards of treatment are necessary.

A limitation to these studies was poor adherence or exclusions to the CDAD treatment pathways (30%, 20%), which resulted in a smaller than expected sample size. In addition, these are retrospective studies and data is limited to what is collected in the normal course of care and entered into the patient's clinical record. Nonetheless, these pathways allowed for evaluation of fidaxomicin use and demonstrate the difficulties of adherence and evaluation of institution-specific pathways across multiple institutions. CDAD scoring tools can aid in identifying severity of disease and allow for modification of treatment regimens to optimize patient outcomes.

Authors' contributions
All authors have contributed in full capacity to this research and manuscript. All authors read and approved the final manuscript.

Author details
[1] College of Pharmacy, The University of Texas at Tyler, 3900 University Blvd., Tyler, TX 75799, USA. [2] Clinical Affairs, T2 Biosystems, Inc., Lexington, MA, USA. [3] Department of Pharmacy, Sarasota Memorial Health Care System, Sarasota, FL, USA. [4] Department of Pharmacy, WellStar Cobb Hospital, WellStar Health System, Austell, GA, USA. [5] Merck & Co., Inc., Kenilworth, NJ, USA.

Acknowledgements
Not applicable.

Previous presentations A portion of the data reported here was presented at ASM New Orleans, LA #265 June, 2017.

Competing interests
JCC serves on the speakers bureau for Allergan. SJE has received research funding from The Medicines Company and Theravance; served as a consultant for Astellas, CutisPharma, Theravance, and The Medicines Company; and served on speakers' bureaus for Allergan, Astellas, Merck, T2Biosystems and The Medicines Company.

Consent for publication
All authors have consented for publication.

Funding
No funding reported.

References

1. Lessa FC, Mu Y, Bamberg WM, et al. Burden of *Clostridium difficile* infection in the United States. N Engl J Med. 2015;372:825–34.
2. Stites SD, Cooblall CA, Aronovits J, Singletary SB, Micklow K, Sjeime M. The tipping point: patients predisposed to *Clostridium difficile* infection and a hospital antimicrobial stewardship programme. J Hosp Infect. 2016;94:242–8.
3. Dubberke ER, Butler AM, Reske KA, et al. Attributable outcomes of endemic *Clostridium difficile*-associated disease in nonsurgical patients. Emerg Infect Dis. 2008;14:1031–8.
4. Cunha BA. Antibiotic essentials. 12th ed. Burlington: Jones and Bartlett Learning; 2013.
5. McDonald LC, Gerding DN, Johnson S, et al. Clinical practice guidelines for *Clostridium difficile* Infection in adults and children: 2017 update by the Infectious Diseases Society of America (IDSA) and Society for Healthcare Epidemiology of America (SHEA). Clin Infect Dis. 2018;66:987–94.
6. Pichenot M, Héquette-Ruz R, Le Guern R, et al. Fidaxomicin for treatment of *Clostridium difficile* infection in clinical practice: a prospective cohort study in a French University Hospital. Infection. 2017;45:425–31.
7. Cornely OA, Crook DW, Esposito R, et al. Fidaxomicin versus vancomycin for infection with *Clostridium difficile* in Europe, Canada, and the USA: a double-blind, non-inferiority, randomised controlled trial. Lancet Infect Dis. 2012;12:281–9.
8. Louie TJ, Miller MA, Mullane KM, et al. Fidaxomicin versus vancomycin for *Clostridium difficile* infection. N Engl J Med. 2011;364(5):422–31.
9. Nelson RL, Suda KJ, Evans CT. Antibiotic treatment for *Clostridium difficile*-associated diarrhoea in adults. Cochrane Database Syst Rev. 2017;3:004610. https://doi.org/10.1002/14651858.cd004610.pub5.
10. McEllistrem MC, McGraw M, Sahud AG, Chan-Tompkins NH, Goswami R, Bhanot N. High frequency of nonadherence to *Clostridium difficile* treatment guidelines. South Med J. 2014;107:597–9.
11. Cohen SH, Gerding DN, Johnson S, et al. Clinical practice guidelines for *Clostridium difficile* infection in adults: 2010 update by the Society for Healthcare Epidemiology of America (SHEA) and the Infectious Diseases Society of America (IDSA). Infect Control Hosp Epidemiol. 2010;315:431–55.
12. Miller MA, Louie T, Mullane K, et al. Derivation and validation of a simple clinical bedside score (ATLAS) for *Clostridium difficile* infection which predicts response to therapy. BMC Infect Dis. 2013;13:148.
13. D'Agostino RB, Collins SH, Pencina KM, Kean Y, Gorbach S. Risk estimation for recurrent *Clostridium difficile* infection based on clinical factors. Clin Infect Dis. 2014;58:1386–93.
14. Mulherin DW, Hutchison AM, Thomas GJ, Hansen RA, Childress DT. Concordance of the SHEA-IDSA severity classification for *Clostridium difficile* infection and the ATLAS bedside scoring system in hospitalized adult patients. Infection. 2014;42:999–1005.
15. Leffler DA, Lamont JT. *Clostridium difficile* infection. N Engl J Med. 2015;372:1539–48.
16. Olsen MA, Yan Y, Reske KA, Zilberberg MD, Dubberke ER. Recurrent *Clostridium difficile* infection is associated with increased mortality. Clin Microbiol Infect. 2015;21(2):164–70.
17. Deshpande A, Pant C, Olyaee M, Donskey CJ. Hospital readmissions related to *Clostridium difficile* infection in the United States. Am J Infect Control. 2018;46(3):346–7.
18. Lofgren ET, Cole SR, Weber DJ, Anderson DJ, Moehring RW. Hospital-acquired *Clostridium difficile* infections: estimating all-cause mortality and length of stay. Epidemiology. 2014;25:570–5.
19. Hebbinckuys E, Marissal JP, Preda C, Leclercq V. Assessing the burden of *Clostridium difficile* infections for hospitals. J Hosp Infect. 2018;98(1):29–35.
20. McDonald LC, Killgore GE, Thompson A, et al. An epidemic, toxin gene—variant strain of *Clostridium difficile*. N Engl J Med. 2005;353:2433–41.

24

Prenatal and postnatal antibiotic exposure influences the gut microbiota of preterm infants in neonatal intensive care units

Zhi-Hui Zou[1,2], Dong Liu[1], Hong-Dong Li[1], Dan-Ping Zhu[1], Yu He[1], Ting Hou[1] and Jia-Lin Yu[1*]

Abstract

Background: To explore the influences of prenatal antibiotic exposure, the intensity of prenatal and postnatal antibiotic exposure on gut microbiota of preterm infants and whether gut microbiota and drug resistant strains in the neonatal intensive care unit (NICU) over a defined period are related.

Methods: Among 28 preterm infants, there were two groups, the PAT (prenatal antibiotic therapy) group (12 cases), and the PAF (prenatal antibiotic free) group (12 cases). Fecal samples from both groups were collected on days 7 and 14. According to the time of prenatal and postnatal antibiotic exposure, cases were divided into two groups, H (high) group (11 cases) and L (low) group (11 cases), and fecal samples on day 14 were collected. Genomic DNA was extracted from the fecal samples and was subjected to high throughput 16S rRNA amplicon sequencing. Bioinformatics methods were used to analyze the sequencing results.

Results: Prenatal and postnatal antibiotic exposure exercised influence on the early establishment of intestinal microflora of preterm infants. *Bacteroidetes* decreased significantly in the PAT group ($p < 0.05$). The number of *Bifidobacterium* significantly decreased in the PAT group and H group ($p < 0.05$). The early gut microbiota of preterm infants with prenatal and postnatal antibiotic exposure was similar to resistant bacteria in NICU during the same period.

Conclusion: Prenatal and postnatal antibiotic exposure may affect the composition of early gut microbiota in preterm infants. Antibiotic-resistant bacteria in NICU may play a role in reshaping the early gut microbiota of preterm infants with prenatal and postnatal antibiotic exposure.

Keywords: Infant, premature, Gastrointestinal microbiome, Anti-bacterial agents, High-throughput nucleotide sequencing, Intensive care unit, neonatal

Background

The human gastrointestinal tract contains diverse, complex, and dynamic communities of microorganisms. Most of these microorganisms are bacteria, the density of which is approximately 10^{13}–10^{14} cells/g fecal matter. Gut microbiota contributes significantly to varied aspects of host health, including immunity, development, and behavior, while major shifts in complex microbial systems are associated with disease [1, 2]. Indeed, epidemiology and laboratory studies have found that gut microbiota imbalances are associated with several infectious diseases, chronic inflammatory bowel diseases, allergic diseases, autoimmune diseases, and some metabolic diseases [3–5].

Prenatal and postnatal periods are critical for the establishment of infant gut microbiota, which is susceptible to maternal factors, delivery mode, and feeding mode [6, 7]. The delay or disorder of preterm infant microbiota has a long-term effect on the physiology of the infant [8, 9].

*Correspondence: yujialin486@126.com
[1] Department of Neonatology, Children's Hospital of Chongqing Medical University, Chongqing 400014, China
Full list of author information is available at the end of the article

Various environmental factors within NICU influence infant microbiota [10, 11]. The routine application of antibiotics in China is very popular, especially in NICU. Due to the high density of inpatients, nosocomial infections caused by resistant bacteria are frequent. However, the effects of antibiotic exposure on the gut microbiota of preterm infants in prenatal and postnatal periods remain undefined.

In this study, high-throughput amplicon sequencing was used to investigate the effects of prenatal antibiotic exposure and its intensity on the development of gut microbiota in preterm infants within 2 weeks of birth. We also explored whether there are similarities between the early gut microbiota and resistant bacteria colonized in the NICU.

Methods

Study population and design

This study was approved by the Ethics Committee of Bo'ai Hospital, Zhongshan, Guangdong Province. Twenty-eight preterm infants were enrolled in the study and the inclusion criteria were as follows: All the pregnant women were admitted to Bo'ai Hospital of Zhongshan before delivery, and the preterm infants were immediately hospitalized in the NICU of Bo'ai Hospital after delivery. Exclusion criteria were as follows: clinical use of probiotics, the presence of asphyxia, congenital malformations, congenital abnormalities, genetic metabolic diseases, or the presence of surgical diseases. For this study, two grouping strategies were established. Firstly, according to whether the infants were exposed to prenatal antibiotic therapy, 28 cases were divided into two groups: PAT (prenatal antibiotic therapy) group and PAF (prenatal antibiotic free) control group; each group had 12 patients. The other four patients were excluded because of difficulty in pairing. Secondly, according to antibiotic exposure intensity, i.e., total time of antibiotic exposure both before and after delivery, there were 11 pairs in two groups, i.e., >7d group (H group) and ≤7d group (L group). These subjects were selected from the same 28 patients. For details on grouping, please refer to Additional files 1: Tables S1, S2 in Additional Materials. Cases and controls were matched by delivery method, gestational age, and feeding pattern. Fecal samples on days 7 (d7) and 14 (d14) were collected.

The antibiotic resistant strains present in Bo'ai Hospital, located in Guangdong, Southern China, were identified. According to the monthly report of drug resistant strains in the NICU, provided by the Infection Control Department of Bo'ai Hospital, the resistant bacteria colonized in the NICU were *Klebsiella pneumoniae* (40%), *Escherichia coli* (28.57%), and *Acinetobacter baumanii* (20%). The main prenatal antibiotics were cefazolin sodium pentahydrate, while the main antibiotics used in the NICU were cefuroxime sodium, cefoperazone-sulbactam, imipenem-cilastatin sodium, and meropenem. The prenatal antibiotic applied to the subjects in this study was exclusively cefazolin sodium pentahydrate, while the postnatal antibiotic was exclusively cefuroxime sodium.

High throughput 16S rRNA amplicon sequencing

Fecal samples were collected with disposable sterile fecal collection tubes from soiled patient diapers, and delivered to the laboratory in an ice box. Then, 250 mg of each sample was put into sterile EP tubes. The samples of d7 and d14 of every infant were put into two to four EP tubes. All samples were stored in the refrigerator at −80 °C. Genomic DNA was extracted from fecal samples using QIAamp FAST DNA Stool Mini Kit (Qiagen, Hilden, Germany), according to the manufacturer's instructions.

The bacterial 16S rRNA gene amplicons (V3+V4 regions) were generated with the following polymerase chain reaction (PCR) primers: Forward, 338F (5′-ACTCCTACGGGAGGCAGCA-3′); reverse, 806R (5′-GGACTACHVGGGTWTCTAAT-3′) [12]. PCRs were completed under the following conditions: 95 °C for 3 min, followed by 27 cycles of 95 °C for 30 s, 55 °C for 30 s, and 72 °C for 45 s, and finally, 72 °C for 10 min. PCR products were analyzed by agarose gel electrophoresis (2% in 0.25 × Tris–acetate-EDTA buffer), and were purified using the AxyPrep kit (AXYGEN, USA), according to the manufacturer's protocol. The DNA amplicons were used to construct the sequencing libraries for the high throughput sequencing on an Illumina MiSeq platform.

Bioinformatic analysis

In order to ensure bioinformatic analysis reliability, the raw sequencing reads were filtered before the biological analysis to assess the quality of the sequence. The specific criteria were as follows: (1) Remove sequences of less than 50 bp; (2) according to the overlap relationship, the sequences were spliced, and the minimum overlap length was 10 bp; (3) the maximum mismatch rate of the splicing sequence overlap region should not be higher than 0.2; (4) the base number of primer mismatches must be less than 2, and the barcode was not allowed to be mismatched.

After the sequences were optimized, operational taxonomic units (OTU) assignment was performed for all sequences at a 97% similarity level. OTU cluster analysis, taxonomy analysis, and species diversity analysis were performed. According to the results of the taxonomy analysis, the differences in the composition of the community structure were analyzed at the phylum and genus levels. The Shannon index and Simpson index were calculated to characterize the community diversity. Rarefaction curves, reflecting the sequencing depth, were calculated using custom R scripts. To characterize the richness in a specific gut community, the custom R scripts were used to obtain the Shannon–Wiener curve, Venn diagrams, and the microbial community bar plots. Principal coordinate analyses (PCoA), using the weighted and unweighted UniFrac distances, were calculated using the PCoA function of the R package Ape [13]. The gut microbial communities of different conditions were further compared using LDA Effect Size (LEfSe; http://huttenhower.sph.harvard.edu/galaxy). The differential features were identified on the OTU level.

Results

Effect of prenatal antibiotic exposure on the development of gut microbiota in preterm infants

In this study, there were no significant differences between the PAT and PAF groups in terms of the gestational age, birth weight, delivery mode, and feeding method ($p > 0.05$; Table 1). Statistically significant differences in gender were observed, and more boys were in the PAT group ($p = 0.009$). The detailed clinical data are shown in Table 1.

The average sequence number of all samples was 448.21 and the sequencing depth reached about 99.5%. The rarefaction curves of different individuals were distinct (Additional file 1: Figure S1), indicating that there were significant inter-individual variations in gut bacterial diversity. The Shannon index of the PAT group was higher on d14 (0.88) than on d7 (0.55), so was that of the PAF group (0.57 on d7, 0.82 on d14). As time went by, there was an increasing trend in gut bacterial diversity. No significant differences were observed between the PAT and PAF groups on both d7 and d14 (Fig. 1a), which indicates the trivial influence of prenatal antibiotic exposure on gut microflora.

The number of OTUs on d7 and d14 in the PAT group was 31 and 81, respectively (Additional file1: Figure S2), with corresponding numbers in the PAF group of 31 and 79, respectively. In the PAT group, the number of shared OTUs between subjects on d7 and d14 was 27, while in the PAF group, it was 26. In both groups, there were more shared OTUs on d7 than on d14, indicating greater diversity in both groups on d14 than on d7 ($p < 0.05$).

At the phylum level on d7, *Proteobacteria* (PAF 79.57%, PAT 92.35%) and *Firmicutes* (PAF 9.73%, PAT 4.69%) were predominant in gut microbiota, followed by *Actinobacteria* (PAF 1.58%, PAT 0.02%) and *Bacteroidetes* (PAF 9.11%, PAT 2.93%). On d14, *Proteobacteria* (PAF 74.78%, PAT 87.22%) and *Firmicutes* (PAF 11.19%, PAT 10.61%) were predominant in gut microbiota, followed by *Actinobacteria* (PAF 8.21%, PAT 1.75%) and *Bacteroidetes* (PAF 5.75%, PAT 0.38%). The relative abundance of *Proteobacteria* was higher in the antibiotic exposure group than in the non-exposure group, on both days, while *Firmicutes* was less abundant in the former group than in the latter one, especially on d7. *Bacteroidetes* in both the PAF and PAT groups were lower on d14 than on d7, with a more marked decrease observed in the PAT group, with a statistically significant difference ($p < 0.05$), further highlighting the prolonged effect of prenatal antibiotic exposure on the establishment and development of neonatal gut microflora.

At the genus level, *Klebsiella* (on d7, PAF 52.17%, PAT 48.96%; on d14, PAF 45.03%, PAT 45.81%) and *Escherichia-Shigella* (on d7, PAF 27.35%, PAT 43.35%; on d14, PAF 29.47%, PAT 40.36%) were predominant. Moreover, in the PAT group, the colonization of *Bifidobacterium* was delayed (0/12 vs. 3/12 on d7; 5/12 vs. 9/12 on d14). By d14, the relative abundance of some bacteria had increased substantially in the gut, such as *Bacteroides*, *Staphylococcus*, *Clostridium_sensu_stricto_1*, *Parabacteroides*, and *Bifidobacterium* (Fig. 2b). Moreover, in the PAT group, the colonization of *Bifidobacterium* was delayed (Fig. 1b). On d7 there was no colonization

Table 1 Clinical data of the PAT and PAF groups

Clinical data	PAT infants	PAF infants	Statistical method	P value
Gestational age (d)	227.6 (mean) ± 7.6 (SD)	229.1 ± 7.3	Student's t test	0.09
Birth weight (g)	1777.08 ± 297.1	1814.16 ± 169.14	Student's t test	0.711
Delivery mode (CS/VD)	3/9	3/9	Chi square test	1
Gender (male/female)	11/1	8/4	Chi square test	0.009
Feeding (premature infant formula/mixed feeding/breastfeeding)	4/3/5	4/3/5	Chi square test	1
Postnatal antibiotic (d)	7 (ranging 3–13)	7 (ranging 3–14)	Non-parametric test	0.671
PROM	12/0	6/6	Chi square test	NA
Histological chorioamnionitis (positive/negative/no. of inspection)	3/6/3	2/6/4	Chi square test	NA

VD vaginally delivered, *CS* cesarean section, *PROM* premature rupture of membranes

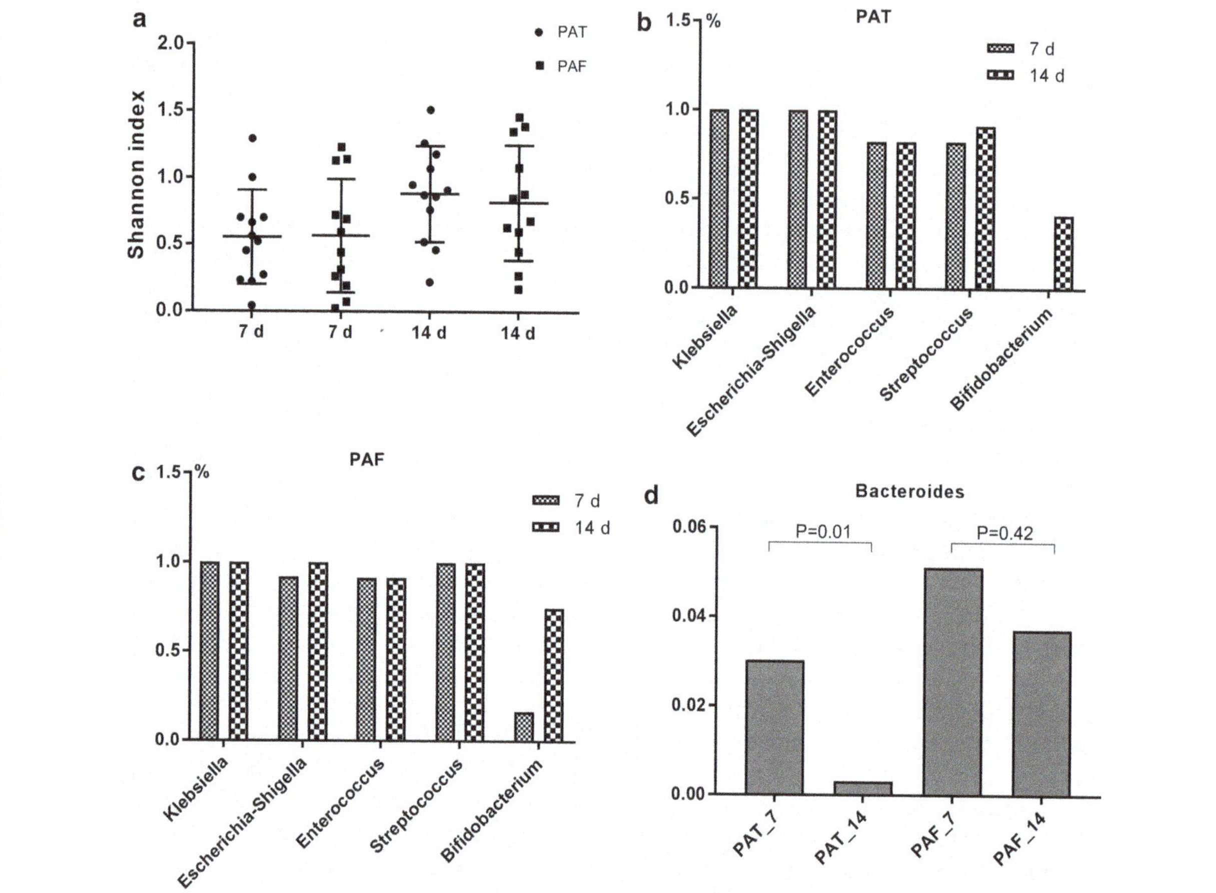

Fig. 1 **a** Shannon index of PAT and PAF groups on postnatal d7 and d14. **b** Colonization percentage of five gut bacteria in the PAT group. **c** Colonization percentage of five gut bacteria in the PAF control group. **d** *Bacteriodetes* in the PAT and PAF groups on d7 and d14

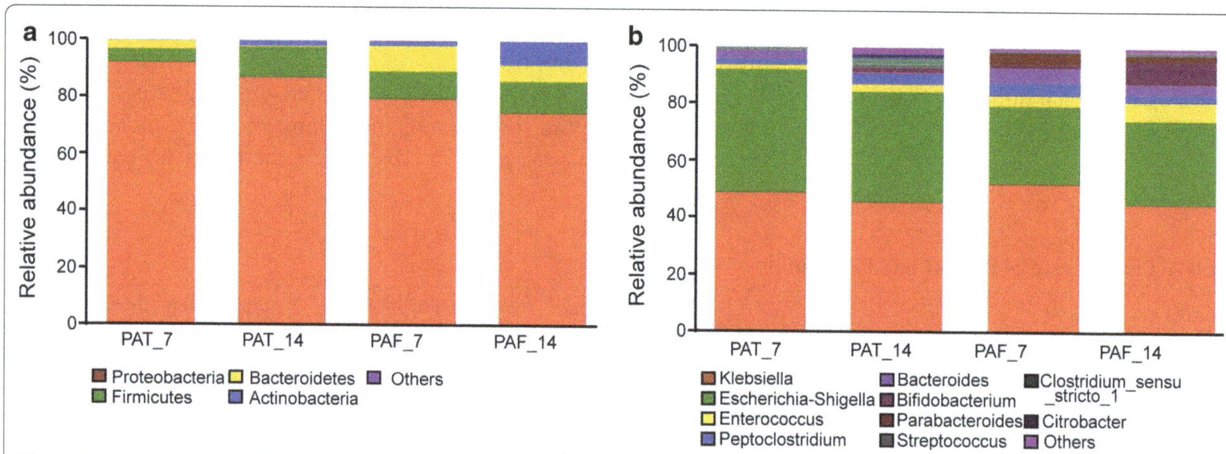

Fig. 2 Relative abundance of the main gut bacterial groups. **a** At the phylum level. **b** At the genus level. On d7 and d14, gut microbiota were generally dominated by the phyla Proteobacteria and Firmicutes, followed by Actinobacteria and Bacteroidetes. At the genus level, *Klebsiella* and *Escherichia-Shigella* were dominant. On d14, bacteria such as *Bacteroides, Staphylococcus, Clostridium_sensu_stricto_1, Parabacteroides*, and *Bifidobacterium* were more abundant than on d7

of *Bifidobacterium*, and by d14 the number of preterm infants colonized by *Bifidobacterium* was significantly lower in the PAT group than in the PAF group (0/12 vs. 3/12 on d7; 5/12 vs. 9/12 on d14; $p<0.05$; Fig. 1b and c). *Bacteroidetes* decreased in both groups with increasing antibiotic exposure time, and this decrease was more significant in the PAT group than the PAF group ($p<0.05$; Fig. 1d).

The predominant bacteria of PAT and PAF groups were similar to the drug resistant strains in NICU of the same period.

The extent of variation within the gut bacteria population in the different samples correlated with the human host, infant growth and development, prenatal/postnatal antibiotic exposure, and so on. In PCoA (Fig. 3), each spot of the PAT and PAF group members were separated well, but neither those of the PAT group nor those of the PAF group clustered together, indicating that antibiotic exposure did not determine the gut microbiota development. As shown in Fig. 3, dots from both datasets were dispersed and intermingled, suggesting that the bacteria community composition of PAF_7 was largely similar to that of PAF_14.

LEfSe is a method for metagenomic biomarker discovery by way of class comparison, tests of biological consistency, and effect size estimation [14]. The differential features were identified on the OTU level. The LEfSe analysis of d7 showed that PAT and PAF groups were not significantly different.

LEfSe analysis of d14 finds the relative abundance of *Saccharicrinis*, *Acteroidia*, *Epsilonproteobacteria*, *Incertae_Sedis*, and *Flavobacteriales* was significantly higher in the PAT group than in the PAF control group, and the relative abundance of *Clostridiales* and *Clostridia* was much lower in the former than in the latter (Fig. 4a and b).

Effects of antibiotic exposure intensity on the development of intestinal microbiota in preterm infants

The preterm infants were divided into two groups according to the antibiotic treatment time: >7d group (H group) and ≤7d group (L group). Delivery modes, gestational age, feeding pattern, and other factors that may affect the intestinal microbiota, were matched between the two groups (Table 2). Twenty-two preterm infants were enrolled. The fecal samples on d14 were collected.

The cut-off was set to 400 sequences per sample and this was the level whereby the rarefaction curves of all samples reached a plateau, indicating that the sequencing depth was sufficient and able to cover most types of bacteria. The Shannon index of the two groups was not significantly different on d14 ($p>0.05$; Fig. 5a). In PCoA, the bacteria community composition of the H group was not similar to that of L group, as six members (H2-6, 9) gathered to form a subgroup of H, which was well separated from L (Fig. 5b–d).

The relative abundance of dominant bacterial phyla and genera was as follows. On d14 the most abundant phylum was *Proteobacteria* (79.35% in group H and 70.66% in group L; Fig. 6a), followed by *Firmicutes* (19.33% in group H and 14.81% in group L). At the genus level, on d14 the microbiota structure was similar between the two groups. The most abundant genus was *Klebsiella* (55.91% in group H and 36.15 in group L), followed by *Enterococcus* (23% in group H and 34.22% in group L). Moreover, the number of *Shigella* and *Streptococcus* tended to decrease in the H group (Fig. 6b). The relative abundance of *Bifidobacterium* significantly decreased (5.47% in H group and 10.24% in L group, $p<0.05$; Fig. 7).

The predominant bacteria of H and L groups were similar to the drug resistant strains in NICU of the same period.

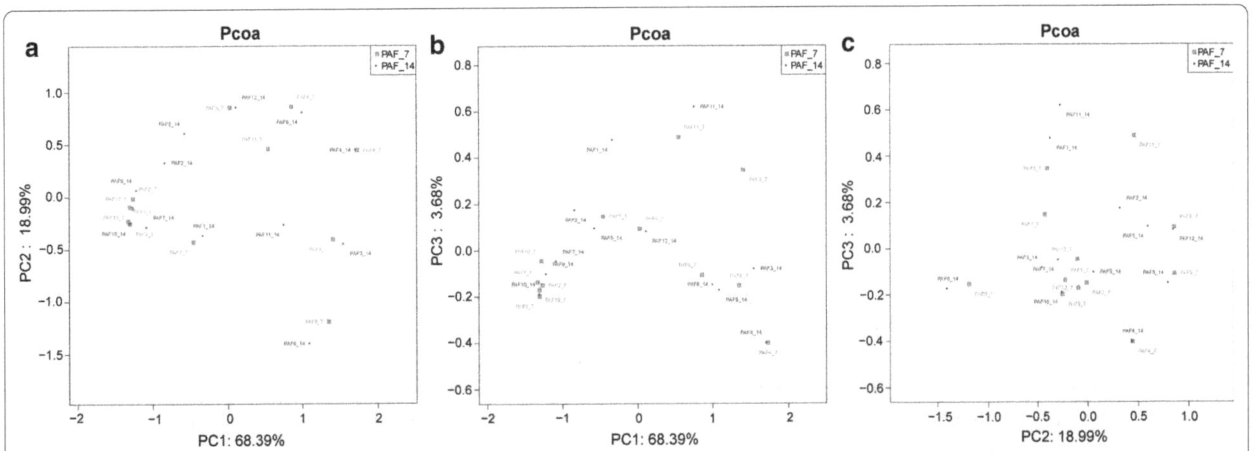

Fig. 3 Comparison of microbial communities by PCoA. PCoA was generated with OTUs (at 97% similarity) present in the different fecal samples. **a** PC1 vs. PC2. **b** PC1 vs. PC3. **c** PC2 vs. PC3

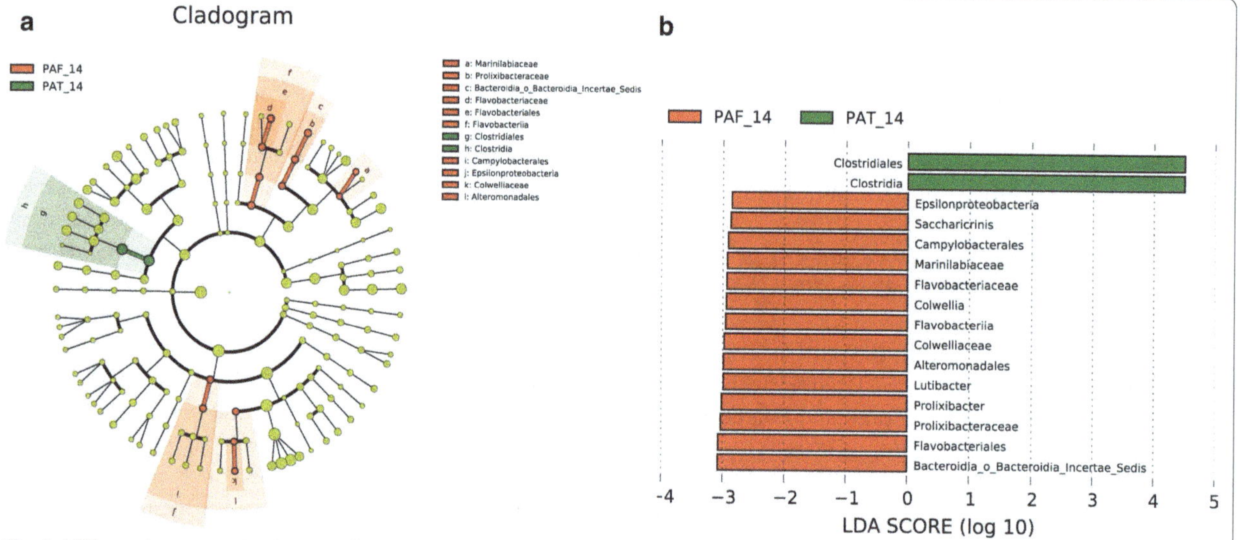

Fig. 4 LEfSe results on gut microbiomes of preterm infants. **a** Clustering tree. Different color areas represent different groups. The yellow nodes represent microbial taxa without significant differences between PAT and PAF groups. The red nodes represent microbial taxa that played an important role in the PAF group, and green nodes represent microbial taxa that played an important role in the PAT group. **b** Histogram showing the distribution of LDA values

Table 2 Clinical data of prenatal antibiotic treatment H group and L group

Clinical data	H group	L group	Statistical method	*P* value
Gestational age (d)	227 (ranging 218–237)	230 (ranging 222–242)	Non-parametric test	0.09
Birth weight (g)	1715 (1050–1955)	1900 (1415–2155)	Non-parametric test	0.101
Delivery mode (CS/VD)	1/10	1/10	Chi square test	1
Gender (male/female)	4/7	4/7	Chi square test	1
Feeding (premature infant formula/mixed feeding/breastfeeding)	3/3/5	3/3/5	Chi square test	1
Duration of antibiotics use (d)	10 (9–16)	6 (3–7)	Non-parametric test	0
Prenatal antibiotic (d)	0 (0–3)	0 (0–4)	Non-parametric test	0.949
Postnatal antibiotic (d)	10 (7–13)	4 (3–7)	Non-parametric test	0
PROM (yes/no)	5/6	5/6	Chi square test	0
Histological chorioamnionitis (positive/negative/no. of inspection)	3/5/3	2/5/4	Chi square test	NA

VD vaginally delivered, *CS* cesarean section, *PROM* premature rupture of membranes

LEfSe analysis of d14 finds the relative abundance of *Betaproteobacteria* was significantly higher in the H group than in the L group; the relative abundance of *Bifidobacterium*, *Bifidobacteriaceae*, and *Bifidobacteriales* was significantly higher in the latter than in the former (Fig. 8).

Discussion

Antibiotics are of significant importance to modern medicine, and their use has played a pivotal role in the maintenance of human health. Despite this, there are ever-increasing concerns about the negative consequences of antibiotic use, including the collateral damage inflicted on the gut microbiota. Prenatal antibiotic exposure resulted in an increase in *Staphylococcus*, *Streptococcus*, *Serratia*, and *Parabacteroides*, constituting potentially pathogenic communities [15]. Fouhy et al. found that postnatal antibiotic subject exposure (ampicillin and gentamicin within 48 h of birth) resulted in significantly lower levels of *Bifidobacterium* and *Lactobacillus* than in untreated controls 4 weeks after the cessation of treatment [16]. Antibiotics are the most commonly prescribed medications in NICUs. The present study addresses an important knowledge gap, as the effects of prenatal and postnatal antibiotic exposure on preterm infant gut microbiota have not, thus far, been characterized by high throughput sequencing methods that provide sufficient coverage of the entire bacterial community.

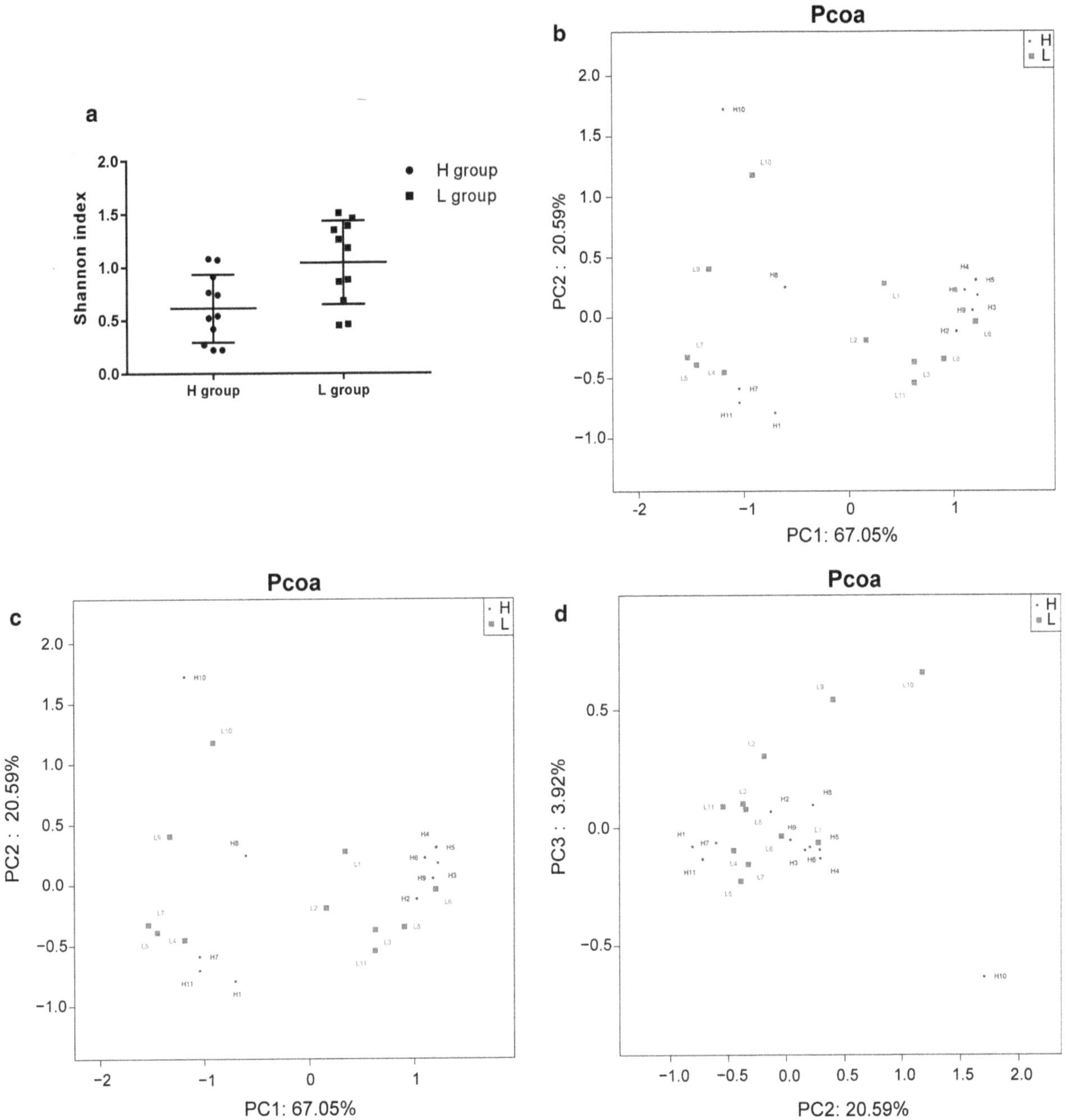

Fig. 5 Comparison of the gut microbial communities in the H and L groups. **a** The Shannon index showed no significant difference between the two groups on d14 ($p > 0.05$). PCoA was generated with OTUs (at 97% similarity) present in the different fecal samples. **b** PC1 vs. PC2. **c** PC1 vs. PC3. **d** PC2 vs. PC3

In this study, at the phylum level, *Proteobacteria* and *Firmicutes* were predominant in gut microbiota, with *Proteobacteria* more abundant than *Firmicutes.* As there are more harmful genera than beneficial ones in Proteobacteria, an increased prevalence of Proteobacteria is a marker of an unstable microbial community, dysbiosis, and a potential diagnostic criterion of disease [17]. In contrast, there are more beneficial genera than harmful ones within the *Firmicutes* phylum [18]. The increase of *Proteobacteria* and the decrease of *Firmicutes* could increase the incidence of necrotizing enterocolitis (NEC) and infectious diseases [19]. At the genus level, *Klebsiella, Escherichia-Shigella* and *Enterococcus* were predominant in gut microbiota, whereas *Bifidobacterium* decreased significantly. It was found that prenatal antibiotic exposure could lead to a reduction in *Bacteroides*

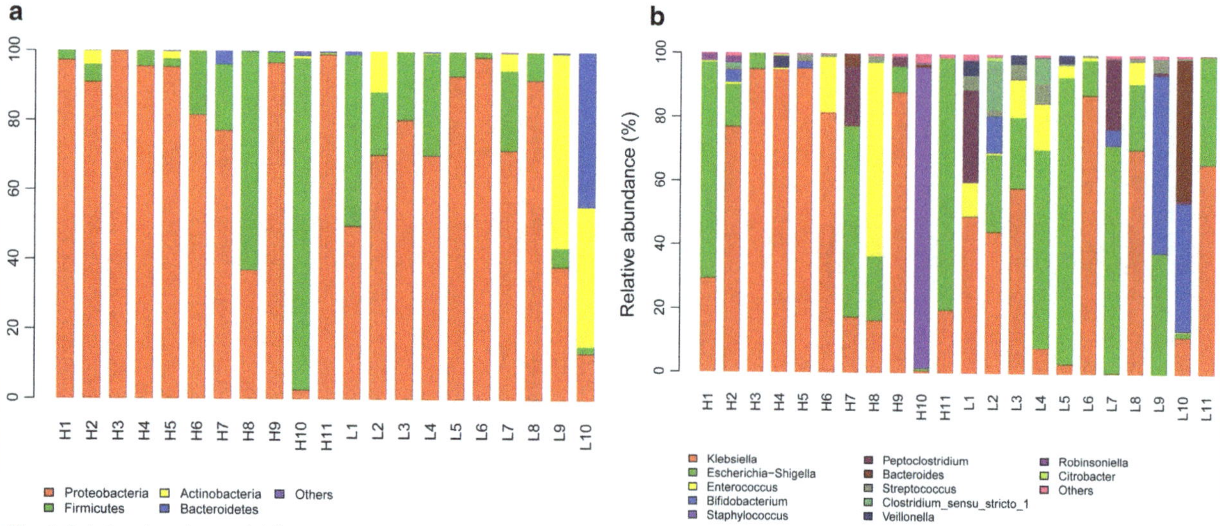

Fig. 6 Relative abundance of different microbial groups in guts of preterm infants undergoing antibiotic prophylaxis at high/low doses. **a** At the phylum level. **b** At the genus level. On d14 gut microbiota were generally dominated by the phyla Proteobacteria (79.35% in the H group vs. 70.66% in the L group) and Firmicutes (19.33% in the H group vs. 14.81% in the L group). At the genus level, on d14 the microbiota structure in both groups was similar. The gut microbiota of the two groups remained predominantly populated with members of *Klebsiella* (55.91% in the H group vs. 36.15% in the L group) and *Enterococcus* (23% in the H group vs. 34.22% in the L group). *Shigella* and *Streptococcus* had a tendency to decrease in the H group

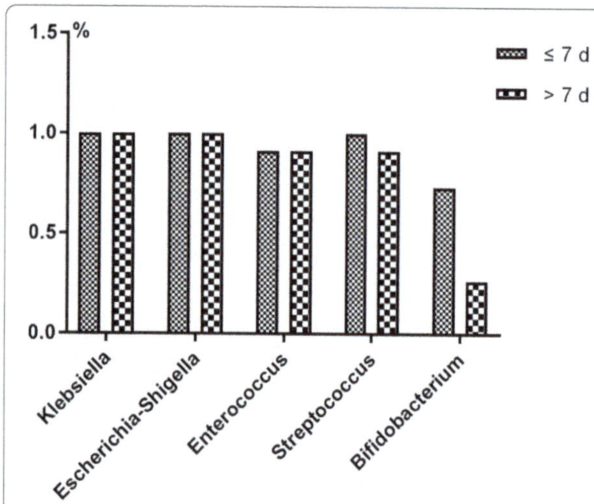

Fig. 7 Colonization percentage of five gut bacteria in the H group (>7d) and L group (≤7d). The colonization of Bifidobacterium decreased more significantly in the H group than in the L group (5.47% in the H group vs. 10.24% in the L group, $p < 0.05$)

and an increase in *Escherichia-Shigella* and *Clostridium* in the intestinal microflora of premature infants. It was also found that high intensity antibiotic exposure led to increases in *Beta-proteobacteria*. *Bacteroides* and *Bifidobacterium* are intestinal protective bacteria, and a decrease in their population could result in NEC; the opportunistic pathogen *Escherichia-Shigella* also results in increased incidence of NEC [19] and increases of *Clostridium* and *Bacteroides* in the intestinal mucosa of NEC cases [20]. It has been found that populations of *Clostridium difficile* increase in NICU environments, which is associated with many intractable infections [21–23]. Therefore, our data implies that preterm infant antibiotic exposure may cause dysbiosis and lead to increased incidences of NEC.

Intriguingly, in both the prenatal antibiotic exposure group and in the high intensity antibiotic exposure group, the colonization of *Bifidobacterium* was delayed and no *Lactobacillus* colonization was observed. *Bifidobacterium* and *Lactobacillus* are very important probiotics. It has been shown that probiotics can restore intestinal micro-ecological balance, repair the intestinal membrane barrier, improve intestinal colonization, and inhibit the excessive growth of opportunistic pathogens [24]. Probiotics help to decrease NEC, late-onset sepsis, and the mortality of preterm infants [25]. It is suggested that the status, the gene phenotype, and the gut microbiota of pregnant women, as well as the delivery mode, could influence the establishment and construction of gut microbiota in newborns [26–29]. Interestingly, microorganisms have also been found in the placenta [30, 31]. Antibiotic treatment for PROM (premature rupture of membranes) pregnant women leads to changes in vaginal microflora, and numbers of *Lactobacillus* have been shown to continuously decline [32]. Further investigations are needed to explore whether or not prenatal

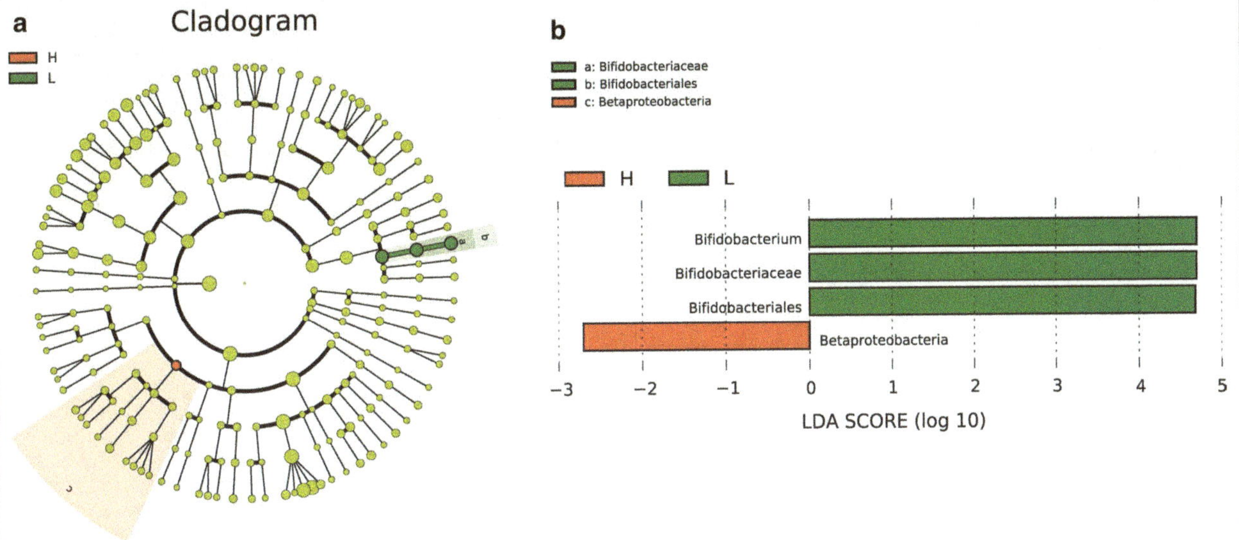

Fig. 8 LEfSe analysis showed significant differences in microbial community structure between the H and L groups. **a** Cladogram. **b** Distribution of LDA scores. Betaproteobacteria played an important role in the H group; in the L group, *Bifidobacterium*, Bifidobacteriaceae, and Bifidobacteriales were the prominent microbes

antibiotic exposure affects the establishment of gut microbiota in preterm infants by influencing the microbiota in the intestines, vagina, and placenta of pregnant women.

The establishment and development of gut microbiota are influenced by environment factors, gestational age, delivery mode, feeding pattern, and antibiotics [10]. In our study no significant differences were found in the Shannon–Wiener Index and PCoA between the PAT and PAF groups, or between the H and L groups, indicating that antibiotic exposure is not dominant in influencing the establishment and development of gut microbiota at an early stage in premature infants. The NICU has its own unique commensal bacteria and pathogens [33, 34]. In our hospital, antibiotic resistant bacteria colonized in the NICU were mainly *Klebsiella pneumoniae* (40%), *Escherichia coli* (28.57%) and *Acinetobacter baumannii* (20%). The incidence of nosocomial infection was 19.4%. Our data showed that these common resistant bacteria were included in the intestinal microflora at an early stage in premature infants, indicating that bacterial colonization in the NICU may play an important role in the development of gut microbiota in preterm infants. It is widely believed that disturbances in gut microbiota are one of the main causes of NEC and late-onset sepsis [35]. Gut microbiota disturbance often occurs before diseases, and changes in gut microbiota could be considered as an early predictor of preterm infant sepsis [36, 37]. Antibiotic exposure influences the establishment of preterm infant gut microbiota, changing its diversity and richness [15, 38]. Additionally, antibiotic exposure could promote the horizontal gene transfer of antibiotic resistance genes [39]. Whether these effects are synergistic is worth further investigation.

Conclusions

In summary, prenatal/postnatal antibiotic exposure and the intensity of antibiotic exposure could affect the composition of gut microbiota in preterm infants. It may be safely assumed that environmental factors (e.g. antibiotic-resistant bacteria in NICU) may have a profound impact on the composition of the early gut microbiota in preterm infants with prenatal and postnatal antibiotic exposure. The gut microbiota of preterm infants includes antibiotic-resistant bacteria in NICU, thus posing a threat to the survival of infants and increasing the possibility of therapy failures.

Abbreviations

NICU: neonatal intensive care units; PAT: prenatal antibiotic therapy; PAF: prenatal antibiotic free; OUT: operational taxonomic units; PCoA: principal coordinate analyses; NEC: necrotizing enterocolitis; PROM: premature rupture of membranes; HC: histological chorioamnionitis; VD: vaginally delivered; CS: cesarean section.

Authors' contributions

ZHZ designed the study. ZHZ collected and analysed the data. JLY and YH advised on analysis. DPZ and TH contributed to sample extraction. ZHZ drafted and wrote the manuscript. ZHZ, JLY, DL, HDL, DPZ, YH, and TH revised the manuscript critically for intellectual content. All authors gave intellectual input to the study. All authors read and approved the final manuscript.

Author details

[1] Department of Neonatology, Children's Hospital of Chongqing Medical University, Chongqing 400014, China. [2] Department of Neonatology, Sichuan Maternal and Child Health Service Hospital, Chengdu 610041, Sichuan, China.

Acknowledgements

Not applicable.

Competing interests

The authors declare that they have no competing interests.

Consent for publication

All data published here are under the consent for publication.

Funding

None.

References

1. Levy M, Blacher E, Elinav E. Microbiome, metabolites and host immunity. Curr Opin Microbiol. 2016;35:8–15.
2. Rodriguez JM, Murphy K, Stanton C, Ross RP, Kober OI, Juge N, et al. The composition of the gut microbiota throughout life, with an emphasis on early life. Microb Ecol Health Dis. 2015;26:26050.
3. Aujnarain A, Mack DR, Benchimol EI. The role of the environment in the development of pediatric inflammatory bowel disease. Curr Gastroenterol Rep. 2013;15(6):326.
4. Goulet O. Potential role of the intestinal microbiota in programming health and disease. Nutr Rev. 2015;73(Suppl 1):32–40.
5. Turta O, Rautava S. Antibiotics, obesity and the link to microbes—what are we doing to our children? BMC Med. 2016;14:57.
6. Marques TM, Wall R, Ross RP, Fitzgerald GF, Ryan CA, Stanton C. Programming infant gut microbiota: influence of dietary and environmental factors. Curr Opin Biotechnol. 2010;21(2):149–56.
7. Patel K, Konduru K, Patra AK, Chandel DS, Panigrahi P. Trends and determinants of gastric bacterial colonization of preterm neonates in a NICU setting. PLoS ONE. 2015;10(7):e0114664.
8. Schulfer A, Blaser MJ. Risks of antibiotic exposures early in life on the developing microbiome. PLoS Pathog. 2015;11(7):e1004903.
9. Tanaka S, Kobayashi T, Songjinda P, Tateyama A, Tsubouchi M, Kiyohara C, et al. Influence of antibiotic exposure in the early postnatal period on the development of intestinal microbiota. FEMS Immunol Med Microbiol. 2009;56(1):80–7.
10. Hartz LE, Bradshaw W, Brandon DH. Potential NICU environmental influences on the neonate's microbiome: a systematic review. Adv Neonatal Care. 2015;15(5):324–35.
11. Ternes YM, Lamaro-Cardoso J, Andre MC, Pessoa VP Jr, Vieira MA, Minamisava R, et al. Molecular epidemiology of coagulase-negative *Staphylococcus* carriage in neonates admitted to an intensive care unit in Brazil. BMC Infect Dis. 2013;13:572.
12. Xu N, Tan G, Wang H, Gai X. Effect of biochar additions to soil on nitrogen leaching, microbial biomass and bacterial community structure. Eur J Soil Biol. 2016;74:1–8.
13. Paradis E, Claude J, Strimmer K. APE: analyses of phylogenetics and evolution in R language. Bioinformatics. 2004;20(2):289–90.
14. Segata N, Izard J, Waldron L, Gevers D, Miropolsky L, Garrett WS, et al. Metagenomic biomarker discovery and explanation. Genome Biol. 2011;12(6):R60.
15. Chernikova DA, Koestler DC, Hoen AG, Housman ML, Hibberd PL, Moore JH, et al. Fetal exposures and perinatal influences on the stool microbiota of premature infants. J Matern Fetal Neonatal Med. 2016;29(1):99–105.
16. Fouhy F, Guinane CM, Hussey S, Wall R, Ryan CA, Dempsey EM, et al. High-throughput sequencing reveals the incomplete, short-term recovery of infant gut microbiota following parenteral antibiotic treatment with ampicillin and gentamicin. Antimicrob Agents Chemother. 2012;56(11):5811–20.
17. Shin NR, Whon TW, Bae JW. Proteobacteria: microbial signature of dysbiosis in gut microbiota. Trends Biotechnol. 2015;33(9):496–503.
18. Hugenholtz F, Ritari J, Nylund L, Davids M, Satokari R, de Vos WM. Feasibility of metatranscriptome analysis from infant gut microbiota: adaptation to solid foods results in increased activity of firmicutes at six months. Int J Microbiol. 2017;2017:9547063.
19. Neu J, Pammi M. Pathogenesis of NEC: impact of an altered intestinal microbiome. Semin Perinatol. 2017;41(1):29–35.
20. Brower-Sinning R, Zhong D, Good M, Firek B, Baker R, Sodhi CP, et al. Mucosa-associated bacterial diversity in necrotizing enterocolitis. PLoS ONE. 2014;9(9):e105046.
21. Forster AJ, Daneman N, van Walraven C. Influence of antibiotics and case exposure on hospital-acquired clostridium difficile infection independent of illness severity. J Hosp Infect. 2017;95(4):400–9.
22. Bacon AE, Fekety R, Schaberg DR, Faix RG. Epidemiology of clostridium difficile colonization in newborns: results using a bacteriophage and bacteriocin typing system. J Infect Dis. 1988;158(2):349–54.
23. Delmee M, Verellen G, Avesani V, Francois G. Clostridium difficile in neonates: serogrouping and epidemiology. Eur J Pediatr. 1988;147(1):36–40.
24. Bertelsen RJ, Jensen ET, Ringel-Kulka T. Use of probiotics and prebiotics in infant feeding. Best Pract Res Clin Gastroenterol. 2016;30(1):39–48.
25. Baucells BJ, Mercadal Hally M, Alvarez Sanchez AT, Figueras Aloy J. Probiotic associations in the prevention of necrotising enterocolitis and the reduction of late-onset sepsis and neonatal mortality in preterm infants under 1,500 g: a systematic review. An Pediatr (Barc). 2016;85(5):247–55.
26. Liu D, Yu J, Li L, Ai Q, Feng J, Song C, et al. Bacterial community structure associated with elective cesarean section versus vaginal delivery in Chinese newborns. J Pediatr Gastroenterol Nutr. 2015;60(2):240–6.
27. Goldsmith F, O'Sullivan A, Smilowitz JT, Freeman SL. Lactation and intestinal microbiota: how early diet shapes the infant gut. J Mammary Gland Biol Neoplasia. 2015;20(3–4):149–58.
28. Mueller NT, Shin H, Pizoni A, Werlang IC, Matte U, Goldani MZ, et al. Birth mode-dependent association between pre-pregnancy maternal weight status and the neonatal intestinal microbiome. Sci Rep. 2016;6:23133.
29. Blaser MJ, Dominguez-Bello MG. The human microbiome before birth. Cell Host Microbe. 2016;20(5):558–60.
30. Aagaard K, Ma J, Antony KM, Ganu R, Petrosino J, Versalovic J. The placenta harbors a unique microbiome. Sci Transl Med. 2014;6(237):237ra65.
31. Kuperman AA, Koren O. Antibiotic use during pregnancy: how bad is it? BMC Med. 2016;14(1):91.
32. Baldwin EA, Walther-Antonio M, MacLean AM, Gohl DM, Beckman KB, Chen J, et al. Persistent microbial dysbiosis in preterm premature rupture of membranes from onset until delivery. PeerJ. 2015;3:e1398.
33. Bokulich NA, Mills DA, Underwood MA. Surface microbes in the neonatal intensive care unit: changes with routine cleaning and over time. J Clin Microbiol. 2013;51(8):2617–24.
34. Hewitt KM, Mannino FL, Gonzalez A, Chase JH, Caporaso JG, Knight R, et al. Bacterial diversity in two neonatal intensive care units (NICUs). PLoS ONE. 2013;8(1):e54703.
35. Young GR, Smith DL, Embleton ND, Berrington JE, Schwalbe EC, Cummings SP, et al. Reducing viability bias in analysis of gut microbiota in preterm infants at risk of NEC and sepsis. Front Cell Infect Microbiol. 2017;7:237.
36. Taft DH, Ambalavanan N, Schibler KR, Yu Z, Newburg DS, Deshmukh H, et al. Center variation in intestinal microbiota prior to late-onset sepsis in preterm infants. PLoS ONE. 2015;10(6):e0130604.
37. Madan JC, Salari RC, Saxena D, Davidson L, O'Toole GA, Moore JH, et al. Gut microbial colonisation in premature neonates predicts neonatal sepsis. Arch Dis Child Fetal Neonatal Ed. 2012;97(6):F456–62.
38. Backhed F, Roswall J, Peng Y, Feng Q, Jia H, Kovatcheva-Datchary P, et al. Dynamics and stabilization of the human gut microbiome during the first year of life. Cell Host Microbe. 2015;17(6):852.
39. Stecher B, Denzler R, Maier L, Bernet F, Sanders MJ, Pickard DJ, et al. Gut inflammation can boost horizontal gene transfer between pathogenic and commensal Enterobacteriaceae. Proc Natl Acad Sci USA. 2012;109(4):1269–74.

Microbial virulence, molecular epidemiology and pathogenic factors of fluoroquinolone-resistant *Haemophilus influenzae* infections in Guangzhou, China

Dingqiang Chen[1†], Shuxian Wen[2†], Donghua Feng[2], Ruirui Xu[3], Junyan Liu[3,4*], Brian M. Peters[4], Danhong Su[2], Yongping Lin[2], Ling Yang[2], Zhenbo Xu[3,5,6*] and Mark E. Shirtliff[6]

Abstract

Background: Fluoroquinolone-resistant *Haemophilus influenzae* (FRHI) has been reported worldwide but remain unclear in China.

Methods: A total of 402 *H. influenzae* isolates collected from 2016 to 2017 were included. Antimicrobial susceptibility on 10 antibiotics was performed, and minimum inhibitory concentration of ciprofloxacin- and nalidixic acid-resistant strains were further determined by E-test strips, with risk factors also evaluated. Strains with resistance or reduced susceptibility to ciprofloxacin were subjected to sequencing of the quinolone resistance-determining regions (QRDR) and plasmid-mediated quinolone resistance genes by sequencing, with multi-locus sequence typing.

Results: 2.2% of *H. influenzae* strains were non-susceptible (7/402, 1.7%) or susceptible (2/402, 0.5%) to ciprofloxacin but NAL-resistant by E-test, and multidrug resistance was more common in fluoroquinolones non-susceptible *H. influenzae* group ($p = 0.000$). Infection risk factors included invasive procedure ($p = 0.011$), catching cold/previous contact with someone who had a cold ($p = 0.019$), fluoroquinolones use during previous 3 months ($p = 0.003$). With none of mutations obtained in *gyrB*, *parE* and other plasmid-mediated quinolone resistance genes, 7 and 4 strains were found for Ser-84-Leu substitutions in *gyrA* and one amino acid substitution in the QRDR of *gyrA* linked with one amino acid substitution in the QRDR of *parC*, respectively. In addition, five sequence types (ST) were identified, with ST1719 firstly found.

Conclusions: For the first time, this study has reported the incidence, risk factors, molecular determinants on fluoroquinolones resistance and ST of FRHI strains in mainland China, representing the first evidence of mutation of gyrA and parC in China and the new ST1719 worldwide.

Keywords: *Haemophilus influenzae*, Fluoroquinolones, Quinolone resistance-determining regions, ST1719

Background

Haemophilus influenzae is a conditional pathogen that commonly colonizes in the nasopharynx of human beings. As a leading cause for community-acquired pneumonia (CAP), *H. influenza* is also a major cause of acute otitis media (AOM) and bronchitis in young children [1], responsible for sever meningitis and septicemia responsible for 371,000 deaths per year globally [2].

Fluoroquinolones (FQs), a frequently used antibiotic for *H. influenzae* infections, was recommended for elderly patients or patients with underlying diseases according to the guidelines for CAP in Japan [3]. After the first report of FQs-resistant *H. influenzae* (FRHI) in 1993, this pathogen has spread worldwide and increased

*Correspondence: yaner0722@hotmail.com; zhenbo.xu@hotmail.com
†Dingqiang Chen and Shuxian Wen contributed equally to this manuscript
[3] School of Food Science and Engineering, South China University of Technology, Guangzhou 510640, China
Full list of author information is available at the end of the article

rapidly [4, 5]. Though a number of previous studies on FRHI from Hong Kong and Taiwan were available, the incidence of FRHI was controversial [4, 6–10]. In Taiwan, resistance rate of fluoroquinolone has increased rapidly over recent years [4, 7], and levofloxacin-resistance *H. influenzae* has been found to spread in the nursing home residents [7, 11] and was related to regional predominance of certain STs [4, 12]. In Hong Kong, the carriage rate of *H. influenzae* was 28.5% in children aged 2–6 years and this was the first report about resistance to quinolones among *H. influenzae* isolates in children [6]. However, despite a regional cross-sectional study recently from Shanghai which reported an 8% *H. influenzae* carriage in healthy children (aged 12–18 months) and sensitivity to all tested antimicrobials except 12.2% ampicillin resistance to ampicillin (with none of FRHI found) [10], surveillance on FRHI still remains significantly limited in mainland China.

Although resistance to FQs in *H. influenzae* remains low, levofloxacin treatment failure in *H. influenzae* pneumonia has been reported [13]. A patient with *H. influenzae* pneumonia died after several days of systemic treatment with levofloxacin and several mutations in the quinolone resistance-determining regions (QRDR) of DNA gyrase and topoisomerase IV genes of the *H. influenzae* strain were detected [14]. Resistance to FQs is due mainly to chromosome-mediated mutations in the QRDRs of the genes encoding DNA gyrase and topoisomerase IV [15], which is including *gyrA*, *gyrB*, *parC* and *parE*. In general, resistance to FQs developed in a stepwise manner. Mutation in DNA gyrase *gyrA*, which was regarded as the first-step mutants, can even occur in *H. influenzae* that FQs MICs remains in the susceptible range according to the current breakpoints in CLSI [6]. Carmen et al. believe that FQ resistance is acquired gradually with increasing numbers of mutations [16]. Nalidixic acid can be used in tests to screen for the detection of decreased susceptibility to quinolones in *H. influenzae* [6, 17, 18], it can find out isolates with QRDR mutant while quinolones MICs were still susceptible according to the breakpoint in CLSI.

In addition to the controversial FRHI incidence in Hong Kong and Taiwan and unavailability on FRHI study in mainland China [6, 7], antimicrobial resistance mechanism and sequence types (ST) of FRHI in mainland China remains unclear. In Guangzhou representative of Southern China, a number of longitudinal surveillances had been previously performed on various bacteria [18–21], including antimicrobial resistance and molecular mechanisms. Conducted in the same location, this study aimed to investigate the molecular epidemiology and risk factors of FRHI infections.

Methods

Species identification

The study was carried out at The First Affiliated Hospital of Guangzhou Medical University, a comprehensive teaching hospital located in Guangzhou representative of Southern China and featured by the leading respiratory diseases study and treatment. *H. influenzae* isolates were recruited from patients during January 2016 to January 2017. The samples were grown on chocolate agars and incubated for 24 h at 37 °C in air with 5% CO_2. Suspicious colonies were removed from the surface of the plate for species identification, meanwhile, colonies (two to three) were homogenized in a reaction tube containing nanopure water (100 μl) [22]. Species identification were performed by matrix-assisted laser desorption ionization time-of-flight mass spectrometry (MALDI-TOF MS, AB biomerieux), and confirmed by 16S rRNA sequencing [23] (Primers were list in Table 1). DNA extracts were performed by boiling the bacterial suspensions [22]. The bacterial suspensions were heated to 100 °C in a boiling water bath for 10 min and centrifuged at 10,000×*g* for 10 min, then DNA was used as template and amplified with the following polymerase chain reactions (PCR) procedure: denaturation at 95 °C for 5 min, followed by 30 cycles of 95 °C for 30 s, 55 °C for 30 s, and 72 °C for 90 s. The samples were then extended at 72 °C for a further 10 min, hold to 4 °C. The sequences of the PCR products were compared with known 16S rRNA gene sequences in the GenBank (http://www.ncbi.nlm.nih.gov) as described previously [23, 24].

Antimicrobial susceptibility

Antimicrobial susceptibility of *H. influenzae* isolates to 10 antibiotics, including ampicillin (AMP), ampicillin–sulbactam (AMS), ciprofloxacin (CIP), levofloxacin (LEV), ceftriaxone (CTR), cefuroxime (ROXH), cefotaxime (TAX), meropenem (MEM), trimethoprim–sulfamethoxazole (SXT), azithromycin (AZT), was determined by Kirby–Bauer disk diffusion test (Oxoid, United Kingdom) on *Haemophilus* test medium (HTM) plates and incubated for 24 h at 37 °C in air with 5% CO_2. All the isolates were tested for the production of β-lactamase by nitrocephin paper disks.

Isolates that showed susceptibility to ciprofloxacin and had an inhibitory zone diameter of 21–28 mm were screened with nalidixic acid (NAL) disks (30 μg). Minimum inhibitory concentrations (MICs) of ciprofloxacin and levofloxacin were detected by E-test method (AB bioMerieux) in isolates resistant to ciprofloxacin or NAL disks. Susceptibility results were interpreted according to CLSI standards 26th Edition except NAL screening. NAL screening was interpreted according to EUCAST criteria [16]. *H. influenzae* was considered decreased

Table 1 Primers used in this study

Genes	Primers	Sequences	References
16S rRNA	*LPW55*	AGTTTGATCCTGGCTCAG	[19]
	LPW56	AGGCCCGGGAACGTATTC AC	
gyrA	*gyrA*-F	CCGCCGCGTACTGTTCT	[21]
	gyrA-R	CCATTTGCTAAAAGTGC	
gyrB	*gyrB*-F	GGAAAATCCTGCAGATGC	[21]
	gyrB-R	AAGCAACGTACGGATGTG	
parC	*parC*-F	TGGTTTAAAACCCGTTCA	[21]
	parC-R	AGCAGGTAAATATTGTGG	
parE	*parE*-F	GAACGCTTATCATCACGCCA	[21]
	parE-R	AGCATCCGCGAGAATACA GA	
qnrA	*QnrA*-F	AGAGGATTTCTCACGCCA GG	[22]
	QnrA-R	TGCCAGGCACAGATCTTG AC	
qnrB	*QnrB*-F	GGMATHGAAATTCGCCAC TG	[22]
	QnrB-R	TTTGCYGYYCGCCAGTCGAA	
qnrS	*QnrS*-F	GCAAGTTCATTGAACAGG GT	[22]
	QnrS-R	TCTAAACCGTCGAGTTCG GCG	
Aac(6′)-Ib-cr	*aac (6′)-Ib-cr*-F	TTGCGATGCTCTATGAGT GGCTA	[22]
	aac (6′)-Ib-cr-R	CTCGAATGCCTGGCGTGTTT	
qepA	*qepA*-F	AACTGCTTGAGCCCGTAGAT	[22]
	qepA-R	GTCTACGCCATGGACCTCAC	
oqxA	*oqxA*-F	AGTCCATACCAACCTCGT CTCC	[22]
	oqxA-R	GCGTGGCTTTGAACTCTGC	
oqxB	*oqxB*-F	CCACCCTTAACTGATCCC TAA	[22]
	oqxB-R	CGCCAGCTCATCCTTCAC	
adk	*adk*-F	GGTGCACCGGGTGCAGGT AA	[23]
	adk-R	CCTAAGATTTTATCTAACTC	
atpG	*atpG*-F	ATGGCAGGTGCAAAA GAGAT	[23]
	atpG-R	TTGTACAACAGGCTTTTGCG	
frdB	*frdB*-F	CTTATCGTTGGTCTTGCCGT	[23]
	frdB-R	TTGGCACTTTCCACTTTTCC	
fucK	*fucK*-F	ACCACTTTCGGCGTGGAT GG	[23]
	fucK-R	AAGATTTCCCAGGTGCCA GA	
mdh	*mdh*-F	TCATTGTATGATATTGCCCC	[23]
	mdh-R	ACTTCTGTACCTGCATTTTG	
pgi	*pgi*-F	GGTGAAAAAATCAATCGTAC	[23]
	pgi-R	ATTGAAAGACCAATAGCTGA	
recA	*recA*-F	ATGGCAACTCAAGAAGAA AA	[23]
	recA-R	TTACCAAACATCACGCCTAT	

susceptibility to ciprofloxacin when MICs of ciprofloxacin were ≥ 0.125 μg/ml. *H. influenzae* ATCC 29247 was used as a quality control strain for susceptibility testing.

Sequencing of QRDRs and plasmid-mediated quinolone resistance genes

Haemophilus influenzae showed decreased susceptibilities to ciprofloxacin were selected for molecular analysis. The isolates were detected for *gyrA*, *gyrB*, *parC* and *parE* mutations by using primers and methods described previously [25]. The amplification condition for QRDRs was as follows: denaturation at 95 °C for 5 min and 30 cycles of 95 °C for 30 s, annealing at 60 °C for 1 min, and polymerization at 72 °C for 90 s; The samples were then extended at 72 °C for 7 min to fully extend the amplicons. The sequences of the PCR products were compared with known sequences *H. influenzae* Rd KW20 complete genome (L42023) in the GenBank. Plasmid mediated quinolone resistance (PMQR) genes *qnrA*, *qnrB*, *qnrS*, *aac(6′)-Ib-cr*, *qepA*, *oqxA*, and *oqxB* were amplified and sequenced as described previously [26] (Table 1).

Nucleotide accession numbers

The sequences of 11 strains with *gyrA* or *parC* mutations have been annotated and submitted to the GenBank under accession number MG694554, MG694555, MG694556, MG694557, MG694558, MG694559, MG694560, MG694561, MG694562, MG694563 and MG694564.

Multilocus sequence typing (MLST)

Seven housekeeping genes fragments including *adk*, *atpG*, *frdB*, *fuck*, *mdh*, *pgi*, *recA* were amplified according to the primers in Table 1. PCR products were obtained with the following PCR amplification procedure, initial denaturation at 95 °C for 4 min, followed by 30 cycles of 95 °C for 30 s, 55 °C for 30 s, and 72 °C for 60 s. The samples were then maintained at 72 °C for 10 min, cooled to 4 °C. Allele numbers and STs were assigned by applying the *H. influenzae* MLST website (http://haemophilus.mlst.net/) [27].

Statistical analysis

Data were analyzed with the Statistical Package for Social Sciences for Windows (SPSSWIN, Chicago, IL, USA, version 19.0). Continuous data, shown as mean ± SD or medians, were compared by Student's t-test or the Mann–Whitney *U*-test. Categorical variables, summarized as numbers and percentages, were compared by Chi square-test or Fisher's exact test. Two sided *p*-values less than 0.05 were considered statistically significant.

Results

Bacterial isolates

As clinical data of the studied 402 nonduplicate *H. influenzae* strains was concerned, male patients accounted for 63.7% (n = 256), and 130 (32.3%), 110 (27.4%) and 162 (40.3%) patients were ≥ 60 (mean: 79.41 ± 8.77), 15–59 (mean: 50.50 ± 15.56) and < 15 (mean: 50.50 ± 15.56) years old, respectively. *H. influenzae* strains were originated from different anatomical sites: sputum (n = 258, 64.1%), throat swab (n = 64, 15.9%), bronchoscope sputum (n = 48, 11.9%), bronchoalveolar lavage fluid (n = 19, 4.7%), secretion (n = 13, 3.2%). *H. influenzae* isolates were obtained from patients admitted to the respiratory department (n = 141, 35.0%), pediatrics department (n = 163, 40.5%), otolaryngology department (n = 12, 3.0%), thoracic surgery (n = 10, 2.5%), nephrology department (n = 8, 2%), allergy department (n = 7, 1.7%), radiotherapy department (n = 7, 1.7%), others (n = 54, 13.4%).

Sensitivity of *H. influenzae* isolates

Of the 402 *H. influenzae* isolates, one hundred and sixty-nine (42.0%) possessed β-lactamases and were resistant to ampicillin. Eighty-nine isolates were β-lactamase negative but resistant to ampicillin which were defined as BLNAR (β-lactamase-negative ampicillin-resistant). Forty isolates were totally susceptible to ten antimicrobials according to Kirby–Bauer disk diffusion test, while 259 (64.4%) strains were resistant to sulfamethoxazole, followed with ampicillin (n = 247, 61.4%), cefuroxime (n = 114, 28.4%), azithromycin (n = 70, 17.4%), cefotaxime (n = 45, 11.2%), ceftriaxone (n = 37, 9.2%), meropenem (n = 21, 5.2%). Multidrug resistant strains accounted for 61 (15.2%).

Ciprofloxacin-nonsusceptible *H. influenzae* isolates

Eleven (2.7%) ciprofloxacin-resistant *H. influenzae* were detected by the Kirby–Bauer disk diffusion test and seven (1.7%) with reduced susceptibilities or resistant to ciprofloxacin (MICs were range from 0.5 to 12 μg/ml) were detected by the E-test method. The MICs of levofloxacin ranged from 0.5 to 3 μg/ml. Among 402 *H. influenzae*, fifteen (3.7%) isolates with ciprofloxacin inhibitory zone diameters of 21–28 mm were screened by the NAL disks, 2 of which were NAL-resistant with inhibitory zone diameters less than 23 mm. The ciprofloxacin MICs of NAL-resistant strains were 0.38 μg/ml and 0.5 μg/ml, respectively. The susceptibility of ciprofloxacin-nonsusceptible *H. influenzae* isolates were shown in Table 3.

Infection risks analysis

The comparison of ciprofloxacin nonsusceptible to susceptible group according to 17 clinical variables is listed in Table 2, which is including sex, underlying diseases, causes, and medical history during previous 3 months. Among the causes, receiving invasive procedure like sputum suction and bronchoscopy ($p = 0.011$), catching cold or previous contact with someone who had a cold ($p = 0.019$) and fluoroquinolones use during previous 3 months ($p = 0.003$) can increased the risks of ciprofloxacin-nonsusceptible *H. influenzae* infection (Table 2). Moreover, multidrug resistant strains were more common to the ciprofloxacin-nonsusceptible group ($p = 0.000$).

Detection of amino acid substitutions in the QRDRs and plasmid-mediated quinolone resistance genes

Seven isolates harbored the amino acid substitution Ser-84-Leu in *gyrA* while four isolates harbored the amino acid substitution Ser-84-ILe in *parC*. Four isolates had both two amino acid substitutions in QRDRs. Three of the isolates with mutations were obtained from young children with 1–3 years of age. The MICs of ciprofloxacin to strains with one or two mutations were of 0.38–1.5 μg/ml, while one strain obtained from an outpatient with MIC of 12 μg/ml did not harbored alterations in QRDRs. No amino acid substitutions were found in *gyrB* and *parE* genes and no plasmid-mediated quinolone resistance genes were found in our investigation (Table 3).

Multilocus sequence typing (MLST)

Nine ciprofloxacin-nonsusceptible isolates were resolved into 5 different sequence types (ST), which displayed high genetic variability. Four STs were previously described in the MLST database and one (ST1791) was a new ST that had not been reported previously. ST408 was the most common ST in our study. However, according to the epidemiological data such as the isolation date and departments, no clonal spread of FRHI was found in our study.

Discussion

This study has provided data of ciprofloxacin-resistant *H. influenzae* incidence in Guangzhou, China. The incidence in our study was closer to the report from Hong Kong [6], which stayed at a very low resistant rate, in contrary to Taiwan's [4, 8]. According to our investigation, the use of fluoroquinolone was not so common in adults, which may explain the low incidence of ciprofloxacin-resistant *H. influenzae* in Guangzhou. Although most of the *H. influenzae* were community-acquired, invasive procedure like sputum suction and bronchoscopy may also increase the infection risks of ciprofloxacin-resistant *H. influenzae* which indicated that nosocomial environment colonization is an important route of ciprofloxacin-resistant *H. influenzae* infection. In addition, medication history of fluoroquinolone during previous 3 months is closely related to ciprofloxacin-resistant *H. influenzae*

Table 2 Clinical characteristics and infection risk factors of *Haemophilus influenzae* with resistance or reduced susceptibility to ciprofloxacin/levofloxacin

Variables[a]	N	Ciprofloxacin[c]		p[d]
		Susceptible	Decreased susceptibility	
Age (years)				
0–14	162 (40.3%)			
5–59	110 (27.4%)			
≥ 60	130 (32.3%)			
Sex				
Male	256 (63.7%)	250 (63.6%)	6 (66.7%)	1.000
Female	146 (36.3%)	143 (36.3%)	3 (33.3%)	1.000
Prevalent seasons (months)				
3–5	138 (34.3%)			
6–8	67 (16.7%)			
9–11	54 (13.4%)			
12–2	143 (35.6%)			
Underlying diseases				
Chronic obstructive pulmonary disease	60 (14.9%)	58 (14.7%)	2 (22.2%)	0.626
Hypertension	70 (17.4%)	68 (17.3%)	2 (22.2%)	1.000
Diabetes	28 (7.0%)	27 (6.9%)	1 (11.1%)	1.000
Chronic kidney disease	33 (8.2%)	33 (8.4%)	0 (0%)	1.000[b]
Cancers	46 (11.4%)	45 (11.5%)	1 (11.1%)	1.000
Interstitial lung Disease	14 (3.5%)	1 3(3.3%)	1 (11.1%)	0.732
Bronchiectasia	27 (6.7%)			
Causes				
Catch cold or be tired	30 (7.5%)	27 (6.9%)	3 (33.3%)	0.019
Invasive procedure	27 (6.7%)	24 (6.1%)	3 (33.3%)	0.011
History of smoking	40 (9.9%)	39 (9.9%)	1 (11.1%)	1.000
Channel of infection				
Community-acquired	372 (92.5%)			
Hospital-acquired	30 (7.5%)			
Hospitalization during previous 3 months	133 (33.1%)	128 (32.6%)	5 (55.6%)	0.147
Fluoroquinolones use during previous 3 months	5 (1.2%)	7 (1.8%)	2 (22.2%)	*0.003*
Antimicrobial use during previous 3 months				
Cephalosporins		144 (36.6%)	4 (44.4%)	0.896
Azithromycin		70 (17.8%)	0 (0%)	0.370[b]
Piperacillin		13 (3.3%)	1 (11.1%)	0.732
Multidrug resistant strains		55 (14.0%)	8 (88.9%)	0.000

[a] Data are presented as mean ± SD or number of patients (%)

[b] Fisher's exact test

[c] Numbers of susceptible and decreased susceptibility are 393 and 9, respectively

[d] Statistically significant data are in italics

infection. Patients who are reinfected with *H. influenzae* should be monitored of fluoroquinolone susceptibility for the isolates may have obtained resistance under antibiotic selective pressure. It is known that fluoroquinolone is not approved for children in most regions of the world now, and children infected with ciprofloxacin-resistant *H. influenzae* in our study were all community-acquired, so we inferred that the acquisition of such *H. influenzae* in children may be attributed to disseminating from community environment and consuming products from food animal previously fed antimicrobial agents of fluoroquinolone. In addition, *H. influenzae* carriage in children should rise our concern in preventing the spread of resistant *H. influenzae*, especially in public areas like daycares [6].

Table 3 Clinical characteristics, resistance and molecular typing of CIP resistant or susceptibility-decreased *H. influenzae* strains

No.	Age	Sex	Date	Department and infection	Causes and underlying diseases	Disk diffusion			E-test		Resistance	During previous 3 months	ST	QRDRs	
						Ci	L	Na	Ci	L		Hospitalization and antimicrobial		*gyrA*	*parC*
38	3	M	17.2.14	Respiratory RI, A	Contact with patient; rhinallergosis	28	25	6	0.38	0.38	AmCfCtST	N; Cf	12	Ser-84-Leu	–
254	70	M	16.5.16	Respiration (4), A	/; interstitial lung disease arthritis deformans	21	19	6	0.5	0.5	AmAsCfS	N; N	836	–	–
179	61	F	16.4.3	Gastrointestinal surgery, B	Radical mastectomy; mammary cancer cholecystolithiasis hypertension	19	21	–	1.5	0.75	CfST	Y; Cf	408	Ser-84-Leu	Ser-84-Ile
187	2	F	16.4.7	Pediatrics, A	Bronchoscopy; acleistocardia	20	6	–	1	0.5	CfS	Y (3); Cf	408	Ser-84-Leu	Ser-84-Ile
197	1	M	16.4.8	Pediatrics, A	Bronchoscopy; tracheostenosis, acleistocardia family history of rhinallergosis	19	23	–	1	0.75	CfS	Y (4); unspecified fluoroquinolone, Cf	408	Ser-84-Leu	Ser-84-Ile
216	62	M	16.4.21	Respiration (2), A	Catch cold, COPD, hypertension	20	21	–	0.5	0.5	AmAsAzS	Y; fluoroquinolone enoxacin, P	422	Ser-84-Leu	--
237	87	F	16.5.3	Respiration (3), A	Mechanical ventilation and catch cold; smoking COPD chronic corpulmonale	19	21	–	0.75	0.5	AmAsAzCfCtST	Y; N	422	Ser-84-Leu	-
291	61	M	16.7.12	Respiration (3), A	/; emphysema	20	6	–	0.75	0.5	AmAsAzCfST	N; N	408	Ser-84-Leu	Ser-84-Ile
387	56	M	16.10.10	Outpatient, A	Catch cold; /	6	18	–	> 12	3	M	/; N	1791	–	–

Figures in brackets after department means different zones of the department. Figures in brackets of column Hospitalization means the frequency of hospitalization during previous 3 months

M male, *F* female, / not mentioned, *Y* yes, *N* no, *A* community-acquired, *B* hospital-acquired, *Am* ampicillin, *As* ampicillin–sulbactam, *Az* azithromycin, *Ci* ciprofloxacin, *Cf* cefuroxime, *Ct* ceftriaxone, *M* meropenem, *Na* nalidixic acid, *L* levofloxacin, *P* piperacillin, *S* trimethoprim–sulfamethoxazole, *T* cefotaxime, *QRDR* quinolone resistance determining regions, *ST* sequence

Although ciprofloxacin-resistant *H. influenzae* remains rare in Guangzhou, nine ciprofloxacin-nonsusceptible. *H. influenzae* isolates were detected in our study (2.2%, including two NAL-resistant strains), which may develop into resistance in a stepwise manner according to the molecular mechanism in QRDRs. Seven of the isolates had developed amino acid substitution in QRDRs, with ciprofloxacin MICs of 0.38 to1.5 μg/ml. *H. influenzae* in our investigation with ciprofloxacin MICs of 0.38–0.75 μg/ml had one amino acid alteration in *gyrA*, and isolates with ciprofloxacin MICs of 0.75–1.5 μg/ml had two amino acid alteration in *gyrA* and *parC*. According to the previous report, isolates with ciprofloxacin MICs of 0.12–0.5 μg/ml had at least one amino acid alteration in a position of the fluoroquinolone targets involved in resistance. It was revealed that the degree of fluoroquinolone-resistance is related to the number of the mutations in QRDRs [16]. Strains presenting one or two mutations in *gyrA* and *parC* have low-level resistance to fluoroquinolone, while those with three or more mutations show high-level resistance [28]. In general, our finding was consistent with the report [16]. However, there were two isolates with ciprofloxacin MICs of 0.5 μg/ml and 12 μg/ml respectively didn't harboring any mutations in QRDRs and plasmid-mediated quinolone resistance genes. We inferred that some other mechanisms may participated in fluoroquinolone-resistance of *H. influenzae*.

Amino acid changes in *gyrA* residue (Ser84) and/or *parC* residue (Ser84) were detected in our study while no substitutions occurred in *gyrB* and *parE*. Ser84Leu in *gyrA* and Ser-84-Ile in *parC* were globally reported according to the current literatures, including Spain, Japan, Taiwan [4, 14, 16, 25, 29]. The similar mutation patterns in QRDRs around different areas indicated that Ser-84-Leu in *gyrA* and Ser-84-Ile in *parC* were one of the most common mutations in QRDRs. Comparing with the mutation profiles in QRDRs from Guangzhou and Taiwan, the latter one had more diverse mutation profiles than Guangzhou [4]. In Taiwan, emergence of fluoroquinolone-resistant isolates may be the results of several clones spreading in the same region. However, according to our investigation, no clone transmitted hospital infection was found which indicated that fluoroquinolone-nonsusceptible *H. influenzae* may occur sporadically in Guangzhou presently. In addition, our investigation reported a relative high genetic diversity among fluoroquinolone-resistant *H. influenzae* isolates. None of the STs published in Taiwan were found in our study, but ST422 and ST408 involved in our study were previously reported in Sichuan, China, where also discovered a series of diverse and novel sequence types as Taiwan [4, 30]. The predominant epidemiological STs in China like ST486 and 480 were not found in our study. The heterogeneous characteristics of the *H. influenzae* strains may be the reason that no outbreak or epidemics occurred in Guangzhou. Moreover, high heterogeneity of *H. influenzae* strains by MLST analysis revealed that the *H. influenzae* strains were regionally varied and evolved independently. One strain was confirmed as novel sequence type (ST1719) in our study, which showed high-level resistance of ciprofloxacin while no mutations in QRDRs was found.

There were two NAL-resistant strains harboring amino acid substitution in QRDRs in our study and both of them were ciprofloxacin-susceptible according to CLSI criteria. It has been argued that, the application of current CLSI criteria may underrecognize the low-level ciprofloxacin-resistant *H. influenzae* with first step mutations in QRDRs [6, 16, 17]. As a screening test for determination of the susceptibilities of gram-negative bacteria to fluoroquinolone, NAL has drawn special attention [6, 16], it can separate strains with reduced quinolone susceptibilities as a result of the acquisition of mutations in the QRDRs. However, NAL screening was not applied routinely in determination of the susceptibilities of *H. influenzae* in clinics which may underrecognize a proportion of strains with decreased fluoroquinolone susceptibilities. In addition, no acceptable criteria for NAL screening was established by CLSI in the current. In order to detect fluoroquinolone non-susceptible strains with first step mutation in QRDRs, screening with NAL as an indicator of resistance was proposed by the EUCAST guidelines. First failure case of oral levofloxacin treatment of community-acquired pneumonia caused by *H. influenzae* had been reported in 2003 [14]. After that, reports on fluoroquinolone treatment failure were occurred globally. An reports from New York declared that persistent stimulation of low concentration fluoroquinolone in fluoroquinolone-susceptible *H. influenzae* may increase the fluoroquinolone resistance of *H. influenzae* isolates which offered experiment evidence for the declaration of avoiding fluoroquinolone treatment in *H. influenzae* close to breakpoints. And they pointed out that the key to preventing fluoroquinolone resistance in *H. influenzae* may be to block enrichment of the first *gyrA* mutation by strictly avoiding low dose fluoroquinolones use [28]. In addition, medication history of fluoroquinolone is related to fluoroquinolone non-susceptible *H. influenzae* infection according to our investigation, so we inferred that a proportion of strains harboring the first step mutation in QRDRs might obtain fluoroquinolone resistance under fluoroquinolone selection pressure. High-level resistance might be induced by repeated treatment with fluoroquinolone in patients with chronic lung diseases like COPD. Treatment failure reminded us that we should pay attention to those *H. influenzae* with resistance or decreased susceptibilities to fluoroquinolone, and should facilitate the laboratory detection of strains with decreased susceptibilities to fluoroquinolone.

In conclusion, as the first study of FRHI in mainland China, reduced susceptibilities to fluoroquinolones had been obtained, despite low incidence of FRHI isolates. Invasive procedure and medication history of fluoroquinolone during previous 3 months can increase the infection risks of FRHI. High genetic diversity in FRHI strains has strongly suggested their sporadic emergence and spread in Guangzhou of Southern China, and amino acid substitutions in QRDRs of strains with decreased susceptibilities to fluoroquinolone have also presented evidence on the initial evolution of fluoroquinolone resistance by mutation in *gyrA*, indicating the potential treatment failure or increase of fluoroquinolone resistance under continuous fluoroquinolone therapy. In addition, this study has for the first time reported the mutation of *gyrA* and *parC* in mainland China and the new ST1719 worldwide, which may further raise clinical concerns regarding the therapeutic efficacy of fluoroquinolone treatment and aid in further investigation on FRHI.

Abbreviations

FRHI: fluoroquinolone-resistant *Haemophilus influenzae*; QRDR: quinolone resistance-determining regions; CAP: community-acquired pneumonia; AOM: acute otitis media; FQs: fluoroquinolones; ST: sequence types; AMP: ampicillin; AMS: ampicillin–sulbactam; CIP: ciprofloxacin; LEV: levofloxacin; CTR: ceftriaxone; ROXH: cefuroxime; TAX: cefotaxime; MEM: meropenem; SXT: trimethoprim–sulfamethoxazole; AZT: azithromycin; HTM: *Haemophilus* test medium; NAL: nalidixic acid; MICs: minimum inhibitory concentrations; PMQR: plasmid mediated quinolone resistance.

Authors' contributions

DC and LY designed the study, SW and DF carried out the experiments, including species identification, antimicrobial susceptibility, YL and DS conducted the experiment of the sequencing of QRDRs and analyzed the plasmid-mediated quinolone resistance genes, etc. ZX, LJ and RX performed the statistical analysis, and wrote the manuscript. All authors read and approved the final manuscript.

Author details

[1] Department of Laboratory Medicine, Zhujiang Hospital, Southern Medical University, Guangzhou 510280, China. [2] Department of Laboratory Medicine, The First Affiliated Hospital of Guangzhou Medical University, Guangzhou Medical University, Guangzhou 510120, China. [3] School of Food Science and Engineering, South China University of Technology, Guangzhou 510640, China. [4] Department of Clinical Pharmacy, College of Pharmacy, University of Tennessee Health Science Center, Memphis, TN 38163, USA. [5] Guangdong Province Key Laboratory for Green Processing of Natural Products and Product Safety, Guangzhou 510640, China. [6] Department of Microbial Pathogenesis, School of Dentistry, University of Maryland, Baltimore, MD 21201, USA.

Acknowledgements

This work was supported by the Natural Science Foundation of Guangdong Province (2018A030310170 and 2018A030313279), the National Key Research and Development Program of China (2016YFD04012021), Guangdong Special Support Program (2016TQ03N682), Pearl River S&T Nova Program of Guangzhou (201710010061), Science and Technology Planning Project of Guangdong Province (2017A050501007), National Outstanding Doctoral Dissertation Funding (201459), and the Fundamental Research Funds for the Central Universities (2017ZD092).

Competing interests

The authors declare that they have no competing interests.

Consent for publication

Not applicable.

References

1. Garcia-Cobos S, Moscoso M, Pumarola F, Arroyo M, Lara N, Perez-vazquez M, et al. Frequent carriage of resistance mechanisms to beta-lactams and biofilm formation in *Haemophilus influenzae* causing treatment failure and recurrent otitis media in young children. J Antimicrob Chemother. 2014;69:2394–9.
2. Watt JP, Wolfson LJ, O'Brien KL, Henkle E, Deloria-Knoll M, Natelie MM, et al. Burden of disease caused by *Haemophilus influenzae* type b in children younger than 5 years: global estimates. Lancet. 2009;374:903–11.
3. Committee for The Japanese Respiratory Society guidelines for the management of respiratory infections. Guidelines for the management of community acquired pneumonia in adults, revised edition. Respirology. 2006;11:S79–133.
4. Kuo S, Chen P, Shiau YR, Wang H, Lai J, Huang IW, et al. Levofloxacin-resistant *Haemophilus influenzae*, Taiwan, 2004–2010. Emerg Infect Dis. 2014;20:1386–90.
5. Li X, Mariano N, Rahal JJ, Urban CM, Drlica K. Quinolone-resistant *Haemophilus influenzae* in a long-term-care facility: nucleotide sequence characterization of alterations in the genes encoding DNA gyrase and DNA topoisomerase IV. Antimicrob Agents Chemother. 2004;48:3570–2.
6. Pak LH, Chow KH, Mak GC, Tsang KW, Lau YL, Ho AY, et al. Decreased levofloxacin susceptibility in *Haemophilus influenzae* in children, Hong Kong. Emerg Infect Dis. 2004;10:1960.
7. Chang C, Lauderdale TL, Lee HC, Lee NY, Wu C, Chen P, et al. Colonisation of fluoroquinolone-resistant *Haemophilus influenzae* among nursing home residents in southern Taiwan. J Hosp Infect. 2010;75:304–8.
8. Hu F, Zhu D, Wang F, Morrissey I, Wang J, Torumkuney D. Results from the survey of antibiotic resistance (SOAR) 2009–11 and 2013–14 in China. J Antimicrob Chemother. 2016;71:33–43.
9. Miao J, Liang Y, Chen L, Wang W, Wang J, Li B, Li L, Chen D, Xu Z. Formation and development of biofilm: with focus on food safety. J Food Saf. 2017;37(4):e12358.
10. Hu J, Sun X, Huang Z, Wagner A, Carlson B, Yang J, et al. *Streptococcus pneumoniae* and *Haemophilus influenzae* type b carriage in Chinese children aged 12–18 months in Shanghai, China: a cross-sectional study. BMC Infect Dis. 2016;16:149.
11. Lin J, Chen X, Chen C, Hu J, Zhou C, Cai X, Wang W, Zheng C, Zhang P, Cheng J, Guo Z, Liu H. Durably antibacterial and bacterially antiadhesive cotton fabrics coated by cationic fluorinated polymers. ACS Appl Mater Interfaces. 2018;10(7):6124–36.
12. Liu J, Chen D, Peters BM, Li L, Li B, Xu Z, Shirliff ME. Staphylococcal chromosomal cassettes mec (SCCmec): a mobile genetic element in methicillin-resistant Staphylococcus aureus. Microb Pathog. 2016;101:56–67.
13. Vila J, Ruiz J, Sanchez F, Navarro F, Mirelis B, de Anta MT, et al. Increase in quinolone resistance in a *Haemophilus influenzae* strain isolated from a patient with recurrent respiratory infections treated with of ofloxacin. Antimicrob Agents Chemother. 1999;43:161–2.
14. Bastida T, Perez-Vazquez M, Campos J, Cortes-Llletget MC, Roman F, Tubau F, et al. Levofloxacin treatment failure in *Haemophilus influenzae* pneumonia. Emerg Infect Dis. 2003;9:475–1478.
15. Georgiou M, Munoz R, Roman F, Canton R, Gomez-Lus R, Campos J, et al. Ciprofloxacin-resistant *Haemophilus influenzae* strains possess mutations in analogous positions of *GyrA* and *ParC*. Antimicrob Agents Chemother. 1996;40:1741–4.
16. Puig C, Tirado-Velez JM, Calatayud L, Tubau F, Garmendia J, Ardanuy C, et al. Molecular characterization of fluoroquinolone resistance in nontypeable *Haemophilus influenzae* clinical isolates. Antimicrob Agents Chemother. 2015;59:461–6.
17. Perez-Vazquez M, Roman F, Aracil B, Canton R, Campos J. Laboratory detection of *Haemophilus influenzae* with decreased susceptibility to nalidixic acid, ciprofloxacin, levofloxacin, and moxifloxacin due to *gyrA* and *parC* mutations. J Clin Microbiol. 2004;42:1185–91.

18. Xu Z, Xie J, Peters BM, Li B, Li L, Yu G, Shirtliff ME. Longitudinal surveillance on antibiogram of important Gram-positive pathogens in Southern China, 2001 to 2015. Microb Pathog. 2017;103:80–6.
19. Xie J, Yang L, Peters BM, Chen L, Chen D, Li B, et al. A 16-year retrospective surveillance report on the pathogenic features and antimicrobial susceptibility of *Pseudomonas aeruginosa* isolates from FAHJU in Guangzhou representative of Southern China. Microb Pathog. 2017;110:37–41.
20. Xie J, Peters BM, Li B, Li L, Yu G, Xu Z, et al. Clinical features and antimicrobial resistance profiles of important *Enterobacteriaceae* pathogens in Guangzhou representative of Southern China, 2001–2015. Microb Pathog. 2017;107:206–11.
21. Liu J, Deng Y, Peters BM, Li L, Li B, Chen L, et al. Transcriptomic analysis on the formation of the viable putative non-culturable state of beer-spoilage *Lactobacillus acetotolerans*. Sci Rep. 2016;6:1–11.
22. McBain AJ, Bartolo RG, Catrenich CE, Charbonneau D, Ledder RG, Gilbert P. Effects of triclosan-containing rinse on the dynamics and antimicrobial susceptibility of in vitro plaque ecosystems. Antimicrob Agents Chemother. 2003;47:3531–8.
23. Lau SKP, Woo PCY, Mok MY, Teng JLL, Tam VKP, Chan KKH, et al. Characterization of *Haemophilus segnis*, an important cause of bacteremia, by 16S rRNA gene sequencing. J Clin Microbiol. 2004;42:877–80.
24. Thompson JD, Higgins DG, Gibson TJ, Clustal W. Improving the sensitivity of progressive multiple sequence alignment through sequence weighting, position-specific gap penalties and weight matrix choice. Nucleic Acids Res. 1994;22:4673–80.
25. Shoji H, Shirakura T, Fukuchi K, Takuma T, Hanaki H, Tanaka K, et al. A molecular analysis of quinolone-resistant *Haemophilus influenzae*: validation of the mutations in quinolone resistance-determining regions. J Infect Chemother. 2014;20:250–5.
26. Al-Agamy MH, Aljallal A, Radwan HH, Shibl AM. Characterization of carbapenemases, ESBLs, and plasmid-mediated quinolone determinants in carbapenem-insensitive *Escherichia coli* and *Klebsiella pneumoniae* in Riyadh hospitals. J Infect Public Health. 2017;731:1–5.
27. Meats E, Feil EJ, Stringer S, Cody AJ, Goldstein R, Kroll JS, et al. Characterization of encapsulated and noncapsulated *Haemophilus influenzae* and determination of phylogenetic relationships by multilocus sequence typing. J Clin Microbiol. 2003;41:1623–36.
28. Li X, Mariano N, Rahal JJ, Urban CM, Drlica K. Quinolone-resistant *Haemophilus influenzae*: determination of mutant selection window for ciprofloxacin, garenoxacin, levofloxacin, and moxifloxacin. Antimicrob Agents Chemother. 2004;48:4460–2.
29. Yokot S, Ohkoshi Y, Sato K, Fujii N. Emergence of fluoroquinolone-resistant *Haemophilus influenzae* strains among elderly patients but not among children. J Clin Microbiol. 2008;46:361–5.
30. Tian G, Zhang L, Li M, Wang X, Zheng Y, Li X, et al. Genotypic characteristics of *Haemophilus influenzae* isolates from pediatric pneumonia patients in Chengdu city, Sichuan, China. J Microbiol. 2009;47:494–7.

26

Molecular characterization of β-lactamase genes in clinical isolates of carbapenem-resistant *Acinetobacter baumannii*

Kevin M. Raible[1,2], Bhaswati Sen[1,2], Nancy Law[1], Tiffany E. Bias[1], Christopher L. Emery[1,6], Garth D. Ehrlich[1,2,3,4,5] and Suresh G. Joshi[1,2,4*]

Abstract

Background: *Acinetobacter baumannii* is a nosocomial pathogen which is establishing as a major cause of morbidity and mortality within the healthcare community. The success of this pathogen is largely due to its ability to rapidly gain resistance to antimicrobial therapies and its capability to persist in an abiotic environment through the production of a biofilm. Our tertiary-care hospital has showed high incidence of carbapenem-resistant *Acinetobacter baumannii* (CRAB) isolates.

Methods: In this study we explore both genotypic and phenotypic properties of 26 CRAB isolates: 16 isolates were collected from January 2010 to March 2011, and 10 were collected between February and May 2015.

Results: We determined that all 26 CRAB isolates possessed multiple β-lactamase genes, including genes from Groups A, C, and D. Specifically, 42% of the isolates possesses the potentially plasmid-borne genes of OXA-23-like or OXA-40-like β-lactamase. The presence of mobile gene element integron cassettes and/or integrases in 88% of the isolates suggests a possible mechanism of dissemination of antibiotic resistance genes. Additionally, the location of insertion sequence (IS) IS*Aba*1 in promotor region of of the OXA-51-like, ADC-7, and ampC genes was confirmed. Multilocus sequence typing (MLST) demonstrated that all 26 CRAB isolates were either sequence type (ST)-229 or ST-2. Interestingly, ST-2 went from being the minority CRAB strain in the 2010–2011 isolates to the predominant strain in the 2015 isolates (from 32 to 90%). We show that the ST-2 strains have an enhanced ability to produce biofilms in comparison to the ST-229 strains, and this fact has potentially led to more successful colonization of the clinical environment over time.

Conclusions: This study provides a longitudinal genetic and phenotypic survey of two CRAB sequence types, and suggests how their differing phenotypes may interact with the selective pressures of a hospital setting effecting strain dominance over a 5-year period.

Keywords: *Acinetobacter baumannii*, β-lactamase, Biofilm, Carbapenem resistance, Colonization, CRAB, Integrase, Integron cassette, Multiple drug resistance, Multilocus sequence typing, MLST, OXA-51, OXA-23, OXA-40, Plasmid

*Correspondence: sgj24@drexel.edu; surejoshi@yahoo.com
[1] Center for Surgical Infections & Biofilms, Institute of Molecular Medicine and Infectious diseases, Drexel University College of Medicine, 245 N. 15th Street, Philadelphia, PA 19102, USA
Full list of author information is available at the end of the article

Background

Acinetobacter baumannii is an opportunistic pathogen that causes a variety of nosocomial infections resulting in considerable morbidity and mortality, and presents a particular threat to intensive care unit (ICU) patients [1–4]. The number of *A. baumannii* infections has been increasing globally over the past three decades; particularly with regard to infections involving multi-drug resistant (MDR) isolates. The rise of MDR bacterial strains is a major cause for concern among healthcare professionals and is prompting changes in both antibiotic regiments and hospital disinfection techniques [5–10]. Genomic studies exploring outbreaks of MDR *A. baumannii* from geographic regions distant from one another shows a high degree of similarity among strains, indicating that most outbreaks may be due to a limited number of clonal lines [11].

The ability of *A. baumannii* to rapidly gain resistance to antimicrobial compounds is an important population-level virulence factor [12] for the successful dissemination of the organism within and among health-care facilities [13, 14]. Most strains of *A. baumannii* are innately resistant to several classes of antibiotics such as first- and second-generation cephalosporins, chloramphenicol, and aminopenicillins; in addition, the ability to both accept exogenous genetic material and overexpress endogenous resistance genes has quickly resulted in the appearance of the MDR phenotype within multiple clonal lineages [6, 15]. Historically the drug of choice to treat severe *A. baumannii* infections has been carbapenems, the clinical use of both meropenem and imipenem increased dramatically in the last 15 years to treat newly emerging MDR strains [1]. Likely as a result of this selective pressure carbapenem-resistant *Acinetobacter baumannii* (CRAB) strains are being reported with greater frequency.

In addition to antibiotic resistance, the ability to adhere and produce biofilm on both biotic and abiotic surfaces has been shown to be a virulence factor in many clinical isolates of *A. baumannii* and other bacterial pathogens [16–19]. The ability of clinical isolates to adhere to lung epithelial cells which is a critical step in the establishment of lung infections, and have also been documented [20–22]. The organism survives even on abiotic surfaces for months, and numerous retrospective epidemiological studies have shown its ability to colonize medical equipment, furniture, and healthcare personnel; this phenomenon provides the organism the capability of causing outbreaks both within and among medical institutions [23–28].

In the present study, we characterize the carbapenem resistance genotypic profile, as well as the colonization-associated phenotypes of 26 CRAB isolates, collected between 2010 and 2015, from a tertiary care hospital in Philadelphia, Pennsylvania. By analyzing these data, we aimed to determine if there was a temporal trend in resistance or colonization among these clinical isolates.

Methods

Bacterial isolates and reference strains

This study included 26 clinical isolates of carbapenem-resistant [minimum inhibitory concentration of meropenem (MIC) $\geq$ 8 mg/L] isolated from Hahnemann Hospital of Drexel University College of Medicine, Philadelphia, PA. Sixteen of the isolates were collected between 2010 and 2011 and were previously partially described by Sen and Joshi [29], (old isolates) and 10 isolates were collected in 2015 (New Isolates) which have not been described to date. The isolates were randomly selected, based on their MIC to meropenem. *A. baumannii* isolates were identified using the Vitek2 system (BioMerieux Vitek Systems Inc., USA), and confirmed by a molecular technique of OXA-51 PCR. Clinical Laboratory Standards Institute (CLSI)—recommended quality control (QC) strains were used as reference strains when necessary. QC strains included: *A. baumannii* ATCC 19606, *A. baumannii* ATCC 17978; *Escherichia coli* ATCC-BAA-2452, NCTC 13476; *Klebsiella pneumoniae* ATCC-BAA-2146, *K. pneumoniae* ATCC-BAA-1705, *K. pneumoniae* NCTC13440, and *Enterobacter cloacae* NCTC 13464. Additional file 1: Table S1 shows the QC strains and the reference gene for which they were used. The study was approved by the Institutional Review Board (IRB) of Drexel University, and a waiver granted.

Determination of minimum inhibitory concentration (MIC)

Carbapenem MIC results were obtained for each CRAB isolate using the VITEK 2 system and the results were confirmed by broth microdilution. All clinical breakpoints recommendations and broth microdilution protocols were followed as per Clinical Laboratory Standards Institute (CLSI) guidelines [30]. The antimicrobial agents tested were ampicillin/sulbactam, imipenem, meropenem, amikacin, levofloxacin, gentamicin, cefepime, tobramycin, trimethoprim/sulfamethoxazole and piperacillin. In routine, our hospital laboratory does not include and report polymyxin and tigecycline for this organism, and hence these agents were not included to study panel.

Polymerase chain reaction (PCR) Amplification and DNA Sequencing

Using DNeasy Blood and Tissue kit (Qiagen, Valencia, CA), genomic DNA was isolated from bacterial cells. All PCR primers targeting resistance genes and mobile elements used in this study are listed in Additional file 2: Table S2. PCR was performed using Thermo Scientific

Dream Taq Green PCR Master Mix (Thermo-Fisher Scientific, Inc, Waltham, MA) using conditions specified by the reference sources. The isolates were tested for each target gene two–four times. Negative controls were included with every PCR setup to monitor for carryover [31] and rule out nonspecific amplification. Appropriate positive control strains were used to confirm the validity of each PCR primer pair (Additional file 1: Table S1). Wherever an appropriate QC strain for a particular gene was unavailable the amplicon present with the approximate size of the predicted product was purified using described method and sequences analyzed, and gene identifications were made using NCBI nucleotide *BLAST* tool (https://blast.ncbi.nlm.nih.gov/Blast/). The presence of IS elements (IS*Aba1*) upstream of target genes following the method described by Sen and Joshi [29].

Meropenem-EDTA double disk synergy test (DDS)

DDS was performed as described previously by Yong et al. using 0.5 McFarland standards, and disks containing Meropenem (10 μg) alone; Meropenem (10 μg) plus 10 μL of 0.5 M EDTA; and 0.5 M EDTA alone. Appropriate control strains were included and synergistic results were interpreted as described [29, 32].

Multi-locus sequence typing (MLST)

MLST assignments were determined using the scheme provided by Pasteur Institute MLST and Whole Genome MLST Database (https://www.pasteur.fr/mlst). MLST target genes, PCR primer sequences, and annealing temperatures were all adopted from the database and optimized. The resulting PCR amplicons were run on a 1% agarose gel to determine the amplicon size and quality, and the PCR product was purified using GeneJet PCR purification kit (ThermoFisher), and sent to GeneWiz, Inc. (GeneWiz) for Sanger sequencing. The allelic identification of the sequences and strain determination was performed using the Pasteur MLST database (http://www.pubmlst.org/abaumannii/).

Biofilm formation assay

Biofilm production was determined using 96-well polystyrene plates as described by O'Toole et al., with minor modifications [33]. Briefly, overnight cultures were grown in LB broth at 37 °C in an aerobic incubator. The following day, 200 μL LB broth diluted cultures (1:100) were added to multiple wells and the plates incubated at 37 °C in a static aerobic incubator for either 24 or 48 h. At the appropriate time the optical density was read at 595 nm, then each well received 30 μL of 0.1% Crystal Violet solution to incubate for 1 h at room temperature. After incubation, the plates were washed with tap water three times and allowed to dry at room temperature for 1 h. Then 250 μL of ethanol:acetone (4:1) solution was added to each well to solubilize the remaining stain. The optical density was then read at 570 nm, and the biofilm production was quantified by taking the OD_{570}:OD_{590} ratio. The ratio was corrected with negative control (LB alone), and biofilm forming capability of the isolates considered if the OD_{570}:OD_{590} ratio was a positive value. Experiments were run in two separate assays with a total of sixteen replicates each.

Results

Characterization of isolates

A total of 26 CRAB isolates were analyzed in this study, all collected from Hahnemann Hospital. Sixteen isolates were collected during 2010–2011 (old isolates), and the additional 10 isolates were collected in 2015 (new isolates). The relevant descriptive features are summarized in Table 1. The average age of all the patients from which the isolates were collected was 50.1 (± 17.7) years, with a range of 19–84 years. Of the 26 total patients 15 (57%) were male. A total of 14 (54%) patients were admitted in the ICU during the time of collection, and the other 12 (46%) patients were being treated for various conditions in non-ICU in-patient rooms in the hospital. A total of 12 (43%) patients' infections were considered nosocomial in origin, in which the first positive *A. baumannii* culture was reported ≥ 48 h post-admission [34].

Antibiotic susceptibility

The findings of the antibiotic susceptibility testing for all isolates are showed in Additional file 3: Table S3. The antibiogram patterns of all 26 CRAB isolates by isolate groups (2010–2011 versus 2015), clinical source, and MLST sequence types are presented in Table 2. All 26 (100%) of the CRAB isolates met the clinical definition of the MDR *A. baumannii* phenotype, defined as being non-susceptible to at least 3 classes of antibiotics [34]. All isolates (100%) were resistant or intermediately resistant to carbapenems (meropenem and imipenem), as well as Levofloxacin (fluoroquinolone). More than 80% of the isolates were resistant or intermediately resistant

Table 1 Demographics of carbapenem-resistant *A. baumannii* positive patients

Features	2010–2011 isolates	2015 isolates
Number of isolates	16	10
Average age of patient (yr)	47.8 ± 19.1	55.6 ± 15.1
Male (%)	62	50
ICU patients (%)	37	50
Nosocomial infections (%)	37	60

Table 2 Antibiogram showing percent resistant isolates of different isolate groups (old and new, clinical source, and clonal lineage) against tested antimicrobial agents

	Ampicillin/sul-bact (%)	Imipinem (%)	Meropenem (%)	Amikacin (%)	Levofloxacin (%)	Gentamicin (%)	Cefepime (%)	Tobramicin (%)	Trimeth-Sul-fametho (%)	Piperacilin (%)
Old (n = 16)	68	100	100	50	100	93	93	88	93	93
New (n = 10)	40	100	100	100	100	60	100	10	90	100
Urine (n = 3)	66	100	100	33	100	100	100	100	100	100
Sp (n = 10)	90	100	100	70	100	100	100	60	90	100
Blood (n = 3)	66	100	100	66	100	100	100	33	100	100
Tx/Wound (n = 10)	40	100	100	80	100	50	90	40	90	90
#229 (n = 12)	75	100	100	50	100	92	100	83	83	92
#2 (n = 14)	57	100	100	85	100	71	92	28	100	100

The antimicrobial agents included were ampicillin/sulbactam, imipenem, meropenem, amikacin, levofloxacin, gentamicin, cefepime, tobramycin, trimethoprim/sulfamethoxazole and piperacillin

to aminoglycosides, cephalosporins, extended-spectrum penicillins, and folate inhibitors.

Multi-locus sequence typing (MLST)

MLST was performed for all 26 CRAB isolates as described in Methods. A total of 12 (46%) isolates were determined to be ST-229 and 14 (54%) were determined to be ST-2. In the 2010–2011 isolate group, 11 (68%) of the 16 isolates were determined to be members of ST-229, while the remaining 5 (32%) isolates were identified as ST-2. In the 2015 isolate group, 9 (90%) of the isolates were identified as strain 2, and only 1 (10%) were determined to be ST 229 (Additional file 4: Figure S1). The isolates and their MLST sequence types are summarized in Table 3.

Extended-spectrum β-lactamase (ESBL) genotypic analysis

Table 3 summarizes all the ESBL genes explored in this study. All CRAB isolates, and *A. baumannii* controls carried the Group D oxacillinase $bla_{\text{OXA-51-like}}$ gene (Additional file 4: Figure S1), while no isolates contained the $bla_{\text{OXA-24}}$ or $bla_{\text{OXA-58-like}}$ gene. Two isolates, one from the 2010–2011 isolate group and one from the 2015 isolate group, possessed the $bla_{\text{OXA-40-like}}$ gene (Fig. 1). Both $bla_{\text{OXA-40-like}}$ positive isolates had the same MLST sequence type with a similar genotypic profile. Similarly, 9 (34%) isolates had $bla_{\text{OXA-23-like}}$ genes (one from the 2010–2011 isolates and eight from the 2015 isolates) had the similar genotypic profiles. All of the CRAB isolates contained the Group A β-lactamase gene bla_{TEM}, and 11 (42%) of the isolates had bla_{SHV}. The bla_{SHV} positive isolates were all ST-229, suggesting a similar clonal linage. All of the isolates were negative for other Group A β-lactamase genes including bla_{PER}, bla_{VEB}, as well as the most commonly reported clinical subtypes of bla_{KPC}, and $bla_{\text{CTX-M}}$. Additionally all isolates were negative for all of the Group B metallo-β-lactamases (MBLs) genes tested which included, bla_{Imp}, bla_{VIM}, bla_{GIM}, bla_{SPM}, bla_{SIM}, bla_{DIM}, and $bla_{\text{NDM-1}}$. All of the CRAB isolates tested contained the Group C cephalosporinase bla_{ampC} gene, while 20 (76%) also possessed the cephalosporinase $bla_{\text{ADC-7}}$ gene.

Mobile genes and insertion sequences

As described by Koeleman et al., the presence of mobile genetic elements is of particular interest as they provide strong evidence for the horizontal dissemination of antibiotic resistance genes [35]. The two mobile gene elements explored in this study were the class 1 integron cassette (ICA1) and three integrase coding genes (*int*123) as described in Hujer et al. [36]. A total of 11 (42%) of the CRAB isolates contained ICA1, and 21 (80%) of the isolates had *int*123. Only two isolates #58 ($bla_{\text{OXA-40-like}}$ positive) and #64 ($bla_{\text{OXA-23-like}}$ positive) from the 2010–2011 isolates were negative for both mobile gene elements, while all 10 (100%) of the 2015 CRAB isolates were positive for one or both of the mobile gene elements (Table 3). These data suggest that the majority of the CRAB isolates in present study may have ability to transfer genetic elements through integrons, and that these mobile elements may contain antibiotic resistance genes.

In addition, we detected IS elements in the promoter regions of several antibiotic resistance genes. A total of 25 (96%) of the CRAB isolates examined in this study were found to have the IS*Aba1* element upstream of OXA-51 (Additional file 5: Figure S2; Table 3), and one negative isolate #58 also carried IS*Aba1* in the non-promoter region of OXA-51 (this isolate also processes the $bla_{\text{OXA-40-like}}$ gene). In addition, IS*Aba1* was found upstream of the ampC cephalosporinases in 92% of the isolates, and upstream of the ADC-7 gene in 76% of the isolates.

Biofilm production

In vitro biofilm production assays were performed on all CRAB isolates (Fig. 1) with 9 of 26 (34%) showing varying degrees of biofilm production. Figure 1a shows the 2015 isolates includes more biofilm producers than the 2010–2011 isolates ($p = 0.03$). There was no significant association found between biofilm production and the source of the isolate (Fig. 1b). Evaluation of biofilm production between the two MLST strain types demonstrated that the ST-2 strains were significantly better biofilm producers than the ST-229 strains ($p = 0.04$) (Fig. 1c).

Discussion

The present study was undertaken to determine whether any patterns of resistance and fitness within our clinical CRAB isolate groups evolved or expanded over time. The unique aspect to this study is the two isolate groups we used were collected 4–5 years apart. This fact allowed us to have a look longitudinally at the genotypes and phenotypes of antibiotic-resistant *A. baumannii* isolates, and to potentially identify traits that make certain isolates successful pathogens under the selective pressures of a hospital setting.

From a clinical perspective, all the isolates examined in this study displayed the MDR phenotype [34]. We aimed to find the genetic mechanisms conferring these resistances in our isolates by exploring the presence of a large number of β-lactamase encoding genes. Metallo-β-lactamase positive *A. baumannii* isolates are rare in the United States, and we did not find isolate carrying MBL gene; however globally, reports detecting their appearance are increasing in frequency [37–39]. The Group A β-lactamases encoded by bla_{TEM} and bla_{SHV} genes has been shown to hydrolyze both penicillins, as well as first- and second- generation cephalosporins [40]. Interestingly

Table 3 PCR results for 26 CRAB isolates

Isolate	Source	MIC	MLST Type	TEM	SHV	PER	KPC	VEB	CTX	MBL	EDTA DDS	ADC-7	ISaba1 + ADC-7	ampC	ISaba1 + ampC	OXA-23	OXA-24	OXA-40	OXA-51	ISaba1 + OXA-51	OXA-58	ICA1	int123
22	Sp	16	229	+	+	–	–	–	–	–	–	–	–	+	+	–	–	–	+	+	–	+	+
25	Sp	16	229	+	+	–	–	–	–	–	–	+	+	+	+	–	–	–	+	+	–	+	+
28	T	8	2	+	–	–	–	–	–	–	–	+	+	+	+	–	–	–	+	+	–	–	+
32	U	32	229	+	+	–	–	–	–	–	–	+	+	+	+	–	–	–	+	+	–	+	+
39	Sp	16	229	+	+	–	–	–	–	–	–	+	+	+	+	–	–	–	+	+	–	+	+
42	T	16	229	+	+	–	–	–	–	–	–	+	+	+	+	–	–	–	+	+	–	+	+
51	T	16	229	+	+	–	–	–	–	–	–	+	+	+	+	–	–	–	+	+	–	+	+
52	U	16	229	+	+	–	–	–	–	–	–	+	+	+	–	–	–	–	+	+	–	+	+
56	U	32	229	+	+	–	–	–	–	–	–	+	+	+	+	–	–	–	+	+	–	+	+
57	U	8	2	+	–	–	–	–	–	–	–	–	–	+	+	–	–	–	+	+	–	–	+
58	T	> 256	2	+	–	–	–	–	–	–	–	+	+	+	–	–	–	+	+	–	–	–	–
61	U	16	229	+	+	–	–	–	–	–	–	–	–	+	+	–	–	–	+	+	–	+	+
62	Sp	16	229	+	+	–	–	–	–	–	–	–	–	+	+	–	–	–	+	+	–	+	+
64	T	32	2	+	–	–	–	–	–	–	–	+	+	+	+	+	–	–	+	+	–	–	–
65	B	16	2	+	+	–	–	–	–	–	–	–	–	+	+	–	–	–	+	+	–	+	+
68	Sp	8	229	+	–	–	–	–	–	–	–	+	+	+	+	–	–	–	+	+	–	–	+
220	T	32	2	+	–	–	–	–	–	–	–	–	–	+	+	+	–	–	+	+	–	–	+
222	B	64	2	+	–	–	–	–	–	–	–	+	+	+	+	+	–	–	+	+	–	–	+
223	Sp	32	2	+	–	–	–	–	–	–	–	+	+	+	+	+	–	–	+	+	–	+	+
224	T	64	229	+	+	–	–	–	–	–	–	+	+	+	+	–	–	–	+	+	–	+	+
225	T	32	2	+	–	–	–	–	–	–	–	+	+	+	+	+	–	–	+	+	–	–	+
226	T	32	2	+	–	–	–	–	–	–	–	+	+	+	+	+	–	–	+	+	–	+	+
229	Sp	32	2	+	–	–	–	–	–	–	–	+	+	+	+	+	–	–	+	+	–	+	+
231	Sp	64	2	+	–	–	–	–	–	–	–	+	+	+	+	+	–	–	+	+	–	–	+
232	T	> 256	2	+	–	–	–	–	–	–	–	+	+	+	+	–	–	+	+	+	–	–	+
235	T	32	2	+	–	–	–	–	–	–	–	+	+	+	+	+	–	–	+	+	–	–	+

Primer sets targeting β-lactamase genes (displayed by Ambler class), insertion sequence (IS*Aba1*), and mobile gene elements. Source (*Sp* sputum, *T* tissue/wound, *U* urine, *B* blood); *MIC* meropenem (≤ 2 µg/mL = Sensitive, ≥ 8 µg/mL = Resistant); KPC (KPC subtypes 1, 2, 5, 10); CTX (CTX-M subtypes 1, 2 8, 9, 25); *MBL* metallo-β-lactamase (DIM, GIM, IMP, NDM, SIM, SPM, VIM); EDTA *DDS* double disk synergy assay, *ICA1* class 1 integron cassette array, *int*123, conserved region of integrases 1, 2, and 3. All PCR reactions run in duplicate with proper control strains

there seems to be a distinction with regard to ST type with regard to possession of the bla_{SHV} gene wherein the bla_{SHV} gene was found in 10 (83%) of ST-229 isolates, and 1 (7%) of the ST-2 isolates. Although bla_{ampC} and bla_{ADC-7} genes encode cephalosporinases were present, the later (bla_{ADC-7} was predominant (in 76% of isolates), which have been shown to be inducible [41, 42].

The $bla_{OXA-51-like}$ allele is chromosomal and has been reported as an intrinsic gene of the *A. baumannii* species [43]. Both the $bla_{OXA-23-like}$ and $bla_{OXA-40-like}$ genes can be either plasmid or chromosome borne, and have an increased risk of horizontal dissemination, resulting in increased rates of resistance in healthcare settings [44, 45]. In our isolate groups, only 2 (7%) isolates contained the $bla_{OXA-40-like}$ gene; interestingly these two isolates display the greatest phenotypic resistance to meropenem (≥ 256 μg/mL), while 9 (34%) of our CRAB isolates possess the $bla_{OXA-23-like}$ gene, and displayed MICs between 32–64 μg/mL. These two oxacillinase genes were only found in ST-2 isolates in among the 2010–2011 isolate group; but seem to have been successfully disseminated into the hospital setting overtime as they were found in 9 (90%) of the 2015 isolate group.

A major concern in the healthcare community is the acquisition of genes such OXA-23-like and OXA-40-like through mobile genetic element transfers [46]. We did not determine whether these mobile elements such as integron-encoded integrase genes flank resistance genes, but their presence in majority (80%) of proposed CRAB suggests that those isolates are capable of acquiring and donating virulence genes by recombination.

An interesting finding from this study was the presence of IS elements upstream of several β-lactamase genes. It has been previously shown that the insertion of the IS element IS*Aba1* upstream of the OXA-51 gene changes the expression level leading to increased antimicrobial resistance [43]. Except isolate #58, which was co-carrying blaOXA-40 like gene), every isolate examined in this study was found to have IS*Aba*1 upstream of the $bla_{OXA-51-like}$ gene (Additional file 5: Figure S2), and suggesting that the isolates may have additional mechanisms resistance against carbopenem. The IS*Aba1* was also present in promoter region of bla_{ampC} gene (92%) and bla_{ADC-7} gene (76%) of the isolates, and suggest the overexpression of the downstream cephalosporinase genes resulting in an enhanced resistance phenotype.

MLST typing showed differing prevalence of the two STs of resistant strains of *A. baumannii* throughout the hospital over time. A comparison suggests that the majority of the isolates of 2010–2011 group were the members of ST-229, and only 5 (32%) isolates were ST-2, whereas interestingly, 90% of the isolates of 2015 group were ST-2, and only (10%) determined as ST-229. These data indicate over the course of 4–5 years that the ST-2 has successfully replaced most of the ST-229 strains to become the predominant resistant type within our hospital.

Why is one strain type more successful than the other when it appears the two strain types share similar genetic resistance mechanisms? It has been previously reported that biofilm production is an important virulence factor for *A. baumannii* as it may aid colonization and survival on abiotic hospital environments [47]. Thus, we explored the ability of our CRAB isolates to produce biofilm on an abiotic (polystyrene) surface, to give an indication of how well these strains might colonize both medical equipment and objects in the clinical environment. We found that there were no significant differences between the clinical source of the isolates or their ability to produce biofilms (Fig. 1b). Other studies using more clonally diverse strains have shown enhanced biofilm producing isolates derived

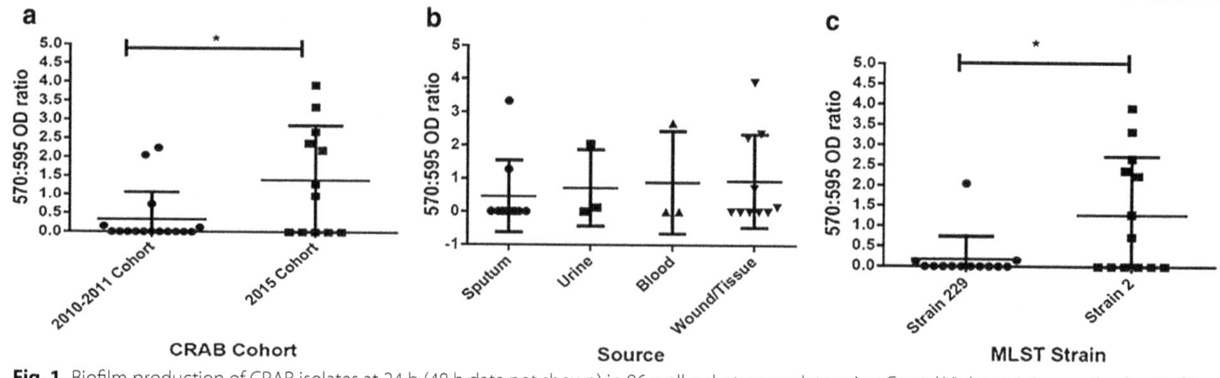

Fig. 1 Biofilm production of CRAB isolates at 24 h (48 h data not shown) in 96-well polystyrene plate using Crystal Violet staining method. **a** Biofilm production with isolates grouped as old and new isolates (*p = 0.03). **b** Isolates grouped by clinical source exhibited non-significant value, may be due to lack of clonal heterogeneity. **c** CRAB isolates showing biofilm production, grouped by MLST sequence type/strain type (*p = 0.04)

from urine and sputum cultures [48, 49]. Therefore, the non-significant result in our isolate group may be due to a lack of clonal heterogeneity. When we grouped our isolates by isolate groups (2010–2011 versus 2015) we found the 2015 isolate group had an enhanced ability to produce biofilm over the old isolates (Fig. 1a). Due to the predominance of ST-2 in the 2015 isolate group we explored biofilm production by MLST strain type, wherein the ST-2 showed an increased biofilm production compared to ST-229 (Fig. 1c). Therefore, a possible explanation for the success of ST-2 over ST-229 may be its enhanced ability to produce biofilms resulting in a more effective colonization within the hospital, even when the two strains exhibit similar antibiotic resistance phenotypes.

Conclusion

The temporal nature of the isolates used in this study provided a unique opportunity to epidemiologically monitor multi-drug-resistant *A. baumannii* isolates from the same hospital over time. We have shown that all of the CRAB isolates in our hospital belong to either MLST strain type ST-2 or ST-229 and that these two strain types most likely share similar mechanisms of resistance with possibly IS*Aba*1-dependent overexpression of β-lactamase genes, resulting in an MDR phenotype. Interestingly over a 4–5 years' timeframe the ST-2 type replaced the ST229 type to become the predominate CRAB strain within the hospital which we believe is due to its enhanced ability to produce biofilms leading to improved colonization and survival on abiotic surfaces. To our knowledge, this is the first study to comparatively characterize the genetic and phenotypic properties of clinical MDR *A. baumannii* isolates from a US hospital over an extended time frame.

Additional files

Additional file 1: Table S1. Quality control (QC) organisms used in this study.

Additional file 2: Table S2. Primer sequences used for *A. baumannii* in present study.

Additional file 3: Table S3. Antimicrobial typing of *A. baumannii* study isolates, showing individual isolates against commonly used drugs.

Additional file 4: Figure S1. Multiplex PCR of CRAB isolates looking at Group D β-lactamases.

Additional file 5: Figure S2. PCR screening of IS*Aba*1 upstream of $ble_{OXA\text{-}51\text{-}like}$ in three representative isolates.

Authors' contributions

The authors KMR and SGJ have hypothesized of mechanisms, designed experiments, analyzed data, and written manuscript. BS, NL, TEB and CLE helped in samples collection, phenotypic verification of some of the members of old isolates, and clinical clubbing for isolate group. KMR, BS and SGJ designed primers and evaluated PCR products, and KMR carried out the experiments, GDE and SGJ verified MLST sequencing data and helped in analyses to KMR. GDE participated in active discussions and data interpretations, and critical editing of the manuscript. All authors read and approved the final manuscript.

Author details

[1] Center for Surgical Infections & Biofilms, Institute of Molecular Medicine and Infectious diseases, Drexel University College of Medicine, 245 N. 15th Street, Philadelphia, PA 19102, USA. [2] Center for Genomic Sciences, Institute of Molecular Medicine and Infectious diseases, Drexel University College of Medicine, 245 N. 15th Street, Philadelphia, PA 19102, USA. [3] Center for Advanced Microbial Processing, Institute of Molecular Medicine and Infectious Diseases, Drexel University College of Medicine, 245 N. 15th Street, Philadelphia, PA 19102, USA. [4] Department of Microbiology and Immunology, Drexel University College of Medicine, 245 N. 15th Street, Philadelphia, PA 19102, USA. [5] Department of Otolaryngology-Head and Neck Surgery, Drexel University College of Medicine, 245 N. 15th Street, Philadelphia, PA 19102, USA. [6] Present Address: Department of Pathology and Lab Medicine, Indiana University School of Medicine, Indianapolis, IN, USA.

Acknowledgements

The research has IRB approval from Drexel University College of Medicine. The technical help provided by clinical laboratory of associated hospital and microbiology immunology department is respectfully acknowledged. This research was a part of graduate (PhD) rotation of Kevin M. Raible in Joshi Laboratory, and was partly presented at American Society for Microbiology-2016 Annual Meeting, and International Symposium of Drexel University.

Competing interests

The authors declare that they have no competing interests.

Consent for publication

All authors have approved this manuscript.

Funding

This research was carried out the intramural support, and as a continuation of Surgical Infection Research Program of the Departments of Surgery, and Microbiology and Immunology.

References

1. Bergogne-Berezin E, Towner KJ. *Acinetobacter* spp. as nosocomial pathogens: microbiological, clinical, and epidemiological features. Clin Microbiol Rev. 1996;9(2):148–65.
2. Seifert H, Strate A, Pulverer G. Nosocomial bacteremia due to *Acinetobacter baumannii*. Clinical features, epidemiology, and predictors of mortality. Medicine (Baltimore). 1995;74(6):340–9.
3. Falagas ME, Bliziotis IA, Siempos II. Attributable mortality of *Acinetobacter baumannii* infections in critically ill patients: a systematic review of matched cohort and case-control studies. Crit Care. 2006;10(2):R48.
4. Peleg AY, Seifert H, Paterson DL. *Acinetobacter baumannii*: emergence of a successful pathogen. Clin Microbiol Rev. 2008;21(3):538–82.
5. Vila J, Marcos A, Marco F, Abdalla S, Vergara Y, Reig R, Gomez-Lus R, Jimenez de Anta T. In vitro antimicrobial production of beta-lactamases, aminoglycoside-modifying enzymes, and chloramphenicol acetyltransferase by and susceptibility of clinical isolates of *Acinetobacter baumannii*. Antimicrob Agents Chemother. 1993;37(1):138–41.
6. Perez F, Hujer AM, Hujer KM, Decker BK, Rather PN, Bonomo RA. Global challenge of multidrug-resistant *Acinetobacter baumannii*. Antimicrob Agents Chemother. 2007;51(10):3471–84.
7. Jones RN, Deshpande L, Fritsche TR, Sader HS. Determination of epidemic clonality among multidrug-resistant strains of *Acinetobacter* spp. and *Pseudomonas aeruginosa* in the MYSTIC Programme (USA, 1999–2003). Diagn Microbiol Infect Dis. 2004;49(3):211–6.

8. Landman D, Quale JM, Mayorga D, Adedeji A, Vangala K, Ravishankar J, Flores C, Brooks S. Citywide clonal outbreak of multiresistant *Acinetobacter baumannii* and *Pseudomonas aeruginosa* in Brooklyn, NY: the pre antibiotic era has returned. Arch Intern Med. 2002;162(13):1515–20.
9. Peleg AY, Franklin C, Bell JM, Spelman DW. Emergence of carbapenem resistance in *Acinetobacter baumannii* recovered from blood cultures in Australia. Infect Control Hosp Epidemiol. 2006;27(7):759–61.
10. Yang HY, Lee HJ, Suh JT, Lee KM. Outbreaks of imipenem resistant *Acinetobacter baumannii* producing OXA-23 beta-lactamase in a tertiary care hospital in Korea. Yonsei Med J. 2009;50(6):764–70.
11. Nemec A, Dijkshoorn L, van der Reijden TJ. Long-term predominance of two pan-European clones among multi-resistant *Acinetobacter baumannii* strains in the Czech Republic. J Med Microbiol. 2004;53(Pt 2):147–53.
12. Hu FZ, Ehrlich GD. Population-level virulence factors amongst pathogenic bacteria: relation to infection outcome. Future Microbiol. 2008;3(1):31–42.
13. Gaynes R, Edwards JR. Overview of nosocomial infections caused by gram-negative bacilli. Clin Infect Dis. 2005;41(6):848–54.
14. Urban C, Segal-Maurer S, Rahal JJ. Considerations in control and treatment of nosocomial infections due to multidrug-resistant *Acinetobacter baumannii*. Clin Infect Dis. 2003;36(10):1268–74.
15. Seifert H, Baginski R, Schulze A, Pulverer G. Antimicrobial susceptibility of *Acinetobacter* species. Antimicrob Agents Chemother. 1993;37(4):750–3.
16. King LB, Swiatlo E, Swiatlo A, McDaniel LS. Serum resistance and biofilm formation in clinical isolates of *Acinetobacter baumannii*. FEMS Immunol Med Microbiol. 2009;55(3):414–21.
17. Gurung J, Khyriem AB, Banik A, Lyngdoh WV, Choudhury B, Bhattacharyya P. Association of biofilm production with multidrug resistance among clinical isolates of *Acinetobacter baumannii* and *Pseudomonas aeruginosa* from intensive care unit. Indian J Crit Care Med. 2013;17(4):214–8.
18. Yun HC, Kreft RE, Castillo MA, Ehrlich GD, Guymon CH, Crouch HK, Chung KK, Wenke JC, Hsu JR, Spirk TL, et al. Comparison of PCR/electron spray ionization-time-of-flight-mass spectrometry versus traditional clinical microbiology for active surveillance of organisms contaminating high-use surfaces in a burn intensive care unit, an orthopedic ward and healthcare workers. BMC Infect Dis. 2012;12:252.
19. Aul JJ, Anderson KW, Wadowsky RM, Doyle WJ, Kingsley LA, Post JC, Ehrlich GD. Comparative evaluation of culture and PCR for the detection and determination of persistence of bacterial strains and DNAs in the *Chinchilla lanigera* model of otitis media. Ann Otol Rhinol Laryngol. 1998;107(6):508–13.
20. Lee JC, Koerten H, van den Broek P, Beekhuizen H, Wolterbeek R, van den Barselaar M, van der Reijden T, van der Meer J, van de Gevel J, Dijkshoorn L. Adherence of *Acinetobacter baumannii* strains to human bronchial epithelial cells. Res Microbiol. 2006;157(4):360–6.
21. Lee HW, Koh YM, Kim J, Lee JC, Lee YC, Seol SY, Cho DT, Kim J. Capacity of multidrug-resistant clinical isolates of *Acinetobacter baumannii* to form biofilm and adhere to epithelial cell surfaces. Clin Microbiol Infect. 2008;14(1):49–54.
22. de Breij A, Gaddy J, van der Meer J, Koning R, Koster A, van den Broek P, Actis L, Nibbering P, Dijkshoorn L. CsuA/BABCDE-dependent pili are not involved in the adherence of *Acinetobacter baumannii* ATCC19606(T) to human airway epithelial cells and their inflammatory response. Res Microbiol. 2009;160(3):213–8.
23. van den Broek PJ, Arends J, Bernards AT, De Brauwer E, Mascini EM, van der Reijden TJ, Spanjaard L, Thewessen EA, van der Zee A, van Zeijl JH, et al. Epidemiology of multiple Acinetobacter outbreaks in The Netherlands during the period 1999–2001. Clin Microbiol Infect. 2006;12(9):837–43.
24. Wilks M, Wilson A, Warwick S, Price E, Kennedy D, Ely A, Millar MR. Control of an outbreak of multidrug-resistant *Acinetobacter baumannii–calcoaceticus* colonization and infection in an intensive care unit (ICU) without closing the ICU or placing patients in isolation. Infect Control Hosp Epidemiol. 2006;27(7):654–8.
25. Catalano M, Quelle LS, Jeric PE, Di Martino A, Maimone SM. Survival of *Acinetobacter baumannii* on bed rails during an outbreak and during sporadic cases. J Hosp Infect. 1999;42(1):27–35.
26. Simor AE, Lee M, Vearncombe M, Jones-Paul L, Barry C, Gomez M, Fish JS, Cartotto RC, Palmer R, Louie M. An outbreak due to multiresistant *Acinetobacter baumannii* in a burn unit: risk factors for acquisition and management. Infect Control Hosp Epidemiol. 2002;23(5):261–7.
27. El Shafie SS, Alishaq M, Leni Garcia M. Investigation of an outbreak of multidrug-resistant *Acinetobacter baumannii* in trauma intensive care unit. J Hosp Infect. 2004;56(2):101–5.
28. Jawad A, Heritage J, Snelling AM, Gascoyne-Binzi DM, Hawkey PM. Influence of relative humidity and suspending menstrua on survival of *Acinetobacter* spp. on dry surfaces. J Clin Microbiol. 1996;34(12):2881–7.
29. Sen B, Joshi SG. Studies on *Acinetobacter baumannii* involving multiple mechanisms of carbapenem resistance. J Appl Microbiol. 2016;120(3):619–29.
30. CLSI. Methods for dilution antimicrobial susceptibility tests for bacteria that grow aerobically; approved standard-ninth edition. In., vol. CLSI document M07-A9. 9th ed. Wayne: Clinical and Laboratory Standards Institute; 2012. p. 697.
31. Ehrlich GD, Greenberg SJ. PCR-based diagnostics in infectious disease. Boston: Blackwell Scientific Publications; 1994. p. 697.
32. Yong D, Lee K, Yum JH, Shin HB, Rossolini GM, Chong Y. Imipenem-EDTA disk method for differentiation of metallo-beta-lactamase-producing clinical isolates of *Pseudomonas* spp. and *Acinetobacter* spp. J Clin Microbiol. 2002;40(10):3798–801.
33. O'Toole GA. Microtiter dish biofilm formation assay. J Vis Exp. 2011;(47). pii: 2437. http://doi.org/10.3791/2437.
34. Magiorakos AP, Srinivasan A, Carey RB, Carmeli Y, Falagas ME, Giske CG, Harbarth S, Hindler JF, Kahlmeter G, Olsson-Liljequist B, et al. Multidrug-resistant, extensively drug-resistant and pandrug-resistant bacteria: an international expert proposal for interim standard definitions for acquired resistance. Clin Microbiol Infect. 2012;18(3):268–81.
35. Koeleman JG, Stoof J, Van Der Bijl MW, Vandenbroucke-Grauls CM, Savelkoul PH. Identification of epidemic strains of *Acinetobacter baumannii* by integrase gene PCR. J Clin Microbiol. 2001;39(1):8–13.
36. Hujer KM, Hujer AM, Hulten EA, Bajaksouzian S, Adams JM, Donskey CJ, Ecker DJ, Massire C, Eshoo MW, Sampath R, et al. Analysis of antibiotic resistance genes in multidrug-resistant Acinetobacter sp. isolates from military and civilian patients treated at the Walter Reed Army Medical Center. Antimicrob Agents Chemother. 2006;50(12):4114–23.
37. Davies TA, Marie Queenan A, Morrow BJ, Shang W, Amsler K, He W, Lynch AS, Pillar C, Flamm RK. Longitudinal survey of carbapenem resistance and resistance mechanisms in Enterobacteriaceae and non-fermenters from the USA in 2007–09. J Antimicrob Chemother. 2011;66(10):2298–307.
38. Chen Y, Zhou Z, Jiang Y, Yu Y. Emergence of NDM-1-producing *Acinetobacter baumannii* in China. J Antimicrob Chemother. 2011;66(6):1255–9.
39. Wei WJ, Yang HF, Ye Y, Li JB. New Delhi metallo-beta-lactamase-mediated carbapenem resistance: origin, diagnosis, treatment and public health concern. Chin Med J (Engl). 2015;128(14):1969–76.
40. Bradford PA. Extended-spectrum beta-lactamases in the 21st century: characterization, epidemiology, and detection of this important resistance threat. Clin Microbiol Rev. 2001;14(4):933–51 **(table of contents)**.
41. Harris PN, Ferguson JK. Antibiotic therapy for inducible AmpC beta-lactamase-producing Gram-negative bacilli: what are the alternatives to carbapenems, quinolones and aminoglycosides? Int J Antimicrob Agents. 2012;40(4):297–305.
42. Hujer KM, Hamza NS, Hujer AM, Perez F, Helfand MS, Bethel CR, Thomson JM, Anderson VE, Barlow M, Rice LB, et al. Identification of a new allelic variant of the *Acinetobacter baumannii* cephalosporinase, ADC-7 beta-lactamase: defining a unique family of class C enzymes. Antimicrob Agents Chemother. 2005;49(7):2941–8.
43. Turton JF, Ward ME, Woodford N, Kaufmann ME, Pike R, Livermore DM, Pitt TL. The role of ISAba1 in expression of OXA carbapenemase genes in *Acinetobacter baumannii*. FEMS Microbiol Lett. 2006;258(1):72–7.
44. Turton JF, Kaufmann ME, Glover J, Coelho JM, Warner M, Pike R, Pitt TL. Detection and typing of integrons in epidemic strains of *Acinetobacter baumannii* found in the United Kingdom. J Clin Microbiol. 2005;43(7):3074–82.
45. Lolans K, Rice TW, Munoz-Price LS, Quinn JP. Multicity outbreak of carbapenem-resistant *Acinetobacter baumannii* isolates producing the carbapenemase OXA-40. Antimicrob Agents Chemother. 2006;50(9):2941–5.
46. Richet H, Fournier PE. Nosocomial infections caused by *Acinetobacter baumannii*: a major threat worldwide. Infect Control Hosp Epidemiol. 2006;27(7):645–6.
47. Badave GK, Kulkarni D. Biofilm producing multidrug resistant *Acinetobacter baumannii*: an emerging challenge. J Clin Diagn Res. 2015;9(1):Dc08–10.

Second-line therapy for *Helicobacter pylori* eradication causing antibiotic-associated hemorrhagic colitis

Kazuyuki Tanaka, Mikihiro Fujiya*, Aki Sakatani, Shugo Fujibayashi, Yoshiki Nomura, Nobuhiro Ueno, Shin Kashima, Takuma Goto, Junpei Sasajima, Kentaro Moriichi and Toshikatsu Okumura

Abstract

Objective: *Helicobacter pylori* (*H. pylori*) eradication rarely develops into antibiotic-associated hemorrhagic colitis (AAHC), in which the etiology of colitis remains unclear. We herein report a rare case of AAHC caused by second-line therapy for *H. pylori* eradication.

Results: A 65-year-old female was administered second-line therapy for *H. pylori* composed of 1500 mg of amoxicillin, 500 mg of metronidazole and 40 mg of vonoprazan for 7 days because of first-line therapy failure. A day after completing second-line therapy, she complained of abdominal pain and hematochezia. Colonoscopy revealed a hemorrhage and edematous mucosa with no transparent vascular pattern in the transverse colon. A bacterial culture detected *Klebsiella oxytoca* (*K. oxytoca*), but no other pathogenic bacteria. A drug-induced lymphocyte stimulation test (DLST) showed positive reactions for both amoxicillin and metronidazole. According to these findings, the patient was diagnosed with AAHC. Bowel rest for 6 days relieved her abdominal pain and hematochezia.

Conclusions: The present case developed AAHC caused by second-line therapy for *H. pylori* eradication. The pathogenesis is considered to be associated with microbial substitution as well as a delayed-type allergy to antibiotics, suggesting that AAHC is a potential adverse event of second-line therapy for *H. pylori* eradication.

Background

Helicobacter pylori (*H. pylori*) infection has been known to cause many gastrointestinal disorders including gastroduodenal ulcers, gastric cancer and lymphoma, and idiopathic thrombocytopenic purpura [1–5]. *H. pylori* eradication is thus recommended to prevent these gastrointestinal disorders [6, 7]. In Japan, treatment for *H. pylori*-associated gastritis is now covered by health insurance [8]. The success rate of first-line therapy for *H. pylori* eradication is considered to be around 70–80% [9]. Second-line therapy for *H. pylori* eradication is needed for the remaining cases. Although *H. pylori* eradication occasionally causes adverse events, such as diarrhea and eruptions, it rarely develops into antibiotic-associated hemorrhagic colitis (AAHC), in which the etiology of colitis remains unclear. We herein report a rare case of AAHC caused by second-line therapy for *H. pylori* eradication.

Case report

A 65-year-old female, who had systemic lupus erythematosus and was taking 5 mg of prednisolone, underwent gastric mucosal resection to remove gastric adenoma. The endoscopic findings of chronic gastritis were confirmed. Histological findings and culture of the gastric specimens obtained from the gastric antrum and body by an endoscopic biopsy procedure detected an *H. pylori* infection. She was therefore administered first-line therapy composed of 1500 mg of amoxicillin, 800 mg of clarithromycin and 60 mg of lansoprazole for 7 days to eradicate *H. pylori* in December 2014. A urea breath test was performed to assess the effect of the

*Correspondence: fjym@asahikawa-med.ac.jp
Division of Gastroenterology and Hematology/Oncology, Department of Medicine, Asahikawa Medical University, 2-1 Midorigaoka-higashi, Asahikawa, Hokkaido 078-8510, Japan

eradication and revealed a positive result for *H. pylori* infection. Seven months after the first-line therapy, the patient was prescribed second-line therapy composed of 1500 mg of amoxicillin, 500 mg of metronidazole and 40 mg of vonoprazan for 7 days to eradicate *H. pylori* in July 2015. A day after completing second-line therapy, she complained of abdominal pain and hematochezia. Blood tests showed increases in neutrophil (6090/μL) and C-reactive protein (1.38 μg/mL) levels, whereas the hemoglobin level was within the normal limits. Colonoscopy revealed a hemorrhage and edematous mucosa with no transparent vascular pattern in the transverse colon (Fig. 1). Histological findings of the biopsy specimens obtained from the transverse colon showed severe infiltrations of neutrophil and lymphocytes and a hemorrhage in the lamina propria (Fig. 2). A bacterial culture detected *Klebsiella oxytoca* (*K. oxytoca*), but not *Clostridium difficile* or other pathogenic bacteria. A drug-induced lymphocyte stimulation test (DLST) showed positive reactions for both amoxicillin and metronidazole. According to these findings, the patient was diagnosed with AAHC.

Bowel rest for 6 days under the oral administration of 5 mg of prednisolone relieved her abdominal pain and hematochezia. Typical symptoms due to SLE have been relieved for 20 months with conservative treatment alone, and no vasculitis was histologically detected in biopsy specimens of the colon. Therefore, lupus enteritis was not thought to be associated with the pathogenesis of the enteric disorder in the patient.

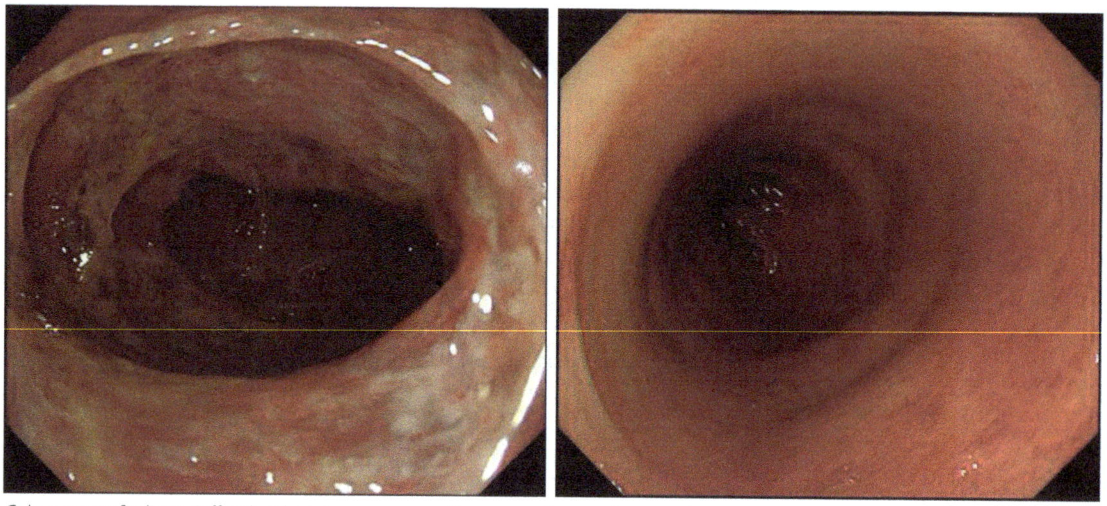

Fig. 1 Colonoscopy findings. Diffusely edematous mucosa with mucus, a hemorrhage and no transparent vascular pattern was detected in the transverse colon

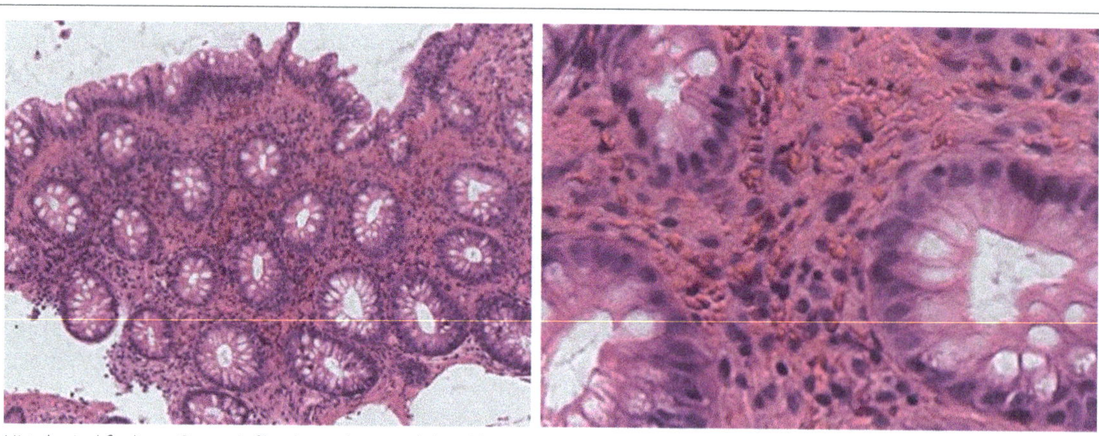

Fig. 2 Histological findings. Severe infiltrations of neutrophil and lymphocytes and a hemorrhage in the lamina propria were detected in the biopsy specimens obtained from the transverse colon (magnifications: 100/400)

Discussion

We herein report a rare case of AAHC that developed after the completion of second-line therapy using amoxicillin, metronidazole and vonoprazan for *H. pylori* eradication. Clinicians must pay careful attention to the possibility of this disorder, even when no side effects develop after the first-line therapy for *H. pylori* eradication.

While the incidence rate of AAHC after the first-line therapy for *H. pylori* eradication has been reported to range from 0.35 to 0.6% [10, 11], the frequency of AAHC after second-line therapy for *H. pylori* eradication is still unclear. A total of five previous cases that exhibited AAHC after completing second-line therapy for *H. pylori* eradication were identified in a literature search on the PubMed and Ichushi databases (Table 1) [12, 13]. Including the present case, there were 2 males and 4 females, and the mean age of the cases was 59.3 years old. Five cases exhibited AAHC after completing second-line *H. pylori* eradication therapy, suggesting that an immediate-type allergy was not a cause of AAHC. In two cases, *K. oxytoca* was isolated from the stool culture. It is known that stool testing reveals *K. oxytoca* in significant amounts in the majority of patients with AAHC [14]. *K. oxytoca* strains isolated from patients with AAHC are known to produce a cytotoxin, which were shown to cause cell death in cultured Hep2, Vero, CHOK1, and HeLa cell lines as well as in an isolated intestinal loop rabbit model [15, 16]. These studies indicated that microbial substitution by amoxicillin- and/or metronidazole-induced overgrowth of *K. oxytoca* could be associated with the development of AAHC in patients with the administration of second-line therapy for *H. pylori* eradication. The DLST was performed only in our case, which detected positive reactions for amoxicillin and metronidazole. Collectively, two mechanisms are thought to be involved in the pathogenesis of AAHC. First, microbial alterations accumulate by repeated antibiotic administration, thereby leading to AAHC at the second-line treatment. Second, amoxicillin sensitization may have been acquired at the time of first-line therapy, and a delayed allergic reaction may have occurred at the time of second-line therapy. Although the delayed-type allergy was a potential cause of AAHC in our case, it is unclear whether this type of allergy is a major cause of AAHC in patients receiving second-line therapy for *H. pylori* eradication. A greater accumulation of cases is warranted to understand the etiology of AAHC due to second-line therapy for *H. pylori* eradication.

Conclusions

In summary, we herein reported a rare case of AAHC caused by second-line therapy for *H. pylori* eradication. Due to the detection of *K. oxytoca* and positive reaction on the DLST for amoxicillin and metronidazole, the pathogenesis of the present case was considered to be associated with microbial substitution as well as a

Table 1 Reported cases of antibiotic-associated hemorrhagic colitis due to the second-line therapy for Helicobacter pylori eradication

Age	Gender	Symptoms	Onset	First-line therapy	Second-line therapy	Fecal bacterial culture	DLST	References
58	F	Abdominal pain, bloody diarrhea	8 days after starting eradication	CAM + AMPC + RPZ	MNZ 500 mg + AMPC 1500 mg + RPZ 20 mg	Pathogenic bacteria was not detected	Not described	#12
54	M	Abdominal pain, bloody diarrhea	7 days after starting eradication	CAM + AMPC + RPZ	MNZ 500 mg + AMPC 1500 mg + RPZ 20 mg	Pathogenic bacteria was not detected	Not described	#12
59	F	Abdominal pain, bloody diarrhea	9 days after starting eradication	CAM + AMPC + RPZ	MNZ 500 mg + AMPC 1500 mg + RPZ 20 mg	Pathogenic bacteria was not detected	Not described	#12
60	F	Abdominal pain, bloody diarrhea	9 days after starting eradication	CAM + AMPC + PPI	MNZ + AMPC + PPI	*Klebsiella oxytoca*	Not described	#13
50	M	Abdominal pain, hematochezia	6 days after starting eradication	CAM + AMPC + PPI	MNZ + AMPC + PPI	Not described	Not described	#13
65	F	Abdominal pain, hematochezia	8 days after starting eradication	CAM 800 mg + AMPC 1500 mg + LPZ 60 mg	MNZ 500 mg + AMPC 1500 mg + Vonoprazan 40 mg	*Klebsiella oxytoca*	Positive for both AMPC and MNZ	Present case

CAM clarithromycin, *AMPC* amoxicillin, *MNZ* metronidazole, *RPZ* rabeprazole, *LPZ* lansoprazole, *PPI* proton pump inhibitor

delayed-type allergy to amoxicillin and/or metronidazole. Clinicians must pay careful attention to the possibility of AAHC, even when administering second-line therapy for *H. pylori* eradication.

Abbreviations

H. pylori: *Helicobacter pylori*; AAHC: antibiotic-associated hemorrhagic colitis; *K. oxytoca*: *Klebsiella oxytoca*; DLST: drug-induced lymphocyte stimulation test; CAM: clarithromycin; AMPC: amoxicillin; MNZ: metronidazole; RPZ: rabeprazole; LPZ: lansoprazole; PPI: proton pump inhibitor.

Authors' contributions

KT and MF contributed equally to this study. KT and MF conceived the report, collected data, and wrote the first draft of the report. KT, AS and YN followed up the patient. SF, NU and SK performed endoscopy and evaluated the disease severity. TG and JS evaluated radiological images including computed tomography. KM and TO supervised the study. All authors contributed to the critical revision of the report for important intellectual content. All authors read and approved the final manuscript.

Acknowledgements

We would like to thank Dr. Masami Ijiri, Dr. Tatsuya Utsumi, Dr. Takuya Iwama, and Dr. Hiroki Sato for significant assistances.

Competing interests

The authors declare that they have no competing interests.

Consent for publication

Written informed consent was obtained from the patient for publication of this case report and accompanying images.

Funding

The authors declare that they have no funding.

References

1. Marshall BJ. *Helicobacter pylori*. Am J Gastroenterol. 1994;89:S116–28.
2. Malfertheiner P, Leodolter A, Peitz U. Cure of *Helicobacter pylori*—associated ulcer disease through eradication. Baillieres Best Pract Res Clin Gastroenterol. 2000;14:119–32.
3. Uemura N, Okamoto S, Yamamoto S, Matsumura N, Yamaguchi S, Yamakido M, et al. *Helicobacter pylori* infection and the development of gastric cancer. N Engl J Med. 2001;345:784–9.
4. Walt RP. Regression of MALT lymphoma and treatment for *Helicobacter pylori*. Lancet. 1996;348:1041–2.
5. Choe YH, Kim SK, Son BK, Lee DH, Hong YC, Pai SH. Randomized placebo-controlled trial of *Helicobacter pylori* eradication for iron- deficiency anemia in preadolescent children and adolescents. Helicobacter. 1999;4:135–9.
6. Gisbert JP, Khorrami S, Carballo F, Calvet X, Gene E, Dominguez-Muñoz E. *Helicobacter pylori* eradication therapy vs. antisecretory non-eradication therapy (with or without long-term maintenance antisecretory therapy) for the prevention of recurrent bleeding from peptic ulcer. Cochrane Database Syst Rev. 2004;2:004062.
7. Fukase K, Kato M, Kikuchi S. Eradication of *Helicobacter pylori* after endoscopic resection of early gastric cancer reduced the incidence of metachronous gastric cancer. Lancet. 2008;372:392–7.
8. Asaka M, Takahashi S, et al. Guidelines for the management of *Helicobacter pylori* infection in Japan: 2009 revised edition. Helicobacter. 2010;15:1–20.
9. Laheij RJ, Rossum LG, Jansen JB, Straatman H, Verbeek AL. Evaluation of treatment regimens to cure *Helicobacter pylori* infection—a meta-analysis. Aliment Pharmacol Ther. 1999;13:857–64.
10. Ishikawa S, Hayami Y, Sugawara K, Tanaka T, Yamamoto N, Hashimoto M, et al. A study on 19 cases of antibiotic-associated hemorrhagic colitis. Progr Dig Endosc. 1998;53:132–3.
11. Kashihara W, Hashimoto A, Kou H, Kin Y, Nishitani H, Okui M, Fukui S, et al. Case of antibiotic-associated hemorrhagic colitis during eradication therapy for *Helicobacter pylori*. Helicobacter Res. 1998;2:580–1.
12. Ikegami R, Kamiya K, Iwashige H. Three cases of antibiotic-associated hemorrhagic colitis after second-line therapy for *Helicobacter pylori*. J Jpn Soc Coloproctol. 2015;68:419–24.
13. Kakinoki K. Two cases of antibiotic-associated hemorrhagic colitis after second-line therapy for *Helicobacter pylori*. J Jpn Assoc Infect Dis. 2015;89:247.
14. Zollner-Schwetz I, Hogenauer C, Joainig M, Weberhofer P, Gorkiewicz G, Valentin T, et al. Role of *Klebsiella oxytoca* in antibiotic-associated diarrhea. Clin Infect Dis. 2008;47:e74–8.
15. Higaki M, Chida T, Takano H, Nakaya R. Cytotoxic component(s) of *Klebsiella oxytoca* on HEp-2 cells. Microbiol Immunol. 1990;34:147–51.
16. Minami J, Katayama S, Matsushita O, Sakamoto H, Okabe A. Enterotoxic activity of *Klebsiella oxytoca* cytotoxin in rabbit intestinal loops. Infect Immun. 1994;62:172–7.

28

Detection of bacterial DNA from central venous catheter removed from patients by next generation sequencing

Ken-ichi Okuda[1,2*†], Yutaka Yoshii[1,2,3†], Satomi Yamada[1], Akio Chiba[1,2], Ippei Hironaka[1,4], Seiji Hori[2,5], Katsuhiko Yanaga[2,4] and Yoshimitsu Mizunoe[1,2]

Abstract

Background: Catheter-related infection (CRI) is one of the serious challenges in clinical practice. This preliminary clinical study aimed to examine whether next-generation sequencing (NGS) targeting 16S rDNA, which was PCR-amplified directly from the tip of a central venous catheter (CVC), can be used to identify causative pathogens in CRI, compared to the culture method.

Methods: Hospitalized patients, from whom a CVC had just been removed, were prospectively enrolled and divided into the CRI-suspected and routine removal groups. DNA was extracted from the sonication fluid of CVC specimens derived from patients. For analysis of bacterial composition by NGS, the V3–V4 fragments of bacterial 16S rDNA were PCR-amplified, followed by index PCR and paired-end sequencing on an Illumina MiSeq device. Conventional culture methods were also performed in the CRI-suspected group.

Results: Of CVCs collected from the 156 enrolled patients (114 men; mean age 65.6 years), a total of 14 specimens [nine out of 31 patients suspected with CRI and five out of 125 patients without infection symptoms (routine removal group)] were PCR-positive. In five patients with definite CRI, *Staphylococcus* was the most frequently detected genus by NGS (4/5 specimens), although no pathogens were detected by NGS in the one remaining specimen. The genera identified by NGS were consistent with those from conventional culture tests. There was high agreement between NGS and the culture method in the CRI-suspected group, with sensitivity and specificity values of 80.0% and 76.9%, respectively; meanwhile, the false-positive rate of NGS was as low as 4.0% in the routine removal group. Moreover, several genera, besides the genus identified by culture test, were detected in each patient with definite CRI and surgical site infection (SSI). Additionally, in one patient with SSI, *Enterococcaceae* were detected not only by NGS but also by abdominal abscess drainage culture.

Conclusions: NGS targeting 16S rDNA was able to analyze the bacterial composition of CVC specimens and detect causative pathogens in patients with CRI and was therefore suggested as a promising diagnostic tool for CRI.

Keywords: Catheter-related infection, Diagnostics, Next-generation sequencing, 16S ribosomal DNA, Staphylococci

*Correspondence: okuda-k@jikei.ac.jp
†Ken-ichi Okuda and Yutaka Yoshii contributed equally to the work
[1] Department of Bacteriology, The Jikei University School of Medicine, 3-25-8 Nishi-Shimbashi, Minato-ku, Tokyo 105-8461, Japan
Full list of author information is available at the end of the article

Background

Catheter-related infection (CRI), one of the major hospital-acquired infections, continues to be associated with morbidity, mortality, and additional medical cost [1–7]. As delayed start of the appropriate antibiotic treatment is a significant risk factor contributing to the worsening of CRI, accurate diagnosis of the causative pathogen is crucial for the survival of the patient. Although culture of blood and catheter samples is the standard process for a definitive diagnosis in clinical practice, catheter-related bloodstream infection frequently occurs despite negative results in blood culture, thereby delaying the relevant treatment [8, 9]. Moreover, if multiple pathogens are present in the specimen, the growth may become a bias in the conventional culture method, thereby rendering it impossible to obtain the true clinical picture. Hence, new diagnostic methods that can complement the limitations of culture testing to enable accurate detection of causative pathogens in CRI may be of clinical importance.

Polymerase chain reaction (PCR)-based methods for detecting causative pathogens in infectious diseases such as CRI have been widely used over the last 20 years since they are more rapid and sensitive than conventional culturing procedures [10, 11]. Nevertheless, there are some disadvantages of using PCR technology alone for detecting pathogens. For example, causative pathogens cannot be detected when specific primer sets are not included. Sanger sequencing of 16S rDNA, amplified using a universal primer set, can be applied when the specimen contains only one species, but it is usually impossible to simultaneously identify more than one species from a polymicrobial specimen without processing mixed chromatograms using a computer program [12]. However, CRI can be caused by various pathogens, such as *Staphylococcus*, *Enterococcus*, and non-fermenting Gram-negative rods, and sometimes appears as a mixed infection [13, 14]. Thus, development of new molecular diagnostic techniques is imperative to comprehensively detect multiple pathogens simultaneously from numerous potential candidates.

Recently, next-generation sequencing (NGS), which gives out millions or billions of sequence reads per instrument run, has attracted attention in molecular diagnosis of infections [15]. NGS enables culture-free and comprehensive detection of pathogens and acquirement of information about the microbiome in the specimens [16, 17]. Moreover, NGS can simultaneously identify all species in a polymicrobial specimen and is superior to Sanger sequencing in this regard [16]. Indeed, several studies have reported that single or multiple bacteria were identified as causative pathogens by NGS using blood [18, 19], urine [20], orthopedic [20], stool [21], pelvic [22], and abscess [23] samples from patients with sepsis, urinary tract infection, orthopedic infections, diarrhea, pelvic infection-induced inflammatory disease, and liver abscess, respectively. Although NGS of clinical samples can be a powerful diagnostic method for detecting causative pathogens, the usefulness of catheter samples from patients with CRI for NGS analysis has not been evaluated. Hence, we thought to apply NGS of catheter tip samples to more accurately detect the bacteria associated with CRI.

In this preliminary clinical study, we attempted to identify pathogens associated with CRI in patients by NGS targeting 16S rDNA. Unlike conventional culture methods, this method enables the identification of bacteria present on the catheter surface without a culture, as bacterial DNA is extracted directly from the catheter surface. Complementing these results with those from conventional methods, more reliable diagnosis may become possible. Moreover, in this study, we also sought to confirm whether this method could detect bacteria in patients with no infection symptom.

Methods

Patients and central venous catheter samples

This preliminary clinical study was prospectively conducted at the Jikei University Hospital from October 2012 to March 2014. Patients (aged 20 years or more), from whom a central venous catheter (CVC) had just been removed using sterile techniques, were eligible along with their CVCs for inclusion in the study. Other inclusion criteria were as follows: (1) the catheter had been inserted using maximal sterile barrier precautions, (2) in case the catheter was removed due to the suspicion of CRI, a culture of either a catheter tip specimen or blood specimen was considered for routine clinical examination. After written informed consent was obtained from each patient, the distal 60-mm segment of the removed catheter tip was cut and preserved in a freezer until the analysis of 16S rDNA PCR assay for targeted NGS was performed. If the catheter tip was already used for the conventional culture examination, the remaining was used for this analysis.

Data collection

Data regarding age, sex, underlying disease, immunosuppressive drug use, body temperature, skin redness at the insertion site, CVC, blood and catheter tip cultures, and antibiotics were obtained from the patients' medical records. Quick sequential (sepsis-related) organ failure assessment (qSOFA) score [24] was also obtained. Moreover, when the catheter was removed due to the suspicion of CRI, the definitive diagnosis was also recorded.

Definition of the confirmed CRI

For the purpose of this study, CRI was originally defined as: (a) positive culture results of catheter tip or blood samples obtained from the peripheral vein or artery when CVC was removed, (b) clinical manifestations of infection (fever and skin redness) that improved following the removal of CVC, and (c) no apparent source of blood stream infection except for the catheter.

Definition of the routine removal group

The patients who were judged as having no infection symptom by the physicians and whose catheter was removed because it was no longer needed were included in the routine removal group.

Culture processing

In case CRI was suspected, blood and catheter tip samples were collected and processed at the clinical laboratory of our hospital. For blood culture, after inoculation of each blood sample in aerobic and anaerobic blood culture bottles (Becton–Dickinson, Sparks, MD, USA), they were incubated in an automated continuous monitoring blood culture system, BACTEC FX (Becton–Dickinson), for a maximum of 5 days. If bacteria had grown, Gram staining of the blood culture fluid was performed. Moreover, if the aerobic culture was positive, a loopful of specimen from the blood culture bottle was inoculated on Twin plate 32 (sheep blood agar + bromothymol blue agar; Kyokuto, Tokyo, Japan) at 37 °C under aerobic conditions for 1 day and on Twin plate 47 (sheep blood agar + chocolate agar; Kyokuto) at 37 °C under 5% CO_2 for 1 day. If the anaerobic blood culture was positive, the specimen was inoculated onto Brucella agar (Kyokuto) at 37 °C under anaerobic conditions for 1 day. Biochemical tests were additionally performed using the Walkaway 96 Plus system (Beckman Coulter, Brea, CA, USA). Based on these results, bacteria were comprehensively identified. The susceptibility testing of antibiotics against identified bacteria was also performed using the Walkaway 96 Plus system (Beckman Coulter).

For catheter tip culture, catheter tips were placed in HK semi-solid medium (Kyokuto) at 37 °C for a maximum of 2 days to culture aerobic and anaerobic microorganisms. If bacteria had grown on the semi-solid medium, Gram staining was performed using the positive sample. Moreover, aliquots of culture were inoculated onto Twin 32 (Kyokuto), Twin 47 (Kyokuto), and Brucella agars (Kyokuto), similarly to the process for identification of positive blood culture samples. Other cultures from wounds, sputum, or drainage were also performed, if considered necessary by the physician.

Extraction and purification of DNA

The tube containing the catheter was filled with purified water until the entire catheter was immersed. Water was passed through the catheter lumen by pipetting. After sonicating the specimen-containing tubes for 15 min in an ultrasonic bath (US-102; SND Co., Ltd., Suwa, Japan), 1 ml of each solution was transferred to clean 1.5-ml Eppendorf tubes. The solutions were concentrated to approximately 100 μl using a SpeedVac (Thermo Fisher Scientific, Waltham, MA, USA). Extraction and purification of DNA was performed using a NucleoSpin® Soil (Macherey–Nagel, Düren, Germany) according to the manufacturer's protocol.

PCR amplification of 16S rDNA

The V3–V4 fragments of 16S rDNA were amplified from DNA extracts as described in the 16S Metagenomic Sequencing Library Preparation Protocol, Part # 15044223 Rev. B (Illumina Inc., San Diego, CA, USA) with the following modifications. PCR was performed in a total volume of 25 μl, containing 9.5 μl of DNA extract, 0.6 μM forward and reverse primers, and 12.5 μl of Tks Gflex™ DNA Polymerase Low DNA (TAKARA BIO INC., Otsu, Japan). PCR reaction conditions were as follows: initial denaturation for 1 min at 94 °C and 30 cycles consisting of 10 s at 98 °C, 15 s at 50 °C, and 15 s at 68 °C. After PCR amplification, 5 μl of reaction mixture was applied to gel electrophoresis using a 1.0% agarose gel and subsequently stained with 0.5 μg/ml of ethidium bromide for 30 min. The gel was analyzed using an ImageQuant LAS-4000 (GE Healthcare, Chalfont St. Giles, UK) under UV trans-illumination. The specimens that showed bands of the target size were regarded as positive. The amplified PCR products were purified using the Agencourt AMPure XP beads (Beckman Coulter) according to the manufacturer's protocol.

Index PCR

Index PCR was performed in a total volume of 25 μl, containing 2 μl of purified DNA sample, 2.5 μl each of index 1 and index 2 primers in the Nextera XT Index Kit (Illumina Inc.), 12.5 μl of Tks Gflex™ DNA Polymerase Low DNA (TAKARA BIO INC.), and 5.5 μl of pure water. PCR reaction conditions were as follows: initial denaturation for 1 min at 94 °C and 8 cycles consisting of 10 s at 98 °C, 15 s at 60 °C, and 15 s at 68 °C. PCR purification was performed as mentioned above. When two bands were observed after electrophoresis, the band of the desired size was purified using a NucleoSpin Gel and PCR Clean-up (Macherey–Nagel). The DNA was finally purified using the AMPure XP beads (Beckman Coulter) according to the manufacturer's protocol. The concentration of DNA was measured using a Qubit 3.0 Fluorometer (Thermo Fisher Scientific) after staining with the Qubit dsDNA HS assay kit (Thermo Fisher Scientific) according to the manufacturer's instructions.

NGS and data analysis

The prepared libraries were subjected to sequencing of paired-end reads of 250 bp using the MiSeq Reagent Kit v3 on the MiSeq (Illumina) at the Biomedical Centre, Takara Bio. The number of reads per sample was between 843,574 and 1,329,426. Processing of the sequencing data, including operational taxonomic unit (OTU) definition and taxonomy assignment, was performed using CD-HIT-OTU 0.0.1 [25] and QIIME ver. 1.8 [26], respectively.

Statistical analysis

Fisher's exact and Mann–Whitney U tests were used for categorical and continuous data, respectively. P value < 0.05 indicated statistical significance in all analyses. Statistical analyses were performed using GraphPad Prism 6 (GraphPad Software, La Jolla, CA, USA).

Results

Patient and CVC characteristics

For the study, 156 patients (114 men; mean age 65.6 years) and their CVCs were enrolled (Fig. 1 and Table 1). In 141 patients (90.4%), catheterization was required for perioperative management. Underlying diseases are summarized in Table 1. In 125 patients (80.1%), catheters were removed because they were no longer needed, whereas in 31 patients (19.9%), catheters were removed due to the suspicion of CRI. There were significant differences in qSOFA score, body temperature, frequency of skin redness, frequency of antibiotic use post-removal, and the defervescence time after catheter removal between the two groups.

Frequency of CRI and other infectious diseases based on the conventional method

Out of the 31 cases in the CRI-suspected group, five patients (16.1% and 3.2% of total) were definitively diagnosed with CRI, based on the positive result of conventional culture tests (Fig. 1 and Table 2). Moreover, surgical site infections (SSIs) were confirmed in 15 (48.4%), based on clinical, radiological, and laboratory findings, followed by pneumonia in six (19.4%).

PCR amplification of 16S rDNA from catheter specimens

Representative results of agarose-gel electrophoresis are shown in Fig. 2. After index PCR, a minor band was observed below the main band in 50% of the samples, probably due to nonspecific amplification.

Summary of cases with positive result from 16S rDNA-targeted NGS

Out of 156 CVC specimens, 14 (9.0%) showed positive results by the 16S rDNA-targeted NGS method. The details of clinical and bacteriological findings are shown in Table 3. Nine out of the above-mentioned 14 patients belonged to the CRI-suspected group, and five belonged to the routine removal group. Bacterial composition is shown in Fig. 3. The genus *Staphylococcus* was the most frequently detected. However, in specimen no. 114, only *Klebsiella pneumoniae* was identified by the culture test, whereas both *Klebsiella* (38.0% of all detected genera) and *Staphylococcus* (42.0%) were detected as the predominant bacteria.

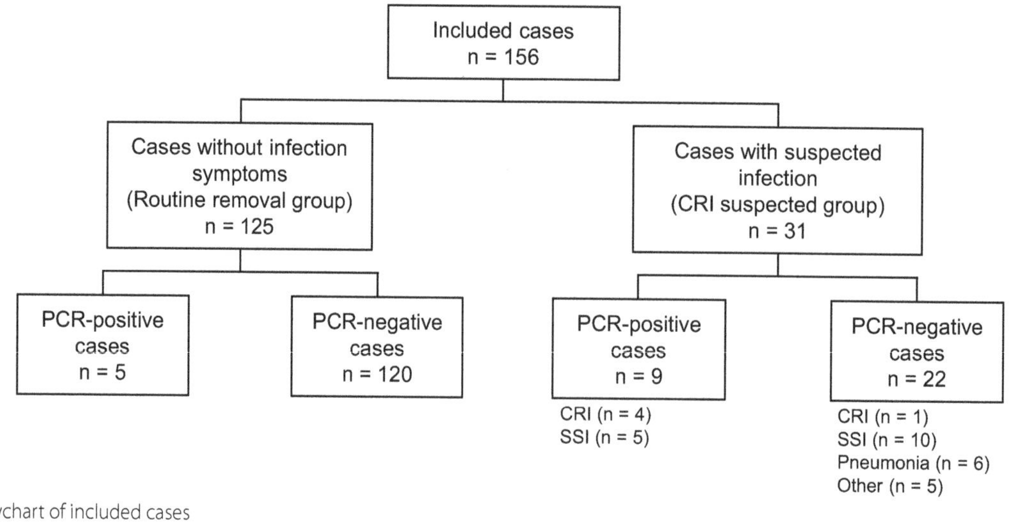

Fig. 1 Flowchart of included cases

Table 1 Patient characteristics (n = 156)

	Total (n = 156)	Routine removal group (n = 125)	CRI-suspected group (n = 31)	*P* value
Age, years (mean ± SD)	65.6 ± 10.8	65.3 ± 10.9	66.5 ± 10.3	0.645
Male, n (%)	114 (73.1%)	93 (74.4%)	21 (67.7%)	0.500
Underlying disease[a]				
Malignancy	126 (80.8%)	101 (80.8%)	25 (80.6%)	1.000
Hepatocellular carcinoma	49 (31.4%)	43 (34.4%)	6 (19.4%)	–
Pancreatic cancer	24 (15.4%)	20 (16.0%)	4 (12.9%)	–
Cholangiocarcinoma	11 (7.1%)	5 (4.0%)	6 (19.4%)	–
Other cancers	42 (26.9%)	33 (26.4%)	9 (29.0%)	–
Diabetes mellitus	40 (25.6%)	33 (26.4%)	7 (22.6%)	0.819
Chronic hepatitis/liver cirrhosis	21 (13.5%)	18 (14.4%)	3 (9.7%)	0.769
Chronic kidney disease	3 (1.9%)	2 (1.6%)	1 (3.2%)	0.488
Other diseases	30 (19.2%)	24 (19.2%)	6 (19.4%)	1.000
Immunosuppressive drug use (yes)	8 (5.1%)	6 (4.8%)	2 (6.5%)	0.659
qSOFA score point (mean and range)	0.2 (0–3)	0.1 (0–1)	0.5 (0–3)	< 0.001
Body temperature, °C (mean ± SD)	36.8 ± 0.8	36.6 ± 0.5	37.7 ± 1.1	< 0.001
Skin redness at the insertion site	5 (3.2%)	0 (0%)	5 (16.1%)	< 0.001
Insertion site of CVC				
Jugular	148 (94.9%)	120 (96.0%)	28 (90.3%)	0.196
Femoral	3 (1.9%)	2 (1.6%)	1 (3.2%)	0.488
Peripherally inserted CVC	5 (3.2%)	3 (2.4%)	2 (6.5%)	0.259
Number of lumen				
3	103 (66.0%)	84 (67.2%)	19 (61.3%)	0.533
2	48 (30.8%)	38 (30.4%)	10 (32.3%)	0.831
1	5 (3.2%)	3 (2.4%)	2 (6.5%)	0.259
Primary purpose for CVC insertion				
Perioperative	141 (90.4%)	114 (91.2%)	27 (87.1%)	0.500
Parenteral nutrition	9 (5.8%)	6 (4.8%)	3 (9.7%)	0.383
Intensive care	6 (3.8%)	5 (4.0%)	1 (3.2%)	1.000
Duration of catheterization, days (mean ± SD)	9.5 ± 9.0	9.0 ± 8.0	11.5 ± 12.2	0.600
Antibiotic use during the catheterization	153 (98.1%)	123 (98.4%)	30 (96.8%)	0.488
Antibiotic use after the removal	47 (30.1%)	22 (17.6%)	25 (80.6%)	< 0.001
Defervescence time from the catheter removal, day (mean ± SD)	0.8 ± 2.4	0.3 ± 0.6	3.4 ± 4.5	< 0.001

Data are presented as the number (percentage) of patients

[a] Some overlap exists

Table 2 Comparison of PCR and conventional culture results in the CRI-suspected group (n = 31)

	Culture results		
	Positive	Negative	Total
PCR results			
Positive	4	6	10
Negative	1	20	21
Total	5	26	31

Comparison of PCR and conventional culture results in the CRI-suspected group

Among the 31 cases in the CRI-suspected group, comparison between the NGS results and conventional culture results for the diagnosis of CRI (blood culture and catheter tip culture) is shown in Table 2. A high level of agreement existed between the two methodologies, with sensitivity, specificity, and accuracy values of 80.0, 76.9,

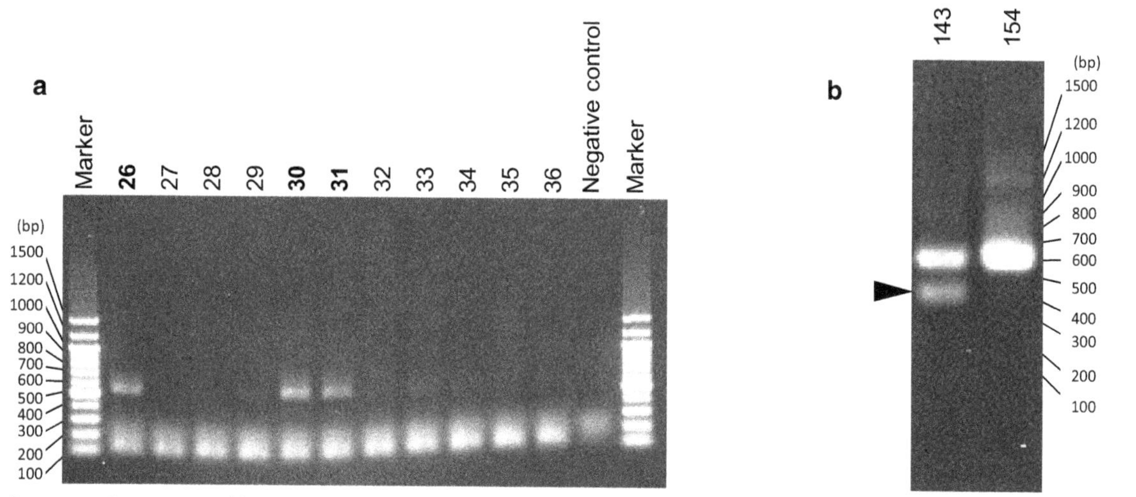

Fig. 2 Representative agarose-gel images. **a** A representative agarose-gel image of PCR-amplified 16S rDNA. The number of specimens regarded as positive are shown in bold. PCR reaction of the negative control sample was performed without any DNA extracted from catheter specimen. The bands around 100 to 200 bp are considered to be primer dimers. **b** A representative agarose-gel image of index PCR products. The minor band, presumably due to nonspecific amplification, is indicated by an arrowhead

and 77.4%, respectively. In the four patients having confirmed CRI, with both 16S rDNA-targeted NGS and culture results positive, pathogens identified by conventional cultures were all detected by the 16S rDNA-targeted NGS method (Table 3).

Discrepant case with culture-positive but NGS-negative outcome in the CRI-suspected group

In one patient with confirmed CRI (no. 112), although *Staphylococcus epidermidis* was identified using the conventional culture method, the NGS method did not detect the pathogen (Table 3).

Discrepant case with NGS-positive but culture-negative outcome in the CRI-suspected group

Five discrepant cases (nos. 13, 26, 92, 107, and 143) with NGS-positive but culture-negative outcomes were obtained; all were diagnosed as SSI. Moreover, in one of the five cases (no. 107), *Enterococcaceae* detected by the NGS method were also identified as *Enterococcus faecalis* in abdominal abscess drainage cultures, although neither blood nor catheter tip cultures were positive.

NGS-positive cases in the routine removal group

Of the 125 patients in the routine removal group, the 16S rDNA-based NGS method showed a false-positive result in five (4.0%); the genus *Staphylococcus* was detected in all (Table 3). There was no clinical evidence of infection in four patients, while *S. capitis* bacteremia had occurred just 9 days before catheter removal in one case (no. 31).

Discussion

In the present study, we have developed a new molecular diagnostic method using targeted NGS of bacterial 16S rDNA extracted from CVC surfaces. To the best of our knowledge, this is the first report demonstrating that NGS can detect causative bacteria in samples obtained from catheter surfaces from patients with CRI. This novel method showed comparable sensitivity with conventional culture methods in the CRI-suspected group and a low false-positive rate in the routine removal group. Hence, we believe that using targeted NGS of bacterial 16S rDNA to detect causative pathogens in catheter tip samples is a clinically promising method.

Staphylococcus was the most frequent causative pathogen of CRI in the present study, consistent with previous reports [13, 14, 27, 28]. In four out of five cases with definitive CRI, there was agreement regarding the causative pathogens between the conventional culture and the 16S rDNA-based NGS method at the genus level. Meanwhile, in the one remaining case with definite CRI (no. 112), *S. epidermidis* was identified by only blood culture, not by the NGS method nor catheter tip culture. It was presumed that both NGS and catheter tip culture were negative because no or a very small amount of bacteria below the detection limit were attached to the segments of catheters used for the assays. Taken together, in cases where a certain amount of bacterial cells are attached to the CVC specimens tested, the NGS method may be

Table 3 Clinical and bacteriological findings in cases with positive result from either NGS or conventional methods (blood and catheter tip culture)

No.	Age	Sex	BT	Skin redness	Bacteria detected by each method				Final diagnosis	Defervescence time (day)	Antibiotic treatment after the catheter removal	Outcome
					NGS (the genera or families account for more than 10% of the leads)	Blood culture	Catheter tip culture	Other cultures				
CRI suspected group												
NGS positive												
6	76	F	36.1	Yes	*Serratia*	NA	*Serratia marcescens*	NA	CRI	–	CMZ	Cure
13	59	M	37.6	No	*Staphylococcus*	NA	Negative	NA	SSI	2	CPFX	Cure
26	59	M	37.0	No	*Staphylococcus*	Negative	Negative	NA	SSI	1	FOM	Cure
30	76	M	40.0	Yes	*Staphylococcus*	*Staphylococcus epidermidis*	*Staphylococcus epidermidis*	NA	CRI	4	PIPC/TAZ	Cure
92	40	F	35.9	No	*Enterococcaceae*	Negative	Negative	NA	SSI	–	LVFX	Cure
107	74	F	37.0	No	*Enterococcaceae*	Negative	Negative	*Enterococcus faecalis* (drain culture)	SSI	1	IPM/CS	Cure
114	65	F	38.7	No	*Staphylococcus, Klebsiella, Enterobacteriaceae*	Negative	*Klebsiella pneumoniae*	NA	CRI	1	CEZ	Cure
135	61	M	39.0	No	*Staphylococcus*	*Staphylococcus aureus*	*Staphylococcus aureus*	NA	CRI	13	VCM	Death[a]
143	62	M	37.0	No	*Staphylococcus*	Negative	Negative	NA	SSI	1	LVFX	Cure
NGS negative												
112	62	M	37.5	Yes	Negative	*Staphylococcus epidermidis*	Negative	NA	CRI	1	VCM	Cure
Routine removal group												
NGS positive												
31	80	F	36.4	No	*Staphylococcus*	NA[b]	NA	NA	Post infection (DNAemia)	–	No	–
54	70	M	36.3	No	*Staphylococcus*	NA	NA	NA	Contamination	–	No	–
88	65	F	36.6	No	*Staphylococcus*	NA	NA	NA	Contamination	–	No	–
104	82	F	35.9	No	*Staphylococcus*	NA	NA	NA	Contamination	–	No	–
154	52	M	36.8	No	*Staphylococcus*	NA	NA	NA	Contamination	–	No	–

BT body temperature, *NA* not applicable, *CEZ* cefazolin, *CMZ* cefmetazole, *CPFX* ciprofloxacin, *FOM* fosfomycin, *IPM/CS* imipenem/cilastatin, *LVFX* levofloxacin, *PIPC/TAZ* piperacillin/tazobactam, *VCM* vancomycin

[a] Although the symptom temporarily improved after catheter removal, CRI finally led to a fatal outcome. An autopsy examination revealed *S. aureus* bacteraemia

[b] *Staphylococcus capitis* was identified 9 days before catheter removal. The catheter was, nevertheless, inserted due to therapeutic requirements

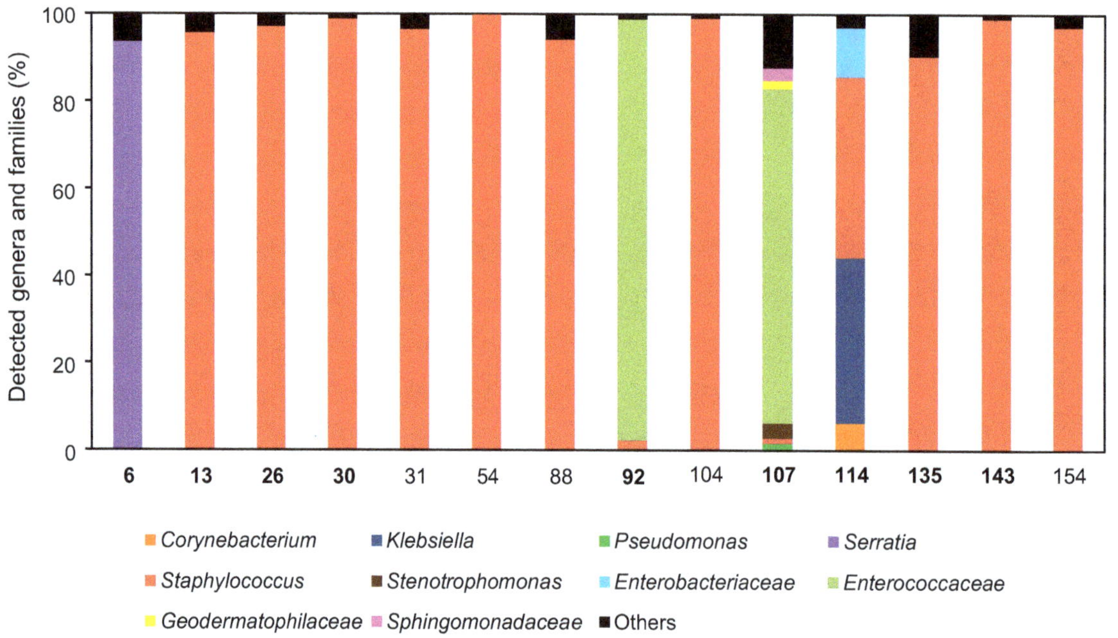

Fig. 3 Bacterial compositions in catheter specimens. "Others" include families and genera that are less than 1%. The final diagnoses of patients from which magenta and blue specimens were derived were of CRI and SSI, respectively

useful as an auxiliary or alternative diagnostic tool for CRI to overcome the limitations of conventional culture tests, such as the low sensitivity of the tests under the influence of antibiotics.

Similar to previous reports [29–31], 83.9% of patients in the suspected group were proven to not have CRI after assessment of catheter tip and blood cultures in the present study. Among the samples, SSI was the most frequent diagnosis in 15 cases. In one such case (no. 107), where *E. faecalis* was identified by the abscess drainage culture, *Enterococcaceae* were also detected in the catheter tip sample based on the NGS method; however, blood and catheter tip culture were both negative. This result suggested that the NGS method has higher sensitivity for detecting an early bloodstream infection than blood culture test.

One advantage of NGS is that one sequence run in a single protocol enables identification of polymicrobial pathogens [16]. Similar to previous studies that revealed the utility of NGS for detecting multiple causative agents in infectious diseases [19, 22, 23], in the present study, multiple causative pathogens were simultaneously detected in CVC specimens by NGS in two cases (nos. 107 and 114) (Fig. 3); meanwhile, the culture method identified only one predominant bacterium detected by NGS (Table 3). This difference might be due to culture conditions. Specifically, the bacteria that can grow under the tested culture conditions are primarily identified, whereas other bacteria for which the culture conditions are not suitable may not be identified. If antibiotic therapy for the bacterial infection identified by culture is ineffective for other undetected bacteria, infection with the latter can worsen, leading to treatment failure. Therefore, the NGS method, which can detect diverse causative bacteria simultaneously, is more useful in selecting appropriate antibiotics, compared to the conventional culture methods.

Among the five NGS-positive cases in the routine removal group, four (nos. 54, 88, 104, and 154) did not show any infectious symptom before and after removal of the catheter, yet *Staphylococcus* was detected. This may be explained by contamination or physiological translocation of bacteria from skin or the nasal cavity, which did not induce bloodstream infection. In the remaining case (no. 31), although *Staphylococcus* was detected, *S. capitis* bacteremia had developed 9 days before the removal. This positive result was surmised as DNAemia. Overall, in the routine removal group, the false-positive rate of the NGS method was as low as 4% (5/125 cases). We believe that the NGS method rarely shows false-positives and thus is a reliable test for the accurate detection of the causative pathogens.

Currently, NGS requires a relatively long turnaround time and high expense [32]. Indeed, our NGS method takes several days for bacterial identification at the genus level, although the method can simultaneously process up to 384 specimens. Combination of our method with a recently reported new technique, which can determine bacterial composition at the species level by sequencing nearly full-length 16S rDNA using a nanopore sequencer within 2 h [33], may enable more rapid and high-resolution identification of causative bacteria from catheter tip samples. In addition, although the cost of NGS is declining, it is still expensive to use for routine diagnosis in clinical settings. To reduce running costs, it would be desirable to examine a large number of samples at the same time. Further cost reduction due to broader application of NGS in clinics is expected.

The present study has some limitations. First, the bacterial 16S rDNA-targeted NGS method is not able to detect fungi such as *Candida*, which is one of the primary causative pathogens of CRI in patients with malignancies [4]. However, in theory, the NGS method can also detect fungi from amplicon libraries composed of internal transcribed spacer (ITS) 1 and 2 lesions, which fungi possess, as previously reported [34]. Second, as the definition and methodology for CRI are slightly different from those recommended by the international guideline for practice [35], the interpretation of our preliminary clinical data might be limited. Nonetheless, the differences did not hinder evaluation of the applicability of the NGS method in this study. Third, in the routine removal group, we did not perform the conventional culture test. Therefore, we cannot distinguish between contamination by NGS or by true colonization. To solve these problems and to confirm the validity of targeted NGS of bacterial 16S rDNA and fungal ITS lesions using catheter tip samples in comparison to conventional methods, further clinical studies that follow the guidelines and include culture methods for the routine removal group are required.

Conclusions

In conclusion, this preliminary clinical study demonstrated that the 16S rDNA-targeted NGS method correctly detected CRI causative pathogens in catheter tip samples. We believe that 16S rDNA-targeted NGS of catheter tip samples is a promising diagnostic tool in patients with CRI. Moreover, since the principle of this molecular diagnostic method can also be applied to detect pathogens on other devices, such as pacemakers, vascular grafts, and orthopedic implants, targeted NGS of bacterial 16S rDNA can contribute to the diagnosis of other device-related infections.

Abbreviations

CRI: catheter-related infection; CVC: central venous catheter; ITS: internal transcribed spacer; NGS: next-generation sequencing; OTU: operational taxonomic unit; PCR: polymerase chain reaction; qSOFA: quick sequential (sepsis-related) organ failure assessment; SSI: surgical site infection.

Authors' contributions

KO, SH, KY, and YM conceived and designed the experiments; KO, IH, and AC collected the clinical samples; KO, YY, and SY performed the experiments; YY analyzed the clinical data; KO, YY, AC, and YM prepared the manuscript. All authors read and approved the final manuscript.

Author details

[1] Department of Bacteriology, The Jikei University School of Medicine, 3-25-8 Nishi-Shimbashi, Minato-ku, Tokyo 105-8461, Japan. [2] Jikei Center for Biofilm Science and Technology, The Jikei University School of Medicine, Tokyo, Japan. [3] Division of Respiratory Diseases, Department of Internal Medicine, The Jikei University School of Medicine, Tokyo, Japan. [4] Department of Surgery, The Jikei University School of Medicine, Tokyo, Japan. [5] Department of Infectious Disease and Control, The Jikei University School of Medicine, Tokyo, Japan.

Acknowledgements

We are grateful to Dr. Tetsuya Horino and Ms. Michie Mishima for supporting clinical sample collection. We also thank the physicians at the Department of Surgery, the Jikei University School of Medicine, for removing the CVCs from patients and diagnosing the infectious disease.

Competing interests

The authors declare that they have no competing interests.

Consent for publication

Not applicable.

Funding

This work was supported by the Ministry of Education, Culture, Sports, Science and Technology (MEXT)-Supported Program for the Strategic Research Foundation at Private Universities, 2012–2016, The Jikei University Research Fund, and Takeda Science Foundation.

References

1. Timsit JF, Rupp M, Bouza E, Chopra V, Kärpänen T, Laupland K, et al. A state of the art review on optimal practices to prevent, recognize, and manage complications associated with intravascular devices in the critically ill. Intens Care Med. 2018;44:742–59.
2. Rupp ME, Karnatak R. Intravascular catheter-related bloodstream infections. Infect Dis Clin North Am. 2018;32:765–87.
3. Nuckols TK, Keeler E, Morton SC, Anderson L, Doyle B, Booth M, et al. Economic evaluation of quality improvement interventions for bloodstream infections related to central catheters: a systematic review. JAMA Intern Med. 2016;176:1843–54.
4. Zakhour R, Chaftari AM, Raad II. Catheter-related infections in patients with haematological malignancies: novel preventive and therapeutic strategies. Lancet Infect Dis. 2016;16:e241–50.
5. Seifert H. The clinical importance of microbiological findings in the diagnosis and management of bloodstream infections. Clin Infect Dis. 2009;48:S238–45.
6. Blot SI, Depuydt P, Annemans L, Benoit D, Hoste E, De Waele JJ, et al. Clinical and economic outcomes in critically ill patients with nosocomial catheter-related bloodstream infections. Clin Infect Dis. 2005;41:1591–8.
7. Wisplinghoff H, Bischoff T, Tallent SM, Seifert H, Wenzel RP, Edmond MB. Nosocomial bloodstream infections in US hospitals: analysis of 24,179 cases from a prospective nationwide surveillance study. Clin Infect Dis. 2004;39:309–17.
8. Rhodes A, Evans LE, Alhazzani W, Levy MM, Antonelli M, Ferrer R, et al. Surviving sepsis campaign: international guidelines for management of sepsis and septic shock: 2016. Intens Care Med. 2017;43:304–77.

9. Fenollar F, Raoult D. Molecular diagnosis of bloodstream infections caused by non-cultivable bacteria. Int J Antimicrob Agents. 2007;30:S7–15.
10. van de Groep K, Bos MP, Savelkoul PH, Rubenjan A, Gazenbeek C, Melchers WJ, et al. Development and first evaluation of a novel multiplex real-time PCR on whole blood samples for rapid pathogen identification in critically ill patients with sepsis. Eur J Clin Microbiol Infect Dis. 2018;37:1333–44.
11. Guembe M, Marín M, Martín-Rabadán P, Echenagusia A, Camúñez F, Rodríguez-Rosales G, et al. Use of universal 16S rRNA gene PCR as a diagnostic tool for venous access port-related bloodstream infections. J Clin Microbiol. 2013;51:799–804.
12. Kommedal O, Karlsen B, Saebo O. Analysis of mixed sequencing chromatograms and its application in direct 16S rRNA gene sequencing of polymicrobial samples. J Clin Microbiol. 2008;46:3766–71.
13. García-Rodríguez JF, Álvarez-Díaz H, Vilariño-Maneiro L, Lorenzo-García MV, Cantón-Blanco A, Ordoñez-Barrosa P, et al. Epidemiology and impact of a multifaceted approach in controlling central venous catheter associated blood stream infections outside the intensive care unit. BMC Infect Dis. 2013;13:445.
14. Timsit JF, L'Hériteau F, Lepape A, Francais A, Ruckly S, Venier AG, et al. A multicentre analysis of catheter-related infection based on a hierarchical model. Intens Care Med. 2012;38:1662–72.
15. Frey KG, Bishop-Lilly KA. Next-generation sequencing for pathogen detection and identification. In: Sails A, Tang YW, editors. Current and emerging technologies for the diagnosis of microbial infections. Cambridge: Academic Press; 2015. p. 525–54.
16. Deurenberg RH, Bathoorn E, Chlebowicz MA, Couto N, Ferdous M, Garcia-Cobos S, et al. Application of next generation sequencing in clinical microbiology and infection prevention. J Biotechnol. 2017;243:16–24.
17. Besser J, Carleton HA, Gerner-Smidt P, Lindsey RL, Trees E. Next-generation sequencing technologies and their application to the study and control of bacterial infections. Clin Microbiol Infect. 2018;24:335–41.
18. Gosiewski T, Ludwig-Galezowska AH, Huminska K, Sroka-Oleksiak A, Radkowski P, Salamon D, et al. Comprehensive detection and identification of bacterial DNA in the blood of patients with sepsis and healthy volunteers using next-generation sequencing method—the observation of DNAemia. Eur J Clin Microbiol Infect Dis. 2017;36:329–36.
19. Grumaz S, Stevens P, Grumaz C, Decker SO, Weigand MA, Hofer S, et al. Next-generation sequencing diagnostics of bacteremia in septic patients. Genome Med. 2016;8:73.
20. Sabat AJ, van Zanten E, Akkerboom V, Wisselink G, van Slochteren K, de Boer RF, et al. Targeted next-generation sequencing of the 16S-23S rRNA region for culture-independent bacterial identification—increased discrimination of closely related species. Sci Rep. 2017;7:3434.
21. Joensen KG, Engsbro ALØ, Lukjancenko O, Kaas RS, Lund O, Westh H, et al. Evaluating next-generation sequencing for direct clinical diagnostics in diarrhoeal disease. Eur J Clin Microbiol Infect Dis. 2017;36:1325–38.
22. Wang Y, Zhang Y, Zhang Q, Chen H, Feng Y. Characterization of pelvic and cervical microbiotas from patients with pelvic inflammatory disease. J Med Microbiol. 2018;67:1519–26.
23. Song YG, Shim SG, Kim KM, Lee DH, Kim DS, Choi SH, et al. Profiling of the bacteria responsible for pyogenic liver abscess by 16S rRNA gene pyrosequencing. J Microbiol. 2014;52:504–9.
24. Singer M, Deutschman CS, Seymour CW, Shankar-Hari M, Annane D, Bauer M, et al. The third international consensus definitions for sepsis and septic shock (Sepsis-3). JAMA. 2016;315:801–10.
25. Li W, Fu L, Niu B, Wu S, Wooley J. Ultrafast clustering algorithms for metagenomic sequence analysis. Brief Bioinform. 2012;13:656–68.
26. Caporaso JG, Kuczynski J, Stombaugh J, Bittinger K, Bushman FD, Costello EK, et al. QIIME allows analysis of high-throughput community sequencing data. Nat Methods. 2010;7:335–6.
27. See I, Freifeld AG, Magill SS. Causative organisms and associated antimicrobial resistance in healthcare-associated, central line-associated bloodstream infections from oncology settings, 2009–2012. Clin Infect Dis. 2016;62:1203–9.
28. Strasheim W, Kock MM, Ueckermann V, Hoosien E, Dreyer AW, Ehlers MM. Surveillance of catheter-related infections: the supplementary role of the microbiology laboratory. BMC Infect Dis. 2015;15:5.
29. Leon C, Alvarez-Lerma F, Ruiz-Santana S, Gonzalez V, de la Torre MV, Sierra R, et al. Antiseptic chamber-containing hub reduces central venous catheter related infection: a prospective, randomized study. Crit Care Med. 2003;31:1318–24.
30. Ranucci M, Isgro G, Giomarelli PP, Pavesi M, Luzzani A, Cattabriga I, et al. Impact of oligon central venous catheters on catheter colonization and catheter-related bloodstream infection. Crit Care Med. 2003;31:52–9.
31. Merrer J, De Jonghe B, Golliot F, Lefrant JY, Raffy B, Barre E, et al. Complications of femoral and subclavian venous catheterization in critically ill patients: a randomized controlled trial. JAMA. 2001;286:700–7.
32. Lefterova MI, Suarez CJ, Banaei N, Pinsky BA. Next-generation sequencing for infectious disease diagnosis and management: a report of the association for molecular pathology. J Mol Diagn. 2015;17:623–34.
33. Mitsuhashi S, Kryukov K, Nakagawa S, Takeuchi JS, Shiraishi Y, Asano K, et al. A portable system for rapid bacterial composition analysis using a nanopore-based sequencer and laptop computer. Sci Rep. 2017;7:5657.
34. Alonso R, Pisa D, Fernández-Fernández AM, Carrasco L. Infection of fungi and bacteria in brain tissue from elderly persons and patients with Alzheimer's disease. Front Aging Neurosci. 2018;10:159.
35. Mermel LA, Allon M, Bouza E, Craven DE, Flynn P, O'Grady NP, et al. Clinical practice guidelines for the diagnosis and management of intravascular catheter-related infection: 2009. Clin Infect Dis. 2009;49:1–45.

Permissions

All chapters in this book were first published in ACMA, by BioMed Central; hereby published with permission under the Creative Commons Attribution License or equivalent. Every chapter published in this book has been scrutinized by our experts. Their significance has been extensively debated. The topics covered herein carry significant findings which will fuel the growth of the discipline. They may even be implemented as practical applications or may be referred to as a beginning point for another development.

The contributors of this book come from diverse backgrounds, making this book a truly international effort. This book will bring forth new frontiers with its revolutionizing research information and detailed analysis of the nascent developments around the world.

We would like to thank all the contributing authors for lending their expertise to make the book truly unique. They have played a crucial role in the development of this book. Without their invaluable contributions this book wouldn't have been possible. They have made vital efforts to compile up to date information on the varied aspects of this subject to make this book a valuable addition to the collection of many professionals and students.

This book was conceptualized with the vision of imparting up-to-date information and advanced data in this field. To ensure the same, a matchless editorial board was set up. Every individual on the board went through rigorous rounds of assessment to prove their worth. After which they invested a large part of their time researching and compiling the most relevant data for our readers.

The editorial board has been involved in producing this book since its inception. They have spent rigorous hours researching and exploring the diverse topics which have resulted in the successful publishing of this book. They have passed on their knowledge of decades through this book. To expedite this challenging task, the publisher supported the team at every step. A small team of assistant editors was also appointed to further simplify the editing procedure and attain best results for the readers.

Apart from the editorial board, the designing team has also invested a significant amount of their time in understanding the subject and creating the most relevant covers. They scrutinized every image to scout for the most suitable representation of the subject and create an appropriate cover for the book.

The publishing team has been an ardent support to the editorial, designing and production team. Their endless efforts to recruit the best for this project, has resulted in the accomplishment of this book. They are a veteran in the field of academics and their pool of knowledge is as vast as their experience in printing. Their expertise and guidance has proved useful at every step. Their uncompromising quality standards have made this book an exceptional effort. Their encouragement from time to time has been an inspiration for everyone.

The publisher and the editorial board hope that this book will prove to be a valuable piece of knowledge for researchers, students, practitioners and scholars across the globe.

List of Contributors

Elahe Tajbakhsh
Department of Microbiology, Faculty of Basic Sciences, Shahrekord Branch, Islamic Azad University, Shahrekord, Iran

Faham Khamesipour
Young Researchers and Elite Club, Shahrekord Branch, Islamic Azad University, Shahrekord, Iran

Reza Ranjbar
Molecular Biology Research Center, Baqiyatallah University of Medical Sciences, Tehran, Iran

Ifeoma Chinyere Ugwu
Department of Veterinary Pathology and Microbiology, University of Nigeria, Nsukka, Enugu State, Nigeria

A. Różańska, J. Wójkowska-Mach and M. Bulanda
Chair of Microbiology, Jagiellonian University Medical College, 18 Czysta Street, 31-121 Krakow, Poland

P. Adamski
Institute of Nature Conservation Polish Academy of Sciences, Krakow, Poland

M. Borszewska-Kornacka
Clinic of Neonatology and Intensive Neonatal Care, Warsaw Medical University, Warsaw, Poland

E. Gulczyńska and M. Nowiczewski
Clinic of Neonatology, Polish Mother's Memorial Hospital-Research Institute, Lodz, Poland

E. Helwich
Clinic of Neonatology and Intensive Neonatal Care, Institute of Mother and Child, Warsaw, Poland

A. Kordek
Department of Neonatal Diseases, Pomeranian Medical University, Szczecin, Poland

D. Pawlik
Clinic of Neonatology, Jagiellonian University Medical College, Krakow, Poland

Rui Zheng
Faculty of Environmental Science and Engineering, Kunming University of Science and Technology, Kunming, Yunnan, China
Faculty of Life Science and Technology, Kunming University of Science and Technology, No. 727 Jing Ming Road, Chenggong District, Kunming, Yunnan, China
Department of Clinical Laboratory, First People's Hospital of Yunnan province, Kunming, Yunnan, China

Yue Feng, Li Liu, Amei Zhang, Yue Zhao, Xiaoyu Yang and Xueshan Xia
Faculty of Environmental Science and Engineering, Kunming University of Science and Technology, Kunming, Yunnan, China
Faculty of Life Science and Technology, Kunming University of Science and Technology, No. 727 Jing Ming Road, Chenggong District, Kunming, Yunnan, China

Qian Zhang
Department of Clinical Laboratory, Kunming City Maternal and Child health Hospital, Kunming, Yunnan, China

Yidan Guo
Yunnan Center for Disease Control and Prevention, Kunming, Yunnan, China

Jun Li, Mingxiang Zou, Yongmei Hu, Haichen Wang, Qun Yan and Wen' en Liu
Department of Clinical Laboratory, Xiangya Hospital, Central South University, No. 87, Xiangya Road; Kaifu District, Changsha 410008, Hunan, China

Qingya Dou
Department of Infection Control Center, Xiangya Hospital, Central South University, Changsha 410008, Hunan, China

Dietmar Enko, Gabriele Halwachs-Baumann, Robert Stolba and Gernot Kriegshäuser
Institute of Clinical Chemistry and Laboratory Medicine, General Hospital Steyr, Sierningerstraße 170, 4400 Steyr, Austria

Ortrun Rössler
Institute of Pathology, General Hospital Steyr, Sierningerstraße 170, 4400 Steyr, Austria

Abdessalam Cherkaoui, Stéphane Emonet and Gesuele Renzi
Bacteriology Lab, Division of Laboratory Medicine, Department of Genetics and Laboratory Medicine, Geneva University Hospitals, 4 rue Gabrielle-Perret-Gentil, 1205 Geneva, Switzerland

Jacques Schrenzel
Bacteriology Lab, Division of Laboratory Medicine, Department of Genetics and Laboratory Medicine, Geneva University Hospitals, 4 rue Gabrielle-Perret-Gentil, 1205 Geneva, Switzerland
Genomic Research Laboratory, Service of Infectious Diseases, Geneva University Hospitals, 4 rue Gabrielle-Perret-Gentil, 1205 Geneva, Switzerland

Paul Cheddie
Department of Medical Technology, University of Guyana, Georgetown, Guyana

Francis Dziva
Faculty of Medical Sciences, The University of the West Indies, St. Augustine, Trinidad and Tobago

Patrick Eberechi Akpaka
Department of Para-Clinical Sciences, Faculty of Medical Sciences, The University of the West Indies, St. Augustine, Trinidad and Tobago

Wanli Li, Yao Liu and Qun Sun
Key Laboratory of Bio-resources and Eco-environment of the Ministry of Education, College of Life Sciences, Sichuan University, 29# Wangjiang Rd., Chengdu, Sichuan 610064, P. R. China

Yinghui Li, Xiaolu Shi, Qian Zhang, Qiongcheng Chen and Qinghua Hu
Shenzhen Major Infectious Disease Control Key Laboratory, Shenzhen Centre for Disease Control and Prevention, Shenzhen, Guangdong 518055, P. R. China

Yarong Wu and Yujun Cui
State Key Laboratory of Pathogen and Biosecurity, Beijing Institute of Microbiology and Epidemiology, Beijing 100071, P. R. China

Yalil T. Bracho-Churio, Ruth A. Martínez-Vega, Ronald G. Díaz-Quijano, María L. Luna-González
Organización Latinoamericana para el Fomento de la Investigación en Salud, Bucaramanga, Santander, Colombia

Alfonso J. Rodriguez-Morales
Organización Latinoamericana para el Fomento de la Investigación en Salud, Bucaramanga, Santander, Colombia
Public Health and Infection Research Group, Faculty of Health Sciences, Universidad Tecnológica de Pereira, Pereira, Risaralda, Colombia

Fredi A. Diaz-Quijano
Department of Epidemiology, Faculdade de Saúde Pública, Universidade de São Paulo, Av. Dr. Arnaldo, 715, São Paulo, SP CEP-01246-904, Brazil

Yaa Difie Osei and Sammy Tawiah Sackey
Department of Biochemistry, Cell and Molecular Biology, School of Biological Sciences, University of Ghana, Legon, Accra, Ghana

Daniel Oduro-Mensah
Department of Biochemistry, Cell and Molecular Biology, School of Biological Sciences, University of Ghana, Legon, Accra, Ghana
Department of Applied Chemistry and Biochemistry, University for Development Studies, Navrongo Campus, Navrongo, Ghana

Kingsley Twum-Danso and Noah Obeng-Nkrumah
Department of Microbiology, University of Ghana Medical School, Korle-Bu, Accra, Ghana

Evelyn Yayra Bonney
Department of Virology, Noguchi Memorial Institute for Medical Research, University of Ghana, Legon, Accra, Ghana

Ebenezer Oduro-Mensah
Adabraka Polyclinic, Ghana Health Service, Accra, Ghana

Malini Shariff
Department of Microbiology, Vallabhbhai Patel Chest Institute, University of Delhi, Delhi 110007, India

Monorama Deb
Vardhaman Mahavir Medical Collegeand Safdarjung Hospital, New Delhi 110029, India

Deepjyoti Paul, Anand Prakash Maurya and Amitabha Bhattacharjee
Department of Microbiology, Assam University, Silchar, India

Dabet Rynga
Department of Microbiology, Vallabhbhai Patel Chest Institute, University of Delhi, Delhi 110007, India
Department of Microbiology, Vardhaman Mahavir Medical College and Safdarjung Hospital, New Delhi, India

Kaisheng Lai, Yanning Ma, Ling Guo, Jingna An, Liyan Ye and Jiyong Yang
Department of Microbiology, Chinese PLA General Hospital, 301 Hospital, 28# Fuxing Road, Beijing 100853, China

Debadatta Dhar and Atanu Chakravarty
Department of Microbiology, Silchar Medical College and Hospital, Silchar, India

Shweta Mishra
Department of Microbiology, Institute of Medical Sciences, Banaras Hindu University, Varanasi, India

Gauri Dutt Sharma
Department of Life Science and Bioinformatics, Assam University, Silchar, India

Ahmed Sahib Abdulamir
Microbiology Department, College of Medicine, Alnahrain University, 14222 Baghdad, Iraq

Sabah A. A. Jassim
Applied Bio Research Inc., Windsor, Canada
Environmental Engineering, University of Windsor, Windsor, Canada

Rand R. Hafidh
Microbiology Department, College of Medicine, Baghdad University, Baghdad, Iraq

Fatimah Abu Bakar
Faculty of Food Science, University Putra Malaysia, Serdang, 43400 Selangor, Malaysia

Essam J. Alyamani, Rayan Y. Booq and Majed A. Majrashi
National Center for Biotechnology, King Abdulaziz City for Science and Technology, Riyadh 11442, Saudi Arabia

Anamil M. Khiyami
College of Medicine, Princess Nora Bint Abdul Rahman University, Riyadh 12484, Saudi Arabia

Fayez S. Bahwerth
Hera Hospital, Makkah, Saudi Arabia

Elena Rechkina
ID Genomics, Seattle, WA, USA

Yao Liu, Wanli Li and Qun Sun
Key Laboratory of Bio-resources and Eco-environment of the Ministry of Education, College of Life Sciences, Sichuan University, 29# Wangjiang Road, Chengdu 610064, Sichuan, People's Republic of China

Shi, Yinghui Li, Qiongcheng Chen, Min Jiang, Yaqun Qiu, Yiman Lin and Yixiang Jiang
Shenzhen Major Infectious Disease Control Key Laboratory, Shenzhen Center for Disease Control and Prevention, Shenzhen 518055, Guangdong, People's Republic of China

Qinghua Hu
Shenzhen Major Infectious Disease Control Key Laboratory, Shenzhen Center for Disease Control and Prevention, Shenzhen 518055, Guangdong, People's Republic of China
School of Life Sciences, Shenzhen University, Shenzhen 518000, Guangdong, People's Republic of China

Biao Kan
Key Laboratory of Surveillance and Early-warning on Infectious Disease, Division of Infectious Disease, Chinese Center for Disease Control and Prevention, Beijing, People's Republic of China

Robert-Jan ten Hove, Mesfin Nigussie and Melaku Tesfaye
International Clinical Laboratories, Addis Ababa, Ethiopia

Witold Frederik ten Hove
HAN University of Applied Sciences, Nijmegen, The Netherlands

Yong Guo and Xiao Deng
Institutes of Biology and Medical Sciences, Medical College of Soochow University, Suzhou 215123, China

Yuan Liang
State Key Laboratory of Genetic Engineering, School of Life Sciences, Fudan University, Shanghai 200433, China

Liang Zhang
Shanghai- MOST Key Laboratory of Health and Disease Genomics, Chinese National Human Genome Center at Shanghai, Shanghai 201203, China

Guo-Ping Zhao and Yan Zhou
State Key Laboratory of Genetic Engineering, School of Life Sciences, Fudan University, Shanghai 200433, China
Shanghai- MOST Key Laboratory of Health and Disease Genomics, Chinese National Human Genome Center at Shanghai, Shanghai 201203, China

Krishus Nepal, Bibhusan Neupane, Ankit Belbase and Rikesh Baidhya
Department of Microbiology, GoldenGate International College, Battisputali, Kathmandu, Nepal

Narayan Dutt Pant
Department of Microbiology, Grande International Hospital, Dhapasi, Kathmandu, Nepal

Ram Krishna Shrestha and Bharat Jha
Department of Laboratory Medicine, OM Hospital and Research Center, Chabahil, Kathmandu, Nepal

Binod Lekhak and Dwij Raj Bhatta
Central Department of Microbiology, Tribhuvan University, Kirtipur, Kathmandu, Nepal

Masomeh Dehshiri, Seyed Sajjad Khoramrooz, Mohammad Zoladl, Seyed Abdolmajid Khosravani Najmeh Parhizgari and Asghar Sharifi
Cellular and Molecular Research Centre, Yasuj University of Medical Sciences, Yasuj, Iran

Mohammad Hossein Motazedian
Department of Parasitology and Mycology, Shiraz University of Medical Sciences, Shiraz, Iran

Soheyla Jahedi
Paradise shahid Bahonar, Farhangian University of Shiraz, Shiraz, Iran

Zahra Farshadzadeh, Masoumeh Mokhtaran and Farhad B. Hashemi
Department of Microbiology, School of Medicine, Tehran University of Medical Sciences, 100 Poursina Ave., 100 Keshavarz Blvd, Tehran 14167-53955, Iran

Maryam Pourhajibagher
Department of Microbiology, School of Medicine, Tehran University of Medical Sciences, 100 Poursina Ave., 100 Keshavarz Blvd, Tehran 14167-53955, Iran
Dental Research Center, Dentistry Research Institute, Tehran University of Medical Sciences, Tehran, Iran

Abbas Bahador
Department of Microbiology, School of Medicine, Tehran University of Medical Sciences, 100 Poursina Ave., 100 Keshavarz Blvd, Tehran 14167-53955, Iran
Dental Research Center, Dentistry Research Institute, Tehran University of Medical Sciences, Tehran, Iran
Laser Research Center, Dentistry Research Institute, Tehran University of Medical Sciences, Tehran, Iran

Reza Raoofian
Legal Medicine Research Center, Legal Medicine Organization, Tehran, Iran
Innovative Research Center, Islamic Azad University, Mashhad Branch, Mashhad, Iran

Babak Pourakbari
Pediatrics Infectious Disease Research Center, Tehran University of Medical Sciences, Tehran, Iran

Yohannes Equar Messele, Shimels Tikuye Yalew, Desiye Tesfaye Tegegne, Bezina Arega Emeru and Gebremeskel Mamu Werid
Ethiopian Institute of Agricultural Research, National Agricultural Biotechnology Research Center, Holeta, Ethiopia

Reta Duguma Abdi
College of Veterinary Medicine and Agriculture, Addis Ababa University, Bishoftu, Ethiopia
University of Tennessee Institute of Agriculture Department of Animal Science, Rivers Drive, Knoxville, TN, USA

Jonathan C. Cho
College of Pharmacy, The University of Texas at Tyler, 3900 University Blvd., Tyler, TX 75799, USA

Sandy J. Estrada
Clinical Affairs, T2 Biosystems, Inc., Lexington, MA, USA

Jamie J. Kisgen
Department of Pharmacy, Sarasota Memorial Health Care System, Sarasota, FL, USA

Angelina Davis
Department of Pharmacy, WellStar Cobb Hospital, WellStar Health System, Austell, GA, USA

Ruirui Xu
School of Food Science and Engineering, South China University of Technology, Guangzhou 510640, China

Laura Puzniak
Merck & Co., Inc., Kenilworth, NJ, USA

Dong Liu, Hong-Dong Li, Dan-Ping Zhu, Yu He, Ting Hou and Jia-Lin Yu
Department of Neonatology, Children's Hospital of Chongqing Medical University, Chongqing 400014, China

Zhi-Hui Zou
Department of Neonatology, Children's Hospital of Chongqing Medical University, Chongqing 400014, China
Department of Neonatology, Sichuan Maternal and Child Health Service Hospital, Chengdu 610041, Sichuan, China

Dingqiang Chen
Department of Laboratory Medicine, Zhujiang Hospital, Southern Medical University, Guangzhou 510280, China

Shuxian Wen, Donghua Feng, Danhong Su, Yongping Lin and Ling Yang
Department of Laboratory Medicine, The First Affiliated Hospital of Guangzhou Medical University, Guangzhou Medical University, Guangzhou 510120, China

Junyan Liu
School of Food Science and Engineering, South China University of Technology, Guangzhou 510640, China
Department of Clinical Pharmacy, College of Pharmacy, University of Tennessee Health Science Center, Memphis, TN 38163, USA

Zhenbo Xu
School of Food Science and Engineering, South China University of Technology, Guangzhou 510640, China
Guangdong Province Key Laboratory for Green Processing of Natural Products and Product Safety, Guangzhou 510640, China
Department of Microbial Pathogenesis, School of Dentistry, University of Maryland, Baltimore, MD 21201, USA

Brian M. Peters
Department of Clinical Pharmacy, College of Pharmacy, University of Tennessee Health Science Center, Memphis, TN 38163, USA

Mark E. Shirtliff
Department of Microbial Pathogenesis, School of Dentistry, University of Maryland, Baltimore, MD 21201, USA

Nancy Law and Tiffany E. Bias
Center for Surgical Infections & Biofilms, Institute of Molecular Medicine and Infectious diseases, Drexel University College of Medicine, 245 N. 15th Street, Philadelphia, PA 19102, USA

Kevin M. Raible and Bhaswati Sen
Center for Surgical Infections & Biofilms, Institute of Molecular Medicine and Infectious diseases, Drexel University College of Medicine, 245 N. 15th Street, Philadelphia, PA 19102, USA
Center for Genomic Sciences, Institute of Molecular Medicine and Infectious diseases, Drexel University College of Medicine, 245 N. 15th Street, Philadelphia, PA 19102, USA

Suresh G. Joshi
Center for Surgical Infections & Biofilms, Institute of Molecular Medicine and Infectious diseases, Drexel University College of Medicine, 245 N. 15th Street, Philadelphia, PA 19102, USA
Center for Genomic Sciences, Institute of Molecular Medicine and Infectious diseases, Drexel University College of Medicine, 245 N. 15th Street, Philadelphia, PA 19102, USA
Department of Microbiology and Immunology, Drexel University College of Medicine, 245 N. 15th Street, Philadelphia, PA 19102, USA

Garth D. Ehrlich
Center for Surgical Infections & Biofilms, Institute of Molecular Medicine and Infectious diseases, Drexel University College of Medicine, 245 N. 15th Street, Philadelphia, PA 19102, USA
Center for Genomic Sciences, Institute of Molecular Medicine and Infectious diseases, Drexel University College of Medicine, 245 N. 15th Street, Philadelphia, PA 19102, USA
Center for Advanced Microbial Processing, Institute of Molecular Medicine and Infectious Diseases, Drexel University College of Medicine, 245 N. 15th Street, Philadelphia, PA 19102, USA
Department of Microbiology and Immunology, Drexel University College of Medicine, 245 N. 15th Street, Philadelphia, PA 19102, USA
Department of Otolaryngology-Head and Neck Surgery, Drexel University College of Medicine, 245 N. 15th Street, Philadelphia, PA 19102, USA

Christopher L. Emery
Center for Surgical Infections & Biofilms, Institute of Molecular Medicine and Infectious diseases, Drexel University College of Medicine, 245 N. 15th Street, Philadelphia, PA 19102, USA
Present Address: Department of Pathology and Lab Medicine, Indiana University School of Medicine, Indianapolis, IN, USA

Kazuyuki Tanaka, Mikihiro Fujiya, Aki Sakatani, Shugo Fujibayashi, Yoshiki Nomura, Nobuhiro Ueno, Shin Kashima, Takuma Goto, Junpei Sasajima, Kentaro Moriichi and Toshikatsu Okumura
Division of Gastroenterology and Hematology/ Oncology, Department of Medicine, Asahikawa Medical University, 2-1 Midorigaoka-higashi, Asahikawa, Hokkaido 078-8510, Japan

Satomi Yamada
Department of Bacteriology, The Jikei University School of Medicine, 3-25-8 Nishi-Shimbashi, Minato-ku, Tokyo 105-8461, Japan

Ken-ichi Okuda, Akio Chiba and Yoshimitsu Mizunoe
Department of Bacteriology, The Jikei University School of Medicine, 3-25-8 Nishi-Shimbashi, Minato-ku, Tokyo 105-8461, Japan
Jikei Center for Biofilm Science and Technology, The Jikei University School of Medicine, Tokyo, Japan

Yutaka Yoshii
Department of Bacteriology, The Jikei University School of Medicine, 3-25-8 Nishi-Shimbashi, Minato-ku, Tokyo 105-8461, Japan
Jikei Center for Biofilm Science and Technology, The Jikei University School of Medicine, Tokyo, Japan
Division of Respiratory Diseases, Department of Internal Medicine, The Jikei University School of Medicine, Tokyo, Japan

Ippei Hironaka
Department of Bacteriology, The Jikei University School of Medicine, 3-25-8 Nishi-Shimbashi, Minato-ku, Tokyo 105-8461, Japan
Department of Surgery, The Jikei University School of Medicine, Tokyo, Japan

Katsuhiko Yanaga
Jikei Center for Biofilm Science and Technology, The Jikei University School of Medicine, Tokyo, Japan
Department of Surgery, The Jikei University School of Medicine, Tokyo, Japan

Seiji Hori
Jikei Center for Biofilm Science and Technology, The Jikei University School of Medicine, Tokyo, Japan
Department of Infectious Disease and Control, The Jikei University School of Medicine, Tokyo, Japan

Index

www.ingramcontent.com/pod-product-compliance
Lightning Source LLC
LaVergne TN
LVHW080714210926
848485LV00003B/464
* 9 7 8 1 6 3 9 2 7 2 5 9 4 *